D0926447

Surgical Pathology of the Salivary Glands

Volume 25 in the Series
MAJOR PROBLEMS IN PATHOLOGY

GARY L. ELLIS, D.D.S.

Department of Oral Pathology
Armed Forces Institute of Pathology
Washington, D.C.

PAUL L. AUCLAIR, D.M.D.

Department of Oral Pathology
Armed Forces Institute of Pathology
Washington, D.C.

DOUGLAS R. GNEPP, M.D.

Professor, Departments of Pathology and
    Otolaryngology–Head & Neck Surgery
St. Louis University School of Medicine
St. Louis, Missouri

Surgical Pathology of the Salivary Glands

Volume 25 in the Series
MAJOR PROBLEMS IN PATHOLOGY

W.B. SAUNDERS COMPANY
Harcourt Brace Jovanovich, Inc.
PHILADELPHIA LONDON TORONTO MONTREAL SYDNEY TOKYO

W. B. SAUNDERS COMPANY
Harcourt Brace Jovanovich, Inc.

The Curtis Center
Independence Square West
Philadelphia, PA 19106

Library of Congress Cataloging-in-Publication Data

Surgical pathology of the salivary glands / [edited by] Gary L.
Ellis, Paul L. Auclair, Douglas R. Gnepp.

p. cm. — (Major problems in pathology; v. 25)

Includes index.

ISBN 0–7216–3224–6

1. Salivary glands—Biopsy. 2. Salivary glands—Cytopathology.
3. Pathology, Surgical. 4. Salivary glands—Cancer—Diagnosis.
5. Salivary glands—Diseases—Diagnosis. I. Ellis, Gary L.
II. Auclair, Paul L. III. Gnepp, Douglas R. IV. Series.

[DNLM: 1. Salivary Gland Neoplasms—pathology. 2. Salivary
Gland Neoplasms—surgery. 3. Salivary Glands—pathology.
4. Salivary Glands—surgery. W1 MA492X v. 25 / WI 230 S961]

RC815.S86 1991

616.99′2316—dc20

DNLM/DLC   91-15029

Editor: Jennifer Mitchell
Designer: Ellen Bodner-Zanolle
Production Manager: Ken Neimeister
Manuscript Editor: Joan Powers
Illustration Coordinator: Brett MacNaughton
Indexer: Nancy Newman

SURGICAL PATHOLOGY OF THE SALIVARY GLANDS   ISBN 0–7216–3224–6

Copyright © 1991 by W. B. Saunders Company.

All rights reserved. No part of this publication may be reproduced or transmitted in any form or
by any means, electronic or mechanical, including photocopy, recording, or any information storage
and retrieval system, without permission in writing from the publisher.

Printed in the United States of America.

Last digit is the print number: 9   8   7   6   5   4   3   2   1

Contributors

PAUL L. AUCLAIR, D.M.D., M.S., CAPTAIN, DC, UNITED STATES NAVY

Chairman, Department of Oral Pathology, Armed Forces Institute of Pathology, Washington, D.C.
Classification of Salivary Gland Neoplasms; Salivary Gland Neoplasms: General Considerations; Ductal Papillomas; Other Benign Epithelial Neoplasms; Mucoepidermoid Carcinoma; Acinic Cell Adenocarcinoma; Adenocarcinoma, Not Otherwise Specified; Primary Squamous Cell Carcinoma; Clear Cell Carcinoma; Basal Cell Adenocarcinoma; Other Malignant Epithelial Neoplasms; Nonlymphoid Sarcomas of the Major Salivary Glands; Malignant Lymphomas

RUSSELL L. CORIO, D.D.S., M.S.D., M.A.

Associate Professor of Dermatology, The Johns Hopkins University School of Medicine, Baltimore, Maryland; Attending Staff, The Johns Hopkins Hospital, Baltimore, Maryland
Epithelial-Myoepithelial Carcinoma

TROY E. DANIELS, D.D.S., M.S.

Professor and Chair, Division of Oral Pathology, School of Dentistry, University of California, San Francisco, California; Attending Dentist, Moffitt-Long Hospitals, University of California, San Francisco, California
Benign Lymphoepithelial Lesion and Sjögren's Syndrome

IRVING DARDICK, M.D., M.Sc., F.R.C.P.(C)

Associate Professor of Pathology and Otolaryngology, University of Toronto, Toronto, Ontario, Canada; Head, Diagnostic Electron Microscopy, The Toronto Hospital, Toronto, Ontario
Histogenesis and Morphogenesis of Salivary Gland Neoplasms

GARY L. ELLIS, D.D.S.

Department of Oral Pathology and Department of Veterans Affairs Special Reference Laboratory for Pathology, Armed Forces Institute of Pathology, Washington, D.C.
Classification of Salivary Gland Neoplasms; Salivary Gland Neoplasms: General Considerations; Ductal Papillomas; Other Benign Epithelial Neoplasms; Mucoepidermoid Carcinoma; Acinic Cell Adenocarcinoma; Adenocarcinoma, Not Otherwise Specified; Primary Squamous Cell Carcinoma; Clear Cell Carcinoma; Basal Cell Adenocarcinoma; Other Malignant Epithelial Neoplasms; Nonlymphoid Sarcomas of the Major Salivary Glands; Malignant Lymphomas

GALEN M. EVERSOLE, M.D., F.C.A.P.

Active Staff, Eastern New Mexico Medical Center, Roswell, New Mexico; Roosevelt General Hospital, Portales, New Mexico; and DeBaca General Hospital, Fort Sumner, New Mexico
Undifferentiated Carcinoma

LEWIS R. EVERSOLE, D.D.S., M.S.D.

Professor, Oral Pathology, University of California Los Angeles School of Dentistry, Los Angeles, California
Undifferentiated Carcinoma

DOUGLAS R. GNEPP, M.D., M.S.

Professor, Departments of Pathology and Otolaryngology–Head & Neck Surgery, St. Louis University School of Medicine, St. Louis, Missouri; Pathologist, St. Louis University Hospital, St. Louis, Missouri
Salivary Gland Neoplasms: General Considerations; Other Benign Epithelial Neoplasms; Malignant Mixed Tumors; Polymorphous Low-Grade Adenocarcinoma of Minor Salivary Glands; Undifferentiated Carcinoma; Other Malignant Epithelial Neoplasms; Metastatic Disease to the Major Salivary Glands

ROBERT K. GOODE, D.M.D., COLONEL, DC, UNITED STATES AIR FORCE

Department of Oral Pathology, Armed Forces Institute of Pathology, Washington, D.C.
Oncocytoma; Other Malignant Epithelial Neoplasms

DENNIS K. HEFFNER, M.D., CAPTAIN, MC, UNITED STATES NAVY

Chairman, Otolaryngic Pathology Department, Armed Forces Institute of Pathology, Washington, D.C.; Adjunct Professor, Department of Otolaryngology, Georgetown University Medical School, Washington, D.C.
Sinonasal and Laryngeal Salivary Gland Lesions

JAMES L. HIATT, B.S., M.S., PH.D.

Associate Professor of Anatomy, Baltimore College of Dental Surgery, Dental School, University of Maryland, Baltimore, Maryland
Embryology and Anatomy of the Salivary Glands

JERALD L. JENSEN, D.D.S., M.S.

Oral Pathologist, Laboratory Service, Department of Veterans Affairs Medical Center, Long Beach, California; Associate Clinical Professor of Pathology, University of California, Irvine, California
Developmental Diseases; Idiopathic Diseases

CHRISTINE G. JANNEY, M.D.

Assistant Professor, St. Louis University School of Medicine, St. Louis, Missouri; Director of Surgical Pathology, St. Louis University Hospital, St. Louis, Missouri
Salivary Gland Neoplasms: General Considerations

BRENT M. KOUDELKA, D.D.S., M.S., COLONEL, DC, UNITED STATES ARMY

Staff Pathologist, Department of Pathology, 196th Station Hospital, Supreme Headquarters Allied Powers Europe (SHAPE), Belgium; Formerly Chairman, Department of Oral Pathology, Armed Forces Institute of Pathology, Washington, D.C.
Obstructive Disorders

FRANK J. KRATOCHVIL, D.D.S., COMMANDER, DC, UNITED STATES NAVY

Professor, Department of Oral Pathology, Naval Dental School, National Naval Dental Center, Bethesda, Maryland; Anatomic Pathology, National Naval Medical Center, Bethesda, Maryland
Developmental Diseases; Canalicular Adenoma and Basal Cell Adenoma

R. KEITH McDANIEL, B.A., D.D.S., M.S.

Professor and Chairman, Department of Oral Diagnostic Sciences, The University of Texas Health Science at Houston, Dental Branch, Houston, Texas
Benign Mesenchymal Neoplasms

JOHN J. SAUK, B.S., D.D.S., M.S.

Professor and Chairman, Department of Pathology, Baltimore College of Dental Surgery, Dental School, University of Maryland, Baltimore, Maryland
Embryology and Anatomy of the Salivary Glands

JAMES J. SCIUBBA, D.M.D., PH.D.

Professor, Oral Biology and Pathology, School of Dental Medicine, State University of New York at Stony Brook, Stony Brook, New York; Chairman, Department of Dental Medicine, Long Island Jewish Medical Center, New Hyde Park, New York
Malignant Lymphomas

CHARLES E. TOMICH, D.D.S., M.S.D.

Professor and Chairman, Department of Oral Pathology, School of Dentistry, Indiana University Medical Center, Indianapolis, Indiana
Adenoid Cystic Carcinoma

CHARLES A. WALDRON, D.D.S., M.S.D.

Professor Emeritus and Consultant, Department of Oral Pathology, Emory University School of Postgraduate Dentistry, Atlanta, Georgia
Mixed Tumor (Pleomorphic Adenoma) and Myoepithelioma

GARY R. WARNOCK, D.D.S., M.S., M.A., M.S., CAPTAIN, DC, UNITED STATES NAVY

Chairman, Oral Pathology, Naval Dental School, National Naval Dental Center, Bethesda, Maryland; Consulting Staff, National Naval Medical Center, Bethesda, Maryland
Developmental Diseases; Papillary Cystadenoma Lymphomatosum (Warthin's Tumor)

BRUCE M. WENIG, M.D., LCDR, MC, UNITED STATES NAVY

Assistant Chairman, Department of Otolaryngic Pathology, Armed Forces Institute of Pathology, Washington, D.C.; Consultant in Pathology, Department of Pathology, National Naval Medical Center, Bethesda, Maryland; Consultant in Pathology, Department of Pathology, Walter Reed Army Medical Center, Washington, D.C.
Salivary Gland Neoplasms: General Considerations; Malignant Mixed Tumors; Polymorphous Low-Grade Adenocarcinoma of Minor Salivary Glands

JOHN T. WERNING, D.D.S., M.S., CAPTAIN, DC, UNITED STATES NAVY (Retired)

Formerly Assistant Chairman, Department of Oral Pathology, Armed Forces Institute of Pathology, Washington, D.C.
Infectious and Systemic Diseases

Preface

The understanding of salivary gland disease has undergone significant expansion and modification in terminology, classification, histogenesis, and pathogenesis since the first book in the series *Major Problems in Pathology* on salivary glands was written by Winston Evans and Alan Cruickshank over 20 years ago. Even though their book was limited to a discussion of tumors of the major salivary glands, it was the state of knowledge at that time, and a comparison of their text with our discussion of salivary gland neoplasms reflects significant change. This current text has been greatly expanded in scope and content over Evans and Cruickshank's original monograph and includes non-neoplastic as well as neoplastic epithelial, mesenchymal, and metastatic diseases that involve the salivary glands. Our hope is that this text will contribute to a more consistent classification of salivary gland disease, which, ultimately, will result in improved patient care.

This in no way suggests that our understanding of salivary gland pathology has reached a culmination. Far from it. This area of pathology is dynamic and evolving. It is our intent in this text to present the current understanding of salivary gland disease in a manner that is readily usable as a reference by surgical pathologists and clinicians.

The histomorphology of salivary gland disease, especially neoplasms, is complex and diverse. In fact, for such a quantitatively limited tissue, pathology of the salivary glands may be one of the most diverse in the body. This diversity, combined with the fact that most surgical pathologists have limited opportunity for experience with salivary glands, is the primary reason these diseases cause difficulty for many pathologists. Experience, of course, is a great teacher. At the Armed Forces Institute of Pathology (AFIP) we have information on over 21,000 salivary gland lesions on file and have the opportunity to review 800 to 900 new cases a year. In part, it is this AFIP experience that we wish to share in this text.

We elicited contributions to this text from several experts in salivary gland pathology. Many of these authors are recognized as well-known oral pathologists, whose specialized field requires them to be experts in this area. Others are general pathologists whose interest, research, and experience have given them special expertise in salivary gland disease. We are most grateful to all our contributors for giving their valuable time and effort to the preparation of this text. We would also especially like to thank the AFIP and the American Registry of Pathology (ARP) for their cooperation and support. This textbook is a cooperative project of the AFIP and the ARP.

We are indebted to the numerous pathologists who submit their interesting and challenging cases to us and often provide photographs and follow-up information. We are thankful for the timely support of the photographic staff of the AFIP, in particular for the efforts of Mr. Luther Duckett, Mr. M. Steven Kruger, and Mr. Gene Griffith. We also thank Mrs. Joyce Manus, who provided her expertise and numerous hours to help us retrieve the data on 21,000 cases from the AFIP computer files. Finally, we thank our families for their enthusiastic support and patience.

GARY L. ELLIS
PAUL L. AUCLAIR
DOUGLAS R. GNEPP

Contents

Normal Development and Non-neoplastic Disease of the Salivary Glands

EMBRYOLOGY AND ANATOMY OF THE SALIVARY GLANDS

James L. Hiatt and John J. Sauk

DEVELOPMENT OF THE SALIVARY GLANDS

All salivary glands develop similarly as initial discrete thickenings of the epithelium of the stomodeum. Although it is not yet clear, the parotid gland is believed to develop from the oral ectoderm, whereas the submandibular and sublingual glands are believed to develop from the endodermal germ layer.[1, 2] These epithelial cells then proliferate as cordlike strands into the underlying ectomesenchyme. They then terminate to form terminal bulbs that are each 10 to 12 cells in diameter. Clefts form in each of the terminal bulbs and deepen until two or more bulbs are formed. These newly formed bulbs then advance into the ectomesenchyme in a fashion similar to their predecessors; however, the bulbs remain attached to a cord of cells that is connected to the original cord, which is contiguous to the oral epithelium. This branching process continues with successive volleys of bulb formation, clefting, and extension through cordlike structures.

Coincident with these epithelial dynamics, adjacent ectomesenchyme increases around the anlage to form concentrations of cells. Classically, this has been termed a condensation of mesenchyme. Interactions between the surrounding ectomesenchyme and the developing glandular anlage have been demonstrated. Recently, it has been shown in rat submandibular gland development that two basement membrane components, i.e., laminin and type IV collagen, are synthesized transiently at certain times by the cells of the terminal cell cluster of the glandular epithelium, thus indicating the role of these components in development.[3] Primary lobule branching is associated with a full complement of basal lamina components, whereas removal of collagens and proteoglycans from an area will promote outgrowth.[4]

The anlage of the parotid gland, the first gland to form in humans, may be observed in the 8-mm embryo as a furrow of tissue that projects dorsally between the maxillary and mandibular processes of the developing mandibular arch. Later, it loses its connection to the entrance of the oral cavity as the developing maxillary and mandibular processes narrow the oral fissure. However, as the gland continues to grow into the cheek, an opening in the oral cavity is maintained in the buccal mucosa.

Identification of the submandibular gland primordium may be observed in the 13-mm embryo as an outgrowth of the floor of the oral cavity at the linguogingival groove. From here, the gland grows rapidly, and its duct is connected to the oral cavity lateral to the tongue. Later, the duct is more medially directed to lie just lateral to the midline beneath the tongue.

The sublingual gland develops in the 20-mm embryo as a complex of several epithelial thickenings both in the linguogingival groove and adjacent to the area where the submandibular gland develops. Its major duct either joins the submandibular duct or opens independently adjacent to it. Several other small ducts that develop open directly into the oral cavity from clusters of the glandular tissue.[5, 6] The minor salivary glands develop later during the third gestational month.[7]

Until this point of development, the glands have

This work was supported in part by grant DE–08648 NIH/NIDR.

no lumina, and the intercellular spaces of the cords and terminal bulbs lack the system of tight junctions, desmosomes, and subplasmalemmal microfilaments that constitutes a terminal web. In the major salivary glands, lumina appear in the branching cords prior to luminization of the terminal bulbs. Subsequent to initial lumen formation, the complexity of the tight junctions increases and ultimately exceeds that of the acini. Redman[8] notes that these observations negate the idea that luminization of the ducts occurs as a result of secretory pressure from the developing acinar or ductal cells. In addition, these findings indicate that degeneration of the inner cells is not a factor in lumen formation.

With the formation of lumina in the terminal bulbs, further clefting occurs in the surrounding cells. As a result, each terminal bulb is divided into a number of subunits called terminal tubules, which are composed of two cell layers that surround a lumen. Luminized terminal units that are insufficiently differentiated to be recognized as acini are known as terminal saccules.

The main and branching cords consequently become excretory ducts. The large striated ducts originate from the distal branched cords, whereas the intercalated and small striated ducts differentiate after the luminization of the terminal bulbs and cords is complete. Structurally, the undifferentiated cells that compose the cords are characterized as irregularly cuboidal, and these cells contain numerous free ribosomes, prominent nucleoli, and underdeveloped Golgi's regions and rough endoplasmic reticulum. Differentiation of the excretory and large striated ducts occurs only after the cords have undergone luminization. Striated ducts are restricted to the major salivary glands only. Although the course of events of striated duct differentiation in humans is not completely clear, it appears that the luminal cells elongate to form columnar cells that possess basal infoldings, which interdigitate intercellularly and contain numerous vertically oriented mitochondria.[7] Microfilaments and vesicles are present in the apical cytoplasm during the last stages of differentiation. The destiny of the peripheral, basal layer of cells has not been elucidated, although it has been speculated that they undergo columnarization or migrate to play a role in other ductal development.

The intercalated and smaller striated ducts differentiate in consort with the acini. Differentiation, as in larger ducts, is distinguished by the presence of moderate amounts of rough endoplasmic reticulum. In addition, small secretory granules appear next to the acinar segments of the intercalated ducts, and these acinar segments expand as the acini differentiate. During this period of development, transitional cells occupy the region between the agranular intercalated duct cells and the striated ducts. Differentiation of the terminal saccules into acini occurs as the cells that border the lumen develop into tubuloacinar or acinar cells and as the peripheral cell layer develops into the myoepithelial cells. The first signs of differentiation of the terminal saccules into acini are the appearance of increased rough endoplasmic reticulum and dilatation of the cisternae with secretory proteins. Later, the Golgi regions become functional, and small angular secretory granules are observed. Progressively, the amounts of rough endoplasmic reticulum, Golgi's complexes, and secretory granules increase to approximate amounts observed in fully formed, mature acini.

As noted previously, the peripheral cells of the terminal saccules eventually develop into myoepithelial cells. These cells can be recognized as primitive myoepithelial cells at the periphery of terminal bulbs, where lumen formation and clefting divide the bulbs into terminal saccules. These primitive contractile cells elongate parallel to the base of the bulb or saccule with an occasional single cilium that projects toward or into an underlying parenchymal cell.[9, 10] Additional myoepithelial differentiation occurs with differentiation of the acini. This is characterized by aggregations of microfilaments and immunohistochemical demonstration of actin, myosin, and prekeratin intermediate filaments as well as by an increase in the intensity of alkaline phosphatase activity that is demonstrated by histochemical staining.

With epithelial ingrowth the ectomesenchyme differentiates to form the connective tissue component that supports the parenchyma of the gland. This component consists of a fibrous capsule and septa that divide the gland into lobes and lobules. The differentiation of this connective tissue component around the parenchyma involves maturation of the primitive ectomesenchyme to fibroblasts. Coincident with these changes is the change in the composition of the extracellular matrix from loose or myxoid to more fibrous. This process continues with maturation as the capsule and adjacent extracellular matrices progressively become more collagenous.

The vascular arrangement of the salivary glands appears to be related to ion transport properties. As such, numerous arterioles run in countercurrent directions around the ducts. These vessels branch as capillaries around the striated ducts, and the distribution of capillaries at the secretory ends appears as arterial arcades. Also found are arteriovenous anastomoses, particularly those related to the acinar circulation. The specific relationship between blood vessel development and gland development is not clear.

The salivary glands receive sensory innervation from branches of the trigeminal nerve. Additionally, it is reported that certain afferent terminals within the glands return to the central nervous system via the parasympathetic and sympathetic nerve roots that serve the glands; however, this phenomenon is not well understood.[11, 12] Motor innervation is provided by both sympathetic and parasympathetic branches of the autonomic nervous system. Parasympathetic stimulation is generally regarded as important in control of overall growth, whereas sympathetic stimulation is implicated in differentiation of the acini.[13] The most important factor for autonomic control of glandular development appears to be the synchronous placement of nerve terminals on or near the parenchymal cells.

ANATOMY AND MORPHOLOGY OF THE SALIVARY GLANDS

As a result of the above developmental processes, the salivary glands take the form of branching structures with terminal secretory end pieces. The main secretory duct of the gland divides into progressively smaller striated ducts. These striated ducts then branch into smaller intercalated ducts, which terminate in the terminal secretory end structures (Fig. 1–1). Terminal end structures vary considerably in size, shape, and cell numbers. They vary from multilobed polygonal structures to tubular or simple circular structures. In general, mucinous glands arrange their end pieces into tubular configurations, whereas serous glands take on spherical forms. The end pieces all consist of collections of cells sitting on a basement membrane that encircles the entire structure. The intercellular spaces technically constitute the beginning of the ductal system because they open into the lumen of the end pieces.

Cell Types

The three primary cell types that are found in the terminal secretory end piece are mucous cells, serous cells, and myoepithelial cells. Several investigators have suggested that there is another cell type, named a seromucous cell, that is intermediate between the serous and mucous cell types. Proponents of this theory base their philosophy on cellular and secretory granule morphology and the method of excretion.[14–17] The evidence for the existence of this seromucous cell type is mounting, and some authorities suggest that the seromucous cell is one of the distinctive cell types that are found in the terminal secretory piece.[5] For some reason, the idea of a seromucous cell has not been universally accepted; however, its morphology is described in this discussion. The distribution of

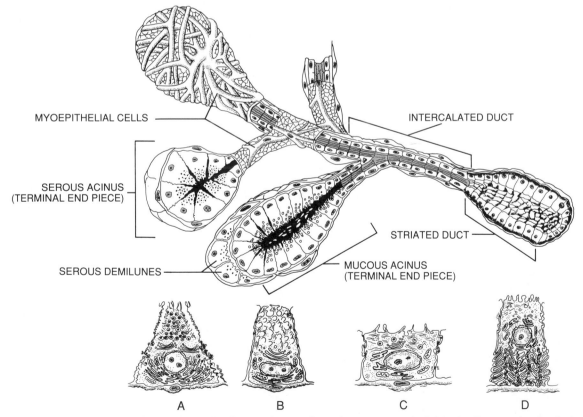

Figure 1–1. Anatomy of the salivary glands. Drawings *A* through *D* represent individual cell types visualized via electron microscopy: *A*, seromucous cell; *B*, mucous cell; *C*, intercalated duct cell; *D*, striated duct cell. (Modified from Williams PL, Warwick R (eds.): Gray's Anatomy, 36th Ed. Philadelphia, WB Saunders Co., 1980.)

these secretory cell types and their numbers vary in each gland and in each end piece. The end piece is also termed the acinus. However, this term has generally been reserved for the spherical structures or the mucus-secreting tubular secretory components. Technically, if the term is to be used, it should be qualified as spherical or tubular acini. Serous and mucous cells have distinct histologic differences, and their secretory products can vary considerably.

Mucous Cells

At the light microscopic level, the mucous cell appears pyramidal with a flattened nucleus that is located at its base. Usually a mucous cell is larger than a serous cell. The apical portion of the cell stains weakly with hematoxylin and eosin and strongly with carbohydrate stains, e.g., mucicarmine stain, which indicates the mucous carbohydrate content of the gland. Secretory materials of these cells are stored as droplets in the apical portion of the cell.

At the ultrastructural level, mucous cells contain a prominent Golgi region with many flattened saccules, which are located adjacent to or between the nucleus and the secretory droplets. In addition, rough endoplasmic reticulum, mitochondria, and other cellular organelles are generally confined to the base and lateral aspects of the cell. Interdigitations between cells are fewer than in seromucous cells. In the major salivary glands, there exists a complex system of basal folds, whereas minor salivary glands exhibit well-developed, lateral interdigitations. There are intercellular secretory canaliculi between mucous cells that lead to serous demilunes. The luminal (apical) plasmalemma normally forms microvilli that are interspersed with pinocytotic vesicles.

Mucous secretory droplets are larger and more irregularly shaped than serous secretory droplets. These also stain very poorly with hematoxylin and eosin and thus appear empty at the light microscopic level. At the ultrastructural level, they are electron lucent and possess a limiting membrane. Occasionally, two droplets may fuse.

Although the method of expelling the mucous droplets may vary, the usual way is for the limiting membrane of the droplet to fuse with the luminal plasmalemma, thus discharging the materials via exocytosis similar to that observed in serous cells. Another method is that several droplets may fuse together, and the large mucous droplet may simply escape through breaks in the plasma membrane.[7, 13, 14] The morphology of mucous cells is complicated by the stage of the functional cycle at which they are observed. At the beginning of a functional cycle, mucous cells resemble seromucous cells in that the Golgi regions of both cell types are poorly developed. This recent recognition of a morphologic dependence on function has led to the reconsideration of previously regarded mixed glands, i.e., labial glands and presumed mixed secretory end pieces in submandibular and sublingual glands, as entirely mucous structures.

Serous Cells

Since human serous cells secrete significant polysaccharide, they may be more properly termed seromucous cells (see previous discussion). These cells appear pyramidal, with the narrow apex of the cell located near the lumen and a spherical nucleus situated near the broad basal one third of the cell. Seromucous cells stain intensely with hematoxylin and eosin stains, and the apical portion of the cell is seen to contain numerous eosinophilic secretory granules.

At the ultrastructural level, an extensive rough endoplasmic reticulum that is arranged in parallel aggregates is noted lateral and basal to the nucleus. There is also a prominent Golgi region located lateral or apical to the nucleus. The secretory granules located in the apical cytoplasm are surrounded by a unit membrane. The end piece of serous cells is supported by a basement membrane that is functionally related and may appear organized in a linear, parallel arrangement. However, when serous cells are not distended with secretory material, the basal plasma membrane may exhibit complex foldings. In the submandibular gland, the structure of the basal portion of these cells is more specialized than in the parotid terminal end pieces. The basal plasma membrane is formed into tall, narrow folds that extend beyond the lateral border of the cell. These foot processes invade deeply into the folds of adjacent cells and significantly enhance the area of the basal regions.

Serous cells are more specialized in their lateral relationships than are mucous cells. Generally, a well-defined intercellular space extends from the lumen of the end piece. The intercellular space or canaliculus terminates in a junctional complex that consists of a tight junction, an intermediate junction, and a desmosome. At various points, adjacent cells contact or join as desmosomal contacts or gap junctions. The surface of these cells manifests microvilli that contact the central lumen and extend into the canalicular space. Although the morphologic character of serous cells is similar in all glands, there is considerable variation in their secretory products, which are morphologically depicted by the variation in the electron density of the secretory granules.

Myoepithelial Cells

Myoepithelial cells are found in relation to the intercalated ducts and the terminal secretory end piece. These cells occupy the space between the basement membrane and the basal plasma membrane. Generally, there is only one myoepithelial cell for each terminal secretory unit. The myoepithelial cells have a flattened central body from which five to eight processes radiate, branch further, and then extend over the long axis of the secretory unit. These cell processes contain numerous microfilaments that frequently show aggregation into dense, dark bodies that resemble the contractile elements of smooth muscle cells, and, indeed, they do contain both actin and myosin as previously discussed. The cytoplasm of myoepithelial cells is segregated into filamentous and nonfilamentous portions, with the normal cellular organelles being located in perinuclear regions. Desmosomes are present between the secretory cells and the myoepithelial cells.

Myoepithelial cells associated with the intercalated ducts are generally more spindle-shaped with fewer cell processes than those associated with the secretory end pieces. On rare occasions, myoepithelial cells located in the intercalated duct region may extend their processes backward to encompass the secretory end piece. In spite of their structural similarity to smooth muscle cells, myoepithelial cells are regarded as epithelial in origin because they are always located between the parenchyma and the basement membrane.

Ductal System

Intercalated Ducts

Secretory products of the terminal end pieces pass first through a system of intercalated ducts. These structures are lined by short cuboidal cells whose nuclei are centrally located and are surrounded by a scant cytoplasm that contains basally situated rough endoplasmic reticulum and more apically positioned Golgi's regions. The cuboidal cells rarely contain granules, except when they are in close proximity to the secretory end pieces. The lateral borders of the cells interdigitate extensively with each other and are connected through junctional complexes. Desmosomal attachments are usually scant and are positioned basal to the junctional complexes. The luminal surfaces of these cuboidal cells have few microvilli. Myoepithelial cells or their processes are usually positioned between the basal lamina and these ductal cells. Intercalated ducts may exhibit great variability in arrangement, location, size, and epithelial structure, depending on their location. Although the simplest ducts are lined by cuboidal epithelium, in such a location as the soft palate they are usually long, highly convoluted structures that consist of mucous cells, simple cuboidal cells, and myoepithelial cells.

Striated Ducts

Striated ducts are the next step in the progressive excretory path for salivary secretions. These ducts are lined by eosinophilic columnar epithelial cells that contain centrally placed nuclei. When visualized via the light microscope, the especially deep indentations of the basal plasma membranes of these cells produce the striated pattern for which these ducts are named. The basal folds extend laterally and interdigitate with adjacent cells in a highly complex manner and, as such, provide an enormous surface area at the basal plasma membrane zone. Contained between these folds are numerous mitochondria arranged in a vertical fashion. The centrally placed nucleus is surrounded by scant amounts of endoplasmic reticulum and Golgi's regions, whereas the apical end contains some free ribosomes, vesicles, small amounts of smooth endoplasmic reticulum, and lysosomes. The luminal surfaces of the cells contain short microvilli, with the cells being joined laterally by junctional complexes and desmosomes. Striated ducts are also often surrounded by numerous blood vessels that are arranged longitudinally to the cross-sectional axis of the ducts.

Terminal Excretory Ducts

Terminal excretory ducts are the final passageway for the secretions destined for the oral cavity. The structure of these ducts is transitional from their junction with the striated ducts to their opening in the oral cavity. Those portions of the excretory ducts closest to the striated ducts are typically lined by a pseudostratified epithelium that consists of columnar cells, which are mingled with small basal cells and goblet cells. As these ducts approach the oral orifice, the epithelial lining becomes stratified squamous in character and merges with the epithelium of the oral mucosa. In some instances, including aging, these ductal cells may become burdened with numerous mitochondria, take on a prominent eosinophilic hue, and be termed oncocytes.

Specific Gland Anatomy and Morphology

The parotid is the largest salivary gland and weighs 15 to 30 g. The gland is enclosed by a capsule from the deep cervical fascia and is positioned in the parotid bed, anterior to the ear and about the ramus of the mandible. A superficial portion of the gland lies over the masseter muscle as far superiorly as the zygomatic arch. Because the gland fills much of the irregularly shaped parotid bed and sends fingerlike projections over the ramus of the mandible, the gland encompasses many structures in this region, including the internal and external carotid arteries and several branches arising from them; the internal jugular vein and some of its tributaries; the retromandibular vein and its tributaries; the facial nerve and the auriculotemporal branch of the trigeminal nerve; and some small parotid lymph nodes.[18] The parotid duct (Stensen's duct) runs forward from the gland over the masseter muscle and dives into the buccal fat pad, where it pierces the buccinator muscle on its way to the oral cavity. The duct opens into the oral vestibule at the parotid papilla opposite the maxillary second molar. The terminal secretory end pieces of the parotid gland are seromucous in character. The gland contains numerous intercalated ducts that are interspersed between the seromucous acini (Fig. 1–2). In elderly individuals, fat can be observed strewn between the parenchyma and the stroma.

The submandibular gland is located in the submandibular triangle, a space bounded by the anterior and posterior bellies of the digastric muscle and the inferior border of the body of the mandible, with the floor formed in part by the mylohyoid muscle. The gland, which weighs about 10 to 15 g, lies in the space of the triangle, nearly filling it. Its deep surface is in contact with the mylohyoid, hyoglossus, styloglossus, and stylohyoid muscles. A fingerlike projection extends into the sublingual space posterior to the mylohyoid muscle. From here, the submandibular duct (Wharton's duct) proceeds anteriorly alongside the mylohyoid, hyoglossus, and genioglossus muscles to open into the oral cavity at the sublingual caruncula lateral to the base of the lingual frenulum.[18] Although the submandibular gland has its own capsule, it is further separated from the parotid gland by a reflection of the deep cervical fascia, the stylomandibular ligament. The submandibular gland contains about 80 percent pure seromucous end pieces, whereas a mixture of mucous and seromucous end pieces make up the remaining gland. These mixed units are characterized by crescent-shaped caps, the demilunes of serous cells at the end of mucus-secreting tubules. Intercalated ducts are shorter and the striated ducts are longer than those ducts in the parotid gland (Fig. 1–3).

The sublingual gland is the smallest of the major salivary glands, weighing about 1.5 to 2.5 g. This gland is housed in the floor of the mouth, covered only by oral mucosa, and lies between the genioglossus muscle of the tongue and the sublingual fossa on the internal aspect of the body of the mandible. Inferiorly, it lies on the superior aspect of the mylohyoid muscle, whereas posteriorly, it is in contact with the submandibular gland. Ducts of this gland may open into the oral cavity proper via tiny ducts (Rivinus's ducts) on the plica sublingualis. However, usually some ducts unite to form a common sublingual duct (Bartholin's duct) that unites with the submandibular duct just prior to its opening into the oral cavity.[18]

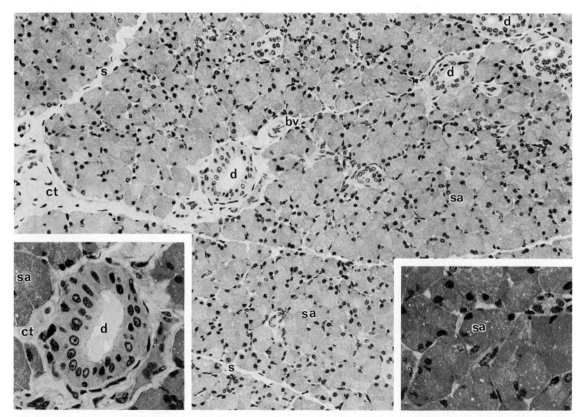

Figure 1–2. Parotid gland. The gland is composed of serous acini (sa) with secretory ducts (d). Septa (s) composed of connective tissue (ct), housing blood vessels (bv), divide the gland into lobes (× 200). *Left inset,* cells composing a salivary duct (× 400). *Right inset,* several acini at higher magnification (× 400).

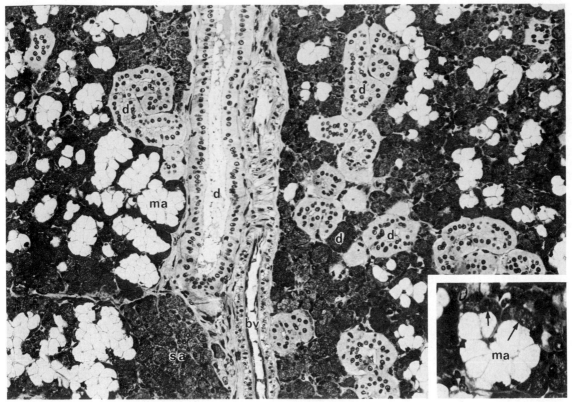

Figure 1–3. Submandibular gland. Both mucous acini (ma) and serous acini (sa) with several ducts (d) and a longitudinal section of a blood vessel (bv) (× 200). *Inset*, a mucous acinus with serous demilunes (arrows) (× 400).

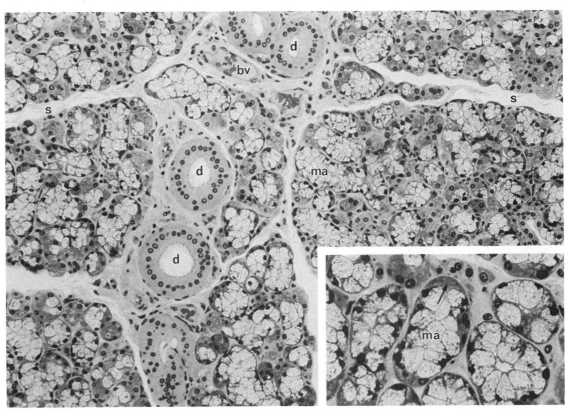

Figure 1–4. Sublingual gland. Observe the preponderance of mucous acini (ma). Many of these glands display serous demilunes. Septa (s) and blood vessels (bv) may also be observed, as can ducts (d) (× 200). *Inset*, several mucous acini with serous demilunes (arrow) (× 400).

In some subjects, the sublingual gland parenchyma may become intermixed with the submandibular gland to form a larger and complex salivary unit. These glands are the most morphologically variable of all glands. Individual acini are known to vary and to contain a mixed collection of cell types. End pieces with few secretory granules can be observed in acini that contain large, mucus-filled cells. Seromucous end pieces are rare; however, mucous tubules with seromucous demilunes are not uncommon. The intercalated ducts are scant and short, as are the striated ducts (Fig. 1–4). Dale[19] notes that even though morphologic distinctions appear to exist, immunocytochemical data suggest that the gland is completely mucous in character.

Except for the gingiva and anterior hard palate, the minor salivary glands are located throughout the submucosa of the oral cavity. There are some 500 to 1000 of these distinct glandular structures present, most of which are mucous glands. The main exception is the Ebner's serous glands, which are located in the circumvallate papillae of the tongue.

REFERENCES

1. Carlson BM: Patten's Foundations of Embryology, 5th Ed. New York, McGraw-Hill Book Co, 1988.
2. Moore KL: The Developing Human: Clinically Oriented Anatomy, 3rd Ed. Philadelphia, WB Saunders Co, 1982.
3. Kadoya Y, Yamashina S: Intercellular accumulation of basement membrane components during morphogenesis of rat submandibular gland. J Histochem Cytochem 1989; 37:1387–1392.
4. Bernfield M, Banerjee SD, Koda JE, Rapraeger AC: Remodeling of the basement membrane as a mechanism of morphogenetic tissue interaction. *In* Trelstad RL (ed.). The Role of Extracellular Matrix in Development. New York, Alan R. Liss, Inc, 1984; 547–572.
5. Williams PL, Warwick R (ed.): Gray's Anatomy, 36th Ed. Philadelphia, WB Saunders Co, 1980.
6. Arey LB: Developmental Anatomy, 7th Ed (revised). Philadelphia, WB Saunders Co, 1974.
7. Hand AR: Salivary glands. *In* Provenza DV, Seibel W: Oral Histology Inheritance and Development, 2nd Ed. Philadelphia, Lea & Febiger, 1986; 388–417.
8. Redman RS: Development of the salivary glands. *In* Sreebrny LM (ed.): The Salivary System. Boca Raton, FL, CRC Press, 1987; 1–20.
9. Tandler B: Ultrastructure of the human submaxillary gland. III. Myoepithelium. Z Zellforsch 1965; 65:852–863.
10. Tandler B, Denning CR, Mandel JD, Kutscher AH: Ultrastructure of human labial salivary glands. III. Myoepithelium and ducts. J Morphol 1970; 130:227–246.
11. Garrett JR: Recent advances in physiology of salivary glands. Br Med Bull 1975; 31:152–155.
12. Garrett JR: Structure and innervation of salivary glands. *In* Cohen B, Kramer JRH (eds.). Scientific Foundations of Dentistry. London, Heineman, 1976; 499–516.
13. Hand AR: Salivary glands. *In* Bhaskar SN (ed.). Orban's Oral Histology and Embryology. St. Louis, The CV Mosby Co, 1980; 336–370.
14. Riva A, Riva-Testa F: Fine structure of acinar cells of human parotid gland. Anat Rec 1973; 176:149–166.
15. Munger BL: Histochemical studies on seromucous and mucous-secreting cells of human salivary glands. Am J Anat 1964; 115:411–429.
16. Shackleford JM, Wilborn WH: Structural and histochemical diversity in mammalian salivary glands. Ala J Med Sci 1968; 5:180–203.
17. Young JA, van Lennep EE: The Morphology of Salivary Glands. New York, Academic Press, 1978.
18. Hiatt JL, Gartner LP: Textbook of Head and Neck Anatomy, 2nd Ed. Baltimore, Williams & Wilkins, 1987.
19. Dale AC: Salivary glands. *In* Ten Cate AR (ed.). Oral Histology, 3rd Ed. St. Louis, CV Mosby Co, 1989; 304–339.

DEVELOPMENTAL DISEASES

2

Gary R. Warnock, Jerald L. Jensen,
and Frank J. Kratochvil

During the normal course of human development, occasional aberrations of the salivary glands occur. It is important that the clinician and pathologist avoid forming an interpretation that is more ominous than that warranted by these conditions. The developmental conditions discussed in this chapter are heterotopic salivary glands, accessory salivary glands, oncocytosis, adenomatoid glandular hyperplasia, and polycystic disease of the parotid gland.

HETEROTOPIC SALIVARY GLANDS

Salivary gland tissue located in sites other than those appropriate for normal anatomic distribution of the major salivary glands, oral mucosa, and pharynx is referred to as heterotopic salivary gland, ectopic salivary gland tissue, or salivary gland choristomas. The embryogenesis of heterotopic salivary gland tissue (HSGT) is often unclear and is related to the anatomic site. Willis[1] has proposed three general explanations for heterotopia: abnormal persistence and development of vestigial structures; dislocation of a portion of a definitive organ rudiment during mass movement of development; and heteroplasia, which is abnormal differentiation of the local tissues. The majority of heterotopic salivary gland tissue has been seen to occur in the head and neck, but such tissue also has been found in remote areas of the body. The most common locations are the paraparotid lymph nodes,[2] the middle ear,[3] and the lower neck.[4] Less frequently recorded are cases involving the upper neck,[5] mandible,[6] external auditory canal,[7] mediastinum,[8] cerebellopontine angle,[9] pituitary gland,[10] prostate gland,[11] vulva,[12] rectum,[13] thyroglossal duct, thyroid gland, and parathyroid capsules.[5]

A survey of over 20,000 salivary gland lesions that are documented in the files of the Armed

Forces Institute of Pathology (AFIP) yielded 110 cases of heterotopic salivary glands; 64 cases specify an exact location. The largest number of the 64 cases involve the lymph nodes (30 cases), including the paraparotid nodes (18 cases) and those specified as neck nodes (12 cases). The second most common site is the lower neck (20 cases), which represents 31 percent of the cases. Other sites recorded in the AFIP series are middle ear (four cases), thyroid gland (two cases), lacrimal gland (two cases), upper neck (one case), stomach (one case), mandible (one case), mediastinum (one case), cerebellopontine angle (one case), and within a thyroglossal duct cyst (one case). HSGT is considered to have given rise to tumors in 13 (12 percent) of the 110 cases. When heterotopia was associated with a salivary gland tumor, the majority (46 percent) were mucoepidermoid carcinomas (six cases). The other tumors were mixed tumor (three cases, 23 percent), Warthin's tumor (three cases, 23 percent), and adenoma, not otherwise specified (one case, 8 percent).

As noted, the vast majority of intranodal heterotopia is seen in the paraparotid area, and the generally accepted explanation for its occurrence at this site is entrapment of salivary gland tissue in lymph nodes during embryonic development. The propensity for HSGT to occur in paraparotid nodes is thought to correlate with latent encapsulation of the parotid gland.[14] Whether salivary gland tissue in paraparotid lymph nodes is true heterotopia rather than a variation of normal tissue is arguable.[15, 16] Histologically, HSGT in paraparotid lymph nodes may contain mixed seromucinous glands but is more likely to consist of serous glands with randomly scattered, well-formed ducts (Fig. 2–1). Salivary gland elements are also seen in association with developmental lesions such as branchial cleft cysts (Fig. 2–2). Care must be taken not to interpret a well-differentiated metastatic tumor in paraparotid nodes as HSGT.

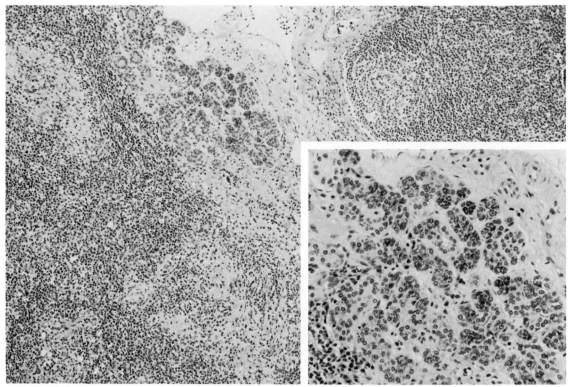

Figure 2–1. Heterotopic salivary gland tissue in a lymph node (× 75). *Inset,* serous acini and ductal structures (× 150).

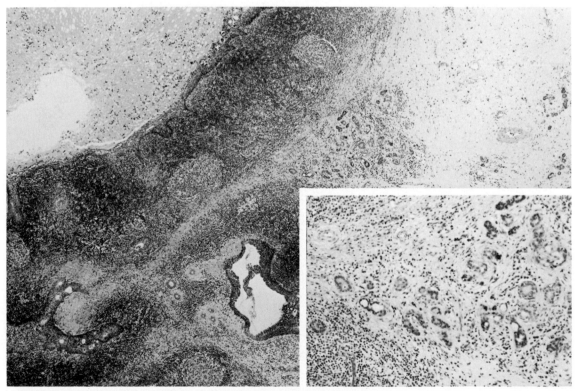

Figure 2–2. Tissue from a benign cervical lymphoepithelial cyst shows small focus of heterotopic salivary gland tissue (HSGT) in wall (× 30). *Inset,* ductal structures and serous acini in fibrous stroma (× 75).

Heterotopic Salivary Gland Tissue of the Lower Neck

Heterotopic salivary gland tissue in the lower neck is unique in its clinical presentation, and its embryogenesis is unexplained. Many cases of heterotopic tissue in the lower neck have been documented,[2, 4, 17–19] including a series of 11 cases reported by Youngs and Scofield[20] and 35 cases reported by Soucy.[21] Clinically, HSGT presents as branchial cleft sinuses in the lower anterolateral neck, medial to the border of the sternocleidomastoid muscle. Bilateral presentation of HSGT is common, as is its existence at birth.[2, 17–19] Swelling may be apparent, but the most frequent clinical expression is presence of a small draining sinus that secretes a mucoid, creamy, or clear salivalike fluid. Drainage is minimal but may increase at mealtime. The gross specimen may contain a perceptible sinus tract. This tract is usually less than 2 cm and emanates from a nodular or lobulated gray or yellow soft tissue mass, which occasionally resembles normal salivary gland tissue. Some lesions present as deep-seated cysts that communicate through the sinus. Microscopically, the sinus may be lined by pseudostratified ciliated columnar epithelium with metaplastic stratified squamous epithelium. The heterotopic salivary gland tissue may be histologically identical with normal oral salivary gland tissue and, thus, may contain serous, mucous, or mixed glandular acini. Lesions that are not associated with draining sinuses are more likely to display disorientated salivary gland tissue elements, including fibrosis, ectatic ducts, and scattered acini (Fig. 2–3). Cartilage may also be present and is possibly attributed to branchial origin.

The pathogenesis of HSGT in the lower neck remains unclear. Youngs and Scofield[20] propose that ectopic salivary gland tissue in the lower neck results from the overgrowth of the second branchial arch, which overlaps the second, third, and fourth branchial clefts, thus forming the precervical sinus of His. This theory of branchiogenic origin is supported by the relationship of HSGT to the sternocleidomastoid muscle and by the presence of cartilage; however, communication to the upper neck has been documented in only one case.[22] Himalstein[23] and Adams and Donahoe[24] have suggested that HSGT is a residuum of the tenth nerve ganglion placodal duct after the sinus of His has dissipated. Soucy[21] has proposed that these lesions would be more properly termed congenital cervical salivary fistula because the origin of these lesions may not be branchial.

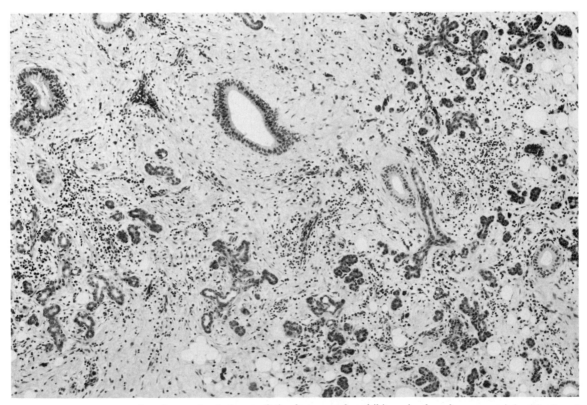

Figure 2–3. Heterotopic salivary gland tissue of the lower neck exhibits mixed and serous acini with ductal structures (× 75).

Heterotopic Salivary Gland Tissue of the Middle Ear

Middle ear salivary gland heterotopia was first reported by Taylor and Martin,[25] and additional cases were reported by Saeger and colleagues,[3] Kartush and Graham,[26] Wine and Metcalf,[27] Moore and colleagues,[28] and Peron and Schuknecht,[29] with reviews of multiple cases by Abadir and Pease[30] and by Quaranta and colleagues.[31] HSGT of the middle ear is quite rare and presents clinically as unilateral conductive hearing loss. The tumor occurs most often in the first and second decades of life, arising in close association with the facial nerve. The ossicles usually involved are the incus and the stapes.[31] In addition to HSGT, many patients display additional middle ear deformities, including ossicle deformities,[26] cholesteatomas,[29] and oval window absence.[32] A single bilateral case of HSGT has been reported in which multiple bilateral auditory anomalies were seen.[29] The high frequency of associated anomalies has promulgated the possibility of a syndrome of conductive hearing loss, HSGT, ossicle anomalies, and facial nerve positioning.[33, 34]

Grossly, the tumor is a gray-to-yellow, lobulated or smooth-surfaced, soft mass that is usually approximal to the facial nerve. Cyst formation has been described in lesions that coexist with cholesteatomas.[29] The microscopic features include mixed serous and mucous glands, and excretory ducts are seen in some, but not in all, cases. The salivary gland elements are intermixed with mature adipose tissue and loosely arranged fibrous connective tissue. The tumor shows little or no propensity for growth, and its recurrence at the site of resection is not expected. Because the HSGT is usually in intimate contact with the facial nerve, careful dissection is recommended to avoid nerve damage. A benign mixed tumor arising from HSGT has been reported in the middle ear.[35]

The pathogenesis of HSGT of the middle ear is thought to be related to errant development of the first and second branchial arches at some time before the fourth month of intrauterine life. Support for this explanation of the pathogenesis is derived from the high percentage of concomitant anomalous ossicles and HSGT, and the embryologic origins of the malleus and incus from the first branchial arch and the stapes from the second branchial arch.[30]

Intraosseous Heterotopic Salivary Gland Tissue

Most salivary gland tissue found in close association with the mandible occurs in cryptlike invaginations of the lingual surface. Technically this tissue does not represent heterotopic tissue because most often it is an extension of indigenous salivary gland tissue that is adjacent to the intraosseous site. The most common location for this type of heterotopic tissue is the posterior mandible, which was originally described by Stafne.[36] The clinical presentation is pathognomonic. A well-defined radiolucency with a sclerotic border is located at the angle of the mandible and below the inferior alveolar canal (Fig. 2–4A). Surgical exploration reveals the presence of salivary gland tissue that is compatible with submandibular gland origin and that often can be visualized as an accessory lobe of the submandibular gland. The salivary gland tissue usually occupies a cortical depression of the lingual surface of the mandible or, rarely, communicates with the medullary bone or is completely enclaved within the body of the mandible. The suggested types of pathogenesis for posterior mandibular lesions include embryonic,[37] congenital,[36] aneurysmal,[38] or developmental.[39] Choukas and Toto[40] suggested the possible entrapment of portions of the submandibular gland secondary to the congenital absence of mandibular bone. Study of postmortem mandibles by Harvey and Noble[39] suggests that the most plausible explanation in some cases is that a gradual development through surface resorption of the lingual cortical bone occurred with eventual inclusion. This concept is supported by the radiographic study of Uemura and colleagues,[41] who did not document any cases involving children.

Osseous inclusions of salivary glands in the anterior mandible are infrequent, with only 12 cases found in the literature.[42] An oval radiolucency with well-defined borders is often seen that mimics a periapical cyst or median mandibular cyst (Fig. 2–4B).[6, 43] Surgical exposure reveals a soft tissue mass that fills an indentation in the lingual mandibular bony plate or may be completely enclaved within the bone. The salivary gland tissue is primarily mucous acini, and some cases are contiguous with the sublingual gland.[44, 45] The consensus regarding pathogenesis of aberrant salivary tissue in the anterior mandible is similar to that for its posterior counterpart.[46, 47] Salivary gland tissue is regularly encountered in the anterior maxilla, in the area of the nasopalatine ducts. However, as pointed out by Abrams and colleagues,[48] 31 percent of nasopalatine duct cysts contain glandular elements, and this finding should be regarded as normal rather than heterotopic.

Heterotopic Salivary Gland Tissue of Other Sites

Several cases of gingival salivary gland choristomas have been reported.[49, 50] Gingival choristomas clinically manifest as yellow swellings at the mucogingival junction and are composed of seromucous or pure mucous glands. An explanation

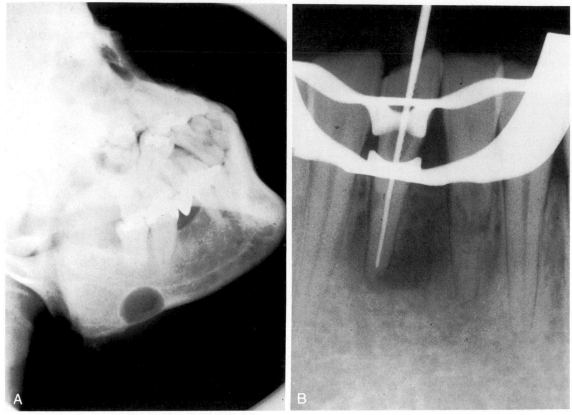

Figure 2–4. *A,* Salivary gland tissue in lingual bony depression causes defect of the posterior mandible that appears as a pathognomonic radiolucency located below the inferior alveolar canal. *B,* Heterotopic salivary gland tissue presents as a periapical lesion in this radiograph of the anterior mandible. The central incisor is undergoing endodontic treatment, but the surgical specimen of the lesion contains normal mucous glands.

for the presence of gingival HSGT is that it arises from pluripotential gingival epithelium or results from a mechanical disturbance during development.[51] A single case of HSGT occurring at the cerebellopontine angle was reported by Curry and colleagues[9] and was associated with an adenoid cystic carcinoma. Like salivary heterotopia located in the ear, the tumor was associated with the seventh and eighth nerves and probably developed from malformation of the branchial pouches. Four cases of HSGT in the external auditory canal are described in the literature.[28] In one of these four cases, HSGT was bilateral and was composed primarily of serous acini with accompanying ducts.[7]

Salivary gland rests are seen so frequently in the posterior lobe of the pituitary that their presence is often regarded as normal. Schochet and colleagues,[10] using triplane sectioning of autospy specimens, found HSGT in 3.4 percent of the cases, but serial sectioning has shown salivary gland elements in virtually all pituitary glands. Histologically, the heterotopic salivary gland rests are tubuloductal structures lined by cuboidal or columnar cells with basally located nuclei and eosinophilic cytoplasm. Oncocytosis was present

in 7 cases of 78 total cases of HSGT of the pituitary gland that were recorded by Schochet and colleagues;[10] this supports speculation that oncocytic tumors of the pituitary may arise from HSGT.

Feigin and colleagues[8] reported a mixed tumor that was theorized to have arisen from heterotopic glandular tissue in a mediastinal lymph node. Three cases of HSGT of the rectum have been documented.[13] Two of the three cases of rectal HSGT were associated with gastric-type mucosa. Marwah and Berman[12] reported a single case of salivary gland tissue in the vulva that contained seromucous glands in addition to respiratory epithelium and cartilage.

Heterotopia and Associated Salivary Gland Tumors

Neoplasms of apparent salivary gland origin that are found at abnormal anatomic sites are usually considered to originate from HSGT. Numerous examples of salivary tumors originating in HSGT have been well documented and include acinic cell carcinoma,[52, 53] adenoid cystic carcinoma,[54] mucoepidermoid carcinoma,[55] adenocarcinoma,[56] monomorphic adenoma,[57] and mixed tumor.[5, 8, 58] The majority of these tumors are thought to arise from heterotopic salivary tissue in lymph nodes. Intraosseous mucoepidermoid carcinomas have been recorded in the posterior mandible; however, many of these tumors are considered to arise from transformation of the lining of odontogenic cysts (see Chapter 16).

The files of the AFIP contain 13 cases of salivary gland tumors that arose from HSGT; 11 of these cases were intranodal. The most common tumor is the mucoepidermoid carcinoma (six cases). Others are mixed tumor (three cases); Warthin's tumor (three cases); and adenoma, not otherwise specified (one case).

ACCESSORY PAROTID GLANDS

The term *accessory parotid gland* refers to lobules of parotid salivary tissue that are separated from the main body of the gland but that drain into Stensen's duct. It is incorrect to refer to the usual intraoral minor salivary glands as accessory salivary glands.

Frommer[59] has shown that 21 percent of a series of 96 cadaver dissections demonstrated accessory parotid salivary gland tissue. He pointed out that anterior extensions of parotid gland tissue along the parotid duct are normal variants of the parotid gland tissue and are not considered accessory salivary gland tissue. Accessory parotid tissue typically ranges from 0.5 to 3.0 cm and may be spherical or oblong. The accessory tissue is usually bound to the fascia of the masseter muscle at an average distance of 6 mm from the anterior edge of the parotid gland, usually on or above the duct. The accessory tissue can be seen anterior to the border of the masseter, resting on the buccal fat pad. This parotid tissue is normally connected to Stensen's duct by a single accessory duct, but there may be two or as many as ten ducts.[60]

The histologic features of accessory parotid tissue are usually identical to those of the primary parotid tissue of the individual.[59] If the main glands exhibit fatty infiltration and mild chronic inflammatory cell infiltrates, then the accessory tissue will display similar features.

It is important to recognize the possible existence of accessory parotid tissue because, for the most part, any pathologic process that can occur in the main gland can also occur in the accessory tissue. If the presence of accessory parotid tissue is not considered in clinical evaluation, inadequate treatment may result. This has been demonstrated by reports of sialadenitis, fibrosis, cysts, and benign and malignant tumors occurring in the accessory parotid tissue.[60–62] Ferguson and MacDonald[61] reported on a patient with parotid sialadenitis that did not resolve after a total parotidectomy was performed because of sialadenitis of an unexcised accessory parotid gland. Polayes

and Rankow[62] reported a series of seven cases involving masses of accessory parotid gland, and they noted one case each of fibrosis, fibromatosis, parotid cyst, and hemangioma. Perzik and White[60] reported that an accessory parotid gland was involved in 46 (7.7 percent) of 591 parotid tumors. Johnson and Spiro[63] found that accessory parotid gland tumors accounted for 1 percent of 2,261 parotid tumors. They noted that 11 of 23 lesions were benign, whereas 12 lesions were malignant. The most common malignant salivary gland neoplasm in accessory parotid tissue has been low-grade mucoepidermoid carcinoma; intermediate and high-grade mucoepidermoid carcinoma, acinic cell carcinoma, malignant mixed tumor, and adenoid cystic carcinoma were also reported.[60–63] The most common benign salivary gland neoplasm has been mixed tumor, although cases of Warthin's tumor and papillary cystadenoma have occurred.[60, 62–64] The histologic character of neoplasms developing in the accessory salivary gland tissue is identical to that seen in lesions arising in the gland proper.

Clinically, lesions of accessory parotid tissue present as masses in the cheek that occur in the central third of a line drawn from the middle of the tragus to a point midway between the ala of the nose and the vermilion border of the upper lip.[60] Some authors[59, 60–62] believe that sialography is useful in the diagnosis of parotid accessory salivary gland lesions, whereas others do not and even consider it misleading.[63] Other investigators have noted that palpation of the area while a lacrimal probe is passed through Stensen's duct can provide as much information as sialography and is less painful and costly.[62]

Failure to recognize and to remove an involved accessory parotid gland during parotidectomy could explain some instances of recurrent lesions. Major considerations in surgical treatment of lesions of accessory parotid tissue are complete removal, acceptable cosmetic result, avoidance of external salivary fistulas, and preservation of the buccozygomatic rami of the facial nerve. Many authors recommend a standard preauriculocervical flap that gives adequate exposure for a superficial or total parotidectomy and that provides an opportunity to preserve facial nerve function.[60, 62, 63, 65] Polayes and Rankow[62] recommend total parotidectomy with excision of the accessory gland for treatment of high-grade malignancy. For inflammatory or benign lesions, they suggest limiting treatment to the excision of the accessory gland or to the excision of the accessory gland and superficial parotidectomy, as clinically indicated.

ONCOCYTOSIS

Oncocytosis is a metaplastic, sometimes hyperplastic, developmental or transformational process that is characterized by focal replacement of normal glandular tissue with enlarged eosinophilic epithelial cells with granular cytoplasm. These swollen epithelial cells were first described by Schaffer,[66] and later the term "onkocyte" was applied by Hamperl.[67] The focal replacement of glandular parenchyma by oncocytes is not exclusive to the salivary glands and may be seen in the bronchial and lacrimal glands, the thyroid and parathyroid glands, the kidney, the breast, the pancreas, the pituitary gland, the testicle, the liver, the stomach, and the esophagus.[68–70] Oncocytosis is seen with greater frequency in older people and is considered a sequela of aging.[71] The majority of cases occur in the parotid, but it may be found in any major or minor gland. Most often oncocytosis is discovered incidentally, particularly in cases of diffuse hyperplastic oncocytosis.[72] When florid, oncocytosis may cause clinical swelling and suggest the presence of a neoplasm. Histologic distinction between oncocytosis and oncocytoma, which is the benign neoplasm of oncocytes, may occasionally be difficult. Multinodular oncocytosis continues to be regarded as a borderline lesion in a conceptually unclear category between a neoplasm and hyperplasia.[73] Most investigators acknowledge focal and diffuse oncocytosis as non-neoplastic but would caution that some oncocytic foci may have the potential for neoplastic growth.[74]

Survey of the AFIP material provided 27 cases of oncocytosis. Many more cases of oncocytosis are included in the AFIP files, but, in most cases, the oncocytosis is a secondary or an incidental finding of insufficient magnitude to warrant coding for later retrieval. The mean age of a patient at the time of diagnosis is 63.9 years with a range of 28.0 to 87.0 years. The distribution of this disorder between males and females is approximately equal. The parotid gland is the most common site (23 cases, 85 percent). Two cases involved the submandibular gland, and one case each involved the buccal mucosa and the tonsil. Oncocytosis was seen in association with a salivary gland tumor in 16 of 27 cases (59 percent). Tumors exhibiting focal oncocytosis included nine cases of oncocytoma, four cases of Warthin's tumor (Fig. 2–5), two cases of acinic cell carcinoma, and one case of mixed tumor.

Histologically, oncocytosis may present as scattered foci of enlarged, eosinophilic epithelial cells (Fig. 2–6) or as a solitary focus of metaplastic oncocytes (Fig. 2–7). The cells may retain an acinar arrangement and form sheets, trabeculae, or duct-like structures surrounded by fine collagen septations. Oncocytosis with a diffuse hyperplastic pattern may show gradual transition from normal cells to oncocytes. The lobular architecture of the glands remains intact. The cytologic features consist of large, eosinophilic, polyhedral epithelial cells with fine granular cytoplasm and a centrally placed pyknotic nucleus. Oncocytes occasionally show transition to clear cells as a result of intracytoplasmic glycogen (Fig. 2–8).[74] Oncocytes stain positive with phosphotungstic acid–hematoxylin

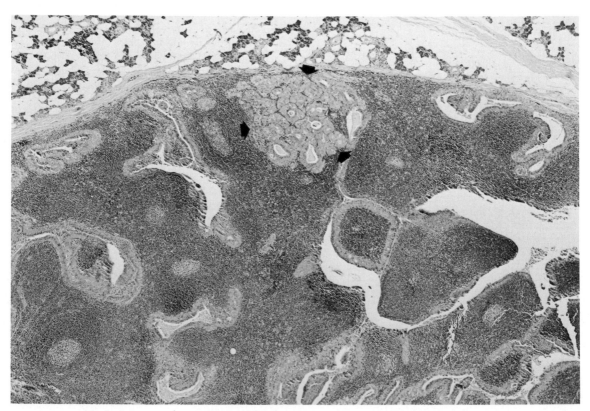

Figure 2–5. Tissue from Warthin's tumor with a focus of oncocytosis (arrows) (× 15).

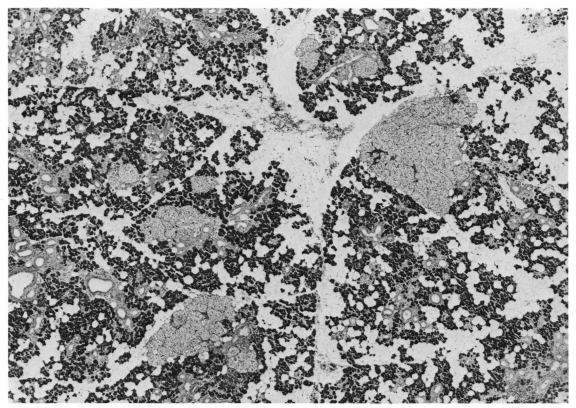

Figure 2–6. Parotid gland tissue with multiple foci of oncocytosis replacing normal acinar tissue (× 15).

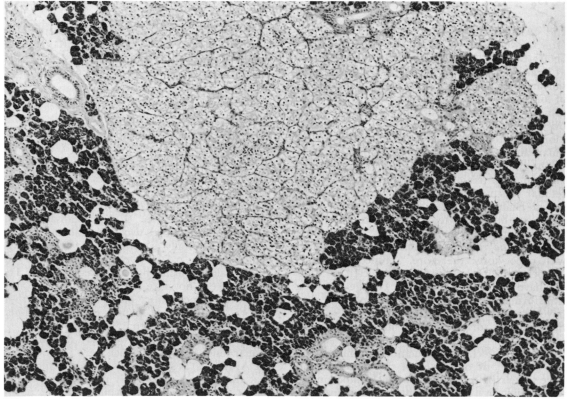

Figure 2–7. Parotid gland tissue with a solitary focus of oncocytes displaying pale-staining granular cytoplasm and centrally placed nuclei (× 30).

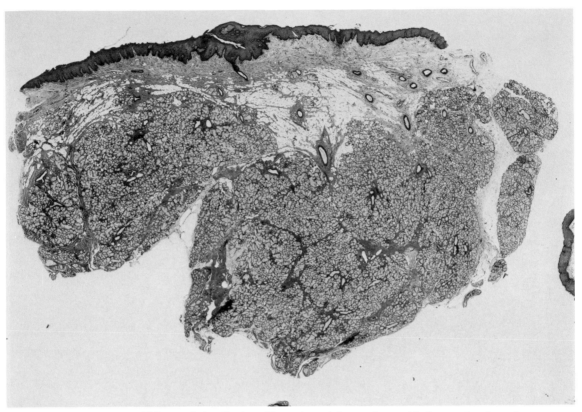

Figure 2–10. Adenomatoid hyperplasia of palate. Normal overlying surface epithelium and enlarged aggregates of mucous acini (× 10). (From AFIP.)

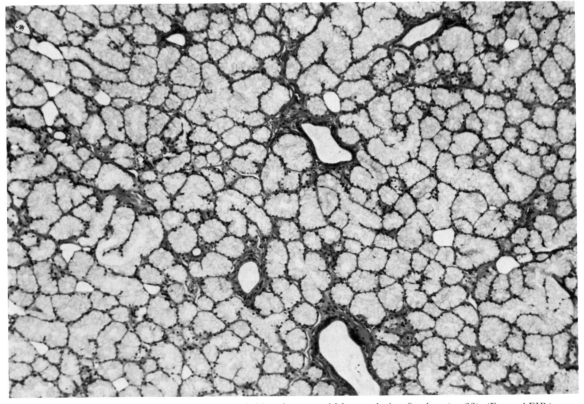

Figure 2–11. Normal-appearing mucous acini in adenomatoid hyperplasia of palate (× 63). (From AFIP.)

tioned that misinterpretation could result in inappropriate treatment.

Treatment for adenomatoid hyperplasia of salivary glands consists of total excision of the lesion.[82, 83, 85–87] Recurrence is not expected.[82–85] Surprisingly, considering the relatively small number of cases published, a possible association with mucoepidermoid carcinoma has been reported. Arafat and coworkers[84] reported on a patient in whom a mucoepidermoid carcinoma developed 12 years after the patient was diagnosed as having mucinous salivary gland hyperplasia on the opposite side of the palate.

POLYCYSTIC (DYSGENETIC) DISEASE OF THE PAROTID GLANDS

Polycystic (dysgenetic) disease is the least common of the benign cystic lesions of the parotid gland and is considered to be a developmental malformation of the duct system. Only six cases have been reported in the literature,[88–90] and two cases are described in the AFIP salivary gland registry.

Clinical Features

The clinical features of polycystic (dysgenetic) disease of the parotid glands are fairly uniform from case to case. All reported lesions in the literature have occurred in females, but one of the two cases from the AFIP involves a male. Five of the six cases reported in the literature were bilateral. The clinical manifestations may be evident during childhood (five of the eight cases) or may be delayed until adulthood. The typical history is that of a recurrent, painless swelling of the involved gland or glands. The swelling is not associated with any clinical abnormality of salivation or with any apparent anomaly of other salivary glands.[88–90] It is not known whether polycystic (dysgenetic) disease of the parotid glands is associated with dysgenetic cysts of the kidney, liver, lung, or pancreas.[88]

Gross Findings

Grossly, the involved glands exhibit an exaggerated lobularity of the subcapsular surface. The cut

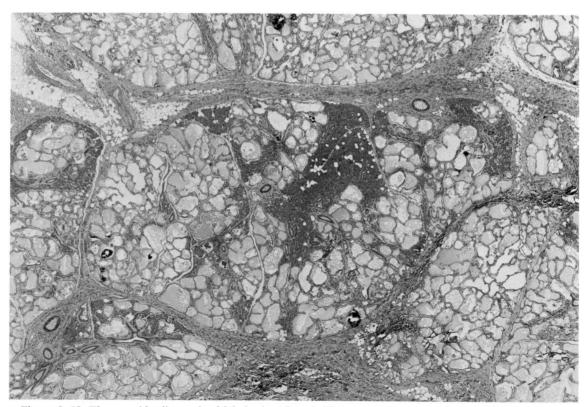

Figure 2–12. The parotid salivary gland lobules in polycystic (dysgenetic) disease are distended by multiple cysts (× 15).

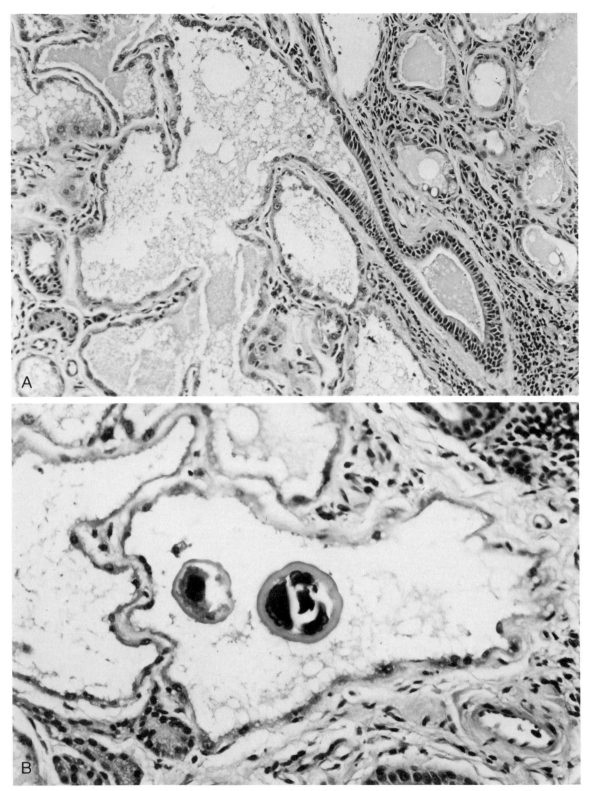

Figure 2–13. Polycystic disease of the parotid gland. *A*, Striated duct is contiguous with cystic dilatation of probable intercalated ducts (× 150). *B*, Microliths with concentric laminar patterns in cyst lumen (× 300).

surface reveals mottled, yellow and ivory nodules, with a fine spongy consistency.[89]

Microscopic Findings

The microscopic features are distinctive. The overall architecture of the glands is preserved; however, the lobules are markedly distended and nearly replaced by epithelum-lined cysts, which impart a honeycombed or latticelike appearance (Fig. 2–12). Small, residual islands of glandular acini are present between the cysts, which vary in size and are variably lined by flattened, cuboidal, or columnar epithelium. The columnar cells have abundant eosinophilic cytoplasm and rounded luminal borders. These features give the appearance of apocrine cells.[88] In some areas, budlike, epithelial proliferations are present; in others, spurlike, incomplete septa occur. Many of the epithelial cells contain striking cytoplasmic vacuolation. Fat stains have confirmed that these vacuoles contain lipid.[89]

Occasional ducts open directly into cysts, and some acinar units communicate with cysts (Fig. 2–13); these features suggest that the cysts arise from intercalated ducts. This suggestion is further supported by the similarity of ultrastructural features of the cuboidal cells to those described in normal intercalated duct epithelium.[89]

Most cyst lumina contain flocculent, eosinophilic material and a few scattered macrophages. In addition, many cysts contain eosinophilic bodies with concentric and radial patterns that are similar to those of spheroliths and microliths (Fig. 2–13). No evidence of sialadenitis in the involved glands is present. In a case reported by Dobson and Ellis,[89] salivary gland tissue in a juxtaparotid lymph node showed cystic changes that were identical to those in the parotid gland.

Differential Diagnosis

Several salivary gland tumors, including mucoepidermoid carcinoma, acinic cell adenocarcinoma, and cystadenocarcinoma, may have a prominent multifocal cystic pattern. However, the widespread involvement of the salivary gland parenchyma, the variable epithelial lining, the presence of spheroliths and microliths, and the relative lack of inflammation are histologic features that separate polycystic (dysgenetic) disease from other cystic lesions of the parotid gland.

REFERENCES

1. Willis RA: Some unusual developmental heterotopias. Br Med J 1968; 3:267–272.
2. Goodman MD, Daly JF, Valenis Q: Heterotopic salivary tissue and branchial cleft sinus. Laryngoscope 1981; 91:260–264.
3. Saeger KL, Gruskin P, Carberry JN: Salivary gland choristoma of the middle ear. Arch Pathol Lab Med 1982; 106:39–40.
4. Stingle WH, Priebe CJ: Ectopic salivary gland and sinus in the lower neck. Ann Otol 1974; 83:379–381.
5. Pesavento G, Ferlito A: Benign mixed tumor of heterotopic salivary gland tissue in the upper neck. J Laryngol Otol 1976; 90:577–584.
6. Stene T, Pedersen KN: Aberrant salivary gland tissue in the anterior mandible. Oral Surg Oral Med Oral Pathol 1977; 44:72–75.
7. Braun GA, Lowry LD, Meyers A: Bilateral choristomas of the external auditory canals. Arch Otolaryngol 1978; 104:467–468.
8. Feigin GA, Robinson B, Marchevsky A: Mixed tumor of the mediastinum. Arch Pathol Lab Med 1986; 110:80–81.
9. Curry B, Taylor CW, Fisher AW: Salivary gland heterotopia. A unique cerebellopontine angle tumor. Arch Pathol Lab Med 1982; 106:35–38.
10. Schochet SS, McCormick WF, Halmi NS: Salivary gland rests in the human pituitary. Arch Pathol 1974; 98:193–200.
11. Dikman SH, Toker C: Seromucinous gland ectopia within the prostatic stroma. J Urol 1973; 109:852–854.
12. Marwah S, Berman ML: Ectopic salivary gland in vulva (choristoma): Report of a case and review of literature. Obstet Gynecol 1980; 56:389–391.
13. Weitzner S: Ectopic salivary gland tissue in submucosa of rectum. Dis Colon Rectum 1983; 26:814–817.
14. Thackray AC, Lucas RB: Tumors of the Major Salivary Glands. Atlas of Tumor Pathology, 2nd Series, Fascicle 10. Washington, DC, Armed Forces Institute of Pathology, 1974; 1–2.
15. Bernier JL, Bhaskar SN: Lymphoepithelial lesions of the salivary glands. Cancer 1978; 11:1156–1178.
16. Azzopardi JG, Hou LT: The genesis of adenolymphoma. J Pathol 1964; 88:213–218.
17. Romano JF, Marino CT: Heterotopic salivary tissue at the base of the neck. Int J Dermatol 1982; 21:42–43.
18. Nash M, Hyun C, Cohen J: Salivary choristomas in the neck. Otolaryngol Head Neck Surg 1982; 90:279–282.
19. Shvero J, Hadar T, Avidor I, Abraham A, Sidi J: Heterotopic salivary tissue and branchial sinuses. J Laryngol Otol 1986; 100:243–246.
20. Youngs LA, Scofield HH: Heterotopic salivary gland tissue in the lower neck. Arch Pathol 1967; 83:550–556.
21. Soucy P: Congenital cervical salivary fistula. Can J Surg 1985; 28:130–131.
22. Mair IWS, Bjorng G, Kearney MS: Heterotopic cervical salivary gland. J Laryngol Otol 1977; 91:35–40.
23. Himalstein MR: Letter to the editor. Laryngoscope 1981; 91:1200–1201.
24. Adams WP, Donahoe PK: Salivary gland heterotopia in the lower part of the neck. Arch Surg 1979; 114:79–81.
25. Taylor G, Martin H: Salivary gland tissue in the middle ear. Arch Otolaryngol 1961; 73:49–51.

26. Kartush JM, Graham MD: Salivary gland choristoma of the middle ear: A case report and review of the literature. Laryngoscope 1984; 94:228–230.

27. Wine CJ, Metcalf JE: Salivary gland choristoma of the middle ear and mastoid. Arch Otolaryngol 1977; 103:435–436.

28. Moore PJ, Benjamin BNP, Kan AE: Salivary gland choristoma of the middle ear. Intern J Pediatr Otolaryngol 1984; 8:91–95.

29. Peron DL, Schuknecht HF: Congenital cholesteatomata with other anomalies. Arch Otolaryngol 1975; 101:498–505.

30. Abadir WF, Pease WS: Salivary gland choristoma of the middle ear. J Laryngol Otol 1978; 92:247–252.

31. Quaranta A, Mininni F, Resta L: Salivary gland choristoma of the middle ear. J Laryngol Otol 1981; 95:953–956.

32. Caplinger CB, Hora JF: Middle ear choristoma with absent oval window. Arch Otolaryngol 1967; 85:39–40.

33. Peel RL, Gnepp DR: Diseases of salivary glands. In Barnes L (ed.): Surgical Pathology of the Head and Neck. New York, Marcel Dekker Inc, 1985; 547.

34. Hociota D, Ataman T: A case of salivary gland choristoma of the middle ear. Arch Otol 1967; 89:1065–1068.

35. Saeed YM, Bassis ML: Mixed tumor of the middle ear. A case report. Arch Otolaryngol 1971; 93:422–434.

36. Stafne EC: Bone cavities situated near the angle of the mandible. J Am Dent Assoc 1942; 29:1969–1972.

37. Jacobs MH: Traumatic bone cyst. Oral Surg Oral Med Oral Pathol 1955; 8:940–949.

38. Thoma KH: Case report of a so called latent bone cyst. Oral Surg Oral Med Oral Pathol 1955; 8:963–966.

39. Harvey W, Noble HW: Defects of the lingual surface of the mandible near the angle. Br J Surg 1968; 6:75–83.

40. Choukas NC, Toto PD: Etiology of static bone defects of the mandible. J Oral Surg 1960; 18:16–20.

41. Uemura S, Fujishita M, Fuchihata H: Radiographic interpretation of so called developmental defect of mandible. Oral Surg Oral Med Oral Pathol 1976; 41:120–128.

42. Strom C, Fjellstrom C: An unusual case of lingual mandibular depression. Oral Surg Oral Med Oral Pathol 1987; 64:159–161.

43. Palladino VS, Rose SA: Salivary gland tissue in the mandible and Stafne's mandibular "cysts." J Am Dent Assoc 1965; 70:388–393.

44. Richard EL, Ziskind J: Aberrant salivary gland in the mandible. Oral Surg Oral Med Oral Pathol 1957; 10:1086–1090.

45. Miller AS, Winnick M: Salivary gland inclusion in the anterior mandible. Oral Surg Oral Med Oral Pathol 1971; 31:790–797.

46. Sandy JR, Williams DM: Anterior salivary gland inclusion in the mandible: Pathological entity or anatomical variant? Br J Oral Surg 1981; 19:223–229.

47. Hayashi Y, Kimura Y, Nagumo M: Anterior lingual mandibular bone concavity. Oral Surg Oral Med Oral Pathol 1984; 57:139–142.

48. Abrams A, Howell F, Bullock W: Nasopalatine cysts. Oral Surg Oral Med Oral Pathol 1963; 16:306–332.

49. Moskow BS, Baden E: Gingival choristoma. Oral Surg Oral Med Oral Pathol 1964; 18:504–516.

50. Ide F, Shimura H, Umemura S: Gingival salivary gland choristoma: an extremely rare phenomenon. Oral Surg Oral Med Oral Pathol 1983; 55:169–172.

51. Brannon RB, Houston GD, Wampler HW: Gingival salivary gland choristoma. Oral Surg Oral Med Oral Pathol 1986; 61:185–188.

52. Perzin KH, Livolsi VA: Acinic cell carcinoma arising in ectopic salivary gland tissue. Cancer 1980; 45:967–972.

53. Yacoub U, Carstens PH, Biscopink RJ, McMurry GT: Acinic cell tumor in ectopic salivary gland tissue (letter). Arch Pathol Lab Med 1981; 105:500–501.

54. Cannon CR, Mclean WC: Adenoid cystic carcinoma of the middle ear and temporal bone. Otolaryngol Head Neck Surg 1983; 91:96–99.

55. Smith A, Winkler B, Perzin KH, Wazen J, Blitzer A: Mucoepidermoid carcinoma arising in an intraparotid lymph node. Cancer 1985; 55:400–403.

56. Ludmer B, Joachims HZ, Ben Aire J, Eliachar I: Adenocarcinoma in heterotopic salivary tissue. Arch Otolaryngol 1981; 107:547–548.

57. Luna MA, Tortoledo ME, Allen M: Salivary dermal analogue tumors arising in lymph nodes. Cancer 1987; 59:1165–1169.

58. Cotelingam JD, Gerberi MP: Parotid heterotopia with pleomorphic adenoma. Arch Otolaryngol 1983; 109:563–565.

59. Frommer J: The human accessory parotid gland: Its incidence, nature, and significance. Oral Surg Oral Med Oral Pathol 1977; 43:671–676.

60. Perzik SL, White IL: Surgical management of preauricular tumors of the accessory parotid apparatus. Am J Surg 1966; 112:498–503.

61. Ferguson MM, MacDonald DG: Persistent sialadenitis in an accessory salivary gland. Oral Surg Oral Med Oral Pathol 1978; 45:696–700.

62. Polayes IM, Rankow RM: Cysts, masses, and tumors of the accessory parotid gland. Plast Reconstr Surg 1979; 64:17–23.

63. Johnson FE, Spiro RH: Tumors arising in accessory parotid tissue. Am J Surg 1979; 138:576–578.

64. Kronenberg J, Horowitz A, Creter D: Pleomorphic adenoma arising in accessory salivary tissue with constriction of Stensen's duct. J Laryngol Otol 1988; 102:382–383.

65. Batsakis JG: Pathology consultation: accessory parotid gland. Ann Otol Rhinol Laryngol 1988; 97:343–435.

66. Schaffer J: Beitrage zur Histologie Menischlicher Organe. IV. Zunge. V. Mundhohle-Schlundkopf. VI. Oesophagus VIII. Cardia. Sitzungsber. d. Kais Akad. d. Wissensch., Math. naturwiss. Classe, Abth.III 1897; 106:353–357.

67. Hamperl H: Onkocyten und Geschwulste der Speicheldrusen. Virchows Arch [A] 1931; 282:724–736.

68. Schwartz IA, Feldman M: Diffuse oncocytoma ("oncocytosis") of the parotid gland. Cancer 1969; 23:636–640.

69. Johns ME, Regezi JA, Batsakis JG: Oncocytic neoplasms of salivary glands: an ultrastructural study. Laryngoscope 1977; 87:862–867.

70. Meza Chavez L: Oxyphilic granular cell adenoma

of the parotid gland (oncocytoma). Am J Pathol 1949; 25:523–538.

71. Martinez-Madrigal F, Micheau C: Histology of the major salivary glands. Am J Surg Pathol 1989; 13:879–899.

72. Tkeda Y: Diffuse hyperplastic oncocytosis of the parotid gland. Int J Oral Maxillofac Surg 1986; 15:765–768.

73. Blanck C, Eneroth CM, Jakobsson PA: Oncocytoma of the parotid gland: neoplasm or nodular hyperplasia? Cancer 1970; 25:919–925.

74. Ellis GL: "Clear cell" oncocytoma of salivary gland. Hum Pathol 1988; 19:862–867.

75. Jaffe RH: Adenolymphoma (onkocytoma) of the parotid gland. Am J Cancer 1932; 16:1415–1423.

76. Becker K, Donath K, Seifert G: Die diffuse onkozytose der parotis. Definition und differentialdiagnose. Laryngol Rhinol Otol 1982; 61:691–701.

77. Batsakis JG: Tumors of the Head and Neck: Clinical and Pathological Considerations, 2nd Ed. Baltimore, Williams & Wilkins, 1979; 58.

78. Schulz H: Electron microscopy of oncocytomas and carcinoid tumors. Recent Results Cancer Res 1974; 44:63–68.

79. Balogh K, Roth SI: Histochemical electron microscopic studies of eosinophilic granular cells (oncocytes) in tumors of the parotid gland. Lab Invest 1965; 44:310–320.

80. Roth RI: Pathology of the parathyroids in hyperparathyroidism. Arch Pathol 1962; 73:85–87.

81. Hendrick JW: The treatment of tumors of minor salivary glands. Surg Gynecol Obstet 1964; 118:101–111.

82. Giansanti JS, Baker GO, Waldron CA: Intraoral, mucinous, minor salivary gland lesions presenting clinically as tumors. Oral Surg Oral Med Oral Pathol 1971; 32:918–922.

83. Devildos LR, Langlois CC: Minor salivary gland lesion presenting clinically as tumor. Oral Surg Oral Med Oral Pathol 1976; 41:657–659.

84. Arafat A, Brannon RB, Ellis GL: Adenomatoid hyperplasia of mucous salivary glands. Oral Surg Oral Med Oral Pathol 1981; 52:51–55.

85. Aufdemorte TB, Ramzy I, Holt GR, Thomas JR, Duncan DL: Focal adenomatoid hyperplasia of salivary glands: a differential diagnostic problem in fine needle aspiration biopsy. Acta Cytol 1985; 29:23–28.

86. Brannon RB, Houston GD, Meader CL: Adenomatoid hyperplasia of mucous salivary glands: A case involving the retromolar area. Oral Surg Oral Med Oral Pathol 1985; 60:188–190.

87. Brown FH, Houston GD, Lubow RM, Sagan MA: Adenomatoid hyperplasia of mucous salivary glands: report of two cases. J Periodontol 1987; 58:125–127.

88. Seifert G, Thomsen ST, Donath K: Bilateral dysgenetic parotid glands. Morphological analysis and differential diagnosis of a rare disease of the salivary glands. Virchows Arch [A] 1981; 390:273–288.

89. Dobson CM, Ellis HA: Polycystic disease of the parotid glands: case report of a rare entity and review of the literature. Histopathology 1987; 11:953–961.

90. Batsakis JG, Bruner JM, Luna MA: Polycystic (dysgenetic) disease of the parotid glands. Arch Otolaryngol Head Neck Surg 1988; 114:1146–1148.

OBSTRUCTIVE DISORDERS

3

Brent M. Koudelka

Obstructive disorders are some of the most common disorders of the major and minor salivary glands. They can occur as a result of traumatic severance of salivary gland ducts, stasis of salivary secretions in ducts, and partial or complete blockage of the excretory ducts. Many conditions may cause enlargement of salivary glands or cessation of salivary flow and, thus, mimic or promote the development of an obstructive disorder. These conditions include congenital malformations and developmental cysts; acute, chronic, and granulomatous inflammation;[1-3] hypersensitivity and autoimmune disorders;[4] drug therapy and chemical exposure;[5, 6] systemic and metabolic disorders;[4] exposure to ionizing radiation;[7] ischemic episodes;[8, 9] and benign and malignant neoplasms.[4]

The primary means by which these disorders cause a reduction or cessation of salivary flow can be attributed to one of two processes: destruction of the secretory elements of the gland, or a mechanical blockage or disruption of the ductal system that leads from the gland to the oral cavity. Infectious processes, autoimmune disorders, drug therapy, ischemic episodes, certain metabolic disorders, and exposure to ionizing radiation can all reduce or eliminate the ability of a gland to produce secretions by altering or destroying the acinar elements of the gland. As such, they are physiologic alterations. Conversely, mechanical methods of obstruction include damage that is caused by trauma, compression by a cyst or a neoplasm, and formation of a mucus plug or sialolith within a duct.

The effects of these disorders are often interrelated. Long-term or recurrent inflammatory processes can cause atrophy of the acinar elements of the gland and can also damage the epithelial lining of the ducts, which results in stenosis, stricture, or both.[4, 7] This can lead to reduction in the

salivary flow, as well as to stasis of glandular secretions, which potentiates the formation of an obstruction. Furthermore, the processes need not be self-limiting. Prolonged stasis can enhance the possibility of recurrent retrograde infections, which may further damage the parenchyma of the gland. Neoplastic processes can also produce a combination of effects. Most benign salivary gland tumors are slow-growing, well-circumscribed lesions that have a primarily compressive effect; however, their malignant counterparts frequently grow more rapidly and infiltrate the parenchyma of the salivary gland. This can lead to mechanical obstruction of the ductal system as well as to physical destruction of the secretory elements of the gland.

In this chapter, emphasis is placed on three of the more common primary mechanical obstructive disorders of salivary glands: mucus escape reactions, mucus retention cysts, and obstructions caused by sialoliths. Of the over 20,000 neoplastic and non-neoplastic salivary gland lesions reported in the registry of salivary gland pathology at the Armed Forces Institute of Pathology (AFIP), 2,731 lesions (13.4 percent) are classified as mucus escape reactions, mucus retention cysts, or sialoliths. Of these, the diagnosis for the vast majority of lesions is mucus escape reaction (85.7 percent), with the remainder nearly equally divided between mucus retention cysts (6.5 percent) and sialoliths (7.8 percent).

MUCUS ESCAPE REACTION

Mucus escape reaction is defined as a pooling of mucus in a cavity within the connective tissue that is not lined by epithelium. This lesion is described by a number of names, including mucus retention phenomena,[10, 11] mucocele,[12] ranula,[13] and mucus retention cyst.[14] Of these, mucocele and mucus retention phenomena are probably the

All material in this chapter is in the public domain with the exception of any borrowed figures or tables.

most frequently used terms. Early investigators believed that the lesion developed as a result of obstruction of the excretory duct of a salivary gland and the subsequent formation of an epithelially lined cyst.[15] However, the findings from Bhaskar and coworkers'[16] study of mice and Standish and Shafer's[17] study of rats did not support this hypothesis. In each of these studies, ligation of excretory ducts of salivary glands leading from the submandibular or sublingual glands failed to produce a lesion similar to the classic mucus escape reaction. Instead, in another study, which used mice and rats, Bhaskar and coworkers[12] demonstrated that severance of the duct leading from a salivary gland and subsequent extravasation of mucin into the surrounding tissues produced a lesion histologically identical to the common mucus escape reaction seen in humans. Based on these studies, it is now generally accepted that traumatic severance of a duct with resultant pooling of mucus within the surrounding tissues is the origin of these lesions.

Clinical Features

The mucus escape reaction may present in association with either a major or a minor salivary gland but is most frequently seen in association with the minor glands. Data collected on 2,339 cases accessioned at the AFIP show the lower lip to be the most common site, followed by the lip (upper or lower, unspecified), the buccal mucosa, the floor of the mouth, and the tongue and palate (Table 3–1). Lesions of the lips account for 64.2 percent of all lesions accessioned. Of lip lesions whose site was specified, 98.8 percent affected the lower lip. These findings are consistent with those of Cataldo and Mosadomi,[18] who reported in a study of 594 cases that 58.6 percent of all lesions were of the lower lip and that 96.9 percent of lip lesions were of the lower lip. Conversely, mucus escape reactions of the parotid, submandibular, or sublingual glands are uncommon in AFIP material; collectively they compose only 2.9 percent of the lesions examined.

Most investigators consider these lesions to be most common in children and young adults.[18, 19] The age range of patients in the AFIP material spans the first through the tenth decades. However, lesions presenting in the first through third decades constitute 70.1 percent of all cases accessioned (Fig. 3–1). The mean age of patients is 25.3 years; the average age of females in this group is 21.6 years, and males 26.7 years. Interestingly, collective review of AFIP cases suggests a nearly 3:1 male predilection for these lesions, a finding that contradicts reported studies, which suggest no significant sex predilection for these lesions.[10, 18] However, when only civilian patients are considered, the difference between the number of males (53.1 percent) and females (46.9

Table 3–1. Distribution by Anatomic Site of 2,339 Cases of Mucus Escape Reaction Reported in the AFIP Registry of Salivary Gland Pathology

Anatomic Site	Number	Percent
Major Glands		
Parotid gland	14	0.6
Submandibular gland	27	1.2
Sublingual gland	25	1.1
Minor Glands		
Lip, Total	1,502	64.2
Lip (not otherwise specified)	(727)	(31.1)
Upper lip	(9)	(0.4)
Lower lip	(766)	(32.7)
Palate, total	82	3.5
Palate (not otherwise specified)	(62)	(2.6)
Hard palate	(4)	(0.2)
Soft palate	(16)	(0.7)
Floor of mouth	148	6.3
Tongue (not otherwise specified)	143	6.1
Buccal Mucosa	179	7.7
Neck	1	<0.1
Gingiva	8	0.3
Tonsillar area	1	<0.1
Uvula	3	0.1
Mandible	9	0.4
Retromolar area	4	0.2
Maxilla	1	<0.1
Minor salivary glands	4	0.2
Oral cavity (not otherwise specified)	73	3.1
Site Not Stated	115	4.9
*Total**	2,339	100

*Numbers in parentheses not included in total.

percent) is not significant. The difference is explained by the fact that only 32 of the 1,048 military cases in the AFIP material were female patients. We believe this reflects the greater proportion of males in the military population rather than a true biologic propensity for males to develop mucus escape reactions.

The clinical presentation of these lesions varies, depending on their depth within the soft tissues. Superficial lesions present as raised soft tissue swellings, often vesicular in appearance and fluctuant upon palpation. If the lesions are very close to the surface, the overlying epithelium may appear thinned, which gives the lesion an overall, translucent, bluish color. They are usually well circumscribed and may vary in size from a few millimeters to more than a centimeter in diameter. Lesions located deeper within the soft tissues are more nodular and lack the vesicular appearance of the superficial lesions. They are normally colored in relation to the surrounding mucosa; however, as with the superficial lesions, they are usually well circumscribed and fluctuant when palpated. The most common clinical course of the mucus escape reaction is of a painless mucosal

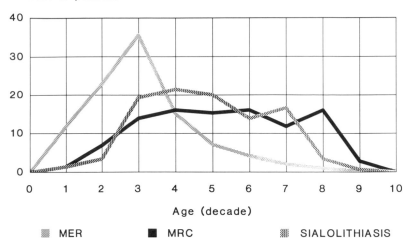

Percent of patients

Age (decade)

MER ■ MRC ▒ SIALOLITHIASIS

Figure 3–1. Graph illustrates distribution by age of patients with mucus escape reaction (MER), mucus retention cyst (MRC), and sialolithiasis according to data from the AFIP registry of salivary gland pathology.

swelling that develops during a period of from a few days to a week and ruptures with apparent resolution, only to recur within a period of from a few weeks to a month. Other lesions may persist for weeks or months and may occasionally increase in size, liberating a viscous, mucinous fluid, if ruptured. As mentioned previously, pain is not a common complaint; however, if the lesion has recently been traumatized or if it becomes secondarily inflamed, mild symptoms may develop. In superficial lesions, recurrent trauma may also result in extravasation of blood into the defect, which produces a reddish color that is suggestive of a vascular lesion (Fig. 3–2).

The ranula is a type of mucus escape reaction that occurs as a swelling in the floor of the mouth (Fig. 3–3).[20, 21] Less common than the small lesions that are associated with minor salivary glands, the ranula is most frequently associated with the sublingual gland, but occasionally it may be associated with the submandibular gland.[10, 13, 20, 22] If the lesion is located above the mylohyoid musculature, it can fill the floor of the mouth and raise the tongue. If it is located below or dissects through the mylohyoid musculature, the swelling is located in the area of the submandibular space and inferior border of the mandible. In rare cases, these lesions may dissect down into the suprahyoid and inframylohyoid regions of the neck. These lesions have been described as "plunging" or cervical ranulas.[13, 22] Like their minor salivary gland counterparts, ranulas present as asymptomatic, fluctuant swellings, with little or no complaint of discomfort by the patient. Superficial ranulas are often translucent, vesicular, and bluish in color. Deeper lesions appear normal in color. Unlike the minor salivary gland lesions, they are usually large lesions that produce a more noticeable swelling and possess the potential for obstruction of the airway.[18, 23]

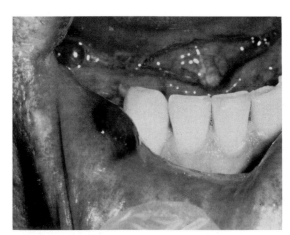

Figure 3–2. Mucus escape reaction of the lower lip, most frequently called a mucocele. Recent trauma resulted in extravasation of blood into the lesion, thus causing erythema.

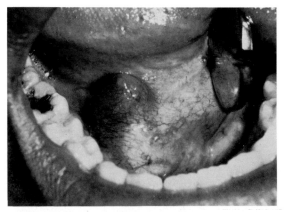

Figure 3–3. Mucus escape reaction of the floor of the mouth, most frequently called a ranula. The lesion appears translucent and bluish in color as a result of its superficial location in relation to the overlying oral mucosa.

Pathologic Features

The histologic features of most mucus escape reactions are similar, with slight variations that depend on the age of the lesion. Common to all lesions is the lack of an epithelial lining. As such, the mucus escape reaction is not a true cyst. Characteristically, an early lesion consists of a moderately well-defined and occasionally circumscribed cavity within the soft tissue that is filled with an eosinophilic material that stains positive for mucin (Fig. 3–4). Within the material, an admixture of acute and chronic inflammatory cells and foamy histiocytes may be found. The tissue surrounding the cavity consists of compressed fibrovascular connective tissue, which on low magnification may be misinterpreted as an epithelial lining (Fig. 3–5A). A variable number of polymorphonuclear leukocytes, lymphocytes, and plasma cells may be seen in the surrounding soft tissue. Salivary gland acini or ductal elements adjacent to the lesion are a frequent finding. As the lesion matures, granulation tissue progressively grows into the cavity and slowly obliterates the defect (Fig. 3–5B). The term *organizing mucocele* is some-times applied to the lesion during this phase. In fact, this granulation process represents an attempted repair of the lesion by the body. Clinically, the ranula is a larger lesion than the mucocele, but they are histologically similar (Fig. 3–6A).

Changes may also be seen in the salivary gland adjacent to the primary lesion. These include a generalized chronic sialadenitis; distention of intralobular and interlobular ducts, with stasis and inspissation of mucus; atrophic changes of the individual acinar elements; proliferation of small ducts; and variable degrees of interstitial fibrosis within the salivary gland lobules (Fig. 3–6B).[16, 17] In addition, the overlying mucosal epithelium may show thinning and flattening of the rete ridges as a result of the circumferential expansion of the lesion.

Differential Diagnosis

Cataldo and Mosadomi[18] reported that over 88 percent of cases of mucus escape reactions in their study were clinically diagnosed as mucoceles by the clinician. This notwithstanding, there are a

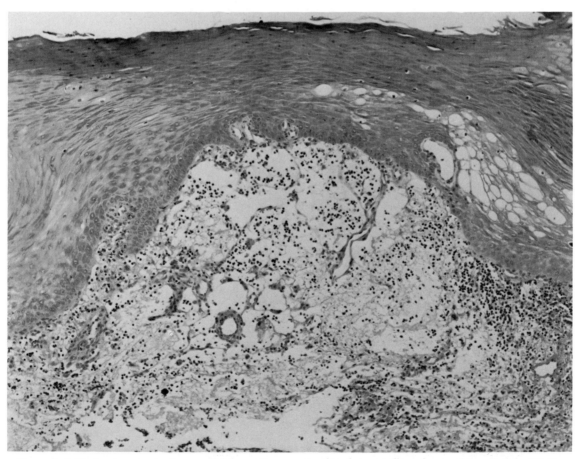

Figure 3–4. Photomicrograph of a superficial mucus escape reaction shows pooling of mucus beneath the epithelium (× 175).

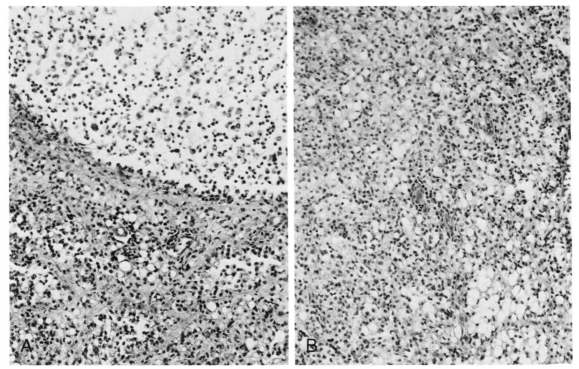

Figure 3–5. *A*, the lumen of the lesion (top) is filled with mucus that contains scattered chronic inflammatory cells and foamy histiocytes. The wall of the lesion (bottom) consists of compressed fibrovascular connective tissue and granulation tissue (× 150). Note the absence of an epithelial lining. *B*, with time, the granulation tissue grows into the cavity and completely obliterates the defect (× 150).

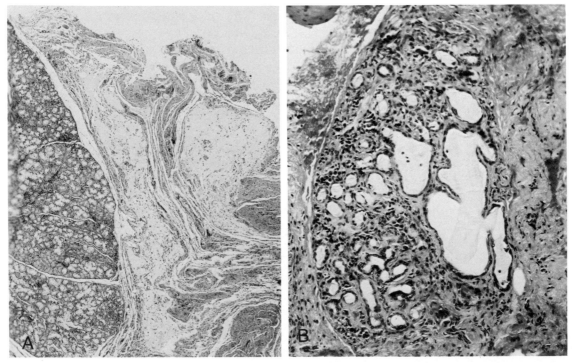

Figure 3–6. *A*, large mucus escape reaction (ranula) of the floor of the mouth (× 30). *B*, adjacent salivary gland lobule shows a chronic inflammatory infiltrate, acinar atrophy, ductal ectasia with stasis of mucus, proliferation of small ducts, and interstitial fibrosis (× 150).

number of conditions that may clinically and histologically mimic mucus escape reactions. These include focal manifestations of a vesiculoerosive disorder, hematoma, lymphangioma, and hemangioma. Deep-seated lesions include developmental cysts and salivary gland adenomas or adenocarcinomas. Cystic processes may usually be excluded histologically because the mucus escape reaction lacks an epithelial lining. However, dilated excretory ducts with metaplastic epithelium are often seen in association with mucoceles. Preparation of sections with a special stain for mucin, such as mucicarmine, Alcian blue, and colloidal iron, is helpful in excluding nonsalivary gland lesions.

Careful histologic examination is essential to exclude several low-grade adenocarcinomas that may have some histologic features similar to those of the mucus escape reactions. First among these adenocarcinomas is low-grade mucoepidermoid carcinoma. These tumors typically are cystic and may contain pools of mucus that dissect through fibrous connective tissue (see Chapter 16, Fig. 16–16); thus they may be misinterpreted as a mucus escape reaction. Any proliferation of epithelium or cells that show intracellular accumulations of mucin should alert the pathologist to the possibility of low-grade mucoepidermoid carcinoma. The mucus filled histiocytes in mucus escape reactions may be mistaken for mucocytes of mucoepidermoid carcinoma. However, the absence of an epithelial lining of the cavity should help differentiate mucus escape reaction from mucoepidermoid carcinoma. Care must also be taken to assure that an acinic cell adenocarcinoma is not misinterpreted as the late stage of a mucus escape reaction. This is because the granular character of the acinar type cells of acinic cell adenocarcinoma can appear similar to the foamy histiocytes of an organizing mucus escape reaction. Acinar cells are mucicarmine negative and possess periodic acid–Schiff–positive granules. Conversely, the foamy histiocytes of a mucus escape reaction are usually mucicarmine positive without periodic acid–Schiff–positive granules.

Swellings below the mylohyoid region or extending into the cervical region require differentiation of plunging or cervical ranula from developmental cysts or neoplastic lesions of the submandibular and thyroid glands.

Treatment and Prognosis

Treatment of mucus escape reactions is most frequently surgical with assured removal of *both* the lesion and the adjacent minor salivary gland and duct. In cases where only the lesion is removed, recurrence is frequently a problem because the involved gland continues to secrete saliva into the connective tissue. When this occurs, retreatment of the lesion is necessary. Exception to this approach may be made for a ranula. Initial

treatment of this lesion may sometimes be limited to the unroofing (marsupialization) of the lesion or the cannulation of the duct.[22, 23] The purpose of these procedures is to salvage the functioning major salivary gland by re-establishing communication with the oral cavity. Unfortunately, in most cases, the cavity does not become lined by epithelium, and the procedure proves unsuccessful. Further treatment, including removal of the salivary gland, is then necessary to avoid subsequent recurrence.[13, 20, 22]

MUCUS RETENTION CYST

An obstructive disorder of the salivary gland that is less common than the mucus escape reaction is the mucus retention cyst. Unlike the mucus escape reaction, the mucus retention cyst is a true cyst that is lined by epithelium. The exact classification of this entity is somewhat in question. Some investigators prefer to simply include it with the more common mucus escape reaction, whereas others would have it stand alone as a separate entity. Harrison[19] suggests using the term *extravasation mucocele* for the common mucus escape reaction and the term *retention mucocele* for the true cyst that is lined by epithelium. Eversole[24] has chosen to classify the mucus retention cyst as an oral sialocyst, thus separating the lesions lined by epithelium from the mucus escape reactions. In fact, there does seem to be justification for separation of these two processes based on the clinical and histologic findings.

There is also some question as to the precise cause of these cystic lesions. Chaudhry and coworkers[14] make reference to the "so-called retention cyst" in their paper on the pathogenesis of the mucocele. In their study, which was designed to confirm the earlier works of Bhaskar and associates[12] and of Standish and Shafer,[10] they noted that ten of their cases showed only markedly dilated ducts, with no evidence of spillage of mucus into the adjacent connective tissue. They interpreted this as suggesting that some "mucus retention cysts" may develop as a result of pinching or partial obstruction of a duct, possibly extraluminal, as opposed to complete severance of the duct as seen in the common mucus escape reaction. They went on to propose that a buildup of pressure in the duct may cause its dilatation without rupture, and they suggested that this increase in intraluminal pressure may be responsible for the proliferation of the ductal epithelium seen in some lesions. Similarly, Standish and Shafer[10] noted in their study of 97 cases of mucus retention phenomenon that occasional lesions, not believed to represent tangentially sectioned dilated ducts adjacent to the pools of extravasated mucus, demonstrated a partial or complete lining of epithelium. Based on these observations, it seems likely that the mucus retention cyst is a distinct entity, the cause of which may be related to epithelial proliferation of a partially obstructed duct of a salivary gland rather than to duct severance, such as occurs in the mucus escape reaction, or in complete obstruction, which is seen with sialoliths.

Clinical Features

In our experience, the mucus retention cyst is a relatively uncommon lesion, representing only 0.9 percent of salivary gland lesions accessioned to the registry of salivary gland pathology at the AFIP. Review of the 178 cases shows the parotid gland to be the most common site (87.6 percent), followed by the submandibular gland, the neck, the sublingual gland, and the buccal mucosa (Table 3–2). Notably, 96.0 percent of all of these lesions occur in one of the major salivary glands. This is in contrast to 70 similar cases studied by Eversole[24] in which the predominant sites were the floor of the mouth (44 percent) and the buccal mucosa (33 percent). The ages of patients reported in the AFIP material ranged from the first through the ninth decades of life, with only 8.3 percent of mucus retention cysts occurring in patients before the age of 20 years (Fig. 3–1).

The mean age of patients is 47.5 years. The average age in this group for females is 46.8 years; for males, it is 47.9 years. Again, the total AFIP data suggest a 2:1 male predilection for this lesion. However, if the cases involving the predominantly male military personnel are excluded, males compose 57.0 percent of the patients and females, 43.0 percent.

The clinical presentation of the mucus retention cyst is usually that of a slowly enlarging, painless, circumscribed, often fluctuant, soft tissue swelling that may persist from months to years (Fig. 3–7). The cysts vary in size, and like the mucus escape reaction, their coloration depends on their depth within the soft tissue. Superficial lesions are more vesicular and bluish, whereas deep lesions are nodular and the same color as the overlying soft tissue.

Table 3–2. Distribution by Anatomic Site of 178 Cases of Mucus Retention Cyst Reported in the AFIP Registry of Salivary Gland Pathology

Anatomic Site	Number	Percent
Major Glands		
Parotid gland	156	87.6
Submandibular gland	14	7.8
Sublingual gland	1	0.6
Minor Glands		
Buccal Mucosa	1	0.6
Neck	3	1.7
Site Not Stated	3	1.7
Total	178	100

Pathologic Features

The key histologic feature of the mucus retention cyst, which sets it apart from the more common mucus escape reaction, is the presence of an epithelial lining. As such, the mucus retention cyst is a true cyst. The lesion is most frequently unilocular, but it may be convoluted, which suggests a multilocular or multicystic pattern (Fig. 3–8). Typically, the lining epithelium consists of a uniform layer of cuboidal-to-low columnar cells.[10, 24, 25] A uniform, thin layer of nonkeratinizing stratified squamous epithelium is common, and occasional mucus secreting cells can be seen within the epithelial lining of the cyst (Fig. 3–9). The lumen of the cyst may be filled with an eosinophilic material that stains positive for mucin. Inflammatory infiltrates within either the cyst contents or the connective tissue that surrounds the cyst are not a notable finding.

Differential Diagnosis

Because of its high frequency and its clinical resemblance to the mucus retention cyst, a mucus escape reaction should be one of the first lesions considered in a differential diagnosis. However, our data show that the mucus retention cyst occurs in an older age group and that it is more likely to be seen in association with a major salivary gland than is the mucus escape reaction. Hemangioma, lymphangioma, developmental cysts, and cystic salivary gland neoplasms must also be considered. Histologically, the presence of an epithelial lining is helpful in excluding the cystlike mucus escape reaction, lymphangioma, and hemangioma. Differentiation from a simple ectatic salivary gland duct is often a matter of degree. However, retention cysts are usually larger than ectatic ducts. The absence of lymphoid aggregates excludes lymphoepithelial (branchial cleft) cysts. The absence of multiple cystic structures and of areas of solid epithelial proliferation helps rule out cystic neoplasms. Careful histologic examination is particularly important to exclude low-grade mucoepidermoid carcinoma because both the mucus retention cyst and the low-grade mucoepidermoid carcinoma may have mucous cells in the epithelial lining. However, mucus retention cysts show no piling up of cells in the wall of the cyst, nor do they show any proliferation or infiltration of islands of epithelium into the connective tissue that surrounds the lumen of the cyst.

Treatment and Prognosis

Treatment of mucus retention cysts is usually conservative surgical excision. Cysts distal to a major salivary gland may be removed while spar-

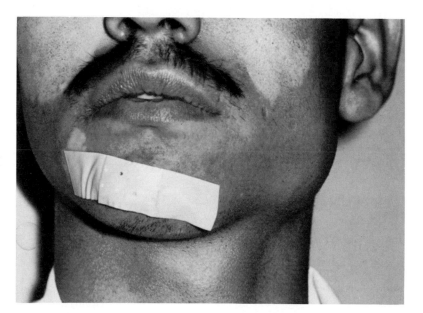

Figure 3–7. Mucus retention cyst of the left parotid gland. These lesions generally present as slowly growing, asymptomatic swellings.

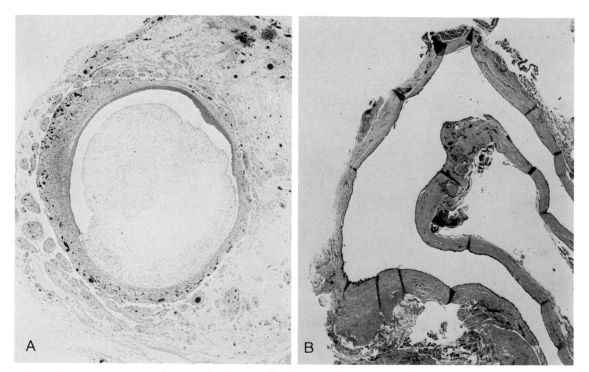

Figure 3–8. *A*, mucus retention cyst showing a well-defined, unilocular cavity that is lined by epithelium (× 15). *B*, tissue of a similar but larger lesion was obtained from a different patient. The lesion is unilocular but convoluted because of the collapse of the specimen during surgical removal (× 15).

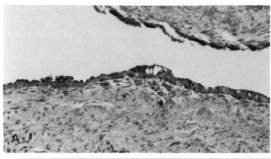

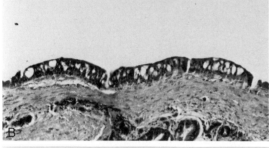

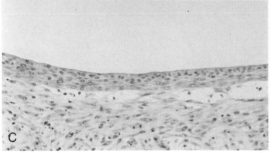

Figure 3–9. Three types of epithelial lining that may be found in mucus retention cysts: *A,* cuboidal epithelium with a focus of mucus cells (× 150); *B,* columnar epithelium with mucous cells (× 150); *C,* squamous epithelium (× 150). Individual cysts may show one or more types of epithelium in the same lesion.

ing the gland. Cysts located within a major salivary gland or in association with a minor salivary gland usually require sacrifice of the gland. Eversole[24] reported an occasional spontaneous resolution of such lesions but noted that there was subsequent recurrence. Prognosis is excellent because these cysts do not tend to recur if completely excised.

SIALOLITHIASIS

Sialoliths are calcified masses that develop in the ductal system of salivary glands. Other terms used to describe these lesions are salivary gland calculi and salivary gland stones. They form as a result of mineralization of debris that has accumulated in the lumen of a duct. This debris may include bacterial colonies, exfoliated ductal epithelial cells, mucus plugs, foreign bodies, or other cellular debris. Chemically, sialoliths are condensations of calcium salts, primarily calcium phos-

phate in the form of hydroxyapatite, with small amounts of magnesium, carbonate, and ammonium.[25] Anneroth and coworkers[26] suggest that sialoliths grow by a rhythmic deposition of inorganic and organic components around a mineralized nucleus. The precise cause of these lesions is not known, but infection or inflammation of the gland or duct, the length and tortuous path of the submandibular duct, and the viscous nature of mucus secretions have all been suggested as predisposing factors for development of salivary gland calculi.[11, 27, 28]

Clinical Features

Sialoliths constitute approximately 1.0 percent of the accessioned AFIP cases considered under the broad heading of obstructive disorders. They may develop in the ductal system of either a major or a minor salivary gland, but most investigators report that the submandibular gland is the most frequent location.[27, 29] AFIP data show the submandibular gland to be the most frequent site, followed by the parotid gland, the buccal mucosa, the upper lip, and the sublingual gland (Table 3–3). Collectively, sialoliths of the major salivary glands comprise 78.6 percent of lesions for which the site was stated. The age range for AFIP material spans 9 decades, but the occurrence of sialoliths in patients younger than 20 or older than age 70 is less common (Fig. 3–1). Of those patients for whom the age is stated, their mean age is 42.8 years; the average age of females in this group is 45.8 years, and for males it is 41.6

Table 3–3. Distribution by Anatomic Site of 214 Cases of Sialolithiasis Reported in the AFIP Registry of Salivary Gland Pathology

Anatomic Site	Number	Percent
Major Glands		
Parotid gland	30	14.0
Submandibular gland	94	43.9
Sublingual gland	5	2.3
Minor Glands		
Lip, total	13	6.1
Lip (not otherwise specified)	(4)	(1.9)
Upper lip	(8)	(3.7)
Lower lip	(1)	(0.5)
Palate (not otherwise specified)	1	0.5
Floor of mouth	3	1.4
Base of tongue	1	0.5
Tongue (not otherwise specified)	1	0.5
Buccal mucosa	12	5.6
Maxilla	1	0.5
Minor salivary glands	3	1.4
Site Not Stated	50	23.3
Total*	214	100

*Numbers in parentheses not included in total.

years. When all reported AFIP data are analyzed, there is a 5:2 male predilection for development of these lesions. However, when the military cases are excluded, the results are reversed, with the data suggesting a 3:2 female predilection for development of these lesions.

Clinical signs and symptoms of a sialolith in a major gland are most frequently swelling and pain in the area of the affected gland. In 180 patients with sialoliths who were studied by Levy and associates,[27] the time from initial presentation of symptoms to the time when the patient sought treatment varied dramatically, ranging from less than 6 months to as long as 30 years. The swelling may be focal or diffuse and is caused by pooling of saliva in an obstructed duct. The severity of the symptoms depends on the degree of obstruction and the amount of pressure caused by the continued secretion of saliva by the gland. If the blockage is incomplete, the symptoms may be mild. Conversely, if the blockage is complete, the symptoms may be quite severe. The episodes of swelling and pain are recurrent and most pronounced at meals. When the obstruction is only partial, the symptoms are generally transient, with resolution between meals. When the obstruction is complete, the swelling and discomfort may persist. Multiple sialoliths in a single duct and multifocal lesions within a single salivary gland have both been reported.[27, 30] A rare case of simultaneous bilateral involvement of the parotid salivary gland ducts has also been reported.[31] Sialoliths of the minor salivary glands are much less common and typically do not cause significant clinical symptoms. Their only presenting feature may be a small, normally colored or yellowish, firm nodule located within the soft tissue.[28]

On clinical examination, sialoliths can frequently be located by bimanual palpation of the affected area (Fig. 3–10). This is particularly true of those lesions located either in the duct of the submandibular gland above the mylohyoid muscle or in the buccal mucosa and lip. Radiographically, sialoliths are usually radiopaque (Fig. 3–11A). However, Langlais and Kasle[32] and Seldin and coworkers[30] reported that not all sialoliths may be visible on standard radiographs or in radiographs using low kilovoltage.

Pathologic Features

Grossly, sialoliths are round, oval, or cylindric calcified masses that vary in color from white to yellow-brown. Their surface texture may be smooth or irregular, and they may vary in size from a few millimeters to several centimeters in diameter (Fig. 3–11B). Salivary gland calculi of the major salivary glands are larger than those of the minor glands; however, the stones of the parotid gland and Stensen's duct are smaller than those of the submandibular gland and Wharton's duct.[25] Microscopically, they consist of concentric laminations of calcification within which may be found foci of organic debris (Fig. 3–12A). On close examination, a thin layer of epithelium representing the compressed wall of the duct may be evident at the periphery of the calcified mass (Fig. 3–12B). Changes in the duct wall may include squamous, oncocytic, and mucous cell metaplasia of the epithelium.[29] Stasis of saliva in a duct can lead to retrograde infections, causing an acute or chronic sialadenitis. This can damage the gland parenchyma, resulting in reduction or complete cessation of salivary flow and, in rare cases, calcification of the entire gland.[33] Long-term obstruction in the absence of infection can also lead to atrophy of the gland, followed by fibrosis and subsequent loss of secretory function.

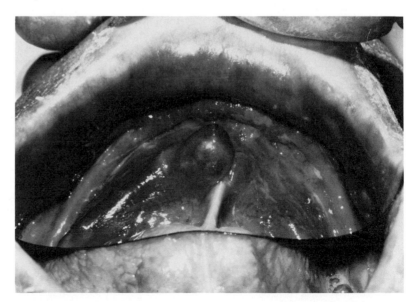

Figure 3–10. Sialolith in the anterior floor of the mouth at the opening of the left submandibular salivary gland duct (Wharton's duct). Erythema is due to secondary inflammation of the duct and soft tissue in the area of the obstruction.

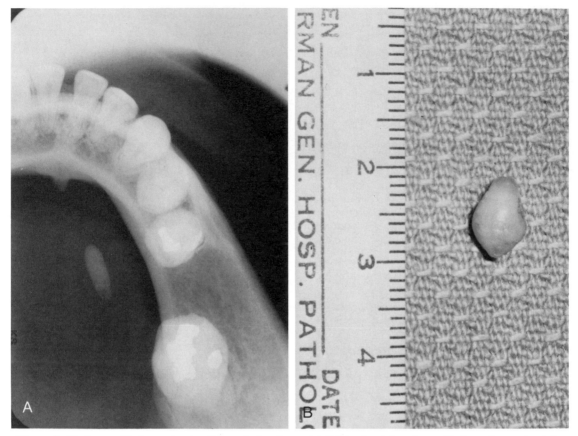

Figure 3–11. *A,* mandibular occlusal radiograph showing a sialolith in the right submandibular salivary gland duct. The submandibular salivary gland ducts are the most common site for sialoliths of the major salivary glands. *B,* gross photograph of a sialolith removed from the submandibular salivary gland duct of another patient. Occasionally, these lesions may grow to be several centimeters in diameter before the patient presents for treatment.

Differential Diagnosis

As with the mucus escape reaction and mucus retention cyst, the sialolith may clinically mimic a number of tumors of the head and neck region. However, given the unique combination of clinical signs and symptoms presented by the sialolith, most cysts and neoplasms can be easily eliminated from consideration. Radiographs are particularly helpful because they assist in separation of the radiopaque sialolith from radiolucent lesions. Two lesions present a radiographic picture similar to that of the sialolth: the phlebolith and the calcified cervical lymph node. Phlebolith formation results from calcification of intravascular thrombi. Calcification of cervical lymph nodes can occur after infections, such as tuberculosis. Cannulation of the salivary gland duct and sialography are valuable diagnostic procedures for excluding phleboliths and calcified cervical lymph nodes and for further identifying the location, size, and shape of a sialolith.[11, 32]

Treatment and Prognosis

Conservative therapy for salivary gland obstruction includes application of moist heat, increased intake of fluids, sialagogues, and gentle massage of the gland toward its opening into the oral cavity to reduce stasis and to enhance salivary flow. Analgesics may be included, if the clinical symptoms are severe. In some cases, this may be all that is necessary to remove a small sialolith and to restore salivary flow. If this fails or if the lesion is large, surgical removal of the stone is necessary. Sialoliths in the ducts that are distal to major salivary glands are often removed, while sparing the gland. However, sialoliths in ducts within a major gland or in association with minor glands usually require sacrifice of the salivary gland. If the gland is secondarily inflamed, massage of the salivary gland sometimes produces a purulent exudate from the duct orifice. This exudate should be cultured and sensitivity tested, because antibiotic therapy may be required. Severe infec-

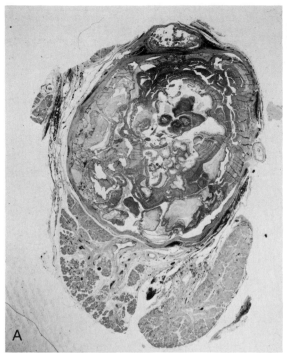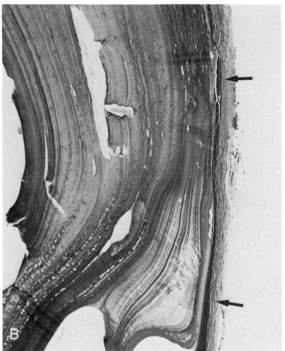

Figure 3–12. *A,* large sialolith removed from the right submandibular salivary gland region of an elderly male. The lesion was grossly 1.5 cm in diameter (× 3). *B,* sialolith shows concentric lamination of calcification and compressed ductal epithelium (arrows) (× 75).

tions may necessitate cannulation and dilatation or incision and surgical drainage of the duct and salivary gland. Follow-up treatment consists of conservative therapy with or without analgesics and antibiotics. Temporary use of drugs, such as pilocarpine, may be included to stimulate salivary flow.[34] However, this will not offer improvement if the secretory elements of the gland have been destroyed as a result of long-term obstruction or inflammation of the gland. If the treatment consists of only removal of the stone from the duct, a new sialolith may develop at a later date. This is not the case if treatment includes sacrifice of the affected salivary gland.[27, 30, 35]

REFERENCES

1. Galili D, Marmary Y: Juvenile recurrent parotitis: Clinicoradiologic follow-up study and the beneficial effect of sialography. Oral Surg Oral Med Oral Pathol 1986; 61:550–556.
2. Doku HC, Shklar G, McCarthy PL: Cheilitis glandularis. Oral Surg Oral Med Oral Pathol 1965; 20:563–571.
3. Schnitt SJ, Antonioli DA, Jaffe B, Peppercorn MA: Granulomatous inflammation of minor salivary gland ducts: a new oral manifestation of Crohn's disease. Hum Pathol 1987; 18:405–407.
4. Blitzer A: Inflammatory and obstructive disorders of salivary glands. J Dent Res 1987; 66:675–679.
5. De Arauyo NS, Tomich CE: Experimental production of mucus-retention phenomenon in animals treated with isoproterenol. Oral Surg Oral Med Oral Pathol 1971; 31:849–860.
6. Rubin MM, Cozzi G: Acute transient sialadenopathy associated with anesthesia. Oral Surg Oral Med Oral Pathol 1986; 61:227–229.
7. Busuttil A: Irradiation-induced changes in human salivary glands. Clin Otolaryngol 1977; 2:199–206.
8. Abrams AM, Melrose RJ, Howell FV: Necrotizing sialometaplasia: a disease simulating malignancy. Cancer 1973; 32:130–135.
9. Grillon GL, Lally ET: Necrotizing sialometaplasia: literature review and presentation of five cases. J Oral Surg 1981; 39:747–753.
10. Standish SM, Shafer WG: The mucus retention phenomenon. J Oral Surg 1959; 17:15–22.
11. Shafer WG, Hine MK, Levy BM: A Textbook of Oral Pathology, 4th Ed. Philadelphia, WB Saunders Co, 1983; 557–560.
12. Bhaskar SN, Bolden TE, Weinmann JP: Pathogenesis of mucoceles. J Dent Res 1956; 35:863–874.
13. Zafarulla MYM: Cervical mucocele (plunging ranula): an unusual case of mucous extravasation cyst. Oral Surg Oral Med Oral Pathol 1986; 62:63–66.
14. Chaudhry AP, Reynolds DH, LaChapelle CF, Vickers RA: A clinical and experimental study of mucocele (retention cyst). J Dent Res 1960; 39:1253–1262.
15. Thoma KH: Oral Pathology, 2nd Ed. St. Louis, CV Mosby Co, 1944; 1290–1291.
16. Bhaskar SN, Bolden TE, Weinmann JP: Experi-

mental obstructive adenitis in the mouse. J Dent Res 1956; 35:852–862.

17. Standish SM, Shafer WG: Serial histologic effects of rat submaxillary and sublingual gland duct and blood vessel ligation. J Dent Res 1957; 36:866–879.

18. Cataldo E, Mosadomi A: Mucoceles of the oral mucous membrane. Arch Otolaryngol 1970; 91:360–365.

19. Harrison JD: Salivary mucoceles. Oral Surg Oral Med Oral Pathol 1975; 39:268–278.

20. Quick CA, Lowell SH: Ranula and the sublingual salivary glands. Arch Otolaryngol 1977; 103:397–400.

21. Rees RT: Congenital ranula. Br Dent J 1979; 146:345–346.

22. McClatchey KD, Appelblatt NH, Zarbo RJ, Merrel DM: Plunging ranula. Oral Surg Oral Med Oral Pathol 1984; 57:408–412.

23. Fein S, Mohnac AM: Submandibular gland extravasation cyst: report of an unusual case. J Oral Surg 1973; 31:551–552.

24. Eversole RL: Oral sialocysts. Arch Otolaryngol Head Neck Surg 1987; 113:51–56.

25. Batsakis JG: Tumors of the Head and Neck: Clinical and Pathological Considerations, 2nd Ed. Baltimore, Williams & Wilkins, 1979; 114–117.

26. Anneroth G, Eneroth CM, Isacsson G: Morphology of salivary calculi: the distribution of the inorganic component. J Oral Pathol 1975; 4:257–265.

27. Levy DM, ReMine WH, Devine KD: Salivary gland calculi: pain, swelling associated with eating. JAMA 1962; 181:1115–1119.

28. Jensen JL, Howell FV, Rick GM, Correll RW: Minor salivary gland calculi: a clinicopathologic study of forty-seven new cases. Oral Surg Oral Med Oral Pathol 1979; 47:44–50.

29. Eversole LR: Clinical Outline of Oral Pathology: Diagnosis and Treatment, 2nd Ed. Philadelphia, Lea & Febiger, 1984; 114–115.

30. Seldin HM, Seldin SD, Rakower W: Conservative surgery for the removal of salivary calculi. Oral Surg Oral Med Oral Pathol 1953; 6:579–587.

31. Kessel LJ, Schow SR, Hunsuck EE: Bilateral parotid duct sialoliths. Oral Surg Oral Med Oral Pathol 1975; 40:164.

32. Langlais RP, Kasle MJ: Sialolithiasis: the radiolucent ones. Oral Surg Oral Med Oral Pathol 1975; 40:686–690.

33. Murphy JB: Dystrophic calcification of the submandibular gland. Oral Surg Oral Med Oral Pathol 1989; 67:362.

34. Fox PC, van der Ven PF: Baum BJ, Mandel ID: Pilocarpine for treatment of xerostomia associated with salivary gland dysfunction. Oral Surg Oral Med Oral Pathol 1986; 61:243–245.

35. Narang R, Dixon RA: Surgical management of submandibular sialadenitis and sialolithiasis. Oral Surg Oral Med Oral Pathol 1977; 43:201–210.

4

INFECTIOUS AND SYSTEMIC DISEASES

John T. Werning

This chapter discusses selected infectious and systemic diseases that may affect the salivary glands. The salivary glands are involved when pathogens or other systemic processes affect the gland parenchyma, its stroma, or intraglandular or paraglandular lymph nodes. Lymph node involvement is a primary factor in many of these diseases, and lymph nodes, of course, are an integral component of the parotid gland. Some of these diseases manifest as masses and may be confused with neoplastic processes.

Non-neoplastic enlargement of salivary glands is usually caused by some form of sialadenosis or sialadenitis. Sialadenosis is discussed later in this chapter. Sialadenitis was classified etiologically by Seifert and Donath[1] (Table 4–1).

TUBERCULOSIS

Tuberculous lymphadenitis is the most common extrathoracic form of this disease, and cervical lymph nodes, including lymph nodes in and around the major salivary glands, are the ones most frequently involved. Since 1964, despite the decline in pulmonary tuberculosis, the number of cases of extrapulmonary tuberculosis reported in the United States has remained fairly constant at approximately 4,000 cases per year.[2] This is due in part to the higher rate of infection in immunocompromised patients. Lowered host resistance in such persons is often caused by old age, renal failure, cirrhosis, malnutrition, hematologic malignancies, or acquired immunodeficiency syndrome (AIDS). Although signs and symptoms of pulmonary infection quickly prompt consideration of tuberculosis, systemic symptoms may be absent in cervical scrofula; this asymptomatic enlargement is likely to be first considered a neoplasm of the lymph nodes or salivary glands.

Infection of the salivary glands and cervical lymph nodes may develop in one of two ways. In the first, a focus of mycobacterial infection in a tonsil, gingival sulcus, or mucosal break liberates bacilli that ascend to the salivary glands via their ducts or pass to their associated lymph nodes via lymphatic drainage. The second pathway involves hematogenous or lymphatic spread from the lungs. This may be followed by healing of the lungs, which leaves calcified pulmonary granulomas and a positive skin test as the only evidence of pulmonary disease.[3] The most common causative agent in cervical tuberculosis is *Mycobacterium tuberculosis*, which has replaced *Mycobacterium bovis* as the leading cause of infection since the identification and elimination of infected dairy cattle and the pasteurization of milk have become standard public health measures.

Clinical Features

The registry of salivary gland disease of the Armed Forces Institute of Pathology (AFIP) includes 20 cases of tuberculous involvement of salivary glands. In 75 percent of these cases, the lymph nodes associated with the parotid gland

Table 4–1. Classification of Sialadenitis According to Cause*

Bacterial sialadenitis
Viral sialadenitis
Radiation sialadenitis
Electrolyte sialadenitis
Chronic sclerosing sialadenitis (Kuttner's tumor)
Immune sialadenitis

*Adapted from Seifert G, Donah K: Classification of the pathohistology of diseases of the salivary glands: Review of 2,600 cases in the salivary gland register. Berichte Path Bd 1976; 159:1–32. Copyright by Springer-Verlag.

were affected. All of the remaining cases were associated with the submandibular gland, with the exception of one case that involved the sublingual gland.

Clinical presentation is not diagnostic. Duration of swelling varies from weeks to years, age range is wide, and the gland is usually painless and contains a cystic or solid nodule that is up to 5 cm in diameter. Preoperatively, a salivary gland tumor or unspecified parotitis is often suspected.[4] In two large series of cases of cervical scrofula, the age of patients ranged from 2 to 64 years, with mean ages of 23 and 35 years, respectively.[5, 6] The number of cases involving females predominated over the number involving males (42:15). Patients are generally free of systemic symptoms and complain only of a painless, firm, discrete enlargement. However, multiple masses are often encountered that may be fixed and adherent to adjacent tissues. Mean size is approximately 3.0 cm. Although a sinus tract is occasionally present, the overlying skin is usually smooth and not erythematous. Chest radiographs are reported as normal in 81 percent of all cases.

The intracutaneous or Mantoux test involves the injection of 0.1 ml of solution containing 5 tuberculin units of purified protein derivative. In the sensitized individual, a reaction of redness, swelling, and induration begins about 6 hours after injection, reaches a maximum intensity some time between 36 and 60 hours, and then fades over a period of several days. A positive result is usually defined as 10 mm or more of induration at 48 hours. The diagnosis of tuberculous sialadenitis or cervical lymphadenitis is most often made on the basis of a combination of findings; the minimum finding necessary for diagnosis is a positive Mantoux test together with the histologic finding of necrotizing granulomas in a gland or lymph node biopsy specimen. Finding acid-fast bacilli in tissue sections is difficult. Therefore, tissue from the suspected lymph node should be submitted for culture on media that support growth of tubercle bacilli, such as Löwenstein-Jensen, Woolley's, or American Thoracic Society medium.[6] Clues helpful in diagnosing tuberculous adenitis include a history of contact with a tuberculous patient and an abnormal chest radiograph. With a parotid or cervical mass, computed tomographic scanning can provide evidence of inflammatory disease and can aid in planning treatment.[7, 8]

Histopathologic Features

The infected gland or lymph node demonstrates multiple granulomas that are often confluent (Fig. 4–1). The classic tuberculous follicle is described as a focus of central necrosis surrounded by concentric bands of giant cells of both Langhans' and foreign body types, epithelioid histiocytes, and lymphocytes (Fig. 4–2). The central necrosis is usually complete in that cellular outlines and nuclear debris are absent. The Langhans giant cell exhibits an arc of peripherally arranged nuclei that is set within a strongly eosinophilic cytoplasm (Fig. 4–3).

Definitive diagnosis of tuberculosis rests on identification of characteristic beaded, rod-shaped, acid-fast bacilli through use of the Fite or Ziehl-Neelsen method of staining.[9] Location of bacilli in tissue sections is quite difficult, but searching efforts are best directed at the periphery of necrotic areas among the epithelioid cells. Rarely are bacilli seen in giant cells. The rapid (48-hour) diagnosis of nasopharyngeal tuberculosis by detection of tuberculostearic acid in formalin-fixed, paraffin-embedded tissue biopsy specimens has been enthusiastically reported by Arnold and coworkers.[10] Their technique showed a sensitivity of 83 percent and a specificity of 98 percent. Use of monoclonal antibodies to detect mycobacterial antigens immunohistochemically in tissue is currently being investigated.[11]

Treatment

The recommended approach to diagnosis and treatment of tuberculous cervical lymphadenitis and sialadenitis is excisional biopsy of a superficial lymph node or lymph nodes for diagnosis by culture and histopathologic staining, which is followed by multidrug antituberculous chemotherapy.[12] Deitel and colleagues[6] found a successful regime involved administration of isoniazid for 9 to 18 months, and rifampin for 9 to 12 months.

Differential Diagnosis

Besides tuberculosis, the differential diagnosis for granulomatous sialadenitis and lymphadenitis includes cat-scratch disease, fungal infections, lymphogranuloma venereum, syphilis, leprosy, tularemia, sarcoidosis, brucellosis, and toxoplasmosis. In addition, it is necessary to rule out the possibility of nontuberculous mycobacterial infection. In adults, mycobacterial infection of lymph nodes is almost always due to *Mycobacterium tuberculosis*, but this does not hold true for children. Instead, the infecting organism is usually one of the atypical mycobacteria, especially *Mycobacterium avium-intracellulare* or *Mycobacterium scrofulaceum*.[12]

CAT-SCRATCH DISEASE

Debre is credited with first recognizing this disease in 1931 and with later reporting his findings in 1950.[13] The cause of cat-scratch disease (CSD) remained a mystery for the following 33 years, until Wear and coinvestigators[14] announced finding pleomorphic, gram-negative, non–acid-

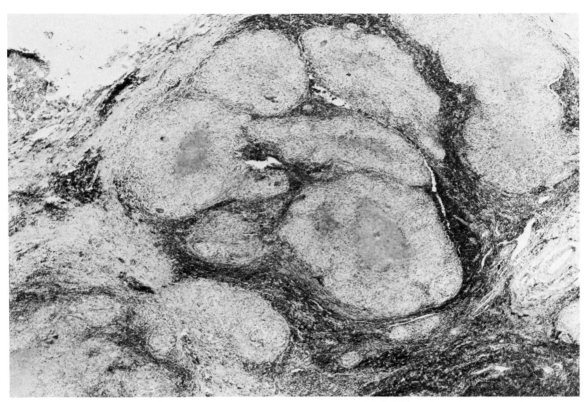

Figure 4–1. Tissue from a parotid intraglandular lymph node shows multiple, sometimes confluent, necrotizing granulomas that are characteristic of tuberculosis (× 30).

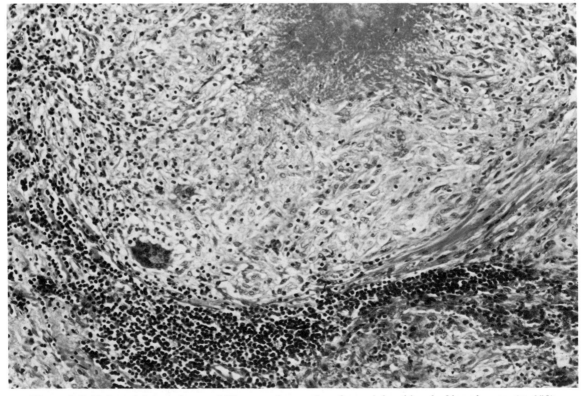

Figure 4–2. Tubercular granuloma exhibits central necrosis and a peripheral band of lymphocytes (× 150).

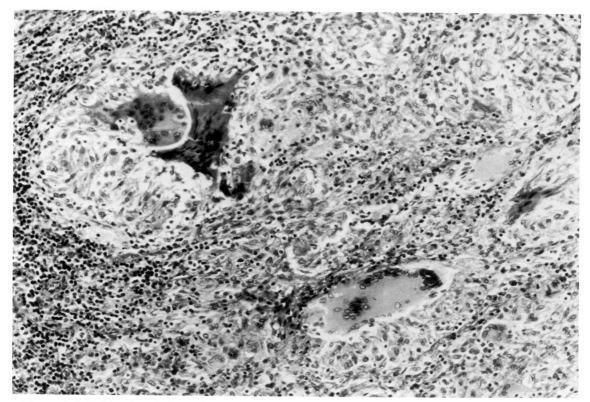

Figure 4–3. Multinucleated giant cells seen with tuberculosis can vary in types from Langhans' type to foreign body type (× 150).

fast bacilli in tissues from patients who met the clinical and histopathologic criteria of the disease. Transmission appears to involve direct contact with a healthy cat, often a kitten, that serves as a mechanical vector for the infective agent, since the cats are not ill and react negatively to the Hangar-Rose antigen.[15] Although about 3,000 patients with CSD have been reported, it is estimated that 2,000 unreported cases occur annually in the United States. Inapparent infection may be rather common since positive findings were obtained with skin tests for cat-scratch antigen in 4 to 8 percent of the general population and 12 to 29 percent of veterinarians.[15, 16] Parotid swelling is a clinical feature in 2 to 3 percent of all patients with CSD.[17, 18]

Clinical Findings

The infection typically occurs in children and young adults. In a series of 706 patients reported by Margileth,[17] 84 percent of these patients were under 21 years of age. In 3 to 10 days after inoculation of the skin—most often the skin of an upper extremity—one or several erythematous papules or pustules develop that persist for 1 to 3 weeks and then heal without scarring. The primary lesion is present on mucous membranes in

7 percent of those cases.[17] Approximately 2 weeks after the scratch, lymphadenopathy that is tender for the first 1 to 2 weeks ensues. The nodes of the head, neck, and axillae are most commonly affected. The adenopathy is usually unilateral and involves a single node or a cluster of nodes. The enlargement measures 1 to 5 cm, occasionally as much as 10 cm, and persists for 2 to 4 months. In 50 percent of the cases, the patient has no other sign or symptom except lymphadenopathy. "The Rule of Five" (Table 4–2) has been suggested by Carithers[19] as an aid in the clinical diagnosis of CSD. Symptoms such as fever, malaise, fatigue, sore throat, headache, and anorexia are present in one third or fewer of the patients. Less common complications include splenomegaly, oculoglan-

Table 4–2. "The Rule of Five"* in the Diagnosis of Cat-Scratch Disease†

Criteria	Points*
Single or regional lymphadenopathy	1.0
Intimate exposure to a cat	2.0
Inoculation site	2.0
Positive skin test	2.0

*Five points = strongly suggestive of disease. Seven points = definite.
†Modified from Carithers HA: Cat-scratch disease. Am J Dis Child 1985; 139:1124–1133. Copyright–1970, American Medical Association.

dular syndrome of Parinaud, central nervous system involvement, and severe chronic systemic disease.[20] Parotid swelling is a clinical feature in 2 to 3 percent of these patients.[17, 18] The salivary gland registry of the AFIP contains reports of 18 cases in which a salivary gland was listed as the site of involvement. The clinical parameters of these cases are presented in Table 4–3.

Histopathologic Features

With CSD, the histopathologic changes in lymph nodes have been divided into three stages.[21] The early stage is nonspecific with little distortion of the general nodal architecture. Reactive follicular hyperplasia is present with proliferation of immunoblasts and macrophages as well as scattered plasma cells and eosinophils. The intermediate stage is characterized by round or stellate granulomas of varying size. A central accumulation of neutrophils is surrounded by a cuff of palisaded spindle or epithelioid cells. The nodal architecture is distorted, and the capsule is often disrupted by granulomas and microabscesses that tend to break into the perinodal fibrofatty tissues. In the late stage, central caseation and colliquative necrosis of granulomata are seen (Fig. 4–4). Special stains

Table 4–3. Clinical Findings of Eighteen Cases of Cat-Scratch Disease Involving the Salivary Glands from the AFIP Registry of Salivary Gland Disease

Features	Number of Patients
*Age (decades of life)**	
1st	2
2nd	7
3rd	6
4th	2
8th	1
Race	
White	9
Asian	1
Unstated	8
Sex	
Male	12
Female	6
Salivary gland	
Parotid	12
Submandibular	6

*Mean age = 21 years.

may be helpful in disclosing the presence of the bacilli. Wear and colleagues[14] used the Warthin-Starry silver impregnation stain to reveal the pleomorphic bacilli that range in size from 0.3 to 1.0

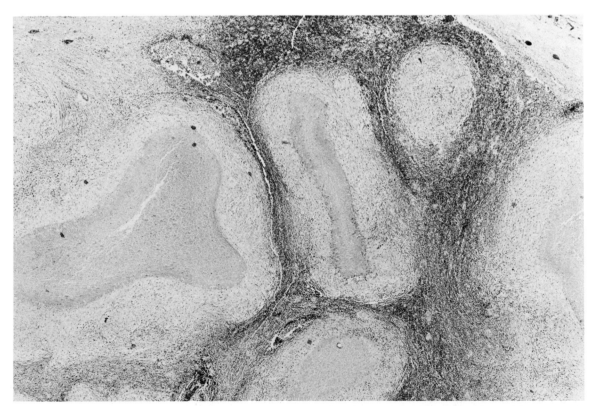

Figure 4–4. Necrotizing granulomas are shown in an intraglandular lymph node of a patient with cat-scratch disease ($\times$ 30).

μm in width by 0.6 to 3.0 μm in length (Fig. 4–5). The microorganisms are found singly in areas of necrosis either free within the necrotic debris or within vacuoles of activated histiocytes. In or near germinal centers, the walls of capillaries and macrophages lining sinuses contain bacilli in chains, clumps, or as single organisms. Wear and colleagues[14] state that bacilli are most easily seen in damaged vessels and microabscesses but are rarely seen in stellate granulomas with central suppuration.

Behavior and Treatment

Once the diagnosis has been established, the best therapy—barring complications—is reassuring the patient that the adenopathy is benign and, in most cases, will resolve spontaneously over a period of 2 to 3 months. Patients with suspected CSD consistently do not respond to treatment with antibiotics; therefore, no antimicrobial drug is recommended. One attack appears to confer life-long immunity.

Differential Diagnosis

Cat-scratch disease is the most common cause of chronic persistent (over 3 weeks) regional lymphadenopathy in children and adolescents. In addition to a thorough patient history, serologic tests and cultures of lymph node aspirate usually rule out other infectious diseases that must be considered. These include infectious mononucleosis, tularemia, brucellosis, toxoplasmosis, cytomegalovirus disease, histoplasmosis, herpes simplex, and atypical mycobacterial disease. If the antigen is available, the cat-scratch (Hangar-Rose) skin test is safe and reliable and was described as "gratifyingly specific" by one investigator.[19] In some cases, in which all clinical studies yield negative results, biopsy of a lymph node is required to rule out neoplasia.

SALIVARY GLAND CYSTS AS MANIFESTATION OF ACQUIRED IMMUNODEFICIENCY SYNDROME

Persistent generalized lymphadenopathy (PGL) is defined as palpable lymphadenopathy (lymph node enlargement of 1 cm or greater) at two or more extrainguinal sites that persists for more than 3 months in the absence of a concurrent illness or condition other than human immunodeficiency virus (HIV) infection.[22] In some cases, the initial manifestation of AIDS or AIDS-related complex may be localized, rather than generalized,

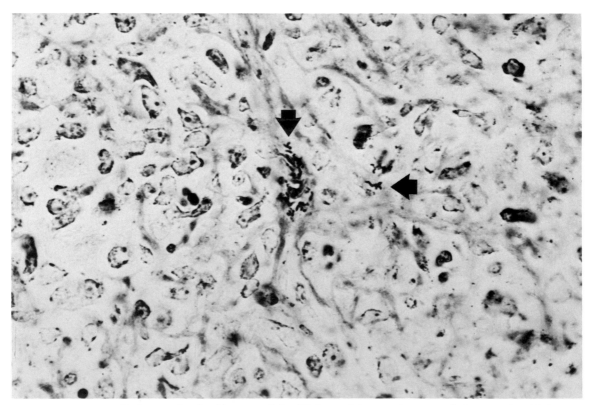

Figure 4–5. A small cluster of stained cat-scratch bacilli (arrows) is seen in a sea of degenerating histiocytes (Warthin-Starry, × 750).

lymphadenopathy that may precede by months or years the more publicized signs of AIDS, such as PGL, opportunistic infections, and neoplasias, especially non-Hodgkin's lymphoma and Kaposi's sarcoma. The histologic findings associated with PGL have been well described.[23-25] Less well appreciated is the proliferation of ductal epithelium that gives rise to cysts and epithelial islands, which are reminiscent of those seen with Sjögren's syndrome, within lymph nodes in and around salivary glands, particularly the parotid gland. These findings are regarded as another manifestation of HIV infection.[26-29]

Clinical Features

Of 16 reported cases of parotid cysts in AIDS or AIDS–related complex patients, all were men whose ages ranged from 29 to 47 years.[26-28] Twelve of them were prison inmates. Eleven of the sixteen patients were intravenous drug abusers, whereas three others stated that they were homosexual or bisexual. Parotid swelling can be unilateral or bilateral. Data available on 11 patients listed bilateral swelling in 5 of those individuals. Swellings had been present in nearly all patients for a period of 1 to 4 years. All 16 patients fulfilled the criteria for PGL. Serologic studies for HIV antibodies were positive in four out of five patients tested.

Holliday and colleagues[29] described a new radiographic manifestation of HIV infection in the head and neck of patients at risk for AIDS prior to the development of opportunistic infections. Using computed tomographic scans of the parotid and cervical areas, these clinicians were able to demonstrate the presence of multiple parotid cysts, which were frequently bilateral (Fig. 4–6), although clinically only a single parotid mass was suspected. Holliday and colleagues believe that the combination of multiple parotid cysts and diffuse cervical adenopathy represents a new computed tomographic finding in individuals who are likely to be HIV-positive. Eleven of twelve patients with this combination were HIV-positive.

Histopathologic Features

In 1983, Guarda and coworkers[23] and Ioachim and colleagues[24] described the histopathologic findings of tissue from persistently enlarged lymph nodes found in homosexual males. Also, Stanley and Frizzera[30] have listed the morphologic features associated with AIDS lymphadenopathy. Florid follicular hyperplasia is the most common pattern encountered, and changes within lymphoid follicles, sinuses, and interfollicular tissue have been emphasized. The follicles are increased in size and number and are irregular in shape (Fig. 4–7). The shapes are serpentine, dumbbell, hourglass, and serrated. The germinal centers house numerous macrophages that bear tingible bodies; mitotic figures are also plentiful. Sinuses are dilated and filled with histiocytes. Monomorphic round cells (clear cells) focally pack medullary sinuses (Fig. 4–8) or form aggregates along blood vessels, fibrous septa, and peripheral lymphocytic mantles of lymphoid follicles. The clear cells are described by Ioachim and colleagues[24] as being larger than immunoblasts and possessing prominent cell borders around fairly abundant clear cytoplasm that contains rounded nuclei with inconspicuous nucleoli. Mitoses are absent. These

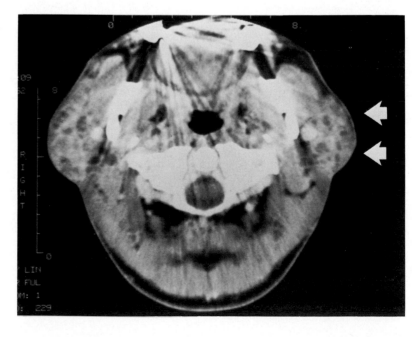

Figure 4–6. Contrast-enhanced axial computed tomographic section through the parotids of a patient in whom human immunodeficiency virus (HIV) seropositivity later developed. Multiple, small, oval radiolucencies (arrows) are present in the abnormally dense left parotid gland. A similar condition is obvious in the right parotid. (Courtesy of Dr. Angelo M. Delbalso, State University of New York at Buffalo, Buffalo, NY.)

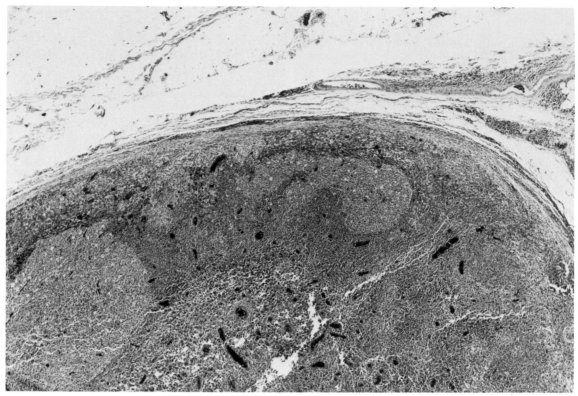

Figure 4–7. Florid follicular hyperplasia and irregularly shaped germinal centers are features of persistent generalized lymphadenopathy (PGL) (× 30).

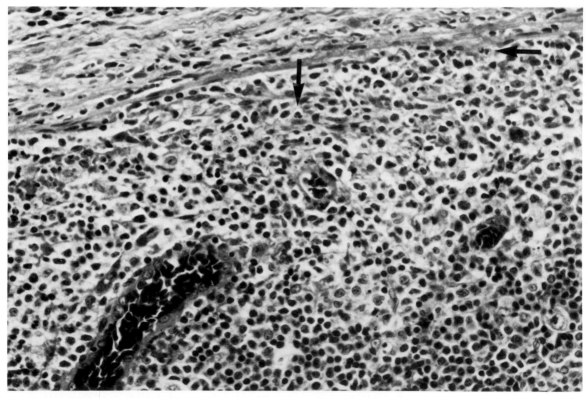

Figure 4–8. Monocytoid ("clear") B-cells that appear in the sinus space are accompanied by occasional neutrophils (arrows) (× 300).

46

clear cells are nearly always accompanied by neutrophils (Fig. 4–8). The interfollicular tissue contains a proliferation of plasma cells and small blood vessels. Brynes and colleagues[31] noted that on occasion an attenuated mantle of small lymphocytes invaginates into the follicle. Burns and associates[32] introduced the term *follicle lysis* to describe this invagination of mantle lymphocytes, which disrupts and segments the germinal centers (Fig. 4–9). In addition, a cohesive clustering of large follicular center cells occurs.

Lymph nodes in and around salivary glands may also contain squamous epithelium-lined cysts and epimyoepithelial islands that are reminiscent of those seen in Mikulicz's disease and Sjögren's syndrome (Fig. 4–10). Such epithelial structures in paraglandular and intraglandular lymph nodes were apparently first publicized by Ryan and colleagues[26] and subsequently elaborated on by others.[27–29]

Behavior

Jaffe and coworkers[33] point out that lymph node biopsies exhibit a spectrum of characteristic, although not specific, changes that roughly correlate with the temporal progression of AIDS. They assign the changes to three stages. The first is florid follicular hyperplasia observed in patients with AIDS-related complex or early AIDS. As described by Holliday and colleagues,[29] it is during the early stage that multiple parotid cysts develop and can be disclosed with computed tomographic scanning. The second stage shows selective paracortical lymphoid depletion, which often heralds the appearance of serious opportunistic infections. The final stage involves severe lymphoid depletion, which is an ominous prognosticator and is frequently seen at autopsy. Patients presenting with persistent lymphadenopathy require excisional biopsy of an enlarged node. As pointed out by Stanley and Frizzera,[30] a variety of diseases have similar, if not identical, clinical and histologic findings.

Differential Diagnosis

Stanley and Frizzera[30] retrospectively studied 50 lymph node biopsies that were obtained prior to the AIDS epidemic and that had been coded as nonspecific follicular hyperplasia. Their purpose was to determine whether the morphologic changes seen with PGL and AIDS were diagnostic or only suggestive of these conditions. They found that PGL had an increased incidence of large, irregularly shaped, germinal centers, mantle zone

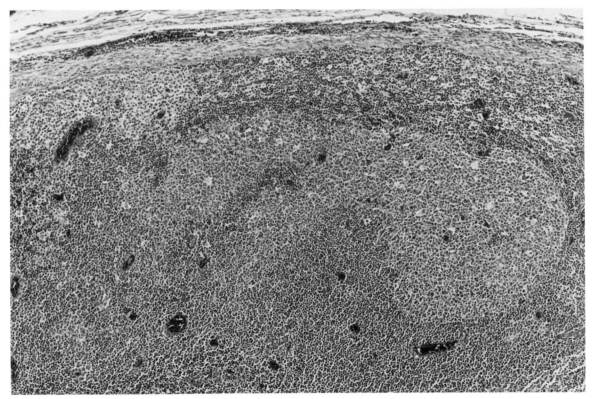

Figure 4–9. Follicle lysis is demonstrated by a focally serrated periphery of germinal center and by segmentation of germinal center by narrow strands of mantle lymphocytes (× 75).

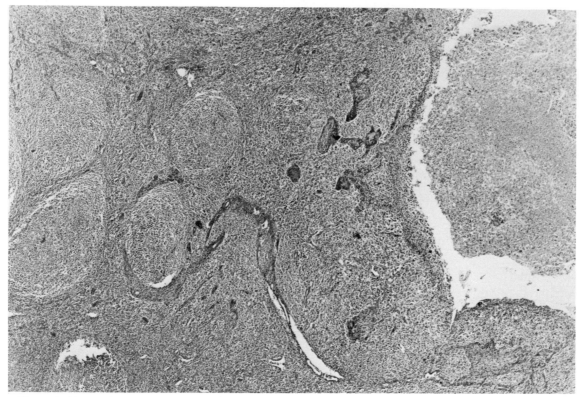

Figure 4–10. Parotid intraglandular lymph node tissue exhibits proliferating nests and strands of ductal epithelium and a lymphoepithelial cyst (× 30).

effacement, and sinusoidal monocytoid cells that was statistically significant. However, these features occurred often enough in nonspecific hyperplastic lymph nodes associated with other conditions that they could not be used for definitive diagnosis of PGL or AIDS. Definitive diagnosis depends on correlation of histologic features with patient history, physical examination, and immunologic and clinical laboratory findings. Studies include the Western blot test and serologic testing for HIV antibodies, gamma globulin level, helper/suppressor T-cell ratio, and spontaneous polyclonal B-cell activation.[27] Immunohistochemical staining of frozen sections from lymph nodes may disclose decreased amounts of helper T cells, increased amounts of suppressor T cells, and the presence of suppressor T cells in germinal centers. Such findings indicate an abnormal immune state and lend support to a diagnosis of PGL or AIDS.[34]

CYTOMEGALOVIRUS

The cytomegalovirus (CMV) is a DNA virus of the Herpesviridae family and measures approximately 113 nm in diameter.[35] Cytomegalovirus is ubiquitous, and over 80 percent of the population of the United States is seropositive for the virus

by the age of 70 years.[36] Like other herpes viruses, it can cause primary, latent, or chronic persistent infection. With the occurrence of approximately 33,000 (10:1,000) infected infants per year in the United States, it is the most common congenital infection.[37] The virus has been isolated from various body fluids or cells, including urine, feces, saliva, semen, cervical secretions, breast milk, and lymphocytes.[38] Most immunologically normal adults and children with antibodies to CMV remain asymptomatic or experience a mild mononucleosislike illness. Serious, even life-threatening, infection occurs in the newborn and in immunocompromised patients, particularly those with AIDS and those undergoing blood transfusions, bone marrow transplants, organ transplants, or chemotherapy for malignant disease. Cytomegalovirus is the most common cause of life-threatening opportunistic viral infection in patients with AIDS.[39]

Clinical Findings

Cytomegalovirus infection is seen in one of four clinical settings: congenital infection, perinatal infection, CMV mononucleosis in nonimmunocompromised patients, and immunocompromised patients.[40] Although salivary glands are involved in cytomegalovirus infection, significant clinical manifestations of this disease involve other organs.

Cytomegalic inclusion disease, as an acute illness in the newborn, occurs in less than 10 percent of congenitally infected infants. Cytomegalic inclusion disease is associated with petechiae, thrombocytopenia, conjugated hyperbilirubinemia, hepatosplenomegaly, chorioretinitis, microcephaly, and cerebral calcifications. Cerebral palsy, sensorineural hearing loss, visual defects, and mental retardation may be present.[37]

In AIDS patients, CMV infection can result in visual loss (retinitis); gastrointestinal distress (gastritis, colitis); nonproductive cough (pneumonitis); altered mentation (encephalitis); and abnormal test results for liver, kidney, and adrenal function.[39] Diagnostic procedures for documentation of the presence of CMV infection involve viral culture of body fluids or cells, seroconversion from negative to positive for specific IgG antibody, presence of serum CMV–specific IgM antibody, detection of CMV antigen in tissue with monoclonal antibodies, detection of CMV nucleic acids by genetic probes, and demonstration of typical CMV inclusions by microscopic examination.[40] Establishing CMV as the cause of a patient's disease is more problematic because of the universality of this infection and because of the other opportunistic microorganisms that are often present. Finding typical CMV inclusion bodies in a tissue biopsy is the best evidence for a causative role. However, this method lacks sensitivity, and the organ involved is not always accessible.

Histopathologic Features

The microscopic hallmark of CMV infection is large cells, 25 to 40 μm in diameter, that exhibit large (9 to 14 μm), central, basophilic nuclear inclusions (Fig. 4–11). Smaller (2 to 4 μm) cytoplasmic inclusions are also present. A chronic inflammatory cell infiltrate that consists primarily of macrophages and lymphocytes is generally elicited.

Treatment and Prognosis

Severe infections of the newborn and immunocompromised patients require antiviral chemotherapy. Agents that have shown activity against CMV include acyclovir, ganciclovir, and foscarnet. Prophylactic administration of specific immunoglobulin may be helpful.[41, 42] Mortality in congenitally infected infants is about 20 to 30 percent. A majority of the survivors develop sequelae, such as sensorineural hearing loss, retardation, sei-

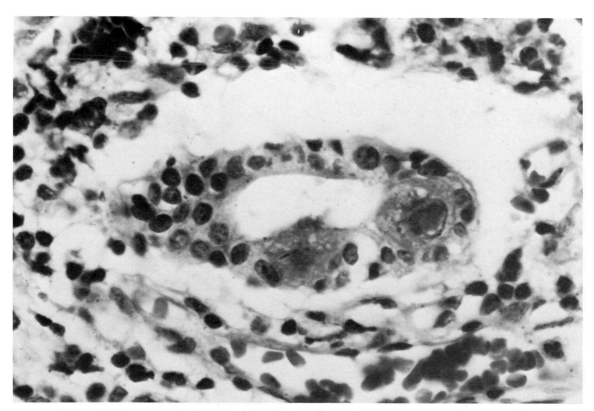

Figure 4–11. Several cells of a parotid intralobular salivary duct contain cytomegalovirus (× 750).

zures, and learning disabilities. Hydrocephalus and intracranial calcifications are indicators of a poor prognosis.[38] Life-threatening opportunistic cytomegalovirus infection is a complication that develops in 7.4 percent or more of patients with AIDS.[39]

Differential Diagnosis

TORCH is a useful acronym for use in differential diagnosis of neonatal infections acquired in utero, natally, or postnatally; it is formed from the first letters of *TO*xoplasmosis, *R*ubella, *C*ytomegalic inclusion disease, and *H*erpes simplex. Kinney and Kumar[43] emphasize that other infections need to be considered in neonates, especially human parvovirus (B19), HIV, and Epstein-Barr virus. They suggest that the letter "O" in the term *TORCH* be used to call attention to these other infections. In the immunocompromised patient, copathogens must be considered, for example, *Pneumocystis carinii* in cases of interstitial pneumonitis and hepatitis A, B, or non-A, non-B hepatitis C viruses in cases of hepatitis. Distinction among participating pathogens is ultimately made on the basis of laboratory studies, which often must be correlated with the clinical setting. Specific gamma M immunoglobulin determinations are available for CMV, toxoplasmosis, rubella, and herpes simplex.[44]

MUMPS (EPIDEMIC PAROTITIS)

A variety of viruses are capable of producing viral sialadenitis, including coxsackieviruses A and B, ECHO virus, Epstein-Barr virus, virus of lymphocytic choriomeningitis, influenza A virus, types 1 and 3 of parainfluenza viruses, cytomegalovirus, and mumps virus.[45] Of these, the mumps virus, an RNA virus of the Paramyxoviridae family, is the most common viral infective agent of salivary glands. It possesses two components that are capable of fixing complement, namely, the soluble (S) antigen that is derived from the nucleocapsid and the viral (V) antigen that is derived from the envelope and contains the hemagglutinin and neuraminidase (HN) and the fusing and hemolyzing (F) proteins. Mumps is an acute, contagious disease that is endemic in all areas of the world and usually spreads from a human reservoir by airborne droplets of infected saliva.

Clinical Findings

School-aged and teen-aged children (from 5 to 19 years old) accounted for 82 percent of all patients with mumps reported in the United States for the 3-year period from 1985 to 1987.[46] Ap-

proximately 9.5 percent of the cases occurred in persons 20 years of age or older. Following the incubation period, usually 16 to 18 days, the onset of the disease becomes manifest as pain and rapid swelling in one or both parotid glands during a period of 1 to 3 days. The subauricular swelling displaces the ear lobe upward and outward. Tasting citrus fruits or other sour liquids that stimulate salivation intensifies the pain. Expressed saliva from Stenson's duct appears normal. The swelling and systemic symptoms gradually subside in 3 to 7 days.

The diagnosis of mumps is generally made on clinical grounds alone; however, in some instances, such as nonparotitis cases, the diagnosis is not readily apparent and viral culture, serologic studies, or enzyme-linked immunosorbent assay may be required. Diagnosis of active disease with the complement-fixation method depends on characteristic specific complement-fixation antibody responses elicited to the S and V antigens. The S antibody develops early and is detected within 2 to 3 days of onset. The titer rises rapidly, often peaking during the first week of symptoms, and then declines to undetectable levels in 8 to 9 months. In contrast, the V antibody rises more slowly and is detected after the first week. The titer peaks in 2 to 3 weeks and then declines, but it ordinarily persists for life. Serum demonstrating elevated S antibody titer suggests acute or very recent disease, whereas serum that shows only V antibody indicates past infection and immunity.[47]

Histopathologic Features

Tissue samples are rarely provided from parotid glands infected with the mumps virus. Available studies indicate that the general architecture of the gland is preserved.[48] The histologic findings can be separated into three sets: interstitial changes, acinar cell changes, and ductal epithelial changes. The interstitium of the periacinar and periductal regions is edematous and densely infiltrated with lymphocytes and plasma cells. Initially, the acinar cells swell and develop cytoplasmic vacuolation. Other features described are dilated ducts with lumina filled with clumps of secretion and desquamated epithelium.

Behavior and Treatment

Mumps is a self-limiting infection, and treatment is entirely symptomatic. A single infection in normal individuals confers permanent immunity against clinically evident infection. Combined measles, mumps, and rubella vaccines were licensed in the United States in 1971, and their use has been quite effective in protecting the population against these diseases, so much so that their virtual elimination from this country has at times been boasted.[49] The viremia that develops with mumps can infect other organs, with or without parotitis, and may cause meningitis, encephalitis, epididymo-orchitis, pancreatitis, and polyarthritis as well as other rarer conditions. Complications of such infections are uncommon but include sterility in males (sequela to orchitis occurring with mumps) and deafness (sequela to encephalitis). Fatalities are extremely rare but have been associated with encephalitis, myocarditis, and nephritis.

SARCOIDOSIS

Sarcoidosis is a multisystem granulomatous disease of unknown cause that occurs in two forms: acute transient (abortive) and chronic persistent (Table 4–4). In the acute type, the patient presents with erythema nodosum in association with hilar lymphadenopathy, fever, migrating polyarthritis, and acute iritis (Löfgren's syndrome). The acute type is self-limiting and subsides in almost all patients within a few months without sequelae. The chronic persistent form is more common in the United States and often involves the lungs, the lymph nodes, the spleen, the skin, and the eyes.

The pathogenesis of sarcoidosis appears to involve some antigenic stimulant that triggers T-cell and B-cell responses that produce peripheral T-cell lymphocytopenia and a normal or increased peripheral B-cell population. This pathogenic mechanism helps explain the cutaneous hyporeactivity these patients have to common antigens, such as *Trichophyton*, mumps virus, pertussis, and purified protein derivative. B-cell proliferation may lead to increased circulating immunoglobulins. Lymphokines are operative in the process of granuloma formation.[50]

Clinical Findings

In their worldwide review of sarcoidosis, James and Williams[51] determined that the acute form of

Table 4–4. Expected Differences Between Acute and Chronic Forms of Sarcoidosis*

Parameter	Acute	Chronic
Onset	Abrupt	Insidious
Age	Under 40 yr	Over 40 yr
Race	Mainly whites	Mainly blacks
Erythema	Present	Absent
Respiratory symptoms	Absent	Present
Ankle periarthritis	Present	Absent
Digital swelling	Absent	Present

*Modified from Katz WA: Sarcoidosis. *In* Rose LF, Kaye D (eds.): Internal Medicine for Dentistry, 2nd Ed. St. Louis, CV Mosby Co, 1990; 64–66.

Table 4–5. Clinical Features of 85 Cases of Sarcoidosis Involving Salivary Glands from the AFIP Registry of Salivary Gland Disease

Feature	Number of Patients	Percent
Age (decades of life)		
1–2	8	12
3–4	42	65
5–6	15	23
Total	65	100
Race		
White	30	60
Black	20	40
Total	50	100
Sex		
Male	39	58
Female	28	42
Total	67	100
Race and Sex		
White male	16	32
White female	14	28
Black male	12	24
Black female	8	16
Total	50	100

this disease is more prevalent and that it presents most often in young to middle-aged, adult, white (79 percent) females (57 percent). In the United States, however, sarcoidosis occurs ten times more frequently among the black population than among the white population, and a female predominance is noted only among black patients. Pulmonary symptoms are present in about 60 percent of reported cases and consist of dyspnea, cough, or nonpleuritic chest pain. Often, the patient is asymptomatic, and the disease is discovered during examination of a chest radiograph that was taken for other purposes. The radiograph usually shows bilateral, symmetric hilar adenopathy, often with either paratracheal adenopathy or reticulonodular parenchymal infiltrates or with both. Cutaneous lesions are present in approximately one third of patients, and typically, they are brownish red or purple-tinted papules or plaques. With central clearing, the skin lesion may acquire an annular or circinate form. When the skin lesions show a predilection for the nose, cheeks, and ears, the term *lupus pernio* has been applied. In some patients, the disease may be entirely confined to the skin.[52] Parotid gland enlargement is present in 4 to 6 percent of cases.[53] The AFIP salivary gland disease registry contains 85 cases of patients with sarcoidosis. The parotid gland and submandibular gland accounted for 65 percent and 13 percent, respectively, of the 77 patients in which a specific gland was identified. Clinical features of these cases are presented in Table 4–5. The data of age and sex distribution among white patients agree with those published. The fact that 65 percent of these patients were in military service accounts for an increased incidence of sarcoidosis in males. A majority of these cases involved white patients, which is an unexpected statistic for such a group from the United States.

The triad of anterior uveitis in conjunction with parotitis and facial nerve palsy has been referred to as Heerfordt's syndrome. Chronic sarcoidosis may also cause hepatosplenomegaly, peripheral and central nervous system lesions (including diabetes insipidus), cardiomyopathy, and renal disease. Because the clinical picture can be quite varied, it is often necessary to employ one or more laboratory studies (Table 4–6) to confidently establish a diagnosis of sarcoidosis, which in certain cases is a diagnosis that is made by exclusion. The Kveim-Siltzbach skin test has been nearly abandoned because of false-positive and false-negative results and the difficulty of obtaining and processing the Kveim antigen. Patients with elevated angiotensin-converting enzyme and a positive gallium scan (sarcoid granulomas actively take up gallium) have a diagnostic specificity for sarcoidosis of 99 percent.[53] Radiographs of distal phalanges may show radiolucencies or punched-out lesions.

Histopathologic Features

Numerous granulomas (Fig. 4–12) may be seen in the affected lymph node and salivary gland.

Table 4–6. Laboratory Procedures Useful in the Evaluation of Sarcoidosis

Procedure or Test	Result in Sarcoidosis
Erythrocyte sedimentation rate	Elevated
Serum calcium	Elevated
Serum alkaline phosphatase	Elevated
Serum angiotensin-converting enzyme	Elevated
Skin test to various allergens	Anergy
1,25-Dihydroxyvitamin D	Elevated
Kveim-Siltzbach skin test	Positive

The typical sarcoid granuloma is noncaseating and consists of a tightly packed central focus of histiocytes that is surrounded at its periphery by lymphocytes and fibroblasts (Fig. 4–13). The histiocytes may be epithelioid and may coalesce to form multinucleated giant cells, often of the Langhans type (Fig. 4–13). Cellular inclusions in the form of asteroid bodies (Fig. 4–14) and Schaumann's bodies may be present and tend to be more frequent in longer standing disease. These histologic features are characteristic but are not pathognomonic of sarcoidosis.

Labial minor salivary gland biopsy has been recommended as an aid in the diagnosis of sarcoidosis.[54] The granulomas in the labial glands tend to be sparse (Fig. 4–15). For this reason, multiple labial glands (3 to 5 glands) ought to be

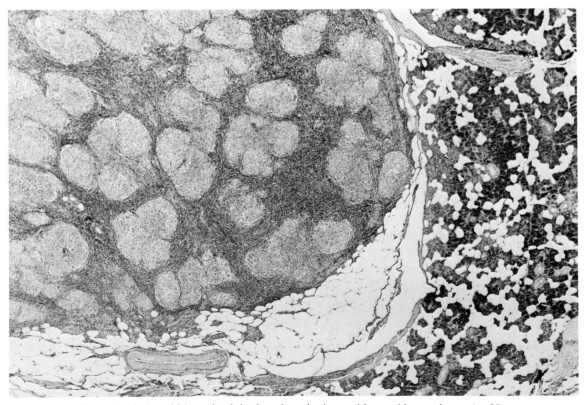

Figure 4–12. Parotid intraglandular lymph node tissue with sarcoid granulomas (× 30).

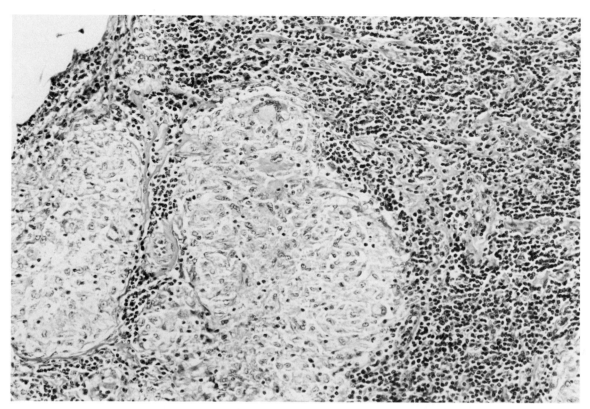

Figure 4–13. Typical noncaseating sarcoid granuloma is surrounded by lymphocytes (× 150).

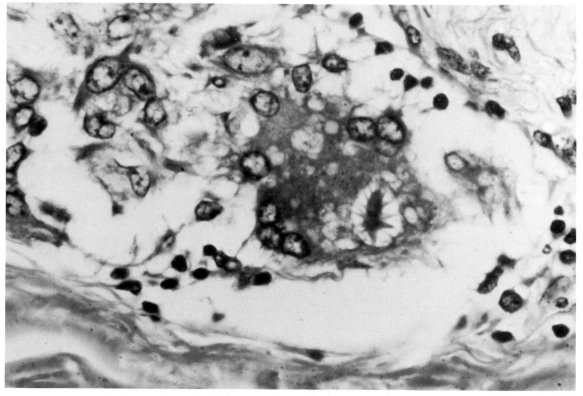

Figure 4–14. Asteroid body in a giant cell of sarcoid granuloma (× 750).

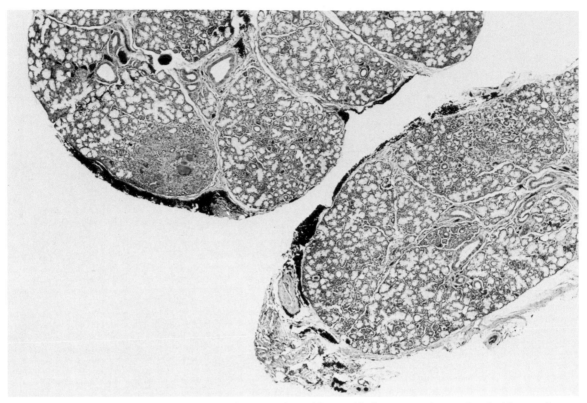

Figure 4–15. Tissue of several labial glands from a patient with sarcoidosis are sparsely populated with granulomas (× 30).

harvested, and multiple sections should be examined to locate granulomas. The granulomas tend to be small and consist primarily of histiocytes and one or several giant cells (Fig. 4–16).

In the attempt to support a clinicoradiographic impression of sarcoidosis, it is desirable to demonstrate noncaseating granulomas in two different organs. The percentage of positive yield varies, depending on the organ biopsied (Table 4–7). In a prospective study by Marx and colleagues,[55] parotid incisional biopsy using the Kraaijenhagen technique was effective in identifying sarcoidosis in 29 of 31 patients. The authors were enthusiastic about use of this technique for suspected inflam-

matory or immune diseases but recommended caution if neoplasia was the prime consideration. For neoplasms, superficial parotidectomy is the minimal recommended procedure.

Behavior and Treatment

The clinical course in the majority of patients is benign, with spontaneous remission being a common event. Because approximately 90 percent of patients with sarcoidosis exhibit radiographic evidence of lung involvement, it is customary to classify intrathoracic disease into one of three stages (Table 4–8). The stages generally parallel disease progression. In approximately 15 percent of patients, stage III disease is present. A majority

Table 4–7. Yield of Sarcoid Granulomas in Biopsies of Various Organs From Patients Suspected of Having Sarcoidosis*

Organ	Percentage Testing Positive to Sarcoidosis
Parotid[55]	93
Bronchial or lung tissue[50]	80
Liver[50]	70
Labial salivary gland[54]	58
Lymph node[51]	47
Conjunctiva[51]	17

*See references 50, 51, 54, 55.

Table 4–8. Staging of Intrathoracic Sarcoidosis

Stage 0	Normal-appearing chest radiogram
Stage I	Hilar lymphadenopathy with or without enlarged right paratracheal nodes but without pulmonary infiltration
Stage II	Hilar lymphadenopathy plus pulmonary infiltration
Stage III	Pulmonary infiltration without hilar lymphadenopathy

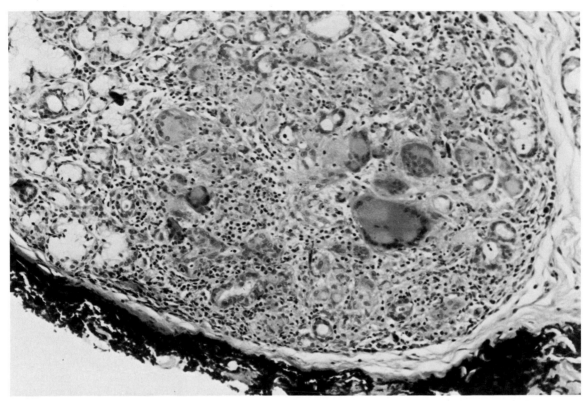

Figure 4–16. Labial gland tissue from a patient with sarcoidosis shows a small granuloma having several giant cells (× 150).

of patients with stages I and II disease experience regression of their disease. Treatment with corticosteroids is reserved for those patients experiencing interference in the function of a vital organ. The most common serious complication is respiratory failure, but myocardial, ocular, and central nervous system involvement and hypercalciuria are additional indications for steroid therapy.

The macrophages in sarcoid granulomas are considered to be the source of excess 1,25–dihydroxyvitamin D that gives rise to hypercalcemia and hypercalciuria. The kidney is the normal source of this hormone, which is responsible for the regulation of intestinal absorption of calcium. Steroid therapy blocks macrophage production of this hormone and prevents hypercalciuria that may lead to renal damage.[56] Despite treatment, sarcoidosis has a mortality rate of 4 percent, usually as a result of pulmonary disease and its sequelae.[53]

Differential Diagnosis

Other granulomatous inflammatory diseases that can afflict the salivary glands must be included in the differential diagnosis. With lung involvement, tuberculosis is the prime consideration. In the absence of pulmonary lesions, other causes are malignancies (especially lymphomas),[57] fungi, and foreign bodies of sarcoid-type granulomas. Detailed clinical history, appropriate clinical laboratory studies, and special histochemical stains should permit exclusion of alternative diagnoses in most cases.

CYSTIC FIBROSIS

Cystic fibrosis is the most common fatal, inherited disease in America, and it is carried as an autosomal recessive gene by about 5 percent of the white population.[58] Although the cystic fibrosis gene has not yet been isolated, it has been localized to the q31 band of the long arm of chromosome 7.[59, 60] In the past few years, new concepts have evolved concerning the cause of cystic fibrosis. Previously thought to be a disease of abnormal mucus production, cystic fibrosis is now considered a disease involving abnormal fluid and electrolyte transport across exocrine gland epithelia, which secondarily affects secretion viscosity.[58] The result of salivary gland involvement is clinically insignificant when compared to pulmonary, gastrointestinal, and pancreatic effects.

Clinical Findings

Cystic fibrosis occurs equally in males and females. A majority of cases are recognized in childhood, although some are not diagnosed until early adulthood. The major clinical manifestations of cystic fibrosis are chronic obstructive pulmonary disease, impaired intestinal digestion and absorption, and elevated concentration of salt in sweat.[61] In the newborn and infant, the occurrence of meconium ileus, the failure to gain weight, the presence of large and frequent bowel movements, the presence of excessive appetite, or a persistent cough may suggest the diagnosis. In clinically suspicious cases, such as patients with some form of malnutrition and chronic pulmonary disease, a positive sweat test result is considered to be confirmatory. This test is positive when the concentration of both sodium and chloride in sweat reaches a level of at least 65 mEq/liter assuming that the standard pilocarpine iontophoresis method is used.[62]

Histopathologic Features

Salivary glands whose acini are mainly mucous in type are most severely affected. Of the major salivary glands, the sublingual gland shows more pathologic alterations than the parotid.[63] The histologic changes are comparable to those seen in chronic obstructive disease and consist of ductal ectasia, inspissated mucin, microliths, and interstitial fibrosis.[64]

Behavior and Treatment

Pulmonary complications include pneumonia, bronchiectasis, atelectasis, empyema, pneumothorax, and hemoptysis. Pulmonary infection with *Staphylococcus aureus* and *Pseudomonas aeruginosa* is common. With the current use of aggressive respiratory and physical therapy as well as administration of appropriate antibiotics, the median age of death has risen to 29 years.[61] Death in cystic fibrosis is primarily due to extensive pulmonary infection that leads to respiratory failure.[62]

SIALADENOSIS

Sialadenosis is the name given to non-neoplastic, noninflammatory enlargement of salivary glands, particularly the parotid gland. The enlargement is usually bilateral and may manifest recurrence or pain or both. The condition is almost always found in association with systemic disorders; this association forms the basis for classification of

Table 4–9. Classification of Sialadenosis*

Hormonal sialadenosis
Sex hormonal sialadenosis
Diabetic sialadenosis
Thyroid sialadenosis
Hypophyseal and adrenal cortical disorders
Neurohumoral sialadenosis
Peripheral neurohumoral sialadenosis
Central neurogenous sialadenosis
Dysenzymatic sialadenosis
Hepatogenic sialadenosis
Pancreatogenic (exocrine) sialadenosis
Nephrogenic sialadenosis
Dysproteinemic sialadenosis
Malnutritional sialadenosis
Mucoviscidosis
Drug-induced sialadenosis

sialadenosis (Table 4–9).[65] Seifert and colleagues[66] believe that a primary neuropathy of the autonomic nervous system leads to disordered secretion in the acinar cell and is the underlying cause of the various forms of sialadenosis. Seifert and colleagues cite ultrastructural changes in the nervous system and the clinical finding of polyneuropathy in the diseases that coexist with sialadenosis as supportive evidence of this hypothesis.

Clinical Findings

Sialadenosis is characterized mainly by the presence of chronic, afebrile salivary gland enlargement, usually of the parotid glands. The enlargement is described as slowly evolving, indolent, undulating, and recurrent. Persons in the later decades of life (4th decade or beyond) are most afflicted. Diminished salivary secretion occurs, and sialochemistry generally demonstrates increased levels of potassium and decreased levels of sodium. Hypertrophy of acinar cells crowds and compresses the finer terminal ducts, thereby yielding the sialographic "leafless tree" pattern.[67]

Histopathologic Features

According to Donath and Seifert,[68] the parotid swelling is due to acinar enlargement. The diameter of the acinar cell increases two to three times that of normal. The nuclei tend to be basally situated, and the cytoplasm tends to be packed with granules. Whether the cytoplasm appears granular, vacuolated, or mixed depends on the optical density of the secretory granules, not on the quantity of granules. In addition, there is little, if any, correlation between these morphologic appearances and any specific clinical type of sia-

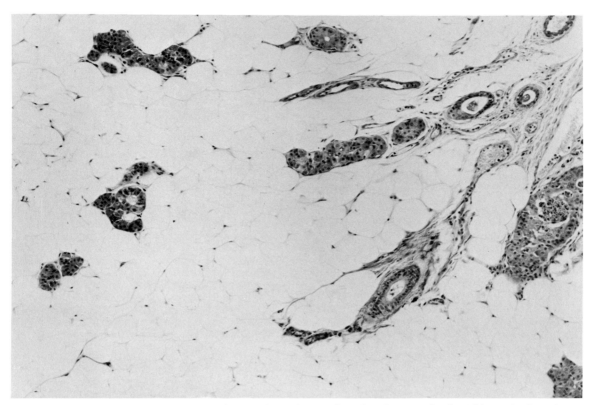

Figure 4–17. Parotid gland tissue exhibiting nearly total parenchymal replacement by fat. This results from long-standing, uncorrected autonomic neuropathy, as in alcoholism or diabetes mellitus (× 75).

ladenosis. Inflammatory cells are absent, but individual fat cells may be seen in the interstitium. Batsakis[69] suggests that unremitting or long-standing uncorrected autonomic neuropathy, such as that which occurs in alcoholism or diabetes mellitus, eventually leads to acinar atrophy and replacement with fat (Fig. 4–17).

Behavior and Treatment

Treatment of sialadenosis is generally unsatisfactory and quite dependent on controlling the underlying cause. In cases of endocrine and neurogenic sialadenosis, the glandular swelling is resistant to treatment. Sialadenosis that is caused by drugs, such as antihypertensive agents, may regress after withdrawal of the drug. If gland swelling persists and becomes cosmetically unacceptable, subtotal parotidectomy may be considered as a last resort.

Differential Diagnosis

Few diseases cause slowly evolving, bilateral, painless swelling of the parotid glands; thus, only a small group of diseases can be confused with

sialadenosis. In this category, however, oncocytosis, benign lymphoepithelial lesion, and bilateral parotid neoplasms must be considered. The neoplasms most likely to present bilaterally are papillary cystadenoma lymphomatosum (Warthin's tumor) and oncocytoma. Biopsy of the mass is the surest method of differentiation.

REFERENCES

1. Seifert G, Donath K: Classification of the pathohistology of diseases of the salivary glands: Review of 2,600 cases in the salivary gland register. Beitr Path Bd 1976; 159:1–32.
2. Wolinsky E: Tuberculosis. *In* Wyngaarden JB, Smith LH (eds.): Cecil Textbook of Medicine, 18th Ed. Philadelphia, WB Saunders Co, 1988; 1682–1692.
3. Stanley RB, Fernandez JA, Peppard SB: Cervicofacial mycobacterial infections presenting as major salivary gland disease. Laryngoscope 1983; 93:1271–1275.
4. Van der Walt JD, Leake J: Granulomatous sialadenitis of the major salivary glands: A clinicopathological study of 57 cases. Histopathology 1987; 11:131–144.
5. Castro JD, Hoover L, Castro DJ, Zuckerbraun L: Cervical mycobacterial lymphadenitis. Arch Otolaryngol 1985; 111:816–819.
6. Deitel M, Bendago M, Krajden S, Ronald AC, Bo-

rowy ZJ: Modern management of cervical scrofula. Head Neck 1989; 11:60–66.

7. Stone DN, Mancuso AA, Rice D, Hanafee WN: Parotid CT sialography. Radiology 1981; 138:393–397.

8. Keusters D, Van de Heyning P, Claes J, Corthouts B, De Schepper A: Cervical tuberculosis: Differential diagnosis and CT imaging. Acta Otorhinolaryngol (Belg) 1987; 41:958–964.

9. Luna LG: Methods for bacteria, fungi, and inclusion bodies. In Manual of Histologic Staining Methods of the Armed Forces Institute of Pathology, 3rd Ed. New York, McGraw-Hill Book Co, 1968; 217–222.

10. Arnold M, Chan CY, Cheung SW, Van Hesselt CA, French GL: Diagnosis of nasopharyngeal tuberculosis by detection of tuberculostearic acid in formalin fixed, paraffin wax embedded tissue biopsy specimens. J Clin Pathol 1988; 41:1324–1336.

11. Barbolini G, Bisetti A, Colizzi V, Damiani G, Migaldi M, Vismara D: Immunohistologic analysis of mycobacterial antigens by monoclonal antibodies in tuberculosis and mycobacteriosis. Hum Pathol 1989; 20:1078–1083.

12. Talmi YP, Cohen AH, Finkelstein Y, Versano I, Zohar Y: Mycobacterium tuberculosis cervical adenitis. Clin Pediatr 1989; 28:408–411.

13. Carithers HA: Cat-scratch disease: Notes on its history. Am J Dis Child 1970; 119:200–203.

14. Wear DJ, Margileth AM, Hadfield TL, Fischer GW, Schlagel CJ, King FM: Cat scratch disease: A bacterial infection. Science 1983; 221:1403–1405.

15. August JR, Loar AS: Zoonotic diseases of cats. Vet Clin N Am 1984; 14:1117–1151.

16. Elliot DL, Tolle SW, Goldberg L, Miller JB: Pet-associated illness. N Engl J Med 1985; 313:985–995.

17. Margileth AM: Cat scratch disease: A therapeutic dilemma. Vet Clin N Amer 1987; 17:91–103.

18. Watkinson JC, Hornung EA, Fagg NLK: Cat-scratch disease: an unusual cause of parotid pain (a case report with a literature review). J Laryngol Otol 1988; 102:562–564.

19. Carithers HA: Cat-scratch disease. Am J Dis Child 1985; 139:1124–1133.

20. Margileth AM: Cat-scratch disease. In Wyngaarden JB, Smith LH (eds.): Cecil Textbook of Medicine, 18th Ed. Philadelphia, WB Saunders Co, 1988; 1679–1681.

21. Strano, AJ: Cat-scratch fever. In Binford CH, Connor DH (eds.): Pathology of Tropical and Extraordinary Diseases. Washington, D.C., Armed Forces Institute of Pathology, 1976; 85–86.

22. Centers for Disease Control. Classification system for human T-lymphotropic virus type III/lymphadenopathy-associated virus infections. MMWR 1986; 35:334–339.

23. Guarda LA, Butler JJ, Mansell P, Hersh EM, Reuben J, Newell GR: Lymphadenopathy in homosexual men: Morbid anatomy with clinical and immunologic correlations. Am J Clin Pathol 1983; 79:559–568.

24. Ioachim HL, Lerner CW, Tapper ML: The lymphoid lesions associated with the acquired immunodeficiency syndrome. Am J Surg Pathol 1983; 7:543–553.

25. Ewing EP Jr, Chandler FW, Spira TJ, Brynes RK, Chan WC: Primary lymph node pathology in AIDS and AIDS–related lymphadenopathy. Arch Pathol Lab Med 1985; 109:977–981.

26. Ryan JR, Ioachim HL, Marmer J, Loubeau JM: Acquired immune deficiency syndrome—related lymphadenopathies presenting in the salivary gland lymph nodes. Arch Otolaryngol 1985; 111:554–556.

27. Ulirsch RC, Jaffe ES: Sjögren's syndrome–like illness associated with the acquired immunodeficiency syndrome–related complex. Hum Pathol 1987; 18(10):1063–1068.

28. Smith FB, Rajdeo H, Panesar N, Bhuta K, Stahl R: Benign lymphoepithelial lesion of the parotid gland in intravenous drug users. Arch Pathol Lab Med 1988; 112:742–745.

29. Holliday RA, Cohen WA, Schinella RA, Rothstein SG, Persky MS, Jacobs JM, Som PM: Benign lymphoepithelial parotid cysts and hyperplastic cervical adenopathy in AIDS–risk patients: a new CT appearance. Radiology 1988; 168:439–441.

30. Stanley MW, Frizzera G: Diagnostic specificity of histologic features in lymph node biopsy specimens from patients at risk for the acquired immunodeficiency syndrome. Hum Pathol 1986; 17:1231–1239.

31. Brynes RK, Chan WC, Spira TJ, Ewing EP Jr, Chandler FW: Value of lymph node biopsy in unexplained lymphadenopathy in homosexual men. JAMA 1983; 250:1313–1317.

32. Burns BF, Wood GS, Dorfman RF: The varied histopathology of lymphadenopathy in the homosexual male. Am J Surg Pathol 1985; 9:287–297.

33. Jaffe ES, Clark J, Steis R, Blattner W, Macher AM, Longo DL, Reichert CM: Lymph node pathology of HTLV and HTLV-associated neoplasms. Cancer Res 1985; 45:4662s–4664s.

34. Said JW, Shintaku IP, Teitelbaum A, Chien K, Sassoon AF: Distribution of T-cell phenotypic subsets and surface immunoglobulin-bearing lymphocytes in lymph nodes from male homosexuals with persistent generalized adenopathy. Hum Pathol 1984; 15:785–790.

35. Hoffman H: Viruses. In Nolte WA (ed.): Oral Microbiology with Basic Microbiology and Immunology, 4th ed. St. Louis, CV Mosby Co, 1982; 463–513.

36. Oh S-H, Starr SE: Diseases caused by viruses. In Rose LF, Kaye D (eds.): Internal Medicine for Dentistry, 2nd Ed. St. Louis, CV Mosby Co, 1990; 107–136.

37. Rudd P, Peckham C: Infection of the fetus and the newborn: prevention, treatment, and related handicap. Baillieres Clin Obstet Gynaecol 1988; 2:55–71.

38. Lesher JL Jr: Cytomegalovirus infections and the skin. J Am Acad Dermatol 1988; 18:1333–1338.

39. Jacobsen MA, Mills J: Serious cytomegalovirus disease in the acquired immunodeficiency syndrome (AIDS). Ann Intern Med 1988; 108:585–594.

40. Drew WL: Diagnosis of cytomegalovirus infection. Rev Infect Dis 1988; 10:S468–S476.

41. Jeffries DJ: The spectrum of cytomegalovirus infection and its management. J Antimicrob Chemother 1989; 23(E):1–10.

42. Fletcher CV, Balfour HH Jr.: Evaluation of ganciclovir for cytomegalovirus disease. DICP 1989; 23:5–12.

43. Kenny JS, Kumar ML: Should we expand the

TORCH complex? Clin Perinatol 1988; 15:727–744.

44. Lang DL: Cytomegalovirus infection. *In* Wyngaarden JB, Smith LH (eds.): Cecil Textbook of Medicine, 18th ed. Philadelphia, WB Saunders Co, 1988; 1784–1786.

45. Myer C, Cotton RT: Salivary gland disease in children: a review. Clin Pediatr 1986; 25:314–322.

46. Centers for Disease Control: Mumps—United States, 1985–1988. MMWR 1989; 38:101–105.

47. Ray CG, Hicks MJ: Laboratory diagnosis of viruses, rickettsia, and chlamydia. *In* Henry JB (ed.): Todd, Sanford, Davidsohn Clinical Diagnosis and Management by Laboratory Methods, 16th ed. Philadelphia, WB Saunders Co, 1979; 1814–1879.

48. Seifert G, Miehlke A, Haubrich J, Chilla R: Diseases of the Salivary Glands: Pathology-Diagnosis-Treatment-Facial Nerve Surgery. Stuttgart, Georg Thieme Verlag Inc, 1986; 110–163.

49. Bart KJ, Orenstein WA, Hinman AR: The virtual elimination of rubella and mumps from the United States and the use of combined measles, mumps, and rubella vaccines (MMR) to eliminate measles. Dev Biol Stand 1986; 65:45–52.

50. Katz WA: Sarcoidosis. *In* Rose LF, Kaye D (eds.): Internal Medicine for Dentistry, 2nd Ed. St. Louis, CV Mosby Co, 1990; 64–66.

51. James DG, Williams WJ: Sarcoidosis and Other Granulomatous Disorders. Philadelphia, WB Saunders Co, 1985; 21–246.

52. Lever WF, Schaumburg-Lever G: Histopathology of the Skin, 6th Ed. Philadelphia, JB Lippincott Co, 1983; 229–233.

53. Winterbauer RH: Sarcoidosis. *In* Petersdorf RG, Adams RD, Braunwald E, Isselbacher KJ, Martin JB, Wilson JD (eds.): Harrison's Principles of Internal Medicine, 10th Ed. New York, McGraw-Hill Book Co, 1983; 1248–1253.

54. Nessan VJ, Jacoway JR: Biopsy of minor salivary glands in the diagnosis of sarcoidosis. N Engl J Med 1979; 301:922–924.

55. Marx RE, Hartman KS, Rethman KV: A prospective study comparing incisional labial to incisional parotid biopsies in the detection and confirmation of sarcoidosis, Sjögren's disease, sialosis, and lymphoma. J Rheumatol 1988; 15:621–629.

56. Burtis WJ, Rasmussen H: Mineral metabolism and metabolic bone disease. *In* Rose LF, Kaye D (eds.): Internal Medicine for Dentistry, 2nd Ed. St. Louis, CV Mosby Co, 1990; 1044–1066.

57. Brinker H: Sarcoid reactions in malignant tumours. Cancer Treat Rev 1986; 13:147–156.

58. Quinton PM: Defective epithelial ion transport in cystic fibrosis. Clin Chem 1989; 35:726–730.

59. Smith DR, Fulton TR, Swain P, Bowcock A, Daneshvar L, Traver C, Gruenert DC, Davis R, Cavalli-Sforza LL, Donis-Keller H: Cystic fibrosis: diagnostic testing and the search for the gene. Clin Chem 1989; 35:B17–B20.

60. Buchwald M, Tsui L-C, Riordan JR: The search for the cystic fibrosis gene. Am J Physiol 1989; 257:L47–L52.

61. Robertson MT: Prolactin, human nutrition and evolution, and the relation to cystic fibrosis. Med Hypothesis 1989; 29:87–99.

62. Shwachman H: Cystic fibrosis. *In* Petersdorf RG, Adams RD, Braunwald E, Isselbacher KJ, Martin JB, Wilson JD (eds.): Harrison's Principles of Internal Medicine, 10th Ed. New York, McGraw-Hill Book Co, 1983; 1542–1544.

63. Tandler B: Salivary gland changes in disease. J Dent Res 1987; 66:398–406.

64. Seifert G, Miehlke A, Haubrich J, Chilla R: Diseases of the Salivary Glands: Pathology-Diagnosis-Treatment-Facial Nerve Surgery. Stuttgart, Georg Thieme Verlag Inc, 1986; 101–109.

65. Rauch S, Gorlin RJ: Diseases of the salivary glands. *In* Gorlin RJ, Goldman HM (eds.): Thoma's Oral Pathology, 6th Ed. St. Louis, CV Mosby Co, 1970; 962–1070.

66. Seifert G, Miehlke A, Haubrich J, Chilla R: Diseases of the Salivary Glands: Pathology-Diagnosis-Treatment-Facial Nerve Surgery. Stuttgart, Georg Thieme Verlag Inc, 1986; 78–84.

67. Hasler JF: Parotid enlargement: a presenting sign in anorexia nervosa. Oral Surg Oral Med Oral Pathol 1982; 53:567–573.

68. Donath K, Seifert G: Ultrastructural studies of the parotid glands in sialadenosis. Virchows Arch [A] 1975; 365:119–135.

69. Batsakis JG: Pathology consultation: Sialadenosis. Ann Otol Rhinol Laryngol 1988; 97:94–95.

Chapter

5

IDIOPATHIC DISEASES

Jerald L. Jensen

Idiopathic diseases of the salivary glands are an unrelated group of lesions for which the causes generally remain unknown. Although, in the broadest sense of the term, salivary gland neoplasms may be considered idiopathic because specific causative factors remain unknown, these neoplasms are thought to fall within the general category of neoplasia and carcinogenesis. Therefore, this chapter is restricted to discussion of nonneoplastic lesions of the salivary glands. Traditionally, necrotizing sialometaplasia has been considered an idiopathic disease, but most investigators now believe that this disease is related to an acute ischemic event. Since in many cases the precipitating cause of the ischemia remains unknown, this chapter provides a convenient place to discuss this interesting and important lesion. Other lesions discussed are benign cysts, angiolymphoid hyperplasia with eosinophilia, Kimura's disease, and cheilitis glandularis. Angiolymphoid hyperplasia with eosinophilia and Kimura's disease are not specifically salivary gland lesions; however, these uncommon lesions most frequently occur in the head and neck and often occur in the parotid gland region.

NECROTIZING SIALOMETAPLASIA

Necrotizing sialometaplasia is a benign, necrotizing, self-healing, inflammatory condition of the salivary glands. It was described as a distinct entity by Abrams and colleagues[1] in 1973. They and others have pointed out that this frightening, but relatively innocuous, condition may be misdiagnosed as carcinoma, particularly mucoepidermoid carcinoma and squamous cell carcinoma.[2-13] This pitfall in diagnosis can be avoided if one is familiar with the clinical and pathologic features of this distinctive condition.

Clinical Features

Necrotizing sialometaplasia most commonly involves the minor salivary glands of the palate, although cases have been described in other locations, including the mucobuccal fold,[14] retromolar trigone,[15] tongue,[16] incisive canal,[16] lip,[9, 17] maxillary sinus,[18] nose,[6, 19] nasopharynx,[6] larynx,[20] and major salivary glands.[21-23] The vast majority of palatal lesions arise spontaneously, whereas most extrapalatal cases appear after operative procedures, trauma, or radiation therapy.[6, 9, 13, 22-25] Some authors have suggested that these iatrogenic lesions do not fulfill all of the criteria originally proposed for the diagnosis of necrotizing sialometaplasia and that the term be reserved for those cases that arise spontaneously.[26, 27]

Necrotizing sialometaplasia of the palate presents most commonly as deep, craterlike ulcers, measuring 1.0 to 3.0 cm in size.[1, 2, 16, 28] The ulcers are usually unilateral but may be bilateral and, rarely, metachronous.[2, 12, 24, 29-32] This condition may also appear as submucosal nodular swellings that may slough and leave characteristic craterlike ulcers.[7, 12, 28, 33-35] Typically, the lesions are asymptomatic; however, patients may complain of numbness and pain or burning.[2, 4, 7, 12, 24, 28, 29, 32, 34-38] The pain may be referred to the ipsilateral side of the face, neck, eye, and ear.[24, 28] The duration of the lesions prior to diagnosis typically varies from a few days to a few weeks.[2, 7] In iatrogenic cases, the time interval between surgery and the development of necrotizing sialometaplasia has ranged from 6 to 53 days (the mean is 18 days).[16] The time required for complete healing depends on the size of the lesion, but in most cases, it varies from 3 to 12 weeks.[2, 7, 28]

The average age of patients with necrotizing sialometaplasia in the Armed Forces Institute of Pathology (AFIP) registry (96 cases) was 47.9 years, with a range of 17 to 80 years. The average age of females was 43.1 years and that of males was 50.3 years. The male to female ratio was 1.8:1.0. These data correspond fairly closely with those of previous reports.[8, 12, 16]

Although the cause of spontaneously occurring necrotizing sialometaplasia is unknown, most authors favor an ischemic pathogenesis.[1, 4, 12, 16, 20, 24, 35, 36] However, some find it difficult to accept this explanation.[3, 5, 39] No viral or fungal pathogens have been cultured from the lesions, and there are no known associations with any systemic disease.[28, 30, 39] Iatrogenic necrotizing sialometaplasia, which accounts for most of the cases involving the major salivary glands and extrapalatal minor salivary glands, appears to be primarily, if not exclusively, a vascular-based lesion.[6, 9, 13, 18, 20, 23] This interpretation is supported by experimental studies, which have shown histologic changes that are similar to those of necrotizing sialometaplasia after ligation of arteries of the major salivary glands.[40–43]

Microscopic Features

The histologic features of necrotizing sialometaplasia are characteristic. The two key features are lobular necrosis with preservation of the lobular architecture of salivary glands and squamous metaplasia of residual acinar and ductal elements (Fig. 5–1). Completely or partially necrotic lobules typically are intermixed with metaplastic lobules (Fig. 5–2). The necrotic lobules are composed of small, acinus-sized pools of mucin that are surrounded by thin, necrotic septa and are frequently ringed by neutrophils. The mucin pools may coalesce and extend into adjacent tissue, where an inflammatory reaction similar to that seen in mucoceles (mucus escape reaction) is elicited. The predominant inflammatory cells in these areas are neutrophils and foamy macrophages. Granulation tissue may be prominent at the periphery of necrotic areas and near ulcers.

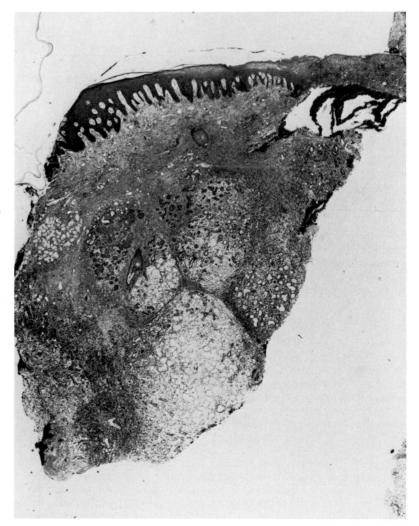

Figure 5–1. Preservation of the lobular pattern of the preexisting salivary glands, as illustrated in this photomicrograph, is the most helpful clue to the diagnosis of necrotizing sialometaplasia. The central, inferior lobule is necrotic, whereas two more superiorly located lobules reveal metaplasia ($\times$ 15).

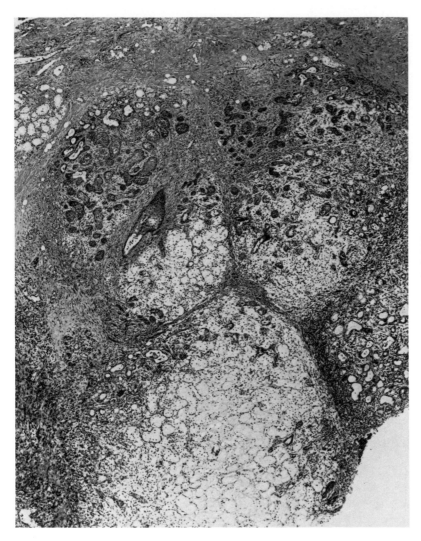

Figure 5–2. Higher magnification of Figure 5–1 illustrates lobular infarction of mucous acini, extrusion of mucus into adjacent tissue with associated intense inflammation, and squamous metaplasia of ducts and acini (× 30).

Squamous metaplasia of the salivary gland ducts and acini is a constant finding. The metaplastic squamous nests typically are bland-appearing, vary moderately in size and shape, have smooth edges, and are arranged in a lobular pattern (Fig. 5–3). These nests are set in a background of granulation tissue and diffuse inflammation. Florid squamous metaplasia may be present in excretory ducts as they approach and merge with the surface epithelium, which results in the ominous picture of pseudoepitheliomatous hyperplasia (Fig. 5–4). Residual ductal lumina may be evident in occasional squamous nests and are clues to the benign nature of the process. In contrast, other nests may contain residual mucous cells and lead to an erroneous diagnosis of mucoepidermoid carcinoma (Fig. 5–3). The majority of the metaplastic nests are composed of squamous cells with abundant pink cytoplasm and uniform bland nuclei. Some metaplastic nests, however, are composed predominantly of basaloid cells with hyperchromatic nuclei (Fig. 5–5). Active regeneration and metaplasia in areas of necrosis may be associated with nuclear enlargement, prominent nucleoli, frequent mitotic figures, and necrosis of either individual cells or small groups of cells. Small biopsy specimens that include only these areas may cause diagnostic problems. In such cases, additional biopsy material may be necessary in order to arrive at the correct diagnosis.

Differential Diagnosis

The presence of florid pseudoepitheliomatous hyperplasia, especially in necrotic, actively regenerating areas of the gland, might lead to confusion of this condition with squamous cell carcinoma. Likewise, metaplastic squamous nests with residual mucous cells might be misinterpreted as mucoepidermoid carcinoma. Separation of necrotizing sialometaplasia from these two malignant neoplasms can be made if attention is paid to the following four points. First, the lobular architec-

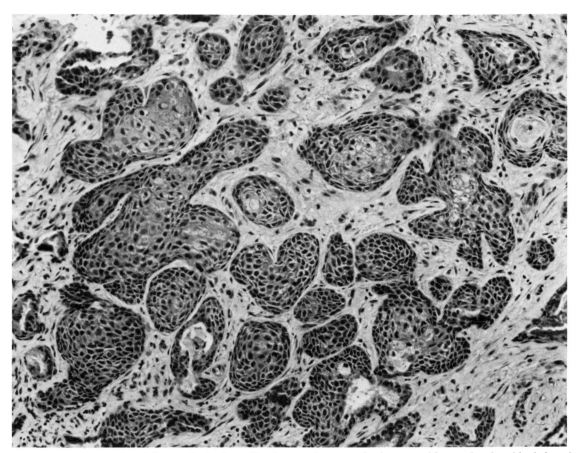

Figure 5–3. Necrotizing sialometaplasia shows bland-appearing metaplastic nests with occasional residual ductal lumina and a few scattered mucous cells (× 150).

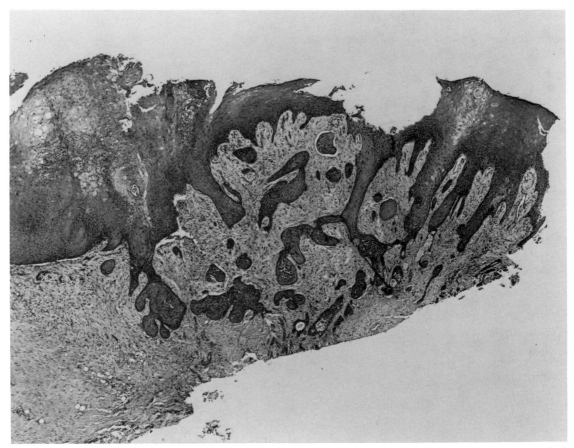

Figure 5–4. As the excretory ducts approach and merge with the surface epithelium, florid, squamous metaplasia of excretory ducts produces the ominous picture of pseudoepitheliomatous hyperplasia in necrotizing sialomctaplasia (× 30).

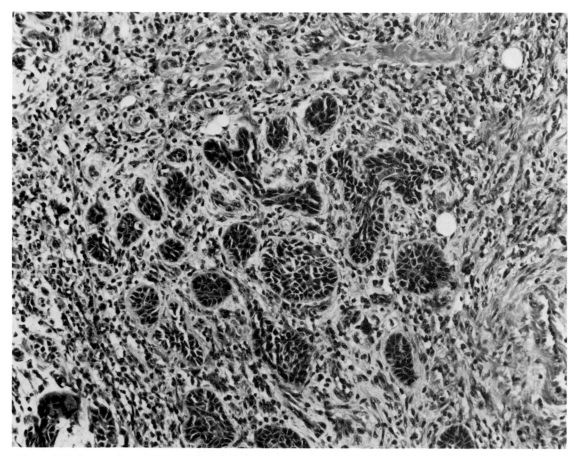

Figure 5–5. A case of necrotizing sialometaplasia shows metaplastic islands composed of basaloid cells with slightly irregular, hyperchromatic nuclei in a background of inflamed granulation tissue (× 150).

ture of the salivary gland is maintained in necrotizing sialometaplasia but not in squamous cell carcinoma or mucoepidermoid carcinoma. Second, necrotizing sialometaplasia is characterized by lobular infarction. Completely or partially necrotic salivary gland lobules are intermixed with metaplastic lobules. This is not a feature of either squamous cell carcinoma or mucoepidermoid carcinoma. Furthermore, necrotizing sialometaplasia lacks the cystic spaces lined by mucous cells that are seen in mucoepidermoid carcinoma. Third, necrotizing sialometaplasia characteristically is associated with an intense, mixed inflammatory reaction. This reaction is typically much more pronounced than that which occurs in either mucoepidermoid carcinoma or squamous cell carcinoma. Finally, other features, such as the generally bland appearance of the squamous cells, the presence of residual glandular lumina in metaplastic nests, and extraglandular mucin pools, are helpful in separating necrotizing sialometaplasia from its simulators.

BENIGN CYSTS OF THE PAROTID GLAND

Most cystic lesions of the major salivary glands are cystic neoplasms.[44] Benign cysts (epithelium-lined cavities usually containing fluid or semisolid material) are much less common and account for approximately 2 to 5 percent of parotid gland lesions.[44–47] They are rare in the other major salivary glands.[48] Benign cysts (sialocysts) of the parotid gland can be conveniently classified into the following three types: lymphoepithelial cysts, salivary duct cysts, and dysgenetic cysts.[48, 49] Polycystic (dysgenetic) disease of the parotid gland is considered a developmental malformation of the ductal system and is discussed in Chapter 2.

Lymphoepithelial Cysts

The histogenesis of these cysts is controversial. Origin from the branchial apparatus[44, 50–59] and origin from salivary gland inclusions in lymph nodes[48, 49, 60–63] are the most widely accepted theories. Since the term brachial cleft cyst implies a specific embryologic origin, it seems more appropriate to use the descriptive term *lymphoepithelial cyst* to designate these lesions.

Clinical Findings

Benign lymphoepithelial cysts of the parotid gland are usually well circumscribed, asymptomatic masses in the superficial portion of the gland.[44, 55, 64–72] However, they occasionally may be tender or painful and, rarely, may be associated with facial paralysis.[57, 59, 70, 73–75] On palpation, these

cysts are firm or rubbery but may be compressible.[55, 64, 66, 68, 71] They range in size from 0.5 to 6.0 cm and average about 2.5 cm in diameter.[73, 75]

Review of 101 cases classified as lymphoepithelial cysts of the parotid gland in the AFIP registry revealed a predilection of this disorder for male patients, with a male to female ratio of 2.9:1.0, which closely corresponds to the 2.7:1.0 predominant occurrence in males that was reported by Fujibayashi and Itoh.[67] However, when only the 58 civilian patients were considered, the predilection of the disease for male patients was only 1.6:1.0. In marked contrast, however, Olsen and coworkers[59] reported a predominant occurrence in females of 5:1.

In the AFIP material, the average age of patients with lymphoepithelial cysts of the parotid gland was 46.6 years, with a range of ages from 18 to 79 years. Reports in the literature closely correspond with these data. For example, Fujibayashi and Itoh[67] reported an average age of 43.1 years with a range of 19 to 69 years, and Gaisford and Anderson[56] reported a median age of 42.5 years with a range of 17 to 71 years.

The vast majority of benign lymphoepithelial cysts are unilateral; however, bilateral lesions have been reported.[59, 71] Occasional cysts are first noted after an upper respiratory tract infection.[71] The average duration of the cysts prior to initial medical consultation was 9 months in the study by Scott.[75] The most common preoperative diagnosis is parotid gland tumor.

Gross Findings

Typically, lymphoepithelial cysts of the parotid gland are sharply circumscribed, ovoid, fluctuant, and unilocular. Multilocular cysts are uncommon.[71] The luminal surface is shiny and varies from yellow-brown to white. Small protrusions are present in many of the cysts and impart a granular appearance to the luminal surface. This appearance is due to reactive lymphoid follicles in the cyst wall. The majority of these cysts contain soft, yellow-white, caseous material. Others, however, are fluid-filled, and after fixation, the contents may be jellylike.

Microscopic Findings

Lymphoepithelial cysts of the parotid gland may be lined by a variety of types of epithelium, including squamous, cuboidal, columnar, and pseudostratified ciliated types. Stratified squamous epithelium is the most common type (Fig. 5–6), but in some cysts it may coexist with flattened or simple squamous, columnar, or respiratory types. Occasional cysts are lined by one to several layers of cuboidal epithelium or by cuboidal and columnar epithelium (Fig. 5–7). Columnar and respiratory epithelium may, in addition, contain inter-

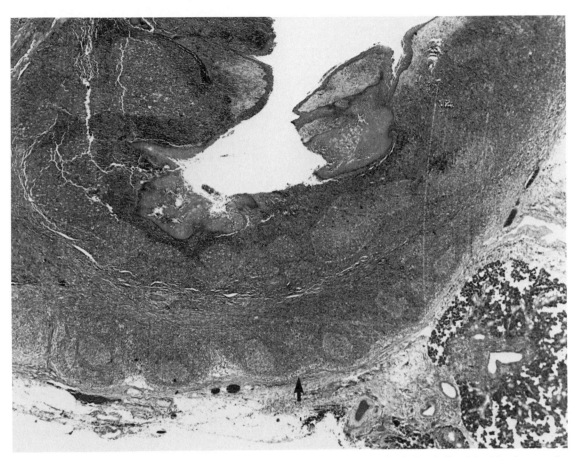

Figure 5–6. Section from a benign lymphoepithelial cyst of the parotid gland that is lined by bland-appearing stratified squamous epithelium. Characteristic features of the abundant lymphoid tissue include prominent germinal centers, sharp circumscription, and separation from the parotid parenchyma. The arrow points to a subcapsular sinus (× 15).

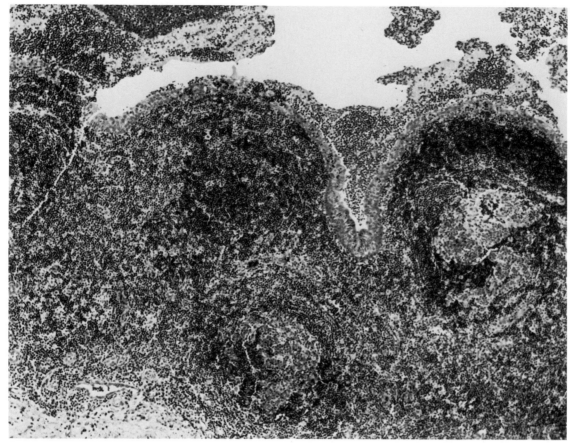

Figure 5–7. Benign lymphoepithelial cyst is lined by several layers of cuboidal epithelium (× 75).

spersed mucous cells (Fig. 5–8). Rarely, these cysts contain sebaceous glands within the stratified epithelial lining or within the lymphoid tissue of the cyst wall.[46, 66]

A highly characteristic feature of lymphoepithelial cysts is the presence of abundant lymphoid tissue in the cyst wall. Typically, the lymphoid tissue contains lymphoid follicles, is fairly sharply circumscribed, and is separated from the parotid parenchyma by a zone of fibrous tissue (Fig. 5–6). Superimposed inflammation, although uncommon, may alter the typical appearance of these cysts.

Differential Diagnosis

Benign lymphoepithelial cysts of the parotid gland have not been known to recur or to metastasize. Therefore, it is important to separate these benign cysts from cystic salivary gland tumors, which include mucoepidermoid carcinoma, acinic cell carcinoma,[76] Warthin's tumor, and metastatic carcinoma.

Features that favor a diagnosis of cystic, low-grade mucoepidermoid carcinoma over that of benign lymphoepithelial cyst include a high proportion of mucin-producing cells relative to squamous cells, the presence of macrocysts and microcysts, and the presence of solid nests of both mucin-producing cells and squamous cells. In addition, most cystic mucoepidermoid tumors are not surrounded by lymphoid tissue. It should be noted, however, that these tumors can arise in intraparotid lymph nodes.[77]

Acinic cell carcinomas may occasionally be almost entirely cystic and lined by deceptively innocuous epithelium.[76] These tumors might be confused with lymphoepithelial cysts that are lined by cuboidal or columnar epithelium. Intracystic papillary projections with a pseudoacinar pattern, multilayered epithelium with a microcystic or follicular pattern, and solid nodules of cells in the wall of the cyst are characteristic features of cystic acinic cell tumors that are not seen in benign lymphoepithelial cysts.

Squamous metaplasia can occur in Warthin's tumors; however, it is usually present in small foci. The predominantly double-layered, granular, eosinophilic epithelium and the papillary cystic pattern separate Warthin's tumors with squamous metaplasia from lymphoepithelial cysts.

Lymphoepithelial cysts with sebaceous differentiation, which are also considered to be cystic variants of sebaceous lymphadenoma,[66] can be separated from branchial cleft duplication anomalies by the presence of skin appendages and cartilage in the branchial cleft duplication anomalies.[45, 59, 66]

The bland nature of the cyst lining epithelium differentiates benign lymphoepithelial cysts from most carcinomas that are metastatic to intraparotid lymph nodes and from malignant lymphoepithelial cysts,[78] although there is serious doubt about the existence of this latter entity. The presence of abundant lymphoid tissue in the walls of lymphoepithelial cysts separates them from other benign cystic lesions of the parotid gland and from epidermoid cysts and cholesteatomas involving the gland.[58]

Occasionally, it might be difficult to differentiate between cystic benign lymphoepithelial lesions and lymphoepithelial cysts. Features that support a diagnosis of cystic benign lymphoepithelial lesion include smaller cyst size; multiple cysts; more diffuse, irregular lymphoid infiltrates; and the presence of epithelial (myoepithelial) islands.

Cystic lesions of the parotid gland have been reported in patients at risk for acquired immunodeficiency syndrome (AIDS) (see Chapter 4).[79–83] The cysts in many of these cases have features of lymphoepithelial cysts but differ from those described before the AIDS epidemic in that they are more frequently multiple and bilateral.[82, 83] Furthermore, in addition to the cysts, the parotid gland (or glands) in many of the patients at risk for AIDS exhibits features suggestive of benign lymphoepithelial lesions.[79–83] Such lesions without associated cysts may also occur in patients at risk for AIDS.[84] The parotid lymphoid tissue in some of these cystic and noncystic lesions may exhibit features seen in the lymph nodes of patients with AIDS-related complex with persistent generalized lymphadenopathy.[80, 84] Moreover, transformation to malignant lymphoma may occur.[80]

Salivary Duct Cysts

Salivary duct cysts may be acquired or congenital.[44, 49] The majority, however, are acquired, and most of these are probably secondary to obstruc-

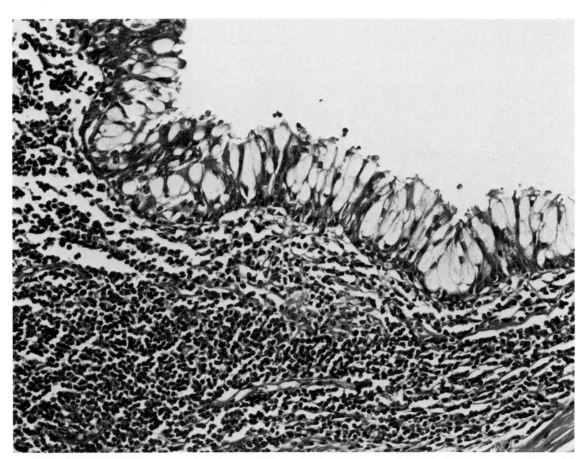

Figure 5–8. Section from a benign lymphoepithelial cyst that is lined by pseudostratified columnar epithelium with interspersed mucous cells (× 200).

tion.[49] Some authors, therefore, prefer the term retention cyst to designate these lesions.[44, 45] Still others prefer the term simple cyst.[47] The obstruction that leads to the formation of these cysts may be due to a variety of causes, including mucous plugs, calculi, postoperative or postinflammatory strictures, neoplasms, and benign lymphoepithelial lesions.

In the major salivary glands, salivary duct cysts primarily involve the parotid glands.[48] A general indication of their prevalence can be gained from several reported series of salivary gland lesions. Seifert and colleagues[49] found 32 salivary duct cysts among 5,739 salivary gland lesions. Eneroth[85] found 15 retention cysts of the parotid gland in a series of 802 parotid gland tumors. Richardson and colleagues[44] reported 5 retention cysts culled from among 708 parotidectomy specimens, and Cohen and colleagues[47] found 4 retention cysts in a review of 137 resected parotid glands. The AFIP registry contains reports of 166 cases of salivary duct cysts occurring in the major salivary glands, 152 cases involving the parotid gland, 13 cases involving the submandibular gland, and 1 case involving the sublingual gland.

Clinical Findings

Clinically, salivary duct cysts of the parotid gland are similar to lymphoepithelial cysts. Typically, they are unilateral painless swellings with no involvement of the facial nerve and no fixation to the overlying skin.[47] The majority of affected patients are over 40 years of age.[46, 47, 86, 87] The cysts range in size from 0.8 to 10.0 cm, with an average size of approximately 1 to 3 cm.[46, 86]

Gross Findings

Grossly, salivary duct cysts are well circumscribed, ovoid, and fluctuant. The cyst contents vary from a serous to a viscid, tan fluid, and the lining is generally smooth and does not exhibit the granular or cobblestone appearance seen in many lymphoepithelial cysts.

Microscopic Findings

Typically, these unilocular cysts are lined by single or multilayered cuboidal or columnar epithelium (Figs. 5–9 and 5–10). Occasional mucus-

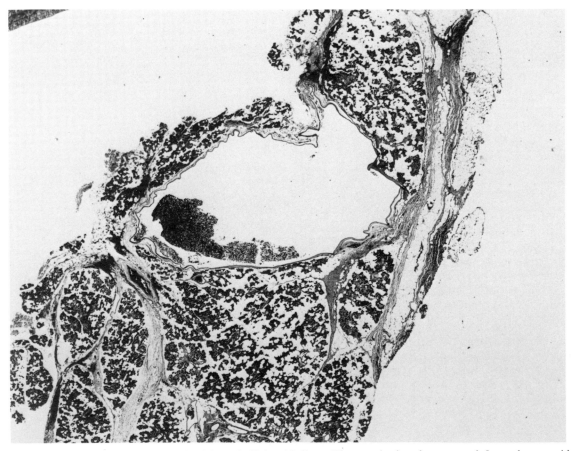

Figure 5–9. Parotid duct cyst is lined by cuboidal epithelium. The cyst is sharply separated from the parotid parenchyma by a thin layer of collagenous tissue (× 7.5).

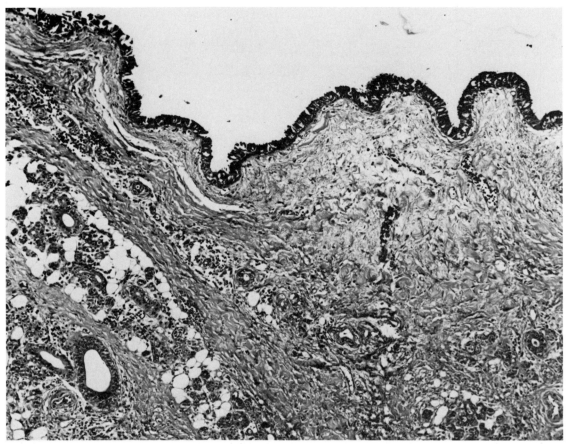

Figure 5–10. Parotid duct cyst is lined by columnar epithelium with a few interspersed mucous cells. The cyst is separated from the parotid parenchyma by dense collagenous tissue of variable thickness (× 75).

containing goblet cells and areas of oncocytic differentiation may be present. Occasional cysts may be completely or partially lined by squamous epithelium (Fig. 5–11). The cyst wall is composed of a layer of collagenous connective tissue of variable thickness, which in most instances is sharply separated from the adjacent parotid gland parenchyma (Fig. 5–9). Occasionally, a sparse to moderate lymphocytic infiltrate is present in the cyst wall (Fig. 5–11). However, the dense lymphoid tissue that characterizes lymphoepithelial cysts is not seen in salivary duct cysts. The adjacent salivary gland tissue may exhibit duct ectasia with inspissated secretions and interstitial and periductal inflammation. The histologic differential diagnosis has been discussed in the section on lymphoepithelial cysts. Simple surgical resection is curative.[44]

ANGIOLYMPHOID HYPERPLASIA WITH EOSINOPHILIA AND KIMURA'S DISEASE

Kimura's disease is a well-defined clinicopathologic entity, which according to Kung and colleagues[88] was first described in China in 1937. It became known as *Kimura's disease* after Kimura reported a similar condition in 1948.[88] Several hundred cases have now been reported in the Chinese and Japanese literature.[88] In 1969, Wells and Whimster[89] reported a condition that they termed *subcutaneous angiolymphoid hyperplasia with eosinophilia*, and they called attention to Kimura's disease. Wells and Whimster proposed that the two conditions were identical or closely related; in many subsequent reports, the two terms were used synonymously.[90–98] This interpretation was based in part on the fact that both conditions share common features, such as a predilection for occurring in the head and neck regions, a tendency to recur, vascular proliferation, and lymphoid and eosinophilic infiltrates. In spite of these similarities, recent reports indicate that Kimura's disease is a distinct entity that is different from angiolymphoid hyperplasia with eosinophilia.[88, 99–104]

Angiolymphoid Hyperplasia with Eosinophilia (Epithelioid Hemangioma)

This unusual but distinctive lesion has been variously called angiolymphoid hyperplasia with

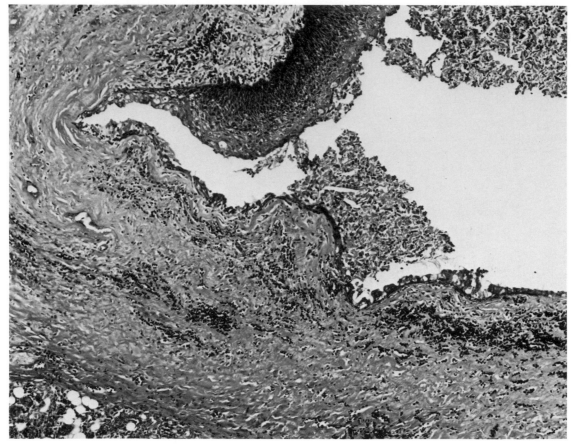

Figure 5–11. Section from a duct cyst that is lined by cuboidal epithelium with interspersed mucous cells and metaplastic, stratified squamous epithelium. Patchy chronic inflammation is present in the thick, fibrous wall (× 75).

eosinophilia,[89] inflammatory angiomatous nodule,[105] pseudopyogenic or atypical pyogenic granuloma,[105, 106] intravenous atypical vascular proliferation,[107] histiocytoid hemangioma,[99] and epithelioid hemangioma.[108]

Clinical Features

Lesions of angiolymphoid hyperplasia occur most commonly in the head and neck region as single or multiple smooth, dull, red papules, plaques, or subcutaneous masses.[100–103, 109] Bleeding and crusting are common secondary features. The most common clinical diagnoses are epidermoid cyst, angioma, and skin adnexal tumor.[103, 109] The duration of the lesions prior to treatment has ranged between 3 weeks and 4 years, with a median duration of 13 months.[109] Women are affected more frequently than men and are typically middle-aged. Regional lymphadenopathy is present in about 20 percent of patients, and, rarely, the lesion may arise within a lymph node in the absence of skin or subcutaneous involvement.[109, 110] The majority of patients have been treated with shave techniques with later excision.

The recurrence rate is around 30 percent.[109] Rarely, lesions regress spontaneously.[89, 109] Peripheral blood eosinophilia is occasionally seen in affected individuals.

Angiolymphoid hyperplasia with eosinophilia may masquerade as a salivary gland tumor; however, judging from the literature, salivary gland involvement is uncommon.[111] A single case involving the parotid gland was found among nine cases listed as angiolymphoid hyperplasia with eosinophilia in the files of the salivary gland registry of the AFIP (Figs. 5–12, 5–13). The remaining eight cases involved soft tissue overlying the gland. The clinical diagnosis in all nine cases was parotid gland tumor.

Pathologic Features

The lesions are well circumscribed, multinodular, and gray-brown. Typically they are composed of ill-defined lobules that are characterized by central parent vessels surrounded by clusters of well-formed capillaries. Large, thick-walled vessels and arteriovenous shunts may also be present. The majority of the vessels are lined by distinctive

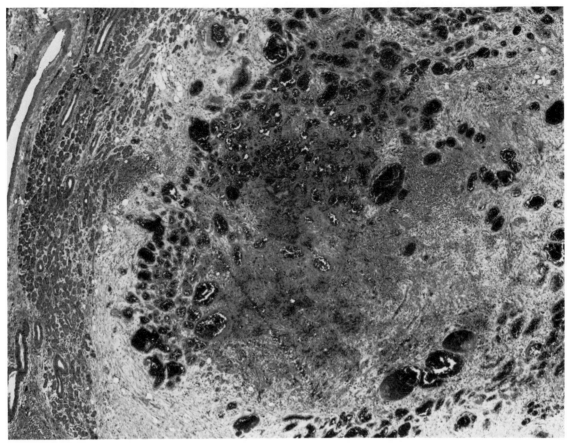

Figure 5–12. The parotid gland parenchyma is compressed by irregular clusters of blood vessels and intermixed lymphocytes and eosinophils in this example of angiolymphoid hyperplasia with eosinophilia ($\times$ 30).

histiocytoid or epithelioid endothelial cells (Fig. 5–13).[99, 100, 108] These cells are ovoid, rounded, or cuboidal and have abundant eosinophilic cytoplasm, which may contain vacuoles that represent primitive lumen formation.[99, 100, 108] The nuclei are centrally located, round, and occasionally folded or reniform, similar to the nuclei of histiocytes. The findings from ultrastructural, histochemical, and immunohistochemical studies support the interpretation that these cells are modified endothelial cells.[100, 102] Epithelioid endothelial cells may project into the lumina of larger vessels, producing a hobnail appearance, and they may form solid nests, occluding smaller vessels. Solid sheets and islands of these cells may be seen in the media and adventitia of traumatized, thick-walled vessels. This appearance could lead to a mistaken diagnosis of squamous cell carcinoma, angiosarcoma, or epithelioid hemangioendothelioma. Occasionally, the lesion may be entirely intravascular. In addition to the vascular component, angiolymphoid hyperplasia with eosinophilia typically contains a diffuse, mixed inflammatory cell infiltrate that is dominated by lymphocytes and eosinophils. Lymphoid follicles are present in many lesions, especially those involving the subcutaneous tissue. Rarely, the germinal centers of these follicles contain polykaryocytes of the Warthin-Finkeldey type.[103]

Behavior

No controversy exists concerning the benign nature of angiolymphoid hyperplasia with eosinophilia. Whether this entity is reactive or neoplastic, however, has not been resolved. Enzinger and Weiss[108] believe that most of these lesions are hemangiomas with epithelioid endothelium (benign neoplasm). However, they acknowledge that some lesions are reactive and suggest that, in spite of many common features, the lesions may be pathogenetically heterogeneous.

Kimura's Disease

Kimura's disease is a chronic inflammatory condition of unknown cause that is endemic in Orientals but may occur sporadically in non-

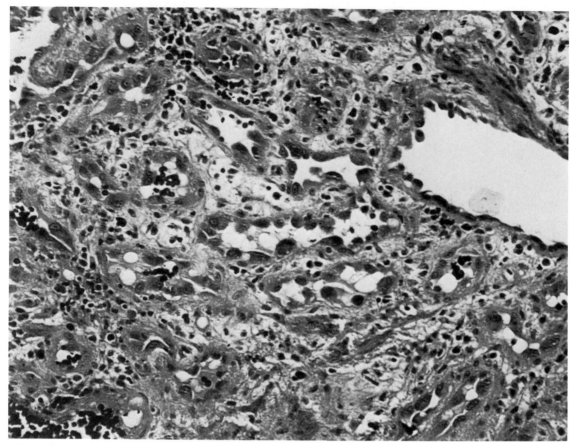

Figure 5–13. Higher power visualization of angiolymphoid hyperplasia with eosinophilia that was shown in Figure 5–12 illustrates the distinctive histiocytoid or epithelioid endothelial cells. A few lymphocytes and eosinophils are present in the stroma (× 200).

Orientals.[101, 104] The disease occurs predominantly in young and middle-aged adults. The median age of onset has been reported to range from 27 to 40 years, and men are more commonly affected than women. The duration of the lesions prior to therapy varies from 1 to 24 years, with a median time period of 4 years.[103] Typically, the lesions are firm, rubbery, subcutaneous, tumorlike nodules or masses, which may reach a size of 11.0 cm, usually over a period of 1 to 2 years.[102, 103, 112] They are most common in the head and neck region, with a predilection for the periauricular area, and they are often misdiagnosed as salivary gland tumors, lymphomas, or Mikulicz's disease.[88, 103, 112] The lesions may be multiple, and there is a fairly high recurrence rate.[88, 101–104, 112] In contrast to angiolymphoid hyperplasia with eosinophilia, the lesions characteristically involve adjacent parotid and submandibular salivary glands, lymph nodes, and muscle.[88, 101–104, 112] In addition to the mass, regional lymphadenopathy is commonly present. Typically, patients with this disease have peripheral blood eosinophilia and elevated immunoglobulin E levels but are usually otherwise healthy.[101]

Pathologic Features

Grossly, the lesions are rubbery and irregular or nodular. The cut surfaces are gray to light brown and may contain embedded lymph nodes and attached salivary gland tissue and muscle. Microscopically, the lesions are unencapsulated and ill defined and are characterized by fibrocollagenous tissue, lymphoid tissue, and a mixed inflammatory cell infiltrate with numerous eosinophils. Some of the reactive lymphoid follicles are infiltrated by eosinophils with resultant eosinophilic microabscesses (Fig. 5–14). Similar extra follicular microabscesses also occur. Polykaryocytes of the Warthin-Finkeldey type are sometimes observed in the germinal centers of the reactive lymphoid follicles. Proliferating capillary-sized blood vessels are a constant feature. Many of these vessels are lined by plump endothelial cells similar to the cells of the so-called high endothelial venules of the interfollicular region of the lymph nodes (Fig. 5–15). In contrast to angiolymphoid hyperplasia with eosinophilia, these vessels do not occur in clusters, and the

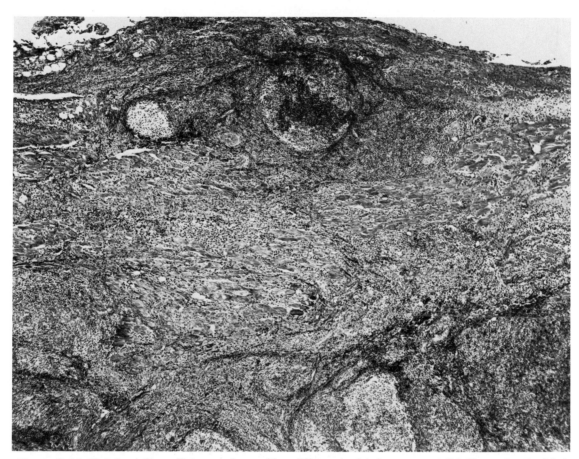

Figure 5–14. Ill-defined fibrocollagenous tissue with a diffuse mixed inflammatory cell infiltrate that is rich in eosinophils and lymphoid follicles with germinal centers is seen in this case of Kimura's disease. The lymphoid follicle at the top of the photomicrograph contains an eosinophilic microabscess (× 100).

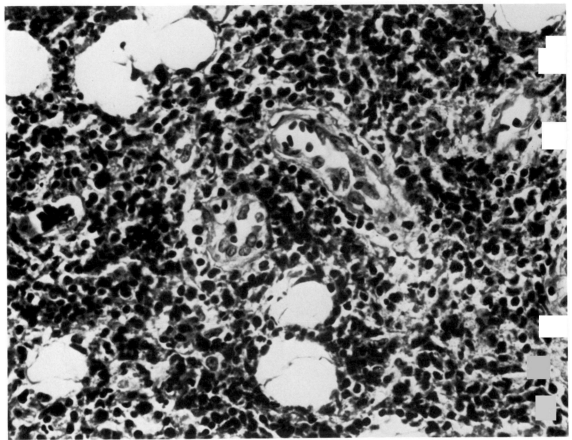

Figure 5–15. Kimura's disease with the characteristic mixed inflammatory cell infiltrate and typical capillary-sized blood vessels lined by plump endothelial cells is illustrated. The endothelial cells never approach the epithelioid proportions that are characteristic of angiolymphoid hyperplasia with eosinophilia (× 400).

endothelial cells never have morphologic features that would justify the designation of "epithelioid" or "histiocytoid." Dense fibrocollagenous tissue is invariably present, even in the early lesions; it may form fibrous bands or septa, and it may extend into adjacent lymph nodes, salivary glands, and muscle.

The enlarged regional lymph nodes in Kimura's disease typically reveal florid follicular hyperplasia, increased postcapillary venules in the paracortex, eosinophilic infiltration, sclerosis, and Warthin-Finkeldey type polykaryocytes.[104] Identical changes may also occur in intraparotid lymph nodes (Fig. 5–16).

The morphologic character of the affected salivary glands is variable. In advanced lesions, the lobules are largely replaced by fibrous tissue that is infiltrated by eosinophils and lymphoid tissue with germinal centers. Occasional ducts that are often surrounded by concentric layers of collagen can be identified along with occasional small nests of ductal and metaplastic squamous epithelium. In minimally affected glands, some of the ducts are surrounded by lymphocytes and variable num-

bers of eosinophils, and some of these cells may extend into the adjacent acini. Lymphoid follicles with germinal centers are occasionally present adjacent to ducts (Fig. 5–17).

Treatment

Surgical excision, radiotherapy, and drug therapy (steroids and oxyphenbutazone) have been used to treat Kimura's disease. Surgical excision appears to be the therapy of choice for large, esthetically objectionable lesions.[112]

Differential Diagnosis

Angiolymphoid hyperplasia with eosinophilia can be differentiated from capillary hemangioma, granuloma faciale, pseudolymphoma, and Kimura's disease by the presence of vascular channels with characteristic epithelioid or histiocytoid endothelial cells. Epithelioid hemangioendothelioma differs from angiolymphoid hyperplasia with eo-

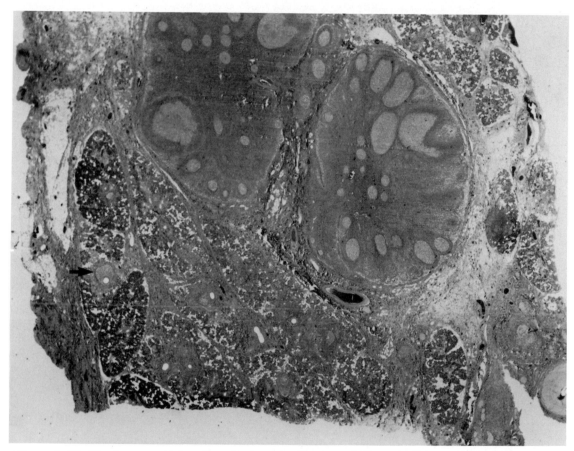

Figure 5–16. The intraparotid lymph node tissue in this case of Kimura's disease exhibits florid follicular hyperplasia. The adjacent gland displays slight focal intralobular and extralobular fibrosis and chronic inflammation. The arrow points to a paraductal lymphoid follicle (× 7.5).

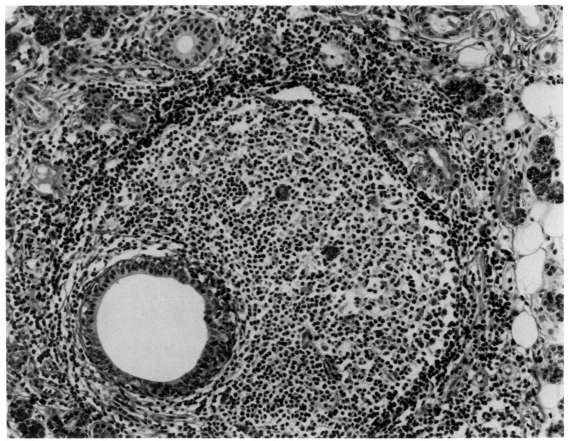

Figure 5–17. Higher magnification of the area that is indicated by an arrow on Figure 5–16 shows a paraductal lymphoid follicle with polykaryocytes of the Warthin-Finkeldey type and an adjacent interstitial mixed inflammatory cell infiltrate with eosinophils (× 150).

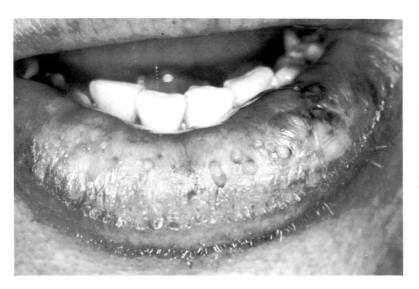

Figure 5–18. Clinical photograph of the lower lip of a middle-aged patient with a soft, painless lip swelling that persisted for many years. Note small droplets of mucinous fluid on the vermilion surface. (Courtesy of Dr. James J. Sciubba, Hillside Medical Center, Long Island, NY).

sinophilia by the presence of solid nests and short strands of epithelioid endothelial cells, many of which contain intracytoplasmic lumina that appear as clear spaces or vacuoles that distort the cells. These cells are typically embedded in a myxoid stroma. Epithelioid hemangioendotheliomas rarely contain large vascular channels, and no evidence of tissue eosinophilia is present. Epithelioid angiosarcomas, in contrast to angiolymphoid hyperplasia with eosinophilia, are composed of sheets of rounded, glassy, eosinophilic endothelial cells with nuclear pleomorphism, mitotic activity, and areas of necrosis. Failure to demonstrate an infectious agent together with the absence of granulomas separates Kimura's disease from the various infectious diseases in which eosinophils are prominent.

CHEILITIS GLANDULARIS

The term *cheilitis glandularis* was introduced by Volkman[113] to describe a condition characterized by a suppurative, inflammatory swelling of the lower lip. After Volkman's paper was published, additional cases of cheilitis glandularis were described, each with a swollen lower lip, with varying degrees of inflammation, and with prominent salivary duct orifices (Fig. 5–18).[114–117] In 1914, Sutton[118] postulated that the swelling was due to enlargement of the labial salivary glands. Authors of many subsequent reports have offered similar interpretations.[119–125] Some authors, however, have considered ductal ectasia and inflammation of minor salivary glands and adjacent tissue to be the essential microscopic features of cheilitis glandularis.[126, 127] In a detailed study of this condition, Swerlick and Cooper[128] found no measurable difference in the size of labial salivary glands in their cases and in their control specimens. Furthermore, the inflammatory infiltrates in the glands of the patients with cheilitis glandularis were sparse and nonspecific. It is apparent from the literature that there exist no consistent morphologic changes in the labial salivary glands on which to base a histologic diagnosis of this condition.

REFERENCES

1. Abrams AM, Melrose RJ, Howell FV: Necrotizing sialometaplasia: A disease simulating malignancy. Cancer 1973; 32:130–135.
2. Dunlap CL, Barker BF: Necrotizing sialometaplasia: Report of five additional cases. Oral Surg Oral Med Oral Pathol 1974; 37:722–727.
3. Myers EN, Bankaci M, Barnes EL Jr: Necrotizing sialometaplasia. Arch Otolaryngol 1975; 101:628–629.
4. Arguelles MT, Viloria JB, Talens MC, McCory TP: Necrotizing sialometaplasia. Oral Surg Oral Med Oral Pathol 1974; 42:86–90.
5. Fechner RE: Necrotizing sialometaplasia: A source of confusion with carcinoma of the palate. Am J Clin Pathol 1977; 67:315–317.
6. Maisel RH, Johnston WH, Anderson HA, Cantrell RW: Necrotizing sialometaplasia involving the nasal cavity. Laryngoscope 1977; 87:429–434.
7. Suckiel JM, Davis WH, Patakas BM, Kamnishi M: Early and late manifestations of necrotizing sialometaplasia. J Oral Surg 1978; 36:902–905.
8. Lynch DP, Cargo CA, Martinez MG Jr: Necrotizing sialometaplasia: A review of the literature and report of two additional cases. Oral Surg Oral Med Oral Pathol 1979; 47:63–69.
9. Gad A, Willén H, Willén R, Thorstensson S, Ekman L: Necrotizing sialometaplasia of the lip simulating squamous cell carcinoma. Histopathology 1980; 4:111–121.
10. Mesa ML, Gertler RS, Schneider LC: Necrotizing sialometaplasia: Frequency of histologic misdiagnosis. Oral Surg Oral Med Oral Pathol 1984; 57:71–73.
11. Poulson TC, Greer RO Jr, Rysner RW: Necrotizing sialometaplasia obscuring an underlying malignancy: Report of a case. J Oral Maxillofac Surg 1984; 44:570–574.
12. Kinney RB, Burton CS, Vollmer RT: Necrotizing sialometaplasia: A sheep in wolf's clothing. Healing as a diagnostic test. Arch Dermatol 1986; 122:208–210.
13. Granick MS, Soloman MP, Benedetto AV, Hannegan MW, Sohn M: Necrotizing sialometaplasia masquerading as residual cancer of the lip. Ann Plast Surg 1988; 21:152–154.
14. Giles AD: Necrotizing sialometaplasia. Br J Oral Surg 1980; 18:45–50.
15. Forney SK, Foley JM, Sugg WE, Otis GW: Necrotizing sialometaplasia of the mandible. Oral Surg Oral Med Oral Pathol 1977; 43:720–726.
16. Fowler CB, Brannon RB, Hartman KS: Necrotizing sialometaplasia: A clinicopathologic study of sixty-seven cases. Abstract 34th Annual Meeting American Academy of Oral Pathology, 1989.
17. Mantilla A, Flores T, Nogales FF, Galera H: Necrotizing sialometaplasia affecting the minor labial glands. Oral Surg Oral Med Oral Pathol 1979; 47:161–163.
18. Johnston WH: Necrotizing sialometaplasia involving the mucous glands of the nasal cavity. Hum Pathol 1977; 8:589–592.
19. Close LG, Cowan DF: Recurrent necrotizing sialometaplasia of the nasal cavity. Otolaryngol Head Neck Surg 1985; 93:422–425.
20. Walker GK, Fechner RE, Johns ME, Kuldeep T: Necrotizing sialometaplasia of the larynx secondary to atheromatous embolization. Am J Clin Pathol 1982; 77:221–223.
21. Donath K: Pathohistologie des Parotisinfarktes (necrotizing sialometaplasia). Laryngol Rhinol Otol (Stuttg) 1979; 58:70–76.
22. Gnepp DR: Warthin's tumor exhibiting sebaceous differentiation and necrotizing sialometaplasia. Virchows Arch [A] 1981; 391:267–273.
23. Batsakis JG, Manning JT: Necrotizing sialometaplasia of major salivary glands. J Laryngol Otol 1987; 101:962–966.
24. Anneroth G, Hansen LS: Necrotizing sialometaplasia: The relationship of its pathogenesis to its clinical characteristics. Int J Oral Surg 1982; 11:283–291.
25. Colquitt WN, Gobetti JP: Necrotizing sialometaplasia: A diagnostic dilemma. J Mich Dent Assoc 1984; 66:23–25.

26. Dunlap CL, Barker BF: Diagnostic problems in oral pathology. Semin Diag Pathol 1985; 2:16–30.
27. Abrams AM: Necrotizing sialometaplasia of the nasal cavity (letter). Otolaryngol Head Neck Surg 1986; 94:416.
28. Gahos F, Enriquez RE, Bahn SK, Ariyans S: Necrotizing sialometaplasia: Report of five cases. Plast Reconstr Surg 1983; 7:650–657.
29. Birkholz H, Minton GA, Yuen YL: Necrotizing sialometaplasia: Review of the literature and report of a nonulcerative case. J Oral Surg 1979; 37:588–592.
30. Grillion GL, Lally ET: Necrotizing sialometaplasia: Literature review and presentation of five cases. J Oral Surg 1981; 39:747–753.
31. Speechley JA, Field EA, Scott J: Necrotizing sialometaplasia occurring during pregnancy: Report of a case. J Oral Maxillofac Surg 1988; 46:696–699.
32. Rossi KM, Allen CM, Burns RA: Necrotizing sialometaplasia: A case report with metachronous lesions. J Oral Maxillofac Surg 1986; 44:1006–1008.
33. Marciani RD, Sabes WR: Necrotizing sialometaplasia: Report of three cases. Oral Surg Oral Med Oral Pathol 1976; 34:722–726.
34. Santis HR, Kabani SP, Roderiques A, Driscoll JM: Necrotizing sialometaplasia: An early nonulcerative presentation. Oral Surg Oral Med Oral Pathol 1982; 53:387–390.
35. Chaudhry AP, Yamane GM, Salman K, Salman S, Saxon M, Pierri LK: Necrotizing sialometaplasia of palatal minor salivary glands: A report of two cases. J Oral Med 1985; 40:2–6.
36. Rye LA, Calhoun NR, Redman RS: Necrotizing sialometaplasia in a patient with Buerger's disease and Raynaud's phenomenon. Oral Surg Oral Med Oral Pathol 1980; 49:233–236.
37. Aversa D, Mock D: Necrotizing sialometaplasia. Ont Dent 1985; 62:17–19.
38. Philipsen HP, Petersen JK, Simonsen BH: Necrotizing sialometaplasia of the palate. Int J Oral Surg 1976; 5:292–299.
39. Dunley RE, Jacoway JR: Necrotizing sialometaplasia. Oral Surg Oral Med Oral Pathol 1979; 47:169–172.
40. Standish SM, Shafer WG: Several histologic effects of rat submaxillary and sublingual salivary gland duct and blood vessel ligation. J Dent Res 1957; 36:866–879.
41. Hanks CT, Chaudhry AP: Regeneration of rat submandibular gland following partial extirpation: A light and electron microscopic study. Am J Anat 1971; 130:195–208.
42. Englander A, Cataldo E: Experimental carcinogenesis in duct-artery ligated rat submandibular gland. J Dent Res 1976; 55(2):229–234.
43. Dardick I, Jeans MTD, Sinnott NM, Wittkuhn JF, Kahn HJ, Baumal R: Salivary gland components involved in the formation of squamous metaplasia. Am J Pathol 1985; 119:33–43.
44. Richardson GS, Clairmont AA, Erickson ER: Cystic lesions of the parotid gland. Plast Reconstr Surg 1978; 61:364–369.
45. Work WP: Cysts and congenital lesions of the parotid gland. Otolaryngol Clin North Am 1977; 10:339–343.
46. Pieterse AS, Seymour AE: Parotid cysts: An analysis of 16 cases and suggested classification. Pathology 1981; 13:225–234.
47. Cohen MN, Rao U, Shedd DP: Benign cysts of the parotid gland. J Surg Oncol 1984; 27:85–88.
48. Batsakis JG, Raymond AK: Sialocysts of the parotid glands. Ann Otol Rhinol Laryngol 1989; 98:487–489.
49. Seifert G, Thomsen ST, Donath K: Bilateral dysgenetic polycystic parotid glands. Morphological analysis and differential diagnosis of a rare disease of the salivary glands. Virchows Arch [A] 1981; 390:273–288.
50. Cunningham WF: Branchial cysts of the parotid gland. Ann Surg 1929; 90:114–119.
51. Little JW, Rickles NH: The histogenesis of the branchial cyst. Am J Pathol 1967; 50:533–547.
52. Rickles NH, Little JW: The histogenesis of the branchial cyst. II. A study of the lining epithelium. Am J Pathol 1967; 50:765–773.
53. Leonard JR, Maran AG, Huffman WC: Branchial cleft cysts in the parotid gland: Facial nerve anomaly. Plast Reconstr Surg 1968; 41:493–496.
54. Paley WG, Kiddie NC: The aetiology and management of branchial cysts. Br J Surg 1970; 57:822–824.
55. Sisson GA, Summers GW: Branchiogenic cysts within the parotid gland: Report of a case. Arch Otolaryngol 1972; 96:165–167.
56. Gaisford JC, Anderson VS: First branchial cleft cysts and sinuses. Plast Reconstr Surg 1974; 55:299–304.
57. Miglets AW: Parotid branchial cleft cyst with facial paralysis: Report of a case. Arch Otolaryngol 1975; 101:637–638.
58. Shaheen NA, Harboyn GT, Nassif RI: Cysts of the parotid gland: Review and report of two unusual cases. J Laryngol Otol 1975; 89:435–444.
59. Olsen K, Margus NE, Weiland LH: First branchial cleft anomalies. Laryngoscope 1980; 90:423–436.
60. Bernier JL, Bhaskar SN: Lymphoepithelial lesions of the salivary glands: Histogenesis and classification based on 186 cases. Cancer 1958; 11:1156–1179.
61. Bhaskar SN, Bernier JL: Histogenesis of branchial cysts: A report of 468 cases. Am J Pathol 1959; 35:407–414.
62. Truong LD, Rangdaeng S, Jordan PH: Lymphoepithelial cyst of the pancreas. Am J Surg Pathol 1987; 11:899–903.
63. Louis DN, Vickery AL, Rosai J, Wang CA: Multiple branchial cleft-like cysts in Hashimoto's thyroiditis. Am J Surg Pathol 1989; 13:45–49.
64. Weitzner S: Lymphoepithelial (branchial) cyst of parotid gland. Oral Surg Oral Med Oral Pathol 1973; 35:85–87.
65. Katz AD: Unusual lesion of the parotid gland. J Surg Oncol 1975; 7:219–235.
66. Gnepp DR, Sporck TF: Benign lymphoepithelial parotid cyst with sebaceous differentiation—cystic sebaceous lymphadenoma. Am J Clin Pathol 1980; 74:683–687.
67. Fujibayashi T, Itoh H: Lymphoepithelial (so-called branchial) cyst within the parotid gland: Report of a case and review of the literature. Int J Oral Surg 1981; 10:283–292.
68. Gerber D, Hugo NE: Branchial cleft cyst in parotid gland. Ann Plast Surg 1982; 9:413–414.
69. Atiyah RA, Wurster CF, Fritsch MA, Sisson GA:

Intraparotid branchial cleft cyst: Pathologic quiz case 1. Arch Otolaryngol 1985; 111:204–207.

70. Weidner N, Geisinger KR, Sterling RT, Miller TR, Benedict TS: Benign lymphoepithelial cysts of the parotid gland: A histologic, cytologic, and ultrastructural study. Am J Clin Pathol 1986; 85:395–401.

71. Morris MR, Moore DW, Shearer GN: Bilateral multiple benign lymphoepithelial cysts of the parotid gland. Otolaryngol Head Neck Surg 1987; 97:87–90.

72. Wyman A, Dunn LK, Talati VR, Rogers K: Lympho-epithelial 'branchial' cysts within the parotid gland. Br J Surg 1988; 75:818–819.

73. Stewart S, Levy R, Karpel J, Stoopack J: Lympho-epithelial (branchial) cyst of the parotid gland. J Oral Surg 1974; 32:100–106.

74. Pensak ML, Casuccio JR, Lesnick TH, Sasaki CT: Facial paralysis resulting from parotid branchial cyst. Otolaryngol Head Neck Surg 1982; 90:676–678.

75. Scott R: Branchial cysts in the parotid gland. J R Coll Surg Edinb 1987; 32:336–338.

76. Hanson TAS: Acinic cell carcinoma of the parotid salivary gland presenting as a cyst: Report of two cases. Cancer 1975; 36:570–575.

77. Smith A, Winkler B, Perzin KH, Wazen J, Blitzer A: Mucoepidermoid carcinoma arising in an intraparotid lymph node. Cancer 1985; 55:400–403.

78. Dwork A, Perzin KH: Carcinoma arising in intra-parotid branchial cleft cyst: Report of a case and review of the literature. Prog Surg Pathol 1982; 4:291–296.

79. Ryan JR, Ioachim HL, Marmer J, Loubeau M: Acquired immune deficiency syndrome-related lymphadenopathies presenting in salivary gland lymph nodes. Arch Otolaryngol 1985; 111:554–556.

80. Ioachim HL, Ryan JR, Blaugrund SM: AIDS-associated lymphadenopathies and lymphomas with primary salivary gland presentation. (abst) Lab Invest 1987; 56:33A.

81. Smith F, Rajdeo H, Panesar N, Stahl R: Benign lymphoepithelial lesion of parotid gland in intra-venous drug users. (abst) Lab Invest 1987; 56:74A.

82. Holliday RA, Cohen WA, Schinella RA, Rothstein SG, Persky MS, Jacobs JM, Som PM: Benign lymphoepithelial parotid cysts and hyperplastic cervical adenopathy in AIDS risk patients: A new CT appearance. Radiology 1988; 168:439–441.

83. Finer MD, Schinella RA, Rothstein SG, Persky MS: Cystic parotid lesions in patients at risk for the acquired immunodeficiency syndrome. Arch Otolaryngol Head Neck Surg 1988; 114:1290–1294.

84. Ulirsch RC, Jaffe ES: Sjögren's syndrome-like illness associated with the acquired immunodeficiency syndrome-related complex. Hum Pathol 1987; 18:1063–1068.

85. Eneroth C-M: Histological and clinical aspects of parotid tumors. Acta Otolaryngol Suppl 1964; 191:1–96.

86. Hooper R, Saxon R, Tropp H: Cysts of the parotid gland. J Laryngol Otol 1975; 89:427–433.

87. Wong PNC, Djamshidi M: Gigantic parotid reten-tion cyst. J Oral Maxillofac Surg 1984; 42:618–620.

88. Kung ITM, Gibson JB, Bannatyne PM: Kimura's disease: A clinico-pathological study of 21 cases and its distinction from angiolymphoid hyper-plasia with eosinophilia. Pathology 1984; 16:39–44.

89. Wells B, Whimster I: Subcutaneous angiolymphoid hyperplasia with eosinophilia. Br J Dermatol 1969; 81:1–5.

90. Mehregan AH, Shapiro L: Angiolymphoid hyper-plasia with eosinophilia. Arch Dermatol 1971; 103:50–57.

91. Reed RJ, Terazakis N: Subcutaneous angioblastic lymphoid hyperplasia with eosinophilia (Kimu-ra's disease). Cancer 1972; 29:489–497.

92. Kim BH, Sithian N, Cucolo GF: Subcutaneous angiolymphoid hyperplasia (Kimura's disease). Arch Surg 1975; 110:1246–1248.

93. Henry PG, Burnett JW: Angiolymphoid hyperpla-sia with eosinophilia. Arch Dermatol 1978; 114:1168–1172.

94. Eveson JW, Lucas RB: Angiolymphoid hyperplasia with eosinophilia. J Oral Pathol 1979; 8:103–108.

95. Buchner A, Silverman S Jr, Ward WM, Hansen LS: Angiolymphoid hyperplasia with eosino-philia (Kimura's disease). Oral Surg Oral Med Oral Pathol 1980; 49:309–313.

96. Rehak A, Bou-Resli M, Mousa AM, Al-Zaid NS: Angiolymphoid hyperplasia with eosinophilia. Dermatologica 1980; 161:157–166.

97. Thompson JW, Colman M, Williamson C, Ward PH: Angiolymphoid hyperplasia with eosino-philia of the external ear canal. Arch Otolaryngol 1981; 107:316–319.

98. Eisenberg E, Lowlicht R: Angiolymphoid hyper-plasia with eosinophilia: A clinico-pathological conference. J Oral Pathol 1985; 14:216–223.

99. Rosai J, Gold J, Landy R: The histiocytoid heman-giomas: A unifying concept embracing several previously described entities of skin, soft tissue, large vessels, bone and heart. Hum Pathol 1979; 10:707–730.

100. Weiss SW, Ishak KG, Dial DH, Sweet DE, Enzinger FM: Epithelioid hemangioendothelioma and re-lated lesions. Semin Diag Pathol 1986; 3:259–287.

101. Googe PB, Harris PB, Mihm MC Jr: Kimura's disease and angiolymphoid hyperplasia with eo-sinophilia: Two distinct histopathological enti-ties. J Cutan Pathol 1987; 14:263–271.

102. Urabe A, Tsuneyoshi M, Enjoji M: Epithelioid hemangioma versus Kimura's disease: A com-parative clinicopathologic study. Am J Surg Pa-thol 1987; 11:758–766.

103. Kuo T-T, Shih L-Y, Chan H-L: Kimura's disease: Involvement of lymph nodes and distinction from angiolymphoid hyperplasia with eosino-philia. Am J Surg Pathol 1988; 12:843–854.

104. Hui PK, Chan JKC, Ng CS, Kung ITM, Gwi E: Lymphadenopathy of Kimura's disease. Am J Surg Pathol 1989; 13:177–186.

105. Wilson-Jones E, Bleehen SS: Inflammatory angi-omatous nodules with abnormal blood vessels occurring about the ears and scalp (pseudo- or atypical pyogenic granuloma). Br J Dermatol 1969; 81:804–816.

106. Peterson WC Jr, Fusaro RM, Goltz RW: Atypical pyogenic granuloma: A case of benign hemangioendotheliosis. Arch Dermatol 1964; 90:197–201.

107. Rosai J, Ackerman LV: Intravenous atypical vascular proliferation: A cutaneous lesion simulating a malignant blood vessel tumor. Arch Dermatol 1974; 109:714–717.

108. Enzinger FM, Weiss SW: Soft Tissue Tumors, 2nd Ed. St. Louis, CV Mosby Co, 1988; 489–532.

109. Olsen TG, Helwig EB: Angiolymphoid hyperplasia with eosinophilia: A clinicopathologic study of 116 cases. J Am Acad Dermatol 1985; 12:781–796.

110. Suster S: Nodal angiolymphoid hyperplasia with eosinophilia. Am J Clin Pathol 1987; 88:236–239.

111. Goldman RL, Klein HZ: Subcutaneous angiolymphoid hyperplasia with eosinophilia: Report of a case masquerading as a salivary gland tumor. Arch Otolaryngol 1976; 102:440–441.

112. Tham K-T, Leung P-C, Saw D, Gwi E: Kimura's disease with salivary gland involvement. Br J Surg 1981; 68:495–497.

113. Volkman R: Einige Falle von Cheilitis Glandularis Apostematosa (Myxadenitis Labialis). Virchows Arch [A] 1870; 50:142–144.

114. Purdon HS: Four cases of cheilitis glandularis. Br J Dermatol 1893; 5:23.

115. Fox H: Cheilitis glandularis. J Cutan Dis 1909; 27:229.

116. Sutton RL: Cheilitis glandularis apostematosa (with case report). J Cutan Dis 1909; 27:151–154.

117. Schamberg JF: Cheilitis glandularis. J Cutan Dis 1911; 29:449.

118. Sutton RL: The symptomatology and treatment of three common diseases of the vermilion border of the lip. Int Clin (series 24) 1914; 3:123–128.

119. Everett FG, Holder TD: Cheilitis glandularis apostematosa. Oral Surg Oral Med Oral Pathol 1955; 8:405–413.

120. Michalowski R: Cheilitis glandularis, heterotopic salivary glands and squamous cell carcinoma of the lip. Br J Dermatol 1962; 74:445–449.

121. Doku HC, Shklar G, McCarthy PL: Cheilitis glandularis. Oral Surg Oral Med Oral Pathol 1965; 20:563–571.

122. Weir TW, Johnson WC: Cheilitis glandularis. Arch Dermatol 1971; 103:433–437.

123. Oliver ID, Pickett AB: Cheilitis glandularis. Oral Surg Oral Med Oral Pathol 1980; 49:526–529.

124. Burwell RK: Cheilitis glandularis. J Assoc Milit Derm 1982; 8:71–72.

125. Cohen DM, Green JG, Diekmann SL: Concurrent anomalies: Cheilitis glandularis and doublelip. Oral Surg Oral Med Oral Pathol 1988; 66:397–399.

126. Rada DC, Koranda FC, Katz FS: Cheilitis glandularis—a disorder of ductal ectasia. J Dermatol Surg Oncol 1985; 11:372–375.

127. Yacobi R, Brown DA: Cheilitis glandularis: A pediatric case report. J Am Dent Assoc 1989; 118:317–318.

128. Swerlick RA, Cooper PH: Cheilitis glandularis: A reevaluation. J Am Acad Dermatol 1984; 10:466–472.

6

BENIGN LYMPHOEPITHELIAL LESION AND SJÖGREN'S SYNDROME

Troy E. Daniels

In the autoimmune diseases known as primary and secondary Sjögren's syndrome (SS), the entire complement of major and minor salivary glands can become infiltrated by lymphocytes. The infiltrating lymphocytes replace the glandular parenchyma, causing gradually decreased salivary secretion, and induce morphologic changes in the glandular epithelium. The affected glands may or may not become enlarged, but when enlarged, they show features of the benign lymphoepithelial lesion (BLL) in almost all cases.

However, BLLs may also occur—occasionally bilaterally—in patients who do not have Sjögren's syndrome or any other identifiable disease. Uncommonly, they may be associated with a variety of other conditions. Furthermore, they do not always remain benign and may be associated with or transform into lymphomas in patients with or without SS (Fig. 6–1). Rarely, they may become carcinomas.

This chapter reviews the clinical features, the pathology, and the immunopathology of the BLL and the salivary component of SS.

BENIGN LYMPHOEPITHELIAL LESION

History

The pathologic entity that we now call *benign lymphoepithelial lesion* was first described at a meeting in 1888 by the German surgeon Johann Mikulicz in a report of a single case. After searching and waiting in vain for similar cases to appear, he

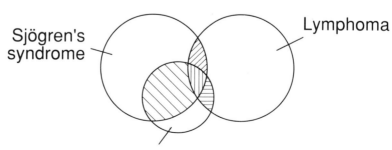

Figure 6–1. Graphic representation of the association between Sjögren's syndrome (SS), benign lymphoepithelial lesion, and lymphoma. One third to one half of patients with SS develop enlarged major salivary glands (benign lymphoepithelial lesions) and a few of these lesions progress to lymphoma. Benign lymphoepithelial lesions also occur in patients without SS, and these lesions may also progress to lymphoma. Infrequently, patients with SS may develop lymphoma in organs other than salivary glands.

reported this one case in a paper in 1892.[1] He described a 42-year-old man who presented with chronic, painless, bilateral enlargement of the lacrimal glands, which grew so large that they interfered with his vision. The lacrimal enlargement was followed by enlargement of the submandibular and parotid glands as well as the sublingual, palatine, labial, and buccal salivary glands. These firmly elastic swellings developed gradually during a period of 7 months. After surgical reduction the tumors returned, necessitating complete removal of the lacrimal and submandibular glands. Lymph node enlargement was not noted at any time. Peritonitis developed in the patient 13 months after the onset of glandular swelling, and he died after a 9-day illness, during which all residual gland enlargement regressed.[2]

Subsequently, in spite of Mikulicz's careful description of the microscopic appearance of his case, the term *Mikulicz's disease* was applied to a variety of cases of bilateral salivary or lacrimal gland enlargement, including those caused by tuberculosis, syphilis, sarcoidosis, or lymphoma. However, Mikulicz refused to accept any cases with known causes as additional instances of the disease he had described.[3]

In 1927, the suggestion was made to divide cases of salivary gland enlargement into two large categories: Mikulicz's disease, if the cause was unknown, and Mikulicz's syndrome, if the enlargement was associated with a known disease.[4] Now, however, these two Mikulicz eponyms are so ambiguous and ill-defined that they should no longer be used.[5]

The name *benign lymphoepithelial lesion* was proposed by Godwin[6] in 1952 to describe parotid gland lesions previously called Mikulicz's disease, adenolymphoma, chronic inflammation, lymphoepithelioma, or lymphocytic tumor. In reviewing clinical and pathologic aspects of 18 cases of "Mikulicz's disease" in 1953, Morgan and Castleman[7] noted many similarities to SS and proposed that Mikulicz's disease is not a distinct clinical and pathologic entity but only one manifestation of the more generalized symptom complex of that syndrome. Morgan[8] then compared the histopathologic findings in these 18 cases with those from the original slides of the salivary gland described by Sjögren[9] in 1933 and found them to be identical. Our current understanding of the relationship between the BLL and SS is discussed in later sections of this chapter.

Pathology

The development of BLLs begins with focal infiltrates of small lymphocytes that expand to replace the glandular epithelium. The infiltration is associated with hyperplasia and metaplasia of ductal epithelium, resulting in the epimyoepithelial islands that characterize the lesion (Figs. 6–2 and 6–3). Lymphoid follicles with germinal centers may or may not be present. Plasma cells and polymorphonuclear leukocytes are usually not a significant component of this infiltrate. The pathologic character of the BLL has been described by Batsakis as a "distinctive, yet not pathognomonic, sialadenopathy."[10]

A cystic variant of this lesion exists. It is not clear whether this variant represents a different pathogenic mechanism or a cystic degeneration of an existing BLL. A recent study describes the pathology and ultrastructure of five cases of benign lymphoepithelial cysts of the parotid gland and distinguishes them from cystic types of the BLL on the basis of differences in the epithelium lining the cystic space.[11] However, the authors pointed out that making this distinction may be difficult in some cases.

Despite the name *epimyoepithelial islands*, the cells making up these structures have not been clearly identified. In an early ultrastructural study of a BLL associated with SS, the authors found several kinds of cells in the islands but no evidence of myoepithelial cells; this led them to suggest that the islands are formed by proliferation and squamous metaplasia of duct cells.[12] Three stages of island formation were described in another ultrastructural study of this lesion, which the authors termed myoepithelial sialadenitis.[13] They suggested that the islands are formed initially from intercalated duct cells around the remains of the duct lumen, with myoepithelial cells arranged peripherally and surrounded by a basement membrane complex. This stage is followed by destruction of duct epithelium, proliferation of myoepithelium, and infiltration by lymphocytes and histiocytes. The final stage involves hyaline transformation.

More recently, one study showed that these islands are composed mainly of keratin-containing epithelial cells and do not contain cells with the immunohistochemical or ultrastructural characteristics of myoepithelial cells.[14] In contrast, in another study, the authors detected myoepithelial cells in the islands by electron microscopy, but the cells were visualized only in the early stages of island development.[15]

An examination of normal parotid glands and BLLs by immunohistochemical methods with five monoclonal antibodies against two classes of intermediate filament proteins (cytokeratins and vimentin) revealed two types of cells in epimyoepithelial islands.[16] One type contained cytokeratins 7, 8, 17, 18, and 19 but no vimentin, which is similar to the profile of normal duct cells; the other type contained the same cytokeratins with vimentin, which is similar to the profile of normal myoepithelial and ductal basal cells. The authors concluded that epimyoepithelial islands are composed of a mixed population of cells that have undergone metaplasia.

At this time, it seems reasonable to assume that the cellular composition of epimyoepithelial islands is heterogeneous and may change during

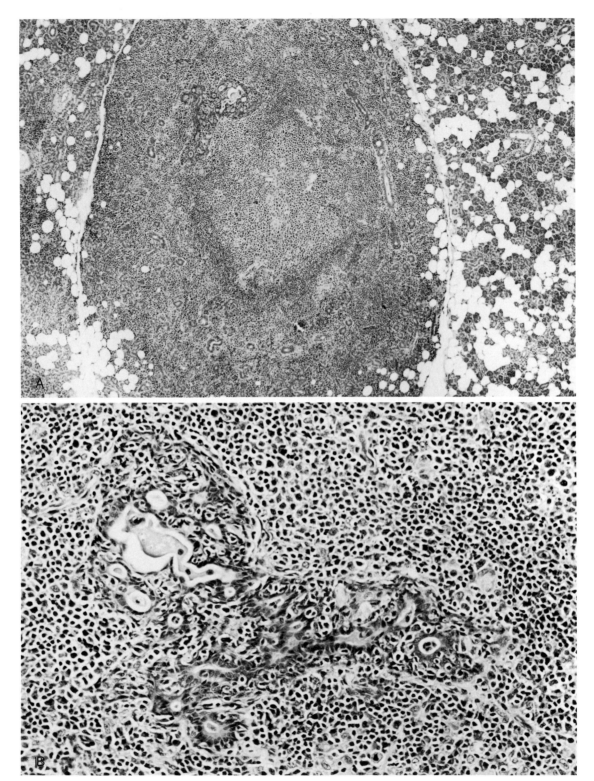

Figure 6–2. *A*, Photomicrograph shows a section of a benign lymphoepithelial lesion from a 67-year-old man with unilateral parotid enlargement present for 5 months. There was no clinical evidence of Sjögren's syndrome. The specimen showed multicentric lesions in most lobes of the gland (× 40). *B*, High magnification of the same section allows visualization of an epimyoepithelial island (× 200).

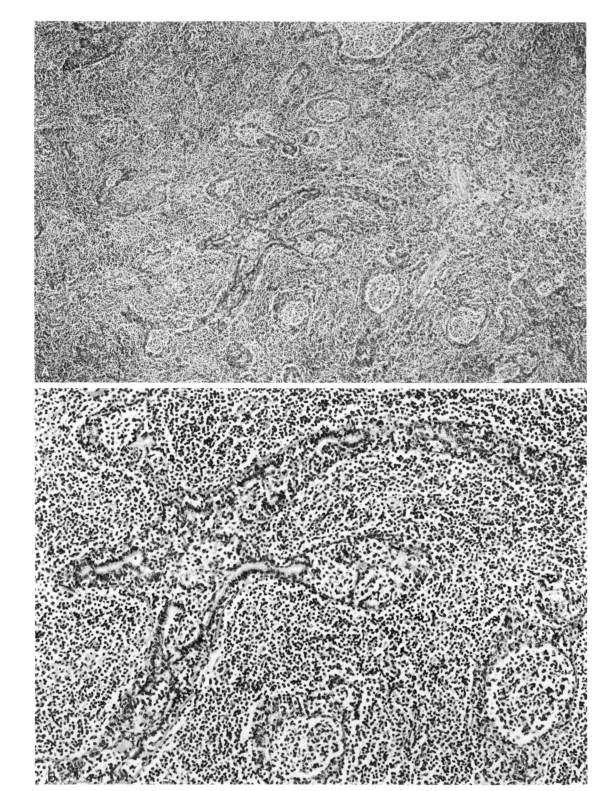

Figure 6–3. Section of a benign lymphoepithelial lesion from a 59-year-old woman with bilateral parotid enlargement, severe clinical xerostomia, absent stimulated parotid flow, focal lymphocytic sialadenitis in a labial salivary gland biopsy (focus score of seven foci/4 mm^2), and severe keratoconjunctivitis sicca. The entire gland had an appearance similar to this field. Few germinal centers were seen, and no normal-appearing parotid epithelium remained in the specimen. Many epimyoepithelial islands are evident. (A, × 40; B, × 100.)

lesion development and that future techniques will allow us to better identify the cells.

Pathogenesis

Like other aspects of this lesion, its pathogenesis remains controversial. Mikulicz[2] suggested that it was the result of an infectious or parasitic process penetrating the gland locally rather than hematogenously. Morgan and Castleman[7] considered it a primary lesion of the salivary duct system with secondary lymphocytic infiltration. Bernier and Bhaskar[17] suggested that BLL is neither a neoplasm nor a lesion in which epithelium plays an aggressive or dominant role; it is primarily a lymphoid lesion that can incidentally involve the salivary glands.

Modern concepts of an immunologically mediated pathogenesis are now evolving through the application of immunohistochemical methods of analysis. Studies have included tissue specimens of enlarged major salivary glands from patients with or without SS and specimens of labial salivary glands from patients with SS. Since, as yet, there are no apparent differences between BLLs from patients with and without SS, this discussion will consider them as representing one pathologic process, which is covered in the section on the immunopathology of Sjögren's syndrome.

Clinical Features

Clinically, the BLL usually presents as a firm swelling in the parotid gland that is asymptomatic or associated with only mild pain. On palpation, no attachment to surrounding structures is apparent, and the enlargement is nontender and either nodular or diffuse in distribution.

To determine some of the clinical features of a large series of BLLs, all cases accessioned by the Armed Forces Institute of Pathology (AFIP) were retrospectively analyzed. Diagnoses of BLLs represent 1.6 percent of the 20,334 AFIP salivary gland diagnoses. There were 333 cases identified, 82 percent of which were cases referred from civilian institutions, and the remaining cases were accumulated by military facilities. The patients ranged in age from 1 to 86 years; 61 percent were female. The average age of female patients was 51 years, whereas the average age of males was 45 years. Eighty-three percent of these cases involved the parotid glands, 11 percent involved the submandibular glands, and 6 percent involved other sites, including the neck and minor salivary glands. Eleven cases (3.3 percent) were cystic; all were located in the parotid gland. Five cases were known to be bilateral, and three cases were known to be recurrent, but this information was not available for most of the cases. A previous survey

of all lymphoepithelial salivary gland lesions examined at the AFIP included detailed discussion of the first 55 cases of BLL reviewed there.[17]

Recently, results from a series of 36 cases of BLL were reported by Gleeson and colleagues[18] and included an average of 5 years of clinical follow-up for 24 of the patients. Eighty percent of these cases occurred in the parotid gland, and 20 percent were bilateral. Eighty-three percent involved female patients, and the average age at onset for all patients was 55 years. The presenting features were firm swelling of the affected gland and, in 40 percent of the patients, localized pain.

Although Mikulicz's patient had enlarged minor salivary glands as well, they were not biopsied; consequently, the occurrence of BLL in minor salivary glands has been infrequently reported. Only four (1.2 percent) of the AFIP cases occurred in minor salivary glands; these were in the lip, palate, soft palate, and mouth floor. Three reports have described the occurrence of BLL in the hard palate,[19-21] and there is one report of its occurrence in the tongue.[22] A recent paper discusses one possible additional case and the potential difficulty in distinguishing benign lymphoid hyperplasia of the palate from a BLL at that site.[23]

Although BLLs usually occur in parotid glands, they can occur in any salivary gland. Clinically, they resemble salivary neoplasms, from which they must be distinguished.

Associations with Other Salivary Gland Diseases

Seventeen (5.2 percent) of the AFIP cases were associated with other pathologic conditions in the same specimen; nine of these cases were found with adenomas, four cases with sialolithiasis, three cases with granulomatous inflammation, and one case with toxoplasmosis. In the series of 36 cases reported by Gleeson and colleagues,[18] the radiographic discovery of heterotopic calcifications in two of the affected glands suggested sialolithiasis.

Malignant lymphoepithelial lesions (lymphoepithelial carcinoma) are discussed at length in Chapter 25, but the frequent association of BLLs with malignant neoplasms and their possible transformation to lymphoma or carcinoma will be briefly mentioned here. Among the AFIP cases reviewed, 22 cases (6.7 percent) showed cellular atypia, and 19 cases (5.8 percent) included morphologic evidence of lymphoma in the same gland. Six (1.8 percent) were associated with other malignant neoplasms, including three mucoepidermoid carcinomas, two primary carcinomas, and one metastatic transitional cell carcinoma. During the period of follow-up in the series of Gleeson and colleagues,[18] lymphoma developed in none of the patients with clinical features of SS; however, among those without SS, a salivary gland lymphoma developed in five patients, extrasalivary lymphoma developed in two, and salivary gland carcinoma developed in one. All of these patients were women.

It is clear that BLLs can be associated with a variety of other primary salivary gland diseases and that these lesions do not always remain benign.

Relationship with Sjögren's Syndrome

Most BLLs appear in association with SS, and in one third to one half of SS patients clinically apparent salivary gland enlargement develops that microscopically shows features of the BLL in almost all cases. It has not been proved whether the pathologic features of BLLs from enlarged salivary glands, with or without SS, differ from the pathologic features of unenlarged but functionally impaired salivary glands in SS. However, they appear to be similar, if not identical. Because major salivary glands that are not enlarged are rarely biopsied, observations are limited; nevertheless, BLL has been observed in parotid biopsies from patients with SS in whom no salivary gland enlargement is present.[24] Furthermore, structures similar to epimyoepithelial islands are occasionally observed in labial salivary glands that are not enlarged.

In patients with SS, those with and those without major salivary gland enlargement have no other noticeably different clinical features. In a scintigraphic study of salivary glands in SS, Daniels and others[25] examined scintigraphy scores, reduction of radionuclide concentration in the parotid glands, stimulated parotid flow rate measurements, and the amount of lymphocytic infiltration in labial salivary gland biopsy specimens. In the 36 patients with SS, there were no significant differences in any of these assessments between the group of 13 patients with bilateral parotid enlargement and the group of 23 patients without enlargement.[26]

Clinical investigation of 19 patients with BLL that was microscopically diagnosed revealed clinical features of SS in 16 patients, as indicated by serologic, sialographic, and ophthalmologic diagnostic criteria.[27] Clinical features of SS were present or developed in half of the 36 patients with BLL reported by Gleeson and colleagues.[18] Of those patients with SS, rheumatoid arthritis was present in 11 patients, and autoimmune thyroiditis was present in 2 patients.

The pathology and clinical features of eight cases leading to lacrimal gland biopsy were reviewed. Four were cases of enlarged glands with the pathologic character of BLL, and four were cases of unenlarged glands from patients with clinical features of SS.[28] Of the latter group, one showed BLL pathology, whereas the other three showed various degrees of lymphocytic infiltration. On follow-up, clinical features of SS developed in two of the patients with enlarged glands.

Thus, in patients with a BLL, SS may or may not be present or develop. But in most patients with SS, the pathologic features of BLL are present or will develop, with or without salivary gland enlargement. The BLL may be a common, relatively uniform inflammatory response to a variety of localized or systemic causes. Etiologic suggestions are discussed in the section on SS later in this chapter.

Imaging

In patients who have swelling or induration in the region of a major salivary gland, the purposes of imaging are to obtain information about tumor structure (solid, cystic, heterogeneous), to determine if the tumor is within the gland or in adjacent structures, and to assess the definition and infiltration at its borders. The techniques for imaging BLLs have included contrast sialography, salivary scintigraphy, computed tomography (CT), computed tomographic sialography, CT with intravenous contrast, magnetic resonance imaging, and ultrasonography. None of these techniques yield histologically specific results, but they often provide valuable information that is helpful in determining whether the lesion is reactive or neoplastic, and some techniques also provide preoperative anatomic assessment of the tumor.

Sialography. For many years, the main technique used to image salivary glands has been contrast sialography. In the case of the BLL, this technique usually reveals diffuse punctate sialectasis.[29] However, this radiographic appearance is not specific and thus often cannot differentiate the BLL from other causes of chronic inflammation. Furthermore, parotid sialectasis has been seen in 15 to 20 percent of a normal population.[30]

Oil-based media, although more sensitive indicators of change in salivary glands than water-based media,[24, 31–34] pose significant hazards. Chronic granulomatous inflammation will result if an oil-based medium extravasates beyond the duct system,[29] and abnormal glands retain the medium for weeks or months, possibly causing further glandular damage. Sialography with water-based media may be relatively insensitive, but it provides a useful and cost-effective means to help distinguish a unilateral inflammatory salivary gland disease, such as BLL, from a neoplasm.[35]

Scintigraphy. Sequential salivary scintigraphy with ^{99m}Tc-pertechnetate is a nuclear imaging technique that can be used to assess the function of all the major salivary glands simultaneously.[36] In patients with SS, uptake of the labeling material by salivary glands is delayed, and secretion of labeled saliva into the mouth is delayed or absent.[25] Salivary scintigraphy reflects the functional status of at least part of the secretory mechanism[37] and is helpful in identifying papillary cystadenoma lymphomatosum (Warthin's tumor),[38, 39] but it provides little anatomic information for assessing enlarged salivary glands.

Computed Tomography and Magnetic Resonance Imaging. Magnetic resonance imaging provides excellent soft tissue resolution and tumor detection that make it, in some ways, superior to CT.[35] One study has suggested that, if a neoplasm is suspected, magnetic resonance imaging is the best choice for imaging; however, if an inflammatory cause is likely, intravenous contrast-enhanced CT is the best choice.[40]

Ultrasonography. Ultrasonography has been used for evaluating salivary glands in patients suspected of having SS. Ultrasonography has revealed decreased parotid gland echogenicity in 69 percent of patients with SS, compared with only 8 percent of those without SS. The echogenicity was not related to the size of the parotid glands as measured by CT.[41] These data suggest that ultrasonography is relatively insensitive and nonspecific, but it is at least as effective as sialography in screening patients for inflammatory salivary gland disease.

Diagnosis

Diagnosis of BLL is by incisional or excisional biopsy. However, because of the close and frequent association of BLL and SS, any histopathologic diagnosis of BLL should be followed by appropriate assessment of the patient for the presence of the ocular or systemic components of SS. These are discussed in later sections of this chapter.

Cytologic examination via fine-needle aspiration of a BLL may reveal rare epithelial cells among a mixed population of lymphocytes and histiocytes, but differentiation of BLL from malignant lymphoma may not be possible.[42] Given the presence of lymphoid tissue in the normal parotid gland, similar aspiration specimens could be obtained from BLLs, normal glands, or glands affected with other forms of chronic sialadenitis. The primary diagnosis of BLL cannot be made from an aspiration specimen, but the technique can provide material for examination by immunohistochemical clonal markers. These markers could be helpful in reexamining a previously diagnosed BLL for possible malignant transformation.

SJÖGREN'S SYNDROME

History

Descriptions of patients with what we now call Sjögren's syndrome began to appear in the medical literature during the latter half of the 19th century.[43, 44] In 1925, Gougerot[45] recognized a generalized condition that involved dryness of the eyes, mouth, larynx, nose, and vulva and could also include thyroid and ovarian hypofunction. In France, this disease is still sometimes called Gougerot's syndrome. The history of SS also overlaps with the history of BLL described previously.

Our understanding of the systemic nature of this disease is largely based on the scholarship of the Swedish ophthalmologist Henrik Sjögren, beginning with his thesis published in 1933.[8] He observed that many patients with a particular form of dry eyes, called keratoconjunctivitis sicca, also had polyarthritis, dry mouth, and elevated erythrocyte sedimentation rates. He microscopically examined lacrimal, parotid, sublingual, and labial glands, as well as conjunctivas and corneas, and observed abundant round cell infiltrates in the glands.[46]

Definitions

Since 1965, SS has been defined as "the triad of keratoconjunctivitis sicca ('dry eyes'), xerostomia ('dry mouth'), and rheumatoid arthritis or other connective tissue disease."[24] The other connective tissue diseases seen in this syndrome include systemic lupus erythematosus, progressive systemic sclerosis (scleroderma), polymyositis/dermatomyositis, mixed connective tissue disease, and polyarteritis nodosa. This definition was based on the comprehensive examination by Bloch and colleagues[24] at the National Institutes of Health Clinical Center of 62 patients with generally severe cases. The authors stated that two of the three major components were sufficient for the diagnosis, and they excluded specific diseases of salivary or lacrimal glands such as lymphoma, sarcoidosis, and tuberculosis. They left the diagnostic criteria for each component unspecified, possibly because in their patients the clinical features of each component were obvious. However, subsequent investigators, in dealing with more diverse patient populations, have applied or have developed various means of objectively assessing and diagnosing the components, especially for the relatively common and nonspecific symptoms of dry eyes and mouth. These means have been reviewed[47, 48] and are discussed below briefly.

Most clinical studies of SS have observed that patients fall into two main categories: those with another connective tissue disease (usually rheumatoid arthritis) and those without another connective tissue disease. The latter condition was called "sicca syndrome" in 1965,[24] but that term has also been used by some as a synonym for SS and by others as a description of patients complaining of dryness. More recently, the names *primary SS*, when another connective tissue disease is absent,[49] and *secondary SS*, when one is present,[50] were introduced; this was soon followed by discussion of clinical and genetic differences between these two forms.[51, 52] The classification of this syndrome into primary and secondary forms has now been widely accepted, making continued use of the terms "sicca syndrome" or "sicca complex" redundant and confusing.

Clinical Features

Between 80 and 90 percent of patients with SS are women. The mean age at diagnosis is about 50 years; however, the age range is wide, and the syndrome can occur in children.[53] The incidence of this disease is unknown, but among the connective tissue diseases, its prevalence is second only to that of rheumatoid arthritis. If extrapolation is made from the 1 or 2 percent prevalence of rheumatoid arthritis[54] and if it is assumed that 25 percent of patients with rheumatoid arthritis have the secondary form of SS and that an equal number of people have the primary form, then the prevalence of SS could be 0.5 to 1.0 percent. A recent epidemiologic study of randomly selected 52- to 72-year-old Swedish adults calculated a 95 percent confidence interval of 1.0 to 4.5 percent for the frequency of primary SS in that group.[55]

Ocular. Symptoms of dry eyes can be caused by many conditions, but the term *keratoconjunctivitis sicca* describes a particular condition that involves both a decrease and qualitative changes in the tear film that can occur alone,[56] can be associated with sarcoidosis[57, 58] or can be the ocular component of SS. The clinical features and diagnosis of keratoconjunctivitis sicca have been reviewed.[59]

Oral Symptoms. The principal oral symptom is dryness, but not all patients complain of dryness per se. Some may describe difficulty in swallowing food, problems in wearing complete dentures, changes in their sense of taste, increase in the incidence of dental caries, chronic symptoms of burning oral mucosa, or inability to eat dry food or to speak continuously for more than a few minutes.[60] Chronic symptoms of dry mouth may be caused by a variety of conditions, but most commonly they are side effects of long-term administration of various drugs.[61] The oral symptoms of SS usually have an insidious onset and may progress gradually.

Oral Signs. The intraoral signs have a wide range of severity and are generally nonspecific, appearing also in chronic xerostomia of other causes. These signs include dry, sticky oral mucosal surfaces; primary or recurrent dental caries in cervical or incisal locations; no saliva, or cloudy saliva, expressible from the major salivary gland ducts; patchy or generalized oral mucosal erythema with dorsal tongue fissuring and papillary atrophy; and angular cheilitis, which indicates chronic erythematous candidiasis[62] (Fig. 6–4).

Salivary Glands. Firm, diffuse, nontender or slightly tender enlargement may develop in the major salivary glands, usually bilaterally (Fig. 6–5). In early or mild cases, there may be slight induration of the glands without enlargement. One third to one half of patients develop salivary gland enlargement during the course of the disease, but patients with more severe gland dysfunction and inflammation are more likely to have enlargement than patients with mild disease.[63] Submandibular glands may be affected before parotids.[63] Many patients report that their salivary gland enlargement occurs in episodes lasting for many weeks or months, whereas other patients have chronic enlargement, with slow fluctuations in size.

A cream-colored exudate may be apparent at a major salivary gland duct orifice, but smear preparations of the exudate usually reveal mostly lymphocytes, with a few polymorphonuclear leukocytes. Superimposed acute bacterial sialadenitis occurs uncommonly, and unless the patient has symptoms and signs of acute sialadenitis, treatment with antibiotics may not be indicated.

Extraglandular. Approximately half of SS patients have the primary form and usually do not develop another connective tissue disease. However, patients with primary SS can develop extraglandular features, including Raynaud's phenomenon, primary biliary cirrhosis,[64] diffuse interstitial lung disease,[65] interstitial nephritis,[66] chronic atrophic gastritis,[64] peripheral neuropathies, and inflammatory vascular disease.[67] The observation of decreased lacrimal and salivary function in patients with central nervous system diseases led to the suggestion that patients with SS may develop central nervous system involvement,[68] but it is not yet clear whether these secretory abnormalities actually represent SS or are another form of dysfunction in patients with central nervous system diseases.

Prognosis. For most patients, the course of SS seems limited, with symptoms and signs reaching a somewhat variable plateau. In other patients, the disease is progressive and can lead to multiorgan involvement and, in a few cases, to malignant transformation, usually to a B-cell lymphoma affecting salivary glands or other organs.[69] The lymphoproliferation in this disease has recently been suggested to have three stages: first, initiation, characterized by glandular infiltrates, serum autoantibodies, and polyclonal hypergammaglobulinemia; second, promotion, with expanding infiltrates, increasing serum autoantibodies, and perhaps pseudolymphoma with monoclonal immunoglobulins; and third, progression to B-cell lymphoma, often with hypogammaglobulinemia.[70]

Histopathology

A common feature of all organs affected by SS is a potentially progressive lymphocytic infiltration. These infiltrates presumably cause the functional changes in affected organs and the diverse clinical features of this disease.

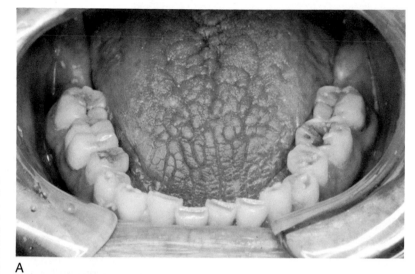

A

Figure 6–4. Intraoral changes in patients with severe chronic xerostomia from primary Sjögren's syndrome. *A,* Note the signs of chronic erythematous candidiasis, including mucosal erythema, papillary atrophy, and fissuring of the dorsal tongue; in addition, note the cervical and incisal dental caries. *B,* Note the erythema and the velvety texture of chronic erythematous candidiasis in the palatal mucosa. The fungal overgrowth and lesions were eliminated by use of topical antifungal drugs, but they recurred when the drugs were discontinued.

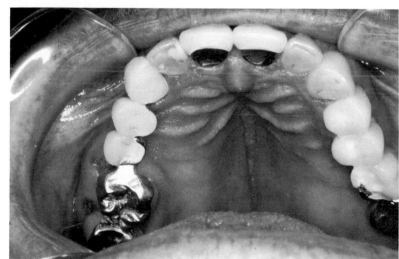

B

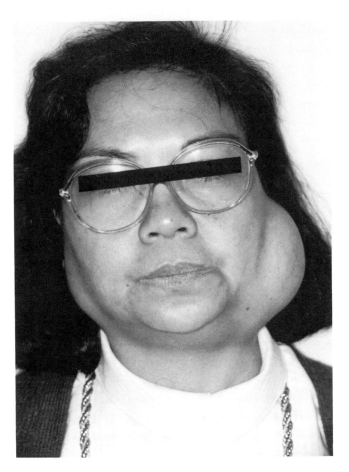

Figure 6–5. A 45-year-old patient with severe primary Sjögren's syndrome and a 14-year history of asymmetric, slowly progressive, bilateral parotid gland enlargement is shown. The swellings have never been more than mildly symptomatic, and the glands are firm and nontender to palpation.

Major Salivary Glands. Microscopic examination of enlarged parotid or submandibular glands usually reveals the BLL, characterized by epimyoepithelial islands in a lymphocytic infiltrate as described previously. However, not all patients show these features. Examination of 22 major salivary gland specimens from SS patients—10 of whom had enlarged salivary glands at the time of biopsy—revealed intact lobular architecture and various degrees of replacement of acini by lymphocytic infiltration.[24] Epimyoepithelial islands were present in only nine (40 percent) of the specimens, four of which were from patients with a history of salivary gland enlargement but in whom there was no enlargement at the time of biopsy.

Minor Salivary Glands. The characteristic histopathologic feature of minor salivary glands in SS is focal lymphocytic sialadenitis.[63, 71] It consists of a primary lymphocytic infiltrate in otherwise generally normal-appearing glands, and includes focal aggregates of 50 or more lymphocytes (a focus) that are adjacent to normal-appearing acini and the consistent presence of these foci in all or most of the glands in the specimen (Fig. 6–6). Plasma cells are often seen interstitially, but few,

if any, are present in the lymphocytic foci. Lymphoid germinal centers are frequently seen within large infiltrates, but the epimyoepithelial islands characteristic of BLLs in major salivary glands occur uncommonly in minor glands.

The microscopic differential diagnosis should exclude a form of mild to moderately severe nonspecific chronic sialadenitis that is commonly seen in the minor glands. It does not appear to be a feature of SS and may occur secondary to glandular obstruction or injury. Nonspecific chronic sialadenitis is characterized by diffuse atrophy of glandular epithelium in lobes or in entire glands, usually with duct dilatation and interstitial fibrosis. It is also characterized by infiltration by lymphocytes, or lymphocytes and plasma cells, in scattered, interstitial, or focal patterns (Fig. 6–7).[71, 72] It occurs in people who have no history of connective tissue disease, increases in frequency with age, and affects females at earlier ages than males.[73]

At the University of California, San Francisco, my colleagues and I have accessioned more than 600 labial salivary gland biopsy specimens since 1971 (Fig. 6–8). Forty-six percent exhibited focal lymphocytic sialadenitis consistent with the sali-

Text continued on page 97

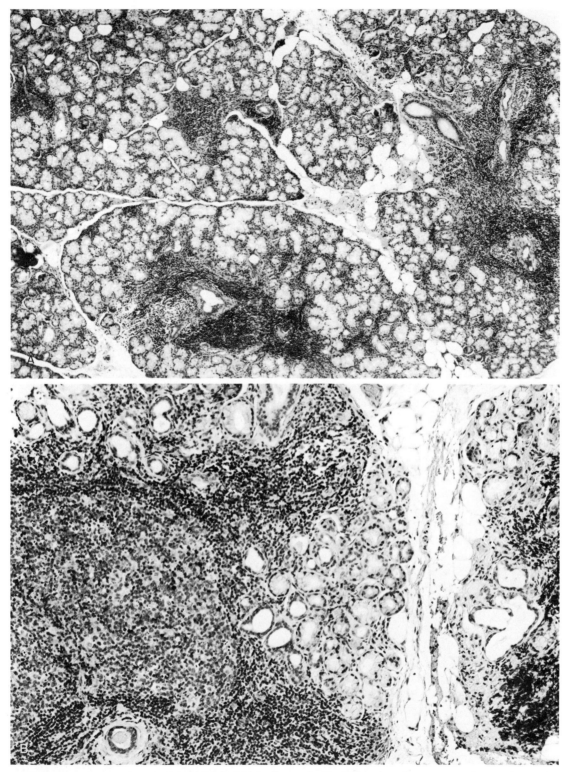

Figure 6–6. Focal lymphocytic sialadenitis in labial salivary glands (LSG). Note the presence of normal-appearing acini adjacent to the infiltrates in *A* to *C*. *A*, Mild inflammation (LSG focus score = two foci/4 mm²) was found in a biopsy specimen from a 37-year-old man with bilateral parotid enlargement and mild keratoconjunctivitis sicca (× 40). *B*, Larger foci of infiltrates with germinal center formation in a biopsy specimen from a 77-year-old patient with rheumatoid arthritis, asymmetric submandibular gland enlargement, LSG focus score of three foci/4 mm², and no keratoconjunctivitis sicca.

Illustration continued on following page

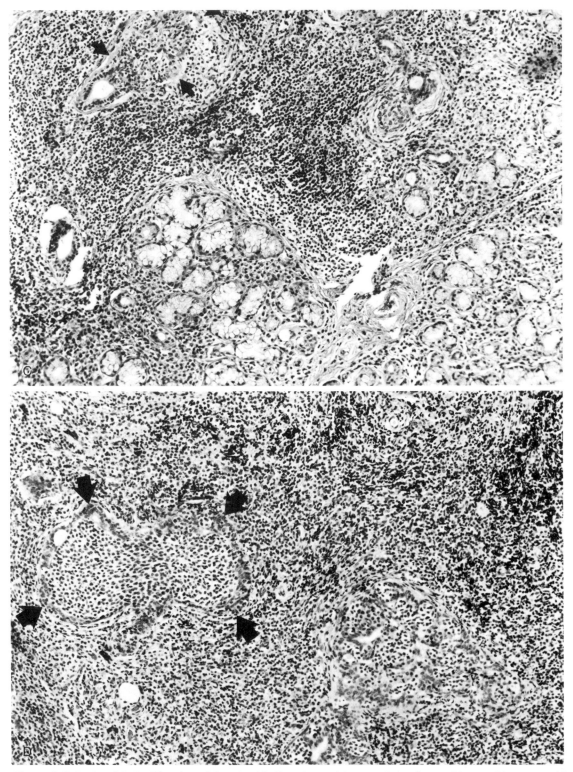

Figure 6–6 *Continued C,* Proliferation of ductal epithelium (arrows) in a specimen from a 28-year-old woman with primary Sjögren's syndrome and LSG focus score of six foci/4 mm² (× 100). *D,* Epimyoepithelial island (arrows) in a specimen from a 70-year-old woman with severe primary Sjögren's syndrome and an LSG focus score of confluent foci. There were few normal-appearing acini or ducts anywhere in the specimen (× 100).

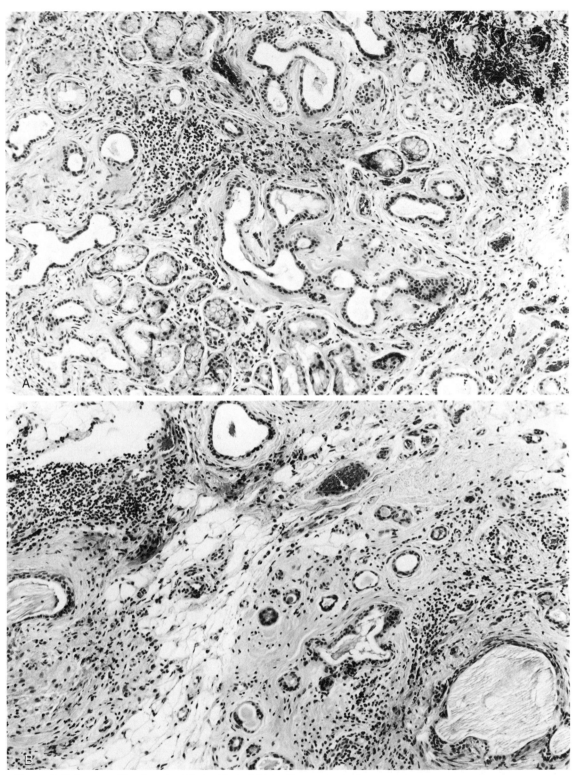

Figure 6–7. Nonspecific chronic sialadenitis in labial salivary glands from two patients, who complained of dry mouth but had no other clinical features of Sjögren's syndrome. Both had normal measurements for stimulated parotid flow rate. Note focal and scattered lymphocytic infiltrations associated with interstitial fibrosis, acinar atrophy, and duct dilatation. *A*, A specimen from a 66-year-old woman is shown (× 100). *B*, A specimen from a 65-year-old man is shown (× 100).

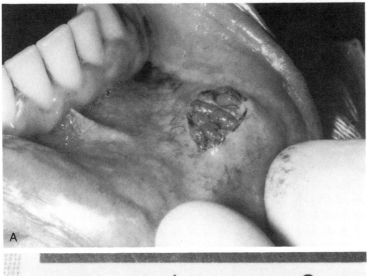

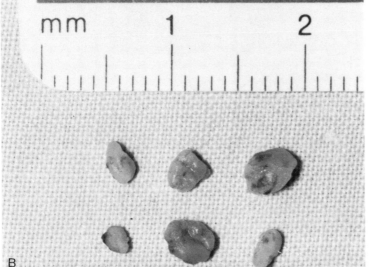

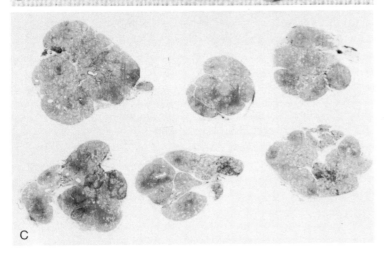

Figure 6–8. Labial salivary gland biopsy. *A,* An incision through mucosal epithelium reveals individual salivary glands. *B,* The glands are separated before fixation and processing. *C,* Midplane section through the glands in *B* from a patient who had primary Sjögren's syndrome with a focus score of 10 foci/4 mm², and keratoconjunctivitis sicca (× 4). (Reprinted from Daniels TE: Labial salivary gland biopsy in Sjögren's syndrome: Assessment as a diagnostic criterion in 362 suspected cases. Arthritis Rheum 1984; 27:147–156. Copyright 1984; used by permission of the American Rheumatism Association.)

vary component of SS (focus scores greater than 1 focus/4 mm²);[63] 9 percent had smaller amounts of focal lymphocytic infiltrates suggestive of the salivary component of SS (focus score = 1 or Chisholm and Mason's[74] grade 3); 43 percent were within normal limits or showed nonspecific chronic sialadenitis; and 2 percent had features of other diseases, such as noncaseating (sarcoid) granuloma, amyloidosis, or hemochromatosis.

Diagnosis

Diagnostic Criteria. Internationally accepted diagnostic criteria for all the components of SS have not yet been established, but one set of criteria has been in use for over 15 years (Table 6–1) and is now widely used.[47] Although the occurrence of xerostomia is part of the traditional definition of the syndrome and is certainly clinically important in most patients, it is not a satisfactory diagnostic criterion because it is perceived subjectively, is nonspecific, and is difficult to assess objectively. An article reviewing the various objective methods for assessing salivary glands in SS and comparing various diagnostic criteria for the salivary component has been published.[48]

Table 6–1. Diagnostic Criteria for Sjögren's Syndrome*

Primary Sjögren's Syndrome
Keratoconjunctivitis sicca
  Characteristic corneal and conjunctival epithelial staining with rose bengal, observed through a slit lamp, *and*
  Reduced tear meniscus and break-up time *or* Unanesthetized Schirmer's test ≤5 mm/5 min
Focal sialadenitis in an adequate labial salivary gland biopsy specimen with a focus score >1 focus/4 mm², after exclusions
Secondary Sjögren's Syndrome
Rheumatoid arthritis or other connective tissue disease diagnosed by established criteria *and*
Either one or both of the criteria for primary Sjögren's syndrome
Possible Sjögren's Syndrome
One of the components of primary Sjögren's syndrome *and*
Presence of any of the following:
  Pulmonary lymphocytic interstitial infiltrates
  Interstitial nephritis and/or renal tubular acidosis
  Purpura (hyperglobulinemic or vasculitic)
  Polymyopathy
  Chronic liver disease (not cirrhosis or infectious)
  Neuropathy
  Hypergammaglobulinemia (polyclonal or monoclonal) with rheumatoid factor or ANA or anti-Ro/SS-A or anti-La/SS-B

*Data from Daniels TE, Talal N: Diagnosis and differential diagnosis of Sjögren's syndrome. *In* Talal N, Moutsopoulos HM, Kassan SS (eds.): Sjögren's Syndrome: Clinical and Immunological Aspects. Berlin, Springer-Verlag, 1987; 193–199.

The use of diverse diagnostic criteria over the years has led to heterogeneous collections of patients being given the diagnosis of SS. Internationally recognized criteria are needed both to provide a common basis for defining patients for studies and to clarify case-by-case clinical diagnosis. Because SS is a chronic, incurable, and potentially progressive disease, assigning the diagnosis inappropriately can cause a patient years of unnecessary concern; but if the disease is not recognized and is not managed early, preventable damage and suffering will go untreated. A Commission of the European Communities has supported the beginning of studies to develop diagnostic criteria for SS.[75]

Sialometry. Unstimulated whole salivary flow rates quantify basal salivary secretion, fairly closely reflect symptoms of dry mouth, and are reduced by diseases affecting salivary glands and by side effects of many drugs, depression,[76] and increasing age.[77] Measuring flow rates under gustatory or masticatory stimulus will estimate the gland's secretory capacity, and thus it can assess damage caused by disease. These stimulated flow rates are less affected by drug side effects and are not significantly affected by aging,[78] but they correlate poorly with a patient's symptoms. Standardized flow rate measurements provide useful quantitative assessment of salivary gland function and a repeatable, noninvasive method to monitor the course of a chronic disease, but they are too variable and nonspecific to serve as a diagnostic criterion for the salivary component of SS.

Sialography. Sialography can examine anatomic changes in the duct system of major glands. It may also be useful in assessing glands in which neoplasia or obstruction is suspected.

Scintigraphy. Changes in sequential salivary scintigraphy correlate with stimulated parotid flow rate measurements,[25, 36] but these changes are not specific to SS.

Sialochemistry. Measurement of chemical and immunologic components in saliva from patients with SS has yielded interesting preliminary observations.[79] However, none are sufficiently sensitive or specific to serve as diagnostic criteria for the salivary component of this disease.

Parotid Biopsy. Diagnosis of the salivary component of SS from biopsy specimens of parotid glands would seem to be a direct route. However, in the past, parotid biopsy has carried the risks of facial nerve damage, of cutaneous fistula, and of scarring, and it has required hospitalization. Recently, however, two studies on outpatients have reported finding no significant postoperative morbidity when an incisional biopsy technique was used in the posteroinferior lobe of the parotid gland.[80, 81]

Investigators in one of these studies compared labial salivary gland and incisional parotid biopsy specimens in 36 patients suspected of having SS, 61 percent of whom had parotid enlargement.[80]

They reported lymphocytic and/or plasmacytic infiltrates in 58 percent of labial and 100 percent of parotid specimens. However, they took the unusual view of confirming the presence or absence of SS only on the results of salivary gland biopsy, and they did not report on the presence or absence of xerostomia, the ocular component of the syndrome, other connective tissue diseases, or serologic changes in their patients.

Authors of the other study, which also compared labial salivary gland and incisional parotid biopsies, examined 24 patients suspected of having SS, but no parotid enlargement was mentioned.[81] They were able to obtain adequate tissue from all labial biopsies but from only 19 of the 24 parotid biopsies. They concluded that findings from parotid gland biopsy added very little to those from the minor gland biopsy. They also observed significantly greater diagnostic sensitivity in the labial specimens; 67 percent of labial and 32 percent of parotid specimens showed evidence of the salivary component of SS. Patients with positive parotid specimens had higher labial gland focus scores, more frequent evidence of ocular involvement, and higher titers or more frequent presence of several serum autoantibodies than those recorded for patients with normal parotid specimens.

Using parotid glands to diagnose SS can present a diagnostic problem because lymphocytic foci may be seen in parotid glands of persons who have no history of any connective tissue disease.[82] This makes it difficult to distinguish persons with early or mild SS from those with normal glands. The two studies just discussed have demonstrated new and safer surgical techniques for parotid biopsy, but as yet, parotid biopsy does not seem to offer a reliable diagnostic alternative to labial salivary gland biopsy, especially in patients without parotid enlargement or for diagnosis of early or mild disease.

Minor Gland Biopsy. Biopsy of minor salivary glands was introduced as a clinical procedure for diagnosis of the salivary component of SS in 1966,[83, 84] and many studies have followed to assess the value of this biopsy procedure. In contrast to postmortem studies of major salivary glands, most similar studies on labial salivary gland specimens confirmed that, after lobes with duct dilatation and extravascular polymorphonuclear leukocytes are excluded, significant focal sialadenitis is not found in these glands unless a connective tissue disease is present.[74, 84–87] Even in those studies that found focal infiltrates in glands from some subjects with no history of connective tissue disease, most of the foci were associated with the nonspecific changes described in the previous section dealing with histopathology.[73]

Using a semiquantitative inflammatory grading method that is similar to that used on parotid and submandibular glands,[82, 88] Chisholm and Mason[74] graded inflammation in labial salivary gland biopsy specimens from patients with various rheumatologic diseases and in postmortem specimens. They found that grade 4 (more than one focus of 50 or more lymphocytes per 4 mm² area of gland) was seen only in patients with SS and was not present in postmortem specimens. The four grades in this scheme were then expanded to a focus score ranging from 0 to 12 to provide more sensitive data for analysis[89] (Fig. 6–9). Subsequent studies showed a positive correlation in the pattern and the extent of inflammation between labial and submandibular glands from 116 postmortem subjects[85] and histopathologic agreement between labial and parotid glands from patients with SS.[90]

Because of its strong association with the presence of SS and because xerostomia is difficult to assess clinically and is not specific to SS, focal sialadenitis in a labial salivary gland biopsy specimen with a focus score of more than 1 focus/4 mm² was proposed as the diagnostic criterion for the salivary component of this disease.[60] This criterion has subsequently been widely adopted.[47, 91, 92]

The observation of significant focal sialadenitis in a labial salivary gland specimen has been shown to be the most disease-specific diagnostic criterion for the salivary component of SS, provided that the specimen is taken from beneath clinically normal mucosa; includes five or more glands that are separated from their surrounding connective tissue; is interpreted after areas of nonspecific chronic sialadenitis are excluded; demonstrates focal sialadenitis in all or most of the glands in the specimen; and has a focus score of greater than 1 focus/4 mm² of gland area, as a threshold for significance (Fig. 6–8).[63, 71]

Immunopathology

The primary immunopathologic process in SS is infiltration of affected organs by lymphocytes. However, during this dynamic process, metabolically active cells affect the surrounding tissue, participate in their own proliferation, and may signal generalized or regional changes in lymphoid regulation.

Infiltrating Lymphocytes. Immunoglobulin synthesis by lymphocytes in salivary glands from patients with SS was described in 1970.[93] Four years later, using indirect immunofluorescence and polyclonal antisera on labial salivary glands, investigators described clusters of B lymphocytes in each specimen.[94] They also found that the proportion of T lymphocytes in infiltrates was greater in the specimens with more and larger infiltrates.

In the early 1980s, with the availability of monoclonal antibodies and more sensitive labeling systems, phenotypic identification of infiltrating cells progressed rapidly. Labial salivary glands from patients with primary SS contained more than

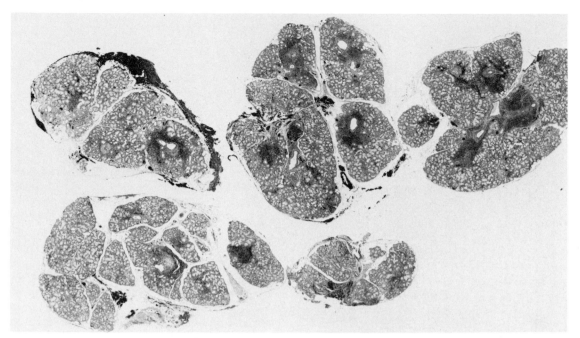

Figure 6–9. Focal lymphocytic sialadenitis is seen in a labial salivary gland biopsy from a 58-year-old woman with primary Sjögren's syndrome. The focus score was five foci/4 mm² (Chisholm and Mason Grade 4) (× 10).

three times as many T-helper cells (CD4 +) as T-suppressor cells (CD8 +) (Fig. 6–10), and this was generally unrelated to the proportion of these cells in the peripheral blood.[95] More than 75 percent of the infiltrating cells were T lymphocytes (mainly T-helper type), only 5 to 20 percent were B lymphocytes, and about 50 percent of the cells expressed lymphocyte activation markers, compared with only 15 percent in the peripheral blood.[96] Natural killer (NK) cells are lymphocytes that can lyse certain tumor cell lines in vitro, and NK activity by peripheral blood mononuclear cells has been shown to be significantly reduced in patients with SS.[97, 98]

A recent study[99] retrospectively examined paraffin-embedded sections of 25 benign lymphoepithelial lesions and identified the following three regions: irregularly shaped "germinal" centers made up of B lymphocytes and macrophages that surround epimyoepithelial islands; mantle regions composed of small B and T lymphocytes; and paracortical (interfollicular) regions composed mainly of T lymphocytes. NK cells were also observed in some of the germinal centers. This study suggests that in the BLL there is a characteristic and consistent distribution of inflammatory cells that resembles the distribution in reactive lymph nodes.

Autoantibodies. Hyperactivity of B lymphocytes in SS causes polyclonal hypergammaglobulinemia and production of a variety of autoantibodies, including rheumatoid factor, organ-specific autoantibodies, and various antinuclear antibodies. Clinical laboratory tests often reflect this B-cell hyperactivity. Rheumatoid factor is present in the serum of most patients with primary or secondary SS, often in high titer. Antinuclear antibody, detected by indirect immunofluorescence, is also present in the serum of most patients, usually in a speckled or homogeneous pattern. Antibodies against nuclear antigens Ro (SS-A) and La (SS-B) are found in many patients by the gel precipitation method, but they are found in virtually all patients if sensitive, solid-phase, immunoadsorbent assays are used.[100]

The presence of anti-Ro or anti-La antibodies in the circulation is not specific to SS, nor is the presence of any other autoantibody, but there is a strong correlation between the amount of these antibodies and the presence of clinical vasculitis, purpura, or leukopenia. The circulating antibodies directed against the Ro and La antigens may be a major portion of the patient's increased gammaglobulin.[101] In most SS patients, significantly more anti-La of the IgA class is found in the saliva than in the serum, which suggests that the antibody is synthesized within the gland.[102]

In addition to antinuclear antibodies, patients may exhibit various organ-specific antibodies, such as anti–salivary-duct antibody, but there is no evidence that any of them are involved in damage to the affected organs. The presence of the antinuclear antibodies further confirms an autoimmune pathogenesis for SS and may be diagnostically helpful to support or reject equivocal clinical findings.

Immunologic Regulation. The organ infiltration by T lymphocytes and hyperactivity of B

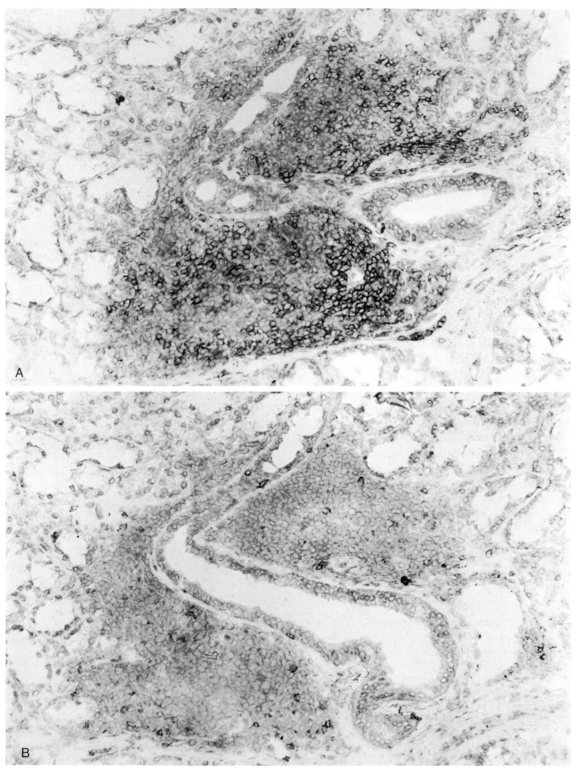

Figure 6–10. Immunohistochemical examination was made of a labial salivary gland biopsy specimen from a patient with primary Sjögren's syndrome. *A*, The majority of the lymphocytes in this small focus express the CD4 (T4) antigen on their membranes (T-helper lymphocytes) (× 150). *B*, Another section of the same focus shows few cells expressing CD8 (T8) antigen (T-suppressor lymphocytes) (× 150).

lymphocytes in SS is generally blamed on a loss of normal immunologic regulation, but specific mechanisms are unknown. The class II major human lymphocyte antigens HLA-DR, HLA-DQ, and HLA-DP have significant roles in regulating the immune response. These antigens are normally seen only on immunocompetent cells, such as B lymphocytes, activated T lymphocytes, monocytes/macrophages, and Langerhans's cells.

However, several investigators have observed that ductal epithelial cells in glands from patients with SS expressed one or more of these HLA antigens.[103–107] Expression of HLA-DR was seen with approximately equal frequency in salivary glands that showed nonspecific chronic inflammation and in salivary glands from patients with SS.[106, 107] However, HLA-DP and HLA-DQ antigens were expressed less frequently and mainly in SS specimens.[106]

Similar examples of this aberrant HLA-DR expression by epithelial cells have been observed in many forms of chronic inflammation, and epithelial cells in vitro can be induced to express HLA-DR under the influence of gamma-interferon.[108] These data suggest that in the presence of chronic inflammation or abnormal localized immune response, epithelial cells may attempt to take over an antigen-processing role.

Interleukin 2 (IL-2), produced by activated lymphocytes, has an important role in regulating lymphocyte proliferation. In patients with SS, IL-2 production by lymphocytes from salivary glands was very high, but it was normal or diminished in peripheral blood lymphocytes.[109] This decreased IL-2 production by peripheral blood lymphocytes was most severe in those patients having extraglandular disease or another connective tissue disease, and it was suggested that qualitative defects in T cells and macrophages may be responsible for the defective IL-2 production.[110]

Recent evidence suggests that the recurrent swelling of salivary glands in SS (benign lymphoepithelial lesions) may be related to clonal expansion of populations of infiltrating T lymphocytes or B lymphocytes.[111, 112] This expansion may represent a step in the progression to lymphoma.

Genetic Susceptibility. Although SS is not an inherited disease in the usual sense, evidence of a genetic susceptibility is emerging. For many years it has been clear that certain histocompatibility antigens occur more frequently than usual in patients with this disease, and the frequency of occurrence differs between the primary and the secondary forms.[52]

HLA-B8 is present in about 20 percent of disease-free persons, but it is present in 60 percent of patients who have primary SS and in 9 percent of those who have the secondary form with rheumatoid arthritis. HLA-DR3 is normally present in about 25 percent of the population, but it occurs in 66 percent of patients with primary SS and with normal frequency in those with secondary SS.[52]

The differences in frequency of occurrence of these gene products identify differences between primary and secondary SS and begin to define a genetic predisposition to the disease.

In a study of the kindreds of patients with SS, there was a strong association between the diagnosis of the disease and the presence of HLA-DR3 and HLA-DR2.[113] It was also observed that 12 percent of 51 patients had at least 1 other relative with the same disease, and primary SS and systemic lupus erythematosus tended to cluster in the same families. The best candidate as the primary genetic marker for SS is HLA-DRw52,[114] whereas HLA-DQ alleles are most likely responsible for the abnormal production of the autoantibodies anti-Ro and anti-La.[115] This suggests that the risk of development of the disease is separate from the risk of development of the autoantibodies.

Etiology

The causes of SS are unknown, but it is generally believed that patients respond abnormally to one or more unidentified antigens, possibly viral antigens or virally altered host antigens. Clues suggesting a viral cause for the connective tissue diseases began to be seen in the 1960s, when elevated titers of anti-viral antibody were detected in patients with rheumatoid arthritis and systemic lupus erythematosus. Cytomegalovirus, paramyxovirus, and Epstein-Barr virus have been implicated in some studies but are unsubstantiated in others.[116–123] Clearly, known viruses have not yet been established as the cause of SS or any other connective tissue disease. However, reactivation of Epstein-Barr virus or another virus may participate in the chronicity or progression of SS. A pathogenesis involving an immunologic response to the presence of viral antigens in a genetically susceptible host remains an intriguing possibility.

Possible Association with Retrovirus Infection

Several investigators have reported a relationship between human immunodeficiency virus (HIV) infection and BLL-like lesions of the salivary glands.[124–129] Symptoms and clinical signs suggestive of SS, including bilateral parotid enlargement and dry mouth and eyes, develop in a small percentage of people infected with HIV.[125–129]

Although some of these reports suggested that these cases represent SS,[125, 127] the consistent absence of serum autoantibodies and the different histopathologic patterns and lymphocytic phenotypes that infiltrate the glands argue against this diagnosis.[124, 130] These cases can be better explained as manifestations of progressive generalized lymphadenopathy associated with HIV infection that, in the parotid gland, can resemble the BLL and can cause infiltration in other glands.

Discussion of a possible relationship between HIV infection and SS is further complicated by the fact that many HIV-infected patients also show evidence of infection with other retroviruses, especially human T-cell leukemia/lymphoma virus I (HTLV-I).[131] HTLV-I has been associated with tropical spastic paraparesis, an uncommon disease affecting the central nervous system. This disease can cause exocrine disease that clinically resembles SS.[132, 133] Furthermore, HTLV-I transgenic mice have been reported to show a unique exocrinopathy that, unlike SS, is characterized by ductal proliferation preceding lymphocytic infiltration.[134] However, the clinical and pathologic differences between retrovirus-associated salivary gland disease and SS do not suggest a common pathogenesis for these conditions.

The most recent evidence of a retroviral link to SS comes from two studies. In one,[135] antibody to the HIV-1 group-specific protein p24 was found in 57 percent of sera from patients with SS but in only 5 percent of normal sera. In the other,[136] T-lymphoblastoid cells were incubated with homogenized labial salivary glands from six SS patients. Cells exposed to two of the six homogenates expressed an HIV-related protein, and electron microscopy demonstrated retroviral particles in some of those cells. These data suggest the presence of an agent that could stimulate production of retrovirus-associated serum antibodies in patients with SS but do not yet identify a viral etiology for SS.

Acknowledgments

The author is grateful to Evangeline Leash for editing the manuscript and to Paul Kolsanoff for the microphotography.

REFERENCES

1. Mikulicz J: Über eine eigenartige symmetrische Erkrankung der Tränen- und Mundspeicheldrüsen. Stuttgart, Beitr z Chir Fetscr f Theodor Billroth, 1892; 610–630.
2. Mikulicz J: Concerning a peculiar symmetrical disease of the lacrimal and salivary glands. Medical Classics 1937; 2:165–186.
3. Ferlito A, Cattai N: The so-called "benign lymphoepithelial lesion." J Laryngol Otol 1980; 94:1189–1197.
4. Schaffer AJ, Jacobsen AW: Mikulicz's disease: A report of ten cases. Am J Dis Child 1927; 34:327–346.
5. Batsakis JG: The pathology of head and neck tumors: The lymphoepithelial lesion and Sjögren's syndrome, Part 16. Head Neck Surg 1982; 5:150–163.
6. Godwin JT: Benign lymphoepithelial lesion of the parotid gland (adenolymphoma, chronic inflammation, lymphoepithelioma, lymphocytic tumor, Mikulicz disease): Report of eleven cases. Cancer 1952; 5:1089–1103.
7. Morgan WS, Castleman B: A clinicopathologic study of "Mikulicz's disease." Am J Pathol 1953; 29:471–503.
8. Morgan WS: The probable systemic nature of Mikulicz's disease and its relation to Sjögren's syndrome. N Engl J Med 1954; 251:5–10.
9. Sjögren H: Zur kenntnis der keratoconjunctivitis sicca (Keratitis filiformis bei Hypofunktion der Tränendrüsen). Acta Ophthalmol (Copenh) 1933; 11(Suppl 2):1–151.
10. Batsakis JG: Lymphoepithelial lesion and Sjögren's syndrome. Ann Otol Rhinol Laryngol 1987; 96:354–355.
11. Weidner N, Geisinger KR, Sterling RT, Miller TR, Yen TSB: Benign lymphoepithelial cysts of the parotid gland: A histologic, cytologic and ultrastructural study. Am J Clin Pathol 1986; 85:395–401.
12. Boquist L, Kumlien A, Östberg Y: Ultrastructural findings in a case of benign lymphoepithelial lesion (Sjögren's syndrome). Acta Otolaryngol 1970; 70:216–226.
13. Donath K, Seifert G: Ultrastruktur und Pathogenese der myoepithelialen Sialadenitis: Über das Vorkommen von Myoepithelzellen bei der benignen lymphoepithelialen Läsion. Virchows Arch [A] 1972; 356:315–329.
14. Saku T, Okabe H: Immunohistochemical and ultrastructural demonstration of keratin in epimyoepithelial islands of autoimmune sialadenitis in man. Arch Oral Biol 1984; 29:687–689.
15. Chaudhry AP, Cutler LS, Yamane GM, Satchidanand S, Labay G, Sunderraj M: Light and ultrastructural features of lymphoepithelial lesions of the salivary glands in Mikulicz's disease. J Pathol 1986; 146:239–250.
16. Kjörell U, Östberg Y, Virtanen I, Thornell L-E: Immunohistochemical analyses of autoimmune sialadenitis in man. J Oral Pathol 1988; 17:374–380.
17. Bernier JL, Bhaskar SN: Lymphoepithelial lesions of salivary glands. Cancer 1958; 11:1156–1179.
18. Gleeson MJ, Cawson RA, Bennett MH: Benign lymphoepithelial lesion: A less than benign disease. Clin Otolaryngol 1986; 11:47–51.
19. Nelson WR, Kay S, Sally JJ: Mikulicz's disease of the palate. Ann Surg 1963; 157:152–156.
20. Clark PM, Gamble JW: Mikulicz disease of a minor salivary gland. J Oral Surg 1978; 36:895–897.
21. Marker P: A case of benign lymphoepithelial lesion of the hard palate. Int J Oral Surg 1983; 12:348–354.
22. Bhaskar SN, Bernier JL: Mikulicz's disease; clinical features, histology, and histogenesis; report of seventy-three cases. Oral Surg Oral Med Oral Pathol 1960; 13:1387–1399.
23. Bradley G, Main JHP, Birt BD, From L: Benign lymphoid hyperplasia of the palate. J Oral Pathol 1987; 16:18–26.
24. Bloch KJ, Buchanan WW, Wohl MJ, Bunim JJ: Sjögren's syndrome: A clinical, pathological and serological study of sixty-two cases. Medicine 1965; 44:187–231

25. Daniels TE, Powell MR, Sylvester RA, Talal N: An evaluation of salivary scintigraphy in Sjögren's syndrome. Arthritis Rheum 1979; 22:809–814.
26. Daniels TE: Unpublished observations.
27. Östberg Y: The clinical picture of benign lymphoepithelial lesion. Clin Otolaryngol 1983; 8:381–390.
28. Font RL, Yanoff M, Zimmerman LE: Benign lymphoepithelial lesion of the lacrimal gland and its relationship to Sjögren's syndrome. Am J Clin Pathol 1967; 48:365–376.
29. Lowman RM, Cheng GK: Diagnostic roentgenology. In Rankow RM, Polayes IM (eds.): Diseases of the Salivary Glands. Philadelphia, WB Saunders Co, 1976; 54–98.
30. Dijkstra PF: Classification and differential diagnosis of sialographic characteristics in Sjögren's syndrome. Semin Arthritis Rheum 1980; 10:10–17.
31. Bertram U: Xerostomia: Clinical aspects, pathology and pathogenesis. Acta Odont Scand 1967; 25(Suppl 49):1–126.
32. Gonzalez L, Mackenzie AH, Tarar RA: Parotid sialography in Sjögren's syndrome. Radiology 1970; 97:91–93.
33. Chisholm DM, Blair GS, Low PS, Whaley K: Hydrostatic sialography as an index of salivary gland disease in Sjögren's syndrome. Acta Radiol [Diagn] (Stockh) 1971; 11:577–585.
34. Whaley K, Williamson J, Chisholm DM, Webb J, Mason DK, Buchanan WW: Sjögren's syndrome. I. Sicca components. Q J Med 1973; 42:279–304.
35. Byrne MN, Spector JG, Garvin CF, Gado MH: Preoperative assessment of parotid masses: A comparative evaluation of radiologic techniques to histopathologic diagnosis. Laryngoscope 1989; 99:284–292.
36. Schall GL, Anderson LG, Wolf RO, Herdt JR, Tarpley TM, Cummings NA, Zeigler LS, Talal N: Xerostomia in Sjögren's syndrome: evaluation by sequential salivary scintigraphy. JAMA 1971; 216:2109–2116.
37. Helman J, Turner RJ, Fox PC, Baum BJ: ^{99m}Tc-pertechnetate uptake in parotid acinar cells by the $Na^+/K^+/Cl^-$ co-transport system. J Clin Invest 1987; 79:1310–1313.
38. Sostre S, Medina L, de Arellano GR: The various scintigraphic patterns of Warthin's tumor. Clin Nucl Med 1987; 12:620–626.
39. Higashi T, Murahashi H, Ikuta H, Mori Y, Watanabe Y: Identification of Warthin's tumor with technetium-99m pertechnetate. Clin Nucl Med 1987, 12:796–800.
40. Casselman JW, Mancuso AA: Major salivary gland masses: Comparison of MR imaging and CT. Radiology 1987; 165:183–189.
41. DeClerck LS, Corthouts R, Francx L, Brussaard C, DeSchepper A, Vercruysse HA, Stevens WJ: Ultrasonography and computer tomography of the salivary glands in the evaluation of Sjögren's syndrome. Comparison with parotid sialography. J Rheumatol 1988; 15:1777–1781.
42. Bedrossian CWM, Martinez F, Silverberg AB: Fine needle aspiration. In Gnepp DR (ed.): Pathology of the Head and Neck. New York, Churchill Livingstone, 1988; 25–99.
43. Bartley AG: Suppression of saliva (letter to the editor). Med Times Gazette 1868; 54:603.
44. Hadden WB: On "dry mouth," or suppression of the salivary and buccal secretions. Trans Clin Soc Lond 1888; 21:176–179.
45. Gougerot H: Insuffisance progressive et atrophie des glandes salivaires et muqueuses de la bouche, des conjonctives (et parfois des muqueuses nasale, laryngée, vulvaire). Bull Soc Franc Derm Syph 1925; 32:376–379.
46. Sjögren H: A New Conception of Keratoconjunctivitis Sicca. JB Hamilton, Translation. Sydney, Australian Medical Publishing Co Ltd, 1943.
47. Daniels TE, Talal N: Diagnosis and differential diagnosis of Sjögren's syndrome. In Talal N, Moutsopoulos HM, Kassan SS (eds.): Sjögren's Syndrome: Clinical and Immunological Aspects. Berlin, Springer-Verlag, 1987; 193–199.
48. Daniels TE: Clinical assessment and diagnosis of immunologically mediated salivary gland disease in Sjögren's syndrome. J Autoimmun 1989; 2:529–541.
49. Ramirez-Mata M, Pena-Ancira FF, Alarcon-Segovia D: Abnormal esophageal motility in primary Sjögren's syndrome. J Rheumatol 1976; 3:63–69.
50. Frost-Larsen K, Isager H, Manthorpe R: Sjögren's syndrome treated with bromhexine: A randomized clinical study. Br Med J 1978; 1:1579–1581.
51. Moutsopoulos HM, Webber BL, Vlagopoulos TP, Chused TM, Decker JL: Differences in the clinical manifestations of sicca syndrome in the presence and absence of rheumatoid arthritis. Am J Med 1979; 66:733–736.
52. Moutsopoulos HM, Mann DL, Johnson AH, Chused TM: Genetic differences between primary and secondary sicca syndrome. N Engl J Med 1979; 301:761–763.
53. Chudwin DS, Daniels TE, Wara DW, Ammann AJ, Barrett DJ, Whitcher JP, Cowan MJ: Spectrum of Sjögren's syndrome in children. J Pediatr 1981; 98:213–217.
54. Utsinger PD, Zvaifler NJ, Ehrlich GE (eds): Rheumatoid Arthritis: Etiology, Diagnosis, Management. Philadelphia, JB Lippincott Co, 1985; 136–141.
55. Jacobsson LTH, Axell TE, Hansen BU, Henricsson VJ, Larsson Å, Lieberkind K, Lilja B, Manthorpe R: Dry eyes or mouth: An epidemiological study in Swedish adults with special reference to primary Sjögren's syndrome. J Autoimmun 1989; 2:521–527.
56. Forstot JZ, Forstot SL, Greer RO, Tan EM: The incidence of Sjögren's sicca complex in a population of patients with keratoconjunctivitis sicca. Arthritis Rheum 1982; 25:156–160.
57. Chisholm DM, Lyell A, Haroon TS, Mason DK, Beeley JA: Salivary gland function in sarcoidosis. Oral Surg Oral Med Oral Pathol 1971; 31:766–771.
58. Tarpley TM, Anderson L, Lightbody P, Sheagren JN: Minor salivary gland involvement in sarcoidosis. Oral Surg Oral Med Oral Pathol 1972; 33:755–762.
59. Whitcher JP: Clinical diagnosis of the dry eye. Int Ophthalmol Clin 1987; 27:7–24.
60. Daniels TE, Silverman S, Michalski JP, Greenspan JS, Sylvester RA, Talal N: The oral component of Sjögren's syndrome. Oral Surg Oral Med Oral Pathol 1975; 39:875–885.
61. Schubert MM, Izutsu KT: Iatrogenic causes of

salivary gland dysfunction. J Dent Res 1987; 66:680–688.

62. Hernandez YL, Daniels TE: Oral candidiasis in Sjögren's syndrome: Prevalence, clinical correlations and treatment. Oral Surg Oral Med Oral Pathol 1989; 68:324–329.

63. Daniels TE: Labial salivary gland biopsy in Sjögren's syndrome: Assessment as a diagnostic criterion in 362 suspected cases. Arthritis Rheum 1984; 27:147–156.

64. Trevino H, Tsianos EB, Schenker S: Gastrointestinal and hepatobiliary features in Sjögren's syndrome. In Talal N, Moutsopoulos HM, Kassan SS (eds.): Sjögren's Syndrome: Clinical and Immunological Aspects. Berlin, Springer-Verlag, 1987; 89–95.

65. Constantopoulos SH, Moutsopoulos HM: The respiratory system in Sjögren's syndrome. In Talal N, Moutsopoulos HM, Kassan SS (eds.): Sjögren's Syndrome: Clinical and Immunological Aspects. Berlin, Springer-Verlag, 1987; 83–88.

66. Kassan SS, Talal N: Renal disease with Sjögren's syndrome. In Talal N, Moutsopoulos HM, Kassan SS (eds.): Sjögren's Syndrome: Clinical and Immunological Aspects. Berlin, Springer-Verlag, 1987; 96–101.

67. Alexander EL: Inflammatory vascular disease in Sjögren's syndrome. In Talal N, Moutsopoulos HM, Kassan SS (eds.): Sjögren's Syndrome: Clinical and Immunological Aspects. Berlin, Springer-Verlag, 1987; 102–125.

68. Alexander EL: Neurovascular complications of primary Sjögren's syndrome. In Talal N, Moutsopoulos HM, Kassan SS (eds.): Sjögren's Syndrome: Clinical and Immunological Aspects. Berlin, Springer-Verlag, 1987; 61–82.

69. Zulman J, Jaffe R, Talal N: Evidence that the malignant lymphoma of Sjögren's syndrome is a monoclonal B-cell neoplasm. N Engl J Med 1975; 299:1215–1220.

70. Tzioufas AG, Moutsopoulos HM, Talal N: Lymphoid malignancy and monoclonal proteins. In Talal N, Moutsopoulos HM, Kassan SS (eds.): Sjögren's Syndrome: Clinical and Immunological Aspects. Berlin, Springer-Verlag, 1987; 129–136.

71. Daniels TE: Salivary histopathology in diagnosis of Sjögren's syndrome. Scand J Rheumatol 1986; 61(Suppl):36–43.

72. Daniels TE, Aufdemorte TB, Greenspan JS: Histopathology of Sjögren's Syndrome. In Talal N, Moutsopoulos HM, Kassan SS (eds.): Sjögren's Syndrome: Clinical and Immunological Aspects. Berlin, Springer-Verlag, 1987; 41 52.

73. Scott J: Qualitative and quantitative observations on the histology of human labial salivary glands obtained postmortem. J Biol Buccale 1980; 8:187–200.

74. Chisholm DM, Mason DK: Labial salivary gland biopsy in Sjögren's syndrome. J Clin Pathol 1968; 21:656–660.

75. Bombardieri S, Moutsopoulos HM (eds.): Workshop on diagnostic criteria for Sjögren's syndrome. Clin Exp Rheumatol 1989; 7:111–220.

76. Brown CC: The parotid puzzle: A review of the literature on human salivation and its application to psychophysiology. Psychophysiology 1970; 7:66–85.

77. Ben-Aryeh J, Miron D, Szargel R, Gutman D: Whole-saliva secretion rates in old and young healthy subjects. J Dent Res 1984; 63:1147–1148.

78. Heft MW, Baum BJ: Unstimulated and stimulated parotid salivary flow rate in individuals of different ages. J Dent Res 1984; 63:1182–1185.

79. Thorn JJ, Prause JU, Oxholm P: Sialochemistry in Sjögren's syndrome: A review. J Oral Pathol Med 1989; 18:457–468.

80. Marx RE, Hartman KS, Rethman KV: A prospective study comparing incisional labial to incisional parotid biopsies in the detection and confirmation of sarcoidosis, Sjögren's disease, sialosis, and lymphoma. J Rheumatol 1988; 15:621–629.

81. Wise CM, Agudelo CA, Semble EL, Stump TE, Woodruff RD: Comparison of parotid and minor salivary gland biopsy specimens in the diagnosis of Sjögren's syndrome. Arthritis Rheum 1988; 31:662–666.

82. Waterhouse JP: Focal adenitis in salivary and lacrimal glands. Proc R Soc Med 1963; 56:911–918.

83. Calman HI, Reifman S: Sjögren's syndrome: Report of a case. Oral Surg Oral Med Oral Pathol 1966; 21:158–162.

84. Cifarelli PS, Bennett MJ, Zaino EC: Sjögren's syndrome: A case report with an additional diagnostic aid. Arch Intern Med 1966; 117:429–431.

85. Chisholm DM, Waterhouse JP, Mason DK: Lymphocytic sialadenitis in the major and minor glands: A correlation in postmortem subjects. J Clin Pathol 1970; 23:690–694.

86. Davies JD, Berry H, Bacon PA, Issa MA, Schofield JJ: Labial sialadenitis in Sjögren's syndrome and in rheumatoid arthritis. J Pathol 1973; 109:307–314.

87. Greenspan JS, Daniels TE, Talal N, Sylvester RA: The histopathology of Sjögren's syndrome in labial salivary gland biopsies. Oral Surg Oral Med Oral Pathol 1974; 37:217–229.

88. Waterhouse JP, Doniach I: Post-mortem prevalence of focal lymphocytic adenitis of the submandibular salivary glands. J Pathol Bacteriol 1966; 91:53–64.

89. Greenspan JS, Daniels TE, Talal N, Sylvester RA: The histopathology of Sjögren's syndrome in labial salivary gland biopsies. Oral Surg Oral Med Oral Pathol 1974; 37:217–229.

90. Bertram U, Hjorting-Hansen E: Punch biopsy of minor salivary glands in the diagnosis of Sjögren's syndrome. Scand J Dent Res 1970; 78:295–300.

91. Skopouli FN, Drosos AA, Papaioannou T, Moutsopoulos HM: Preliminary diagnostic criteria for Sjögren's syndrome. Scand J Rheumatol 1986; 61(Suppl):22–25.

92. Fox RI, Robinson CA, Curd JG, Kozin F, Howell FV: Sjögren's syndrome: Proposed criteria for classification. Arthritis Rheum 1986; 29:577–585.

93. Talal N, Asofsky R, Lightbody P: Immunoglobulin synthesis by salivary gland lymphoid cells in Sjögren's syndrome. J Clin Invest 1970; 49:49–54.

94. Talal N, Sylvester RA, Daniels TE, Greenspan JS, Williams RC: T and B lymphocytes in peripheral blood and tissue lesions in Sjögren's syndrome. J Clin Invest 1974; 53:180–189.

95. Fox RI, Carstens SA, Fong S, Robinson CA, Howell

F, Vaughan JH: Use of monoclonal antibodies to analyze peripheral blood and salivary gland lymphocyte subsets in Sjögren's syndrome. Arthritis Rheum 1982; 25:419–426.

96. Adamson TC, Fox RI, Frisman DM, Howell FV: Immunohistologic analysis of lymphoid infiltrates in primary Sjögren's syndrome using monoclonal antibodies. J Immunol 1983; 130:203–208.

97. Miyasaka N, Seaman W, Bakshi A, Sauvezie B, Strand V, Pope R, Talal N: Natural killing activity in Sjögren's syndrome. Arthritis Rheum 1983; 26:954–960.

98. Fox RI, Hugli TE, Lanier LL, Morgan EL, Howell F: Salivary gland lymphocytes in primary Sjögren's syndrome lack lymphocyte subsets defined by Leu-7 and Leu-11 antigens. J Immunol 1985; 135:207–214.

99. Andrade RE, Hagen KA, Manivel JC: Distribution and immunophenotype of the inflammatory cell population in the benign lymphoepithelial lesion (Mikulicz disease). Hum Pathol 1988; 19:932–941.

100. Harley JB, Alexander EL, Bias WB, Fox OF, Provost TT, Reichlin M, Yamagata H, Arnett FC: Anti-Ro (SS-A) and anti-La (SS-B) in patients with Sjögren's syndrome. Arthritis Rheum 1986; 29:196–206.

101. Harley JB: Autoantibodies in Sjögren's syndrome. In Talal N, Moutsopoulos HM, Kassan SS (eds.): Sjögren's Syndrome: Clinical and Immunological Aspects. Berlin, Springer-Verlag, 1987; 218–234.

102. Horsfall AC, Rose LM, Maini RN: Autoantibody synthesis in salivary glands of Sjögren's syndrome patients. J Autoimmun 1989; 2:559–568.

103. Lindahl G, Hedfors E, Klareskog L, Forsum U: Epithelial HLA-DR expression and T lymphocyte subsets in salivary glands in Sjögren's syndrome. Clin Exp Immunol 1985; 61:475–482.

104. Fox RI, Bumol T, Fantozzi R, Bone R, Schreiber R: Expression of histocompatibility antigen HLA-DR by salivary gland epithelial cells in Sjögren's syndrome. Arthritis Rheum 1986; 29:1105–1111.

105. Jonsson R, Klareskog L, Bäckman K, Tarkowski A: Expression of HLA-D-locus (DP, DQ, DR)-coded antigens, beta 2-microglobulin, and the interleukin 2 receptor in Sjögren's syndrome. Clin Immunol Immunopathol 1987; 45:235–243.

106. Thrane PS, Brandtzaeg P: Differential expression of epithelial MHC class II determinants (HLA-DR, -DP, and -DQ) and increased class I expression in inflamed salivary glands. Adv Exp Med Biol 1988; 237:681–688.

107. Speight PM, Cruchley A, Williams DM: Epithelial HLA-DR expression in labial salivary glands in Sjögren's syndrome and non-specific sialadenitis. J Oral Pathol Med 1989; 18:178–183.

108. Basham TY, Nickoloff BJ, Merigan TC, Morhenn VB: Recombinant gamma interferon induces HLA-DR expression on cultured human keratinocytes. J Invest Dermatol 1984; 83:83–90.

109. Fox RI, Theofilopoulos AN, Altman N: Production of interleukin 2 (IL 2) by salivary gland lymphocytes in Sjögren's syndrome: Detection of reactive cells by using antibody directed to synthetic peptides of IL 2. J Immunol 1985; 135:3109–3115.

110. Miyasaka N, Murota N, Yamaoka K, Sato K, Yamada T, Nishido T, Okuda M: Interleukin-2 defect in the peripheral blood and the lung in patients with Sjögren's syndrome. Clin Exp Immunol 1986; 65:497–505.

111. Fishleder A, Tubbs R, Hesse B, Levine H: Uniform detection of immunoglobulin-gene rearrangement in benign lymphoepithelial lesions. N Engl J Med 1987; 316:1118–1121.

112. Freimark B, Fantozzi R, Bone R, Bordin G, Fox R: Detection of clonally expanded salivary gland lymphocytes in Sjögren's syndrome. Arthritis Rheum 1989; 32:859–869.

113. Reveille JD, Wilson RW, Provost TT, Bias WB, Arnett FC: Primary Sjögren's syndrome and other autoimmune diseases in families. Ann Int Med 1984; 101:748–756.

114. Arnett FC, Bias WB, Reveille JD: Genetic studies in Sjögren's syndrome and systemic lupus erythematosus. J Autoimmun 1989; 2:403–413.

115. Harley JB, Reichlin M, Arnett FC, Alexander EL, Bias WB, Provost TT: Gene interaction at HLA-DQ enhances autoantibody production in primary Sjögren's syndrome. Science 1986; 232:1145–1147.

116. Shillitoe EJ, Daniels TE, Whitcher JP, Strand CV, Talal N, Greenspan JS: Antibody to cytomegalovirus in patients with Sjögren's syndrome. Arthritis Rheum 1982; 25:260–265.

117. Venables PJN, Ross MGR, Charles PJ, Melsom RD, Griffiths PD, Maini RN: A seroepidemiological study of cytomegalovirus and Epstein-Barr virus in rheumatoid arthritis and sicca syndrome. Ann Rheum Dis 1985; 44:742–746.

118. Thorn JJ, Oxholm P, Anderson HK: High levels of complement fixing antibodies against cytomegalovirus in patients with primary Sjögren's syndrome. Clin Exp Rheumatol 1988; 6:71–74.

119. Daniels TE, Sylvester RA, Silverman S, Polando V, Talal N: Tubuloreticular structures within labial salivary glands in Sjögren's syndrome. Arthritis Rheum 1974; 17:593–597.

120. Cremer NE, Daniels TE, Oshiro LS, Marcus F, Claypool R, Sylvester RA, Talal N: Immunological and virological studies of cultured labial biopsy cells from patients with Sjögren's syndrome. Clin Exp Immunol 1974; 18:213–224.

121. Wolf H, Haus M, Wilmes E: Persistence of Epstein-Barr virus in the parotid gland. J Virol 1984; 51:795–798.

122. Fox RI, Pearson G, Vaughan JH: Detection of Epstein-Barr virus-associated antigens and DNA in salivary gland biopsies from patients with Sjögren's syndrome. J Immunol 1986; 137:3162–3168.

123. Daniels TE, deSouza YG, Hartzog GA, Felton JR, Greenspan JS: Absence of Epstein-Barr virus DNA in Sjögren's syndrome. J Dent Res 1987; 66:184.

124. Smith FB, Rajdeo H, Panesar N, Bhuta K, Stahl R: Benign lymphoepithelial lesion of the parotid gland in intravenous drug users. Arch Pathol Lab Med 1988; 112:742–745.

125. Gordon JJ, Golbus J, Kurtides ES: Chronic lymphadenopathy and Sjögren's syndrome in a homosexual man. N Engl J Med 1984; 311:1441–1442.

126. Couderc L-J, D'Agay M-F, Danon F, Harzic M, Brocheriou C, Clauvel J-P: Sicca complex and infection with human immunodeficiency virus. Arch Intern Med 1987; 147:898–901.

127. Ulirsch RC, Jaffe ES: Sjögren's syndrome-like illness associated with the acquired immunodeficiency syndrome-related complex. Hum Pathol 1987; 18:1063–1068.
128. Schiødt M, Greenspan D, Daniels TE, Nelson J, Leggott PJ, Wara DW, Greenspan JS: Parotid gland enlargement and xerostomia associated with labial sialadenitis in HIV-infected patients. J Autoimmun 1989; 2:415–425.
129. Itescu S, Brancato LJ, Winchester R: A sicca syndrome in HIV infection: association with HLA-DR5 and CD8 lymphocytosis. Lancet 1989; 2:466–468.
130. Kornstein MJ, Parker GA, Mills AS: Immunohistology of the benign lymphoepithelial lesion in AIDS-related lymphadenopathy: A case report. Hum Pathol 1988; 19:1359–1361.
131. Robert-Guroff M, Weiss SH, Giron JA, Jennings AM, Ginzburg HM, Margolis IB, Blattner WA, Gallo RC: Prevalence of antibodies to HTLV-I, -II, and -III in intravenous drug abusers from an AIDS endemic region. JAMA 1986; 255:3133–3137.
132. Gessain A, Barin F, Vernant JC, Gout O, Maurs L, Calender A, de Thé G: Antibodies to human T-lymphotropic virus type-I in patients with tropical spastic paraparesis. Lancet 1985; 2:407–410.
133. Vernant JC, Buisson G, Magdeleine J, De Thore J, Jouannelle A, Neisson-Vernant C, Monplaisir N: T-lymphocyte alveolitis, tropical spastic paresis, and Sjögren's syndrome. Lancet 1988; 1:177.
134. Green JE, Hinrichs SH, Vogel J, Jay G: Exocrinopathy resembling Sjögren's syndrome in HTLV-I tax transgenic mice. Nature 1989; 341:72–74.
135. Talal N, Dauphinée MJ, Dang H, Alexander SS, Hart DJ, Garry RF: Detection of serum antibodies to retroviral proteins in patients with primary Sjögren's syndrome (autoimmune exocrinopathy). Arthritis Rheum 1990; 33:774–781.
136. Garry RF, Fermin CD, Hart DJ, Alexander SS, Donehower LA, Hong LZ: Detection of a human intracisternal A-type retroviral particle antigenically related to HIV. Science 1990; 250:1127–1129.

PART

II

Neoplastic Disease of Salivary Glands

7

HISTOGENESIS AND MORPHOGENESIS OF SALIVARY GLAND NEOPLASMS

Irving Dardick

Of all the tissues in the human body, perhaps the salivary glands have the most histologically heterogeneous group of tumors and the greatest diversity of morphologic features among their cells and tissue. This is the main reason that those interested in salivary gland pathology have been intrigued by the developmental and morphogenetic processes responsible for the unusual histologic characteristics of these tumors. Although the salivary, sweat, apocrine, and mammary glands all have similar phylogeny and cellular phenotypes, many lesions are unique to the salivary glands. Many of the tumors that form the basic spectrum of common or relatively common salivary gland tumors are quite infrequent in the various adnexal glands of the skin or the breast.

Classification of neoplasms of any organ should be predicated on patterns of differentiation that reflect the organization and cell types of the parental tissue. In the tumors of some tissues, this method of classification is easier to apply than in others. Certain neoplastic processes have obvious histologic, functional, immunohistochemical, and/or ultrastructural markers that allow pathologists to assemble nosologic groupings that function somewhat like a taxonomic system. Good examples are endocrine tumors of the pituitary gland and pancreas and the spectrum of epithelial and stromal tumors of the ovary. Unfortunately, as witnessed by published classifications of salivary gland tumors, such an approach has not been applied with any degree of success to salivary glands;[1-4] current classifications involve listing diagnostic terms in two categories: benign and malignant.

There is a particular need to investigate various developmental processes, the cell types, and the forms of differentiation involved in salivary gland tumors and to produce improved criteria for the segregation of individual types of tumors. Recent advances, particularly in the recognition of various forms of adenocarcinoma with markedly different prognoses,[5-7] highlight the essential nature of such clinicopathologic correlates.

HISTOGENETIC CONCEPTS

Bases for the classification of salivary gland tumors have usually relied on histologic observations of the fetal salivary gland and the cellular differentiation involved in particular segments of the duct system.[1, 8-10] A variety of histogenetic concepts for salivary gland tumors have evolved (for reviews see the reports by Attie and Sciubba[11] and by Dardick and colleagues[12]), but the concept usually cited as central to the induction of these tumors is the semipluripotential bicellular reserve cell hypothesis.[1, 8, 9] It is generally accepted that specific reserve or basal cells of the excretory and intercalated ducts or both are responsible for replacement of all types of cells in the normal gland and hence are the sole source for neoplastic transformation;[1, 9] however, it should be realized that direct evidence for this concept is not available. Indeed, in autoradiographic assessments of adult rat parotid glands after ligation of the main excretory duct, Walker and Gobe[13] have clearly shown that cells in the striated and intercalated ducts are capable of DNA synthesis on both the ligated and unligated sides and that the main cells dividing on the unligated side are striated duct and acinar cells. Such findings negate the reserve cell hypothesis.[1, 8, 9] The nature and function of basal cells in the salivary ducts are also unclear, and evidence exists that they are a complex and heterogeneous population of cells.[14–18] Their potential roles during fetal development of the salivary glands and in the mature glands require further investigation.

The morphology of the prenatal and postnatal salivary gland, principally in the rat,[19, 20] has served as a model for subtyping various salivary gland tumors.[1, 10, 21] Not unexpectedly, embryologically based concepts for the classification of salivary gland tumors are inextricably intertwined with the semipluripotential bicellular reserve cell hypothesis. However, as illustrated by certain tumors[22–26] and morphologic concepts,[12, 27] there likely are basic structural patterns in the developing and mature salivary gland that are reflected in salivary gland tumors in general and in the various differentiation patterns within any one subgroup specifically. The importance of this concept is that it relates the histology of neoplastic processes directly to the classification of salivary gland tumors rather than designating a specific cell or cells of origin that generally are impossible to precisely identify once the tumor is clinically overt and, therefore, remain speculative. If, as seems probable, all types of cells in the mature salivary gland are capable of mitosis,[12] current histogenetic concepts will require reevaluation.

In order to improve current classification of salivary gland tumors, it is essential to extract information from a variety of techniques, such as tissue culture, immunohistochemistry, electron microscopy, and basic research. This helps to determine the processes responsible for the development of histologic patterns and the various types of cells involved, along with their structural modifications in salivary gland tumors. Some aspects of such information will be reviewed prior to outlining a working classification of these neoplasms.

PROLIFERATIVE CAPACITY OF SALIVARY GLANDS

Although it is true that the primary functional unit of the normal salivary gland, the acinus and its associated intercalated duct, has an embryologic origin from simple branching ductal structures,[28] this does not necessarily imply that such ductal cells remain the only source for self-renewal in the mature gland or that the mechanisms for renewal and regeneration in the adult gland are the same as those operating in the immature gland. Judging from the atrophy associated with ductal obstruction, radiation, chronic sialadenitis, expanding tumor, and benign lymphoepithelial

lesion, the salivary glands may have only limited regenerative capacity. Furthermore, many of these insults result in metaplastic alterations of duct epithelium and proliferation of myoepithelial/basal cells.[29–38] Because a cell capable of replicating its DNA has the potential to express genes associated with neoplastic alteration, it is essential to catalog the cell types in salivary glands that retain their capacity to divide.

There is accumulating evidence that acinar cells of the mature gland readily divide under a number of physiologic and nonphysiologic conditions.[12, 13, 39–46] Luminal epithelial cells of breast lobules can also divide.[47, 48] However, in the parotid salivary gland of the adult human, the large majority of cells are noncycling, just as in breast tissue[48] and in tissue of the liver,[49] and the few detectable cycling cells are not confined to the intercalated duct. In surveying the salivary glands of the postnatal rat[12]—the model most often used to support the semipluripotential bicellular reserve cell hypothesis—it is evident that mitotic figures are more frequently seen in luminal than basal cells, that acinar cells (whether serous or mucinous) divide, and that luminal epithelial cells with mitotic figures are present at all levels of the duct system; this even includes the striated duct,[12] a segment that is excluded in the semipluripotential reserve cell theory.[1, 9] In terms of tumor induction, it should be appreciated that differentiated cells are capable of metaplastic alterations. For example, epidermoid metaplasia has been demonstrated in acinar and myoepithelial cells of the salivary gland of the rat[35] and in secretory cells of hamster tracheal mucosa.[50] These data suggest that any of the various cells found in the normal salivary gland could serve as a precursor for neoplasia; thus, this is a multicellular histogenetic concept.[11, 12]

PATTERNS OF DIFFERENTIATION IN SALIVARY GLAND NEOPLASMS

Regardless of the cell of origin for salivary gland tumors, it is essential to appreciate the role of tumor cell organization, the type or types of cell differentiation, and the materials synthesized by the cells and their placement within the tumor. Each of these factors has a bearing on the histologic pattern that is central to categorization of salivary gland tumors.[27, 51]

Batsakis has been instrumental in emphasizing the bicellular constitution (luminal and neoplastically modified myoepithelial cells) of certain of the salivary gland tumors; these include pleomorphic adenoma, adenoid cystic carcinoma, epithelial-myoepithelial carcinoma, and terminal duct carcinoma.[23] This feature has been extended to additional types of salivary gland tumors,[26] such as certain monomorphic adenomas[52] and acinic cell carcinomas,[53, 54] mucoepidermoid carcinoma,[55, 56] malignant mixed tumor,[57] and Warthin's tumor.[58] In fact, the categories of salivary gland tumors in which more than one type of tumor cell is recognized are increasing. The variety of differentiated tumor cells and the neoplasms with myoepithelial/basal cells that are reported in the literature are summarized in Table 7–1. Inherent in this bicellular aspect of these tumors has been the acceptance that the neoplastic myoepithelial cell component can assume a variety of cytologic forms as exemplified by ultrastructural studies of pleomorphic adenoma,[59–61] adenoid cystic carcinoma,[62–64] and epithelial-myoepithelial carcinoma.[65–68] In salivary gland tumors, the myoepithelial cell component rarely has structural features approaching those of the normal cell.[27, 54, 69, 70] This even applies to myoepitheliomas in which there is a range of structural modifications resulting in a variety of cell forms, such as spindle,[26, 71, 72] plasmacytoid, epithelial,[72] and clear.[71–76] The form, numbers, and distribution of luminal epithelial cells are also variable in salivary gland tumors, and these aspects, along with the ratio of ductoid or gland-like structures to myoepithelial cells, are major reasons for the wide spectrum of histologic features in any one salivary gland tumor class.

Modification of the myoepithelial cell component of salivary gland tumors is also evident from immunohistochemical studies. Although the intermediate filaments vimentin and glial fibrillary acidic protein are not expressed in the normal myoepithelium (glial fibrillary acidic protein can be detected in myoepithelial cells of acini undergoing atrophy adjacent to tumors[77]), both are readily detected in the modified myoepithelial cells of pleomorphic adenomas and myoepitheliomas.[74–80] A variety of cytokeratin filaments are also present in normal salivary gland myoepithelium and ductal basal cells, but a few of these, such as cytokeratins 4, 5, 6, and 14, are not expressed in acinar or luminal epithelial cells of the ducts.[14–18, 36, 79] However, cytokeratin 14 is infrequently detected in the myoepithelial cell population of pleomorphic adenoma[78] or in myoepithelioma;[72] yet, in both tumor types, microfilaments and muscle-specific action may occasionally be expressed.[72, 75, 76, 81] Such alterations should not be unexpected in tumors, and the lack of expression of specific markers of myoepithelium in normal salivary glands does not necessarily imply the absence of differentiation of a modified form of myoepithelium as a component of such tumors. A broader view of tumor differentiation is required; this view must take into account both the placement of certain tumor cells in relation to the luminal cells and the fact that abluminal cells may be the neoplastic counterpart of basal cells of the striated or excretory duct (some of which lack muscle-specific actin; see below) in certain cases and myoepithelial cells in others.

The deposition of certain extracellular secretory products is a characteristic histologic feature of salivary gland tumors such as pleomorphic adenoma and adenoid cystic carcinoma, which accounts for the myxoid "stroma" and the pseudolumina (cribriform spaces), respectively. There is some evidence that neoplastic myoepithelial cells are involved in the production of these extracellular materials.[82–84] Ultrastructural[59, 60, 84] and immunohistochemical studies, primarily using antibodies to laminin and collagen IV,[85, 86] have shown that basal lamina (often in excessive amounts), elastic and collagen fibers, and glycosaminoglycans are the main secretory products. Using pleomorphic adenoma as a model, it is evident that the formation of variably sized, discrete basal lamina-lined and glycosaminoglycan-containing spaces that are located between and surrounded by modified myoepithelial cells and their cytoplasmic processes (Fig. 7–1) is the initial phase in the development of the myxoid stroma that is characteristic of this lesion. Subsequent stages involve increasing enlargement of many of these specialized intercellular spaces (presumably as a result of ongoing synthesis of basal lamina, collagens, and glycosaminoglycans) with gradual sep-

Table 7–1. Neoplastic Myoepithelial/Basal Cell Participation in Salivary Gland Tumors*

Neoplasm	Types of Cells
Pleomorphic adenoma[23, 26, 59–61, 76, 80]	Luminal Acinar Myoepithelial
Myoepithelioma[69, 71, 72, 75, 91, 96]	Myoepithelial Rare luminal
Basal cell adenoma[52, 87, 98–100]	Luminal Myoepithelial/basal Acinar
Warthin's tumor[58, 101]	Luminal Basal/myoepithelial
Epithelial-myoepithelial carcinoma[5, 23, 65–68, 102]	Luminal Myoepithelial
Adenoid cystic carcinoma[26, 62–64, 82]	Luminal Myoepithelial
Acinic cell carcinoma[53, 54]	Acinar Intercalated duct Myoepithelial
Mucoepidermoid carcinoma[26, 55, 56, 103–106]	Goblet Luminal Squamous Myoepithelial/basal
Salivary duct carcinoma[107, 108]	Luminal Myoepithelial
Polymorphous low-grade adenocarcinoma[5, 6, 23, 87]	Luminal Myoepithelial
Adenocarcinoma, not otherwise specified[109]	Luminal Myoepithelial
Malignant mixed tumor[57]	Luminal Squamous Myoepithelial

*Based on ultrastructural and/or immunocytochemical evidence.

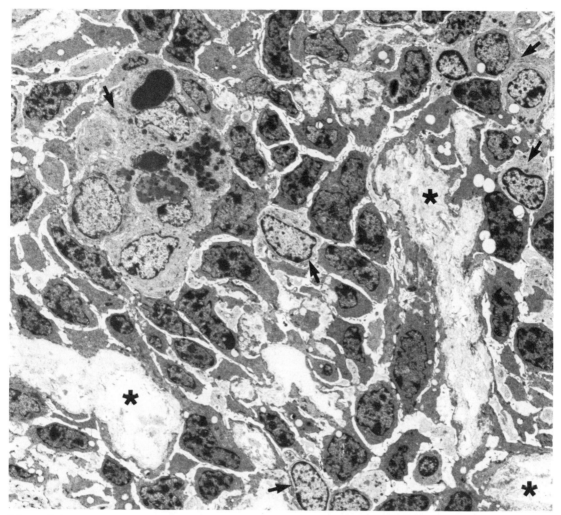

Figure 7–1. Tissue from a pleomorphic adenoma visualized in a survey-type transmission electron micrograph. The tumor is composed of collections (arrows) of ductal luminal epithelial cells (some of which form obvious lumina) that are scattered among the more numerous and slightly to considerably separated modified myoepithelial cells with many narrow cytoplasmic processes. Note the many intercellular spaces (asterisks) that are completely or partially surrounded by modified myoepithelial cells or their processes. At higher magnification, these spaces can be shown to contain excess basal lamina, glycosaminoglycans, and elastic fibers (× 2,300).

aration of the modified myoepithelial cells, fusion of adjacent intercellular spaces, isolation of individual or small groups of tumor cells, and eventual formation of the myxochondroid "stroma."[27, 59, 60] A similar process is involved in the development of the cribriform pattern in adenoid cystic carcinoma,[62–64] but in this case, the spheroidal intercellular spaces continue to be surrounded by an intact boundary of neoplastic myoepithelial cells (Fig. 7–2). Collections of such materials and redundant basal lamina can also be seen in certain monomorphic adenomas,[52, 87] malignant mixed tumor,[57] myoepithelioma,[72, 74] terminal duct carcinoma,[70] epithelial-myoepithelial carcinoma,[65, 67] and an adenoma[22] that is prototypical for salivary gland tumors in general. Perhaps the role of basal lamina

and proteoglycans in determining the histologic patterns of many salivary gland tumors is a reflection of the control of the morphology of developing salivary gland by these cell-surface–associated materials.[88, 89]

It is essential to appreciate these highly controlled developmental processes, because they are a factor bearing on the diagnosis of individual tumors and the classification of salivary gland tumors in general. They also assist in explaining such aspects as the diversity of histologic features within many of the classes of these tumors, the overlap in histologic features between various subtypes, and the formation of multiple growth patterns in a lesion, some of which are characteristic of another type of tumor that may have a different

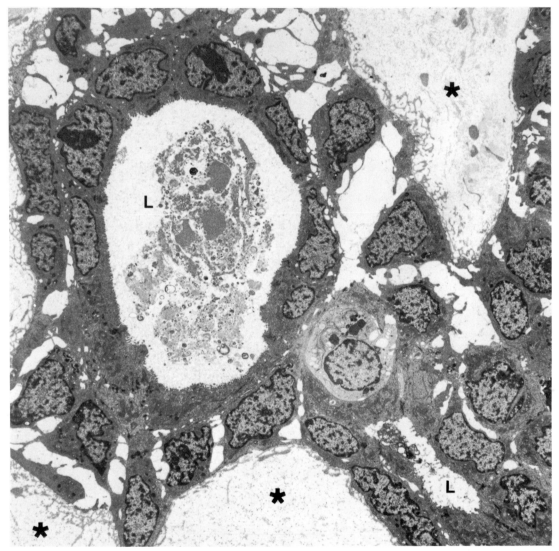

Figure 7–2. Section from an adenoid cystic carcinoma. There are basic structural similarities in this electron micrograph as compared with features seen in Figure 7–1. Duct- or gland-type lumina (L) are formed by flattened to cuboidal epithelial cells that bear microvilli on their apical surfaces. These cells are, in turn, surrounded by slightly separated, irregularly shaped tumor cells, with surfaces that may have multiple, narrow, cytoplasmic projections. The latter cells are again responsible for enclosing the basal lamina-lined intercellular spaces (asterisks) that account for the development of the cribriform growth pattern of this tumor (× 3,300).

biologic behavior. Many of these situations are responsible for the frequent problems in differential diagnosis of salivary gland tumors.

Thus, the form of myoepithelial cells and possibly basal cells, the relative proportion of luminal to myoepithelial cells, and the amounts and localization of basal lamina and glycosaminoglycans are all independent, but highly integrated, factors operating both between the various types of salivary gland tumors and within any one subtype. This type of information has been developed into a centralized concept to assist in explaining the plethora of subtypes of salivary gland tumors, the varied histologic appearances within any one subtype, and the relationship of the various subtypes.[27] Such a morphogenetic approach has more practical applications to the classification of these tumors than a histogenetic one. A summary of the key features of such a concept and accompanying model diagrams of the principal classes are provided below.

MORPHOGENESIS OF SALIVARY GLAND NEOPLASMS

Current studies have revealed the previously unrecognized complexity of the salivary ductal epithelium,[14, 16–18, 79] and some aspects of the cellular organization of these ducts are represented in Figure 7–3. It is now apparent that acini and ducts, including excretory, striated, and intercalated ducts, are associated with some form of basal and/or myoepithelial cell.[17, 18] If one considers the combination of ductal luminal or acinar cells and basal or myoepithelial cells, such as those that might be seen in a cross-section of a duct or acinus (Fig. 7–4), as a basic unit of the normal salivary gland, then neoplasia in this gland might also reflect the cellular makeup of this unit or any individual component.[27] Cellular regions from a typical pleomorphic adenoma provide an example of the application of this concept in a low-power electron micrograph (Fig. 7–1). Multiple ductlike structures composed of luminal cells (occasionally with evidence of acinar cell differentiation) are surrounded by a proliferation of abluminal cells, i.e., modified myoepithelial cells; each duct and a proportion of the surrounding myoepithelial cells in this tumor become the counterpart of the normal ductoacinar unit. As illustrated in the model diagram of Figure 7–4, such a concept envisages the potential development of three principal types of tumors: those composed of luminal and/or acinar cells plus myoepithelial cells; those composed primarily of ductal luminal cells or

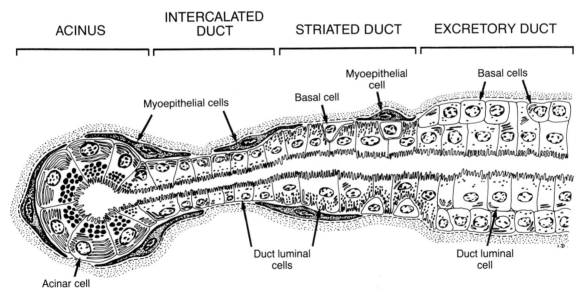

Figure 7–3. Diagram illustrates the cellular organization of the acinus and ducts of a normal salivary gland. Recent ultrastructural and immunohistochemical studies have shown the increasing complexity and heterogeneity of cell types that are associated with all levels of the duct system in this organ (see text). Because the differentiation and organization of cells in salivary gland tumors often appear to reflect those of a normal salivary gland, it is essential to appreciate the general distribution of normal cells. Myoepithelial cells associated with acini and intercalated and striated ducts contain muscle-specific actin and are cytokeratin 14-positive.[16–18] As noted in the diagram, actin-containing myoepithelial cells are also present at the basal aspects of at least a proportion of intralobular striated ducts.[17] In addition, cytokeratin 14-positive basal cells that are actin-negative are found in association with both striated and excretory ducts. Thus all levels of this system can have a basic unit formed by a combination of acinar or ductal luminal and myoepithelial or basal cells. (From Burns BR, Dardick I, Parks WR: Intermediate filament expression in normal parotid glands and pleomorphic adenoma. Virchows Arch [A] 1988; 413:103–112. With permission, Heidelberg, Springer-Verlag.)

DUCTOACINAR UNIT

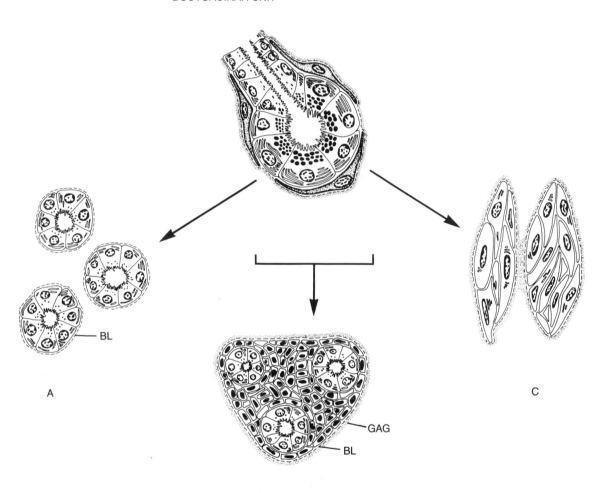

Figure 7–4. Model diagram illustrating the pattern of tumor cell differentiation and tumor cell organization in salivary gland tumors. Using the acinar/intercalated duct unit as a model, three basic types of tumor can develop. *A*, One type is composed entirely or primarily of acinar or luminal epithelial cells; *B*, another type is composed of both luminal and myoepithelial/basal cells; and *C*, a third type is composed of only myoepithelial cells. Dashed lines externally represent basal lamina (BL), and the dotted zone represents glycosaminoglycans (GAG). (Dardick I, van Nostrand AWP. Morphogenesis of salivary gland tumors: A prerequisite to improving classification. Pathol Annu 1987; 22(1):1–53. With permission, Appleton-Century-Crofts.)

acinar cells; and those composed almost solely of myoepithelial/basal cells. Superimposed on these three basic patterns of differentiation is the lack of or production of extracellular materials by the neoplastic myoepithelium, either alone or in association with ductal luminal cells.[27]

Some examples from the literature illustrate certain aspects of such morphologic concepts and the mechanisms responsible for the histologic patterns that are inherent in certain subtypes of salivary gland tumors. Acinic cell carcinoma, if it is well differentiated, can be composed almost entirely of tumor cells that closely resemble the normal serous cell. However, intercalated duct-like cells may be the predominant component,[90] and lumina lined by flattened intercalated duct cells are responsible for the microcystic pattern in this tumor.[54] In addition, myoepithelial cells have been identified ultrastructurally in a few examples.[53, 54] Thus, the tissue of this tumor exemplifies differentiation of cell types predicted in the first two classes of the above model and illustrates the interplay of acinar, ductal, and myoepithelial cells

in their production of the final histologic product and the histologic spectrum within this type of tumor.

By definition, adenoid cystic carcinoma falls within the first model class, that is, the diagnosis requires identification of small duct-type structures within the bulk of modified myoepithelial cells that form the basal lamina-lined "pseudocysts" in the cribriform subclass.[1] The development of the full range of histologic patterns in adenoid cystic carcinoma with or without pseudocysts is readily predicted by the ductoacinar unit model and is illustrated by the diagram in Figure 7–5. Basic similarities of adenoid cystic carcinoma to pleomorphic adenoma have been noted previously.[27, 64] However, the common mechanisms and cell types involved can be appreciated in electron micrographs from typical examples of pleomorphic adenoma (Fig. 7–1) and adenoid cystic carcinoma (Fig. 7–2). Without reference to the accompanying figure legends or light microscopy (Fig. 7–6), it would not be possible to distinguish between the two lesions ultrastruc-

Normal ducts

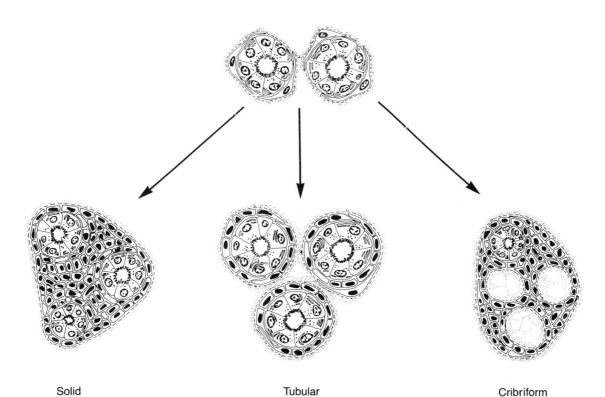

Solid   Tubular   Cribriform

Figure 7–5. Model diagram depicts the development of histologic patterns in adenoid cystic carcinoma. The combination of luminal and myoepithelial/basal cells of the normal ductoacinar unit is replicated in the tubular variant, whereas there is preferential differentiation of myoepithelial/basal cells in the solid form of this tumor. The production of excess basal lamina and glycosaminoglycans in association with the myoepithelial/basal cell component is responsible for development of the cribriform variant. Ductal structures are required for the diagnosis of the solid and cribriform types. (From Dardick I, van Nostrand AWP. Morphogenesis of salivary gland tumors: A prerequisite to improving classification. Pathol Annu 1987; 22(1):1–53. With permission, Appleton-Century-Crofts.)

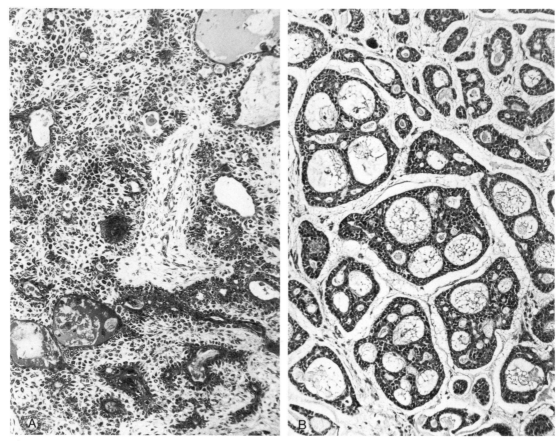

Figure 7–6. *A*, Section from a pleomorphic adenoma. The electron micrograph of Figure 7–1 is representative of the cellular regions seen in this example. In histologic sections, the duct and modified myoepithelial cell components are easily identified, but the development of the extracellular spaces (so essential to the formation of the myxochondroid stroma) is difficult to appreciate (× 120). *B*, Adenoid cystic carcinoma is shown. In this type of tumor, the cribriform spaces and the modified myoepithelial cells predominate, and it is more difficult to observe the small duct-type structures (× 120). The features described in *A* and *B* serve to diagnostically differentiate these two lesions despite the underlying similarities of the structural differentiation processes (compare Figs. 7–1 and 7–2).

turally. The model diagram for adenoid cystic carcinoma (Fig. 7–5) should be compared to the diagram of the formation of the diverse histologic patterns in pleomorphic adenoma (Fig. 7–7). The main difference between these two tumors is the eventual disruption of the basal lamina-lined intercellular spaces, the ragged margins of persisting cellular areas, and the eventual overt formation of the myxochondroid "stroma" in pleomorphic adenomas.[27] Development of cellular pleomorphic adenomas with numerous ducts surrounded by one or more layers of modified myoepithelial cells can be appreciated in this scheme (Fig. 7–7), as can the formation of pleomorphic adenomas with a predominance of myoepithelial cells.[91] Similar morphogenetic processes operate to produce the histologic variants of adenoid cystic carcinoma (Fig. 7–5). Such schemata also assist in understanding the problems of differentiation between these two tumors and how foci resembling adenoid cystic carcinoma can form in pleomorphic adenomas and foci resembling pleomorphic adenoma can form in adenoid cystic carcinoma.

Mucoepidermoid carcinoma is a lesion that has been assiduously excluded from those salivary gland tumors associated with myoepithelial differentiation. This exclusion was based mainly on the assumption that this tumor has a histogenesis from the excretory duct, which is a part of the tissue devoid of myoepithelial cells. It is true that the excretory duct can undergo goblet cell metaplasia and have cytologic features similar to those seen in better differentiated mucoepidermoid carcinomas (Fig. 7–8A). However, it should also be appreciated that such metaplastic alterations can be accompanied by basal cell hyperplasia (Fig. 7–8A) and that basal cells of the excretory duct can express cytokeratin 14 (Fig. 7–8B) similar to the myoepithelium of acini and intercalated ducts as well as the basal cells of some striated ducts.[18, 36] There is histochemical[56] and ultrastructural[55] evidence that at least some mucoepidermoid carcinomas have regions in which basal cells, with features similar to those of modified myoepithelial cells in other tumors, can be identified in association with mucus-secreting or squamous cells. Elec-

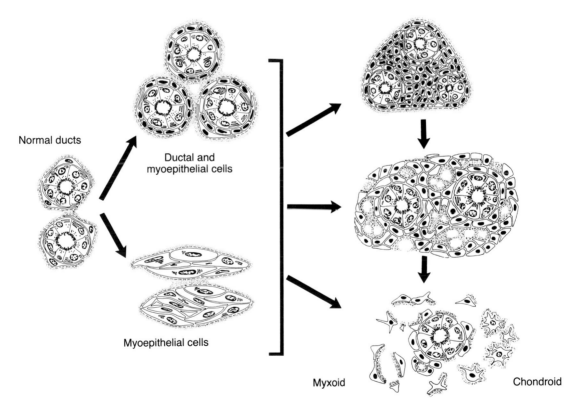

Figure 7–7. Diagram for pleomorphic adenoma is shown. The plethora of histologic patterns and cytologic features in this tumor stems from the multiplicity of differentiation pathways. Some regions or tumors can be composed principally of ducts with associated myoepithelial cells, others are composed largely of modified myoepithelial cells, and still others are composed of a combination of the two cell types, forming solid or cellular zones. Variable production of basal lamina and glycosaminoglycans leads to the gradual separation of the tumor cells and to the formation of the myxoid regions in different degrees, both within each pleomorphic adenoma and between different examples. Metaplastic processes associated with the development of myxomatous areas results in the chondroid component. (From Dardick I, van Nostrand AWP: Recent contributions of electron microscopy to salivary gland pathology. *In* Motta PN, Riva A [eds.]: Ultrastructure of the Extraparietal Glands of the Digestive Tract. Norwell, MA, Klüwer Academic Publishers, 1989; pp. 75–98. With permission, Klüwer Academic Publishers.)

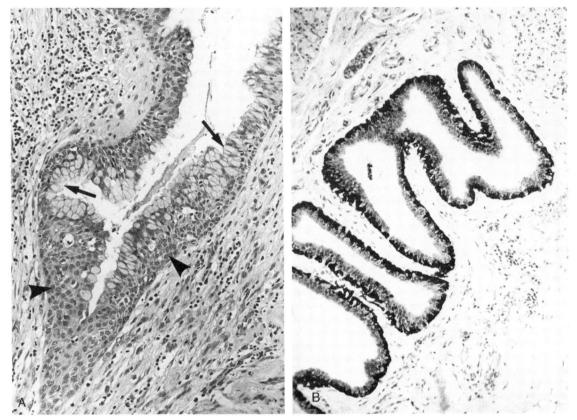

Figure 7–8. Salivary gland excretory ducts are shown. *A*, Goblet cell metaplasia (arrows) occurring in an excretory duct of the superficial lobe of a parotid gland resected for an undifferentiated carcinoma. Note also the considerable hyperplasia of the ductal basal cells (arrowheads) (× 120). *B*, Basal cells of the excretory duct, like the myoepithelium of acini and intercalated ducts, contain cytokeratin 14 as detected by monoclonal antibody 312C8–1[94, 95] (immunoperoxidase with hematoxylin counterstain, × 120).

tron microscopy in two recent cases of well-differentiated mucoepidermoid carcinomas has also revealed an inner layer of mucous granule-containing, microvillus-bearing tumor cells and an outer layer of more loosely arranged cells (Fig. 7–9). In some areas, the more loosely arranged cells contained tonofilaments and developed desmosomes and intercellular bridges, and the basal aspects of the tumor cells developed complex infoldings associated with basal lamina (Fig. 7–9). In other areas, these nonluminal tumor cells were distinctly squamous in their differentiation (Fig. 7–10). Again, these morphologic patterns are reminiscent of the basic ductoacinar unit of the salivary gland, and the arrangement and general features of the nonluminal cells are similar to this component in pleomorphic adenoma (Fig. 7–1) and adenoid cystic carcinoma (Fig. 7–2). Because development of squamous metaplasia in pleomorphic adenomas has many parallel features,[59] perhaps these two lesions are more closely related than has been indicated previously. Like some pleomorphic adenomas and myoepitheliomas,[74, 78] certain mucoepidermoid carcinomas can simultaneously express vimentin, glial fibrillary acidic protein, and cytokeratins.[92] The spectrum and admixture of tumor cell differentiation in mucoepidermoid carcinoma are, however, more complex in both the luminal and myoepithelial/basal cell components;[27] this differentiation is illustrated diagrammatically in Figure 7–11.

The monomorphic adenoma group of neoplasms involves an equally complicated morphology[21, 52, 87] and a confusing terminology.[93] The potential spectrum of histologic types in this class (Fig. 7–12) and the close relationship of monomorphic adenomas to both pleomorphic adenoma (Figs. 7–1 and 7–7) and adenoid cystic carcinoma (Figs. 7–2 and 7–5) are apparent from the figure models. Because of the varied histology and close relationships, it becomes pointless to argue whether myoepitheliomas are a variant of pleomorphic adenoma or a subtype of monomorphic adenomas. All are part of a spectrum and continuum of differentiation in these types of benign salivary gland tumors.[27]

SUMMARY

Based on the discussion in this chapter, development of two types of classification schemes for salivary gland tumors is possible; each type has a different purpose. One scheme can be considered taxonomic in form (Table 7–2) and is organized

Text continued on page 124

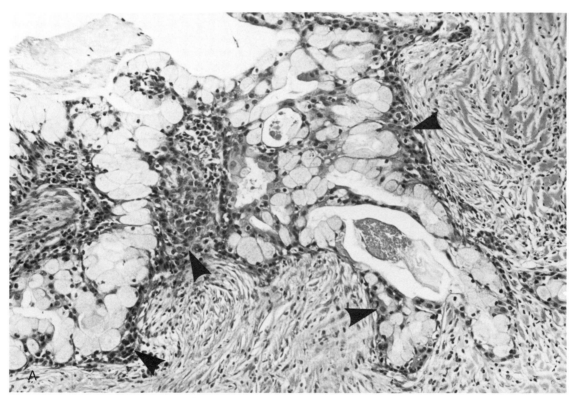

Figure 7–9. Mucoepidermoid carcinoma. *A,* In a well-differentiated example, there are one or more layers of darkly staining, intermediate-type cells (arrowheads) below the goblet cells (× 120).

Illustration continued on following page

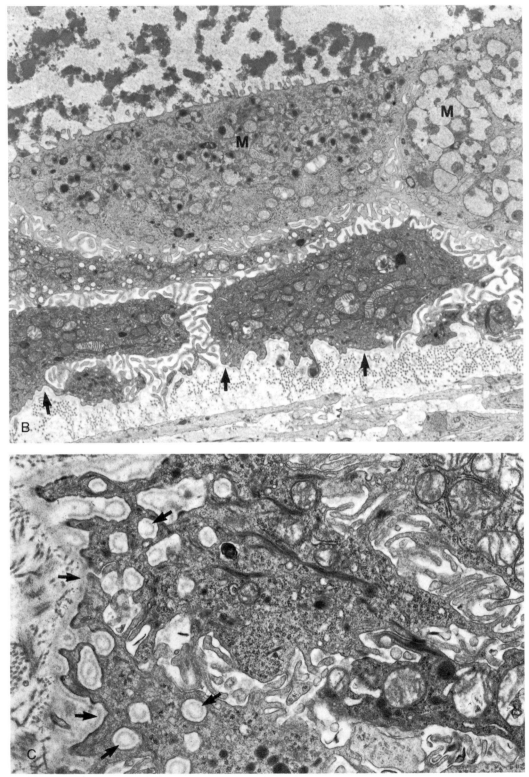

Figure 7–9 *Continued* Transmission electron micrographs from this case reveal the following: *B,* An inner layer of microvillus-bearing and mucous granule-containing *(M)* luminal cells and an outer layer of more angular and loosely arranged tumor cells with multiple cell-surface processes that lie within the basal lamina (arrows). This pattern of differentiation has similarities to that seen in pleomorphic adenoma (Fig. 7–1) and adenoid cystic carcinoma (Fig. 7–2), except for the multiplicity of modified myoepithelial cells in these two types of tumors (× 8,800). *C,* Outer cells that occasionally have complicated arrangements of the basal cell surface associated with distinct basal lamina (arrows) (× 20,000).

120

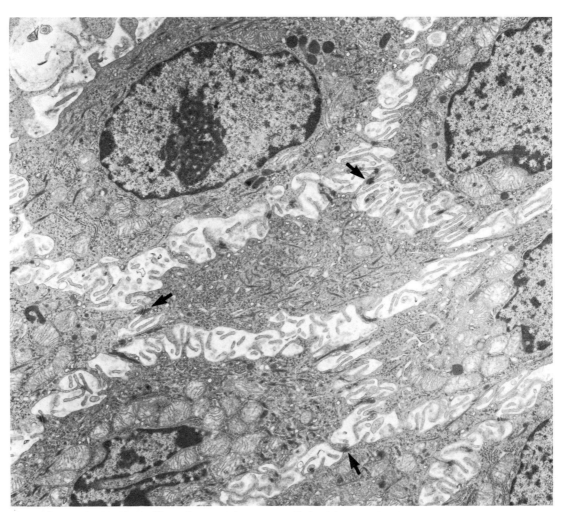

Figure 7–10. Mucoepidermoid carcinoma. Ultrastructurally in this example, the outer type cells (the modified myoepithelial cells) became multilayered, and the prominent desmosomes (arrows), intercellular bridges, and tonofilaments indicate squamous differentiation (× 9,800).

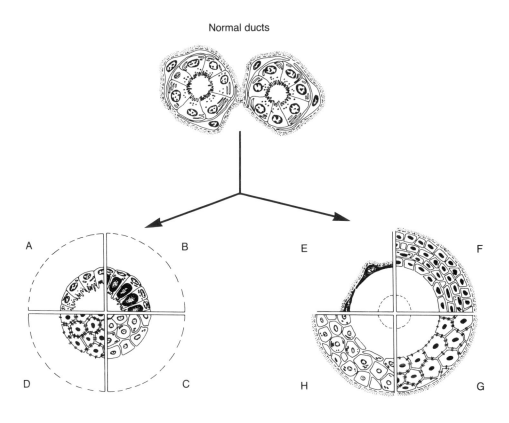

Figure 7–11. Diagram that illustrates potential tumor cell differentiation in mucoepidermoid carcinoma. As a result of the multiplicity of differentiation pathways, morphologic patterns in this tumor can be as complex as in pleomorphic adenoma. Reflections of the primary ductoacinar unit and the varied histologic pattern development are understandable if the luminal cell component differentiates as *(A)* cuboidal, *(B)* goblet, *(C)* clear, or *(D)* squamoid cells, and if the myoepithelium can differentiate as *(E)* myoepithelial, *(F)* intermediate, *(G)* squamoid, or *(H)* clear cells. (From Dardick I, van Nostrand AWP. Morphogenesis of salivary gland tumors: A prerequisite to improving classification. Pathol Annu 1987; 22(1):1–53. With permission, Appleton-Century-Crofts.)

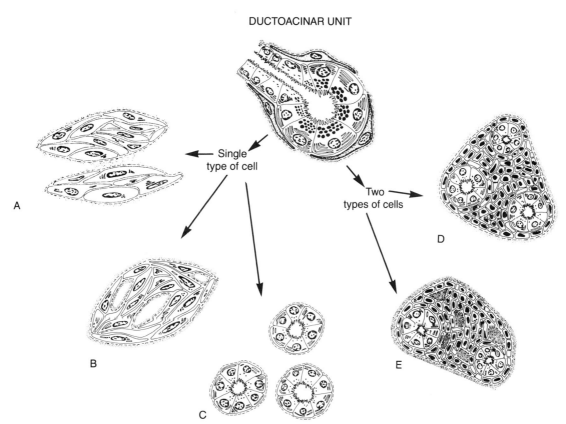

DUCTOACINAR UNIT

Single
type of cell

A

Two
types of cells

D

B

C

E

Figure 7–12. Diagram illustrates possible tumor cell differentiation in monomorphic adenomas. Development of histologic patterns in this tumor group reflects two potential pathways. One involves differentiation of a single type of tumor cell, either myoepithelial (*A* and *B*) or luminal *(C)*, and the other involves a combination of tumor cells: luminal cells and myoepithelial/modified myoepithelial cells (*D* and *E*). In both of these basic patterns, the histologic features can be altered by the production of localized stromal materials by the myoepithelial cell component, as represented in *B* and *E*. (From Dardick I, van Nostrand AWP: Morphogenesis of salivary gland tumors: A prerequisite to improving classification. Pathol Annu 1987; 22(1):1–53. With permission, Appleton-Century-Crofts.)

Table 7–2. Taxonomy of Salivary Gland Neoplasms*

Classification of Neoplasm	Subclassification of Neoplasm	Specific Neoplasms	
		Benign	*Malignant*
Neoplasms composed of luminal and modified myoepithelial cells	Histologically with apparent proteoglycan and basal lamina production	Pleomorphic adenoma Basal cell adenoma	Malignant mixed tumor Adenoid cystic carcinoma (cribriform)
	Histologically lacking obvious proteoglycan and basal lamina production	Basal cell adenoma Cellular pleomorphic adenoma Warthin's tumor	Basal cell adenocarcinoma Adenoid cystic carcinoma (solid/tubular) Epithelial-myoepithelial carcinoma Mucoepidermoid carcinoma Polymorphous low-grade adenocarcinoma
Neoplasms composed primarily of myoepithelial/basal cells	—	Myoepithelioma	Myoepithelial carcinoma
Neoplasms composed primarily of luminal/acinar cells	—	Canalicular adenoma Ductal papillomas Cystadenoma Oncocytoma	Acinic cell carcinoma Salivary duct carcinoma Adenocarcinoma, not otherwise specified Oncocytic carcinoma
Neoplasms composed of undifferentiated cells	—	—	Undifferentiated carcinoma Small cell carcinoma

*Not necessarily inclusive of all salivary tumors listed in the usual classification schemes.

to focus on the interrelationships of many of the various subtypes of salivary gland tumors and developmental processes responsible for the morphologic nature of each subtype. This is the main purpose in designing the series of model diagrams for each of the major salivary gland tumor subtypes. These illustrate the potential cell or types of cells, their organization, and the amounts and placement of cellular synthetic products involved in defining the histology of salivary gland tumors. Perhaps such a classification will assist in emphasizing that lesions such as pleomorphic adenoma, basal cell adenoma, and myoepithelioma are interrelated and that histologic diagnoses only result from subtle differences in the differentiation processes underlying salivary gland tumors. As well, this type of approach is critical to understanding the extraordinary histologic features of these tumors, to establishing well-defined diagnostic criteria for individual subtypes of salivary gland neoplasms, and to improving diagnostic skills.

Previously, in classifying salivary gland tumors, certain subtypes were selected and specifically designated on the basis of unique histologic features and biologic behavior. This has resulted in what might be considered a "working" classification format (see Chapter 8). It should be apparent that the taxonomic chart (Table 7–2) and the generally accepted classification scheme complement each other. Only by reassessing current classification

systems will they become increasingly workable and lead to improved accuracy and consistency of diagnoses by oral and general surgical pathologists in this relatively infrequent and fundamentally complicated group of tumors.

REFERENCES

1. Batsakis JG, Regezi JA: The pathology of head and neck tumors: Salivary glands. Part 1. Head Neck Surg 1978; 1:59–68.
2. Thackray AC, Lucas RB: Tumors of the Major Salivary Glands. Atlas of Tumor Pathology, 2nd Series, Fascicle 10. Washington, DC, Armed Forces Institute of Pathology, 1974; 14.
3. Seifert G, Miehlke A, Haubrich J, Chilla R: Diseases of the Salivary Glands. Pathology-Diagnosis-Treatment-Facial Nerve Surgery. Stuttgart, Georg Thieme Verlag, 1986; 171–180.
4. Ellis GL, Gnepp DR: Unusual salivary gland tumors. *In* Gnepp DR (ed.): Pathology of the Head and Neck. New York, Churchill Livingstone, 1988; 586.
5. Luna MA, Batsakis JG, Ordonez NG, Mackay B, Tortoledo ME: Salivary gland adenocarcinomas: A clinicopathologic analysis of three distinctive types. Sem Diagn Pathol 1987; 4:117–135.
6. Gnepp DR, Chen JC, Warren C: Polymorphous low-grade adenocarcinoma of minor salivary gland: An immunohistochemical and clinicopathologic study. Am J Surg Pathol 1988; 12:461–468.

7. Seifert G, Schulz JP. Das Adenokarzinom der SpeicheldrÜsen: Pathohistologie und Subklassifikation von 77 Fallen. HNO 1985; 33:433–442.

8. Eversole LR: Histogenic classification of salivary gland tumors. Arch Pathol 1971; 92:433–443.

9. Regezi JA, Batsakis JG: Histogenesis of salivary gland neoplasms. Otolaryngol Clin North Am 1977; 10:297–307.

10. Batsakis JG: Salivary gland neoplasia: An outcome of modified morphogenesis and cytodifferentiation. Oral Surg Oral Med Oral Pathol 1980; 49:229–232.

11. Attie JN, Sciubba JJ: Tumors of major and minor salivary glands: Clinical and pathologic features. In Current Problems in Surgery. Vol. 18. Chicago, Year Book Medical Publishers Inc, 1981; 80–83.

12. Dardick I, Byard RW, Carnegie JA: A review of proliferative capacity of major salivary glands and the relationship to current concepts of neoplasia in salivary gland. Oral Surg Oral Med Oral Pathol 1990; 69:53–67.

13. Walker NI, Gobe GC: Cell death and cell proliferation during atrophy of the rat parotid gland induced by duct obstruction. J Pathol 1987; 153:333–344.

14. Geiger S, Geiger B, Leitner O, Marshak G: Cytokeratin polypeptide expression in different epithelial elements in human salivary glands. Virchows Arch [A] 1987; 410:403–414.

15. Leoncini P, Cintorino M, Vindigni C, Leoncini L, Armellini D, Bugnoli M, Skalli O, Gabbiani G: Distribution of cytoskeletal and contractile proteins in normal and tumour bearing salivary and lacrimal glands. Virchows Arch [A] 1988; 412:329–337.

16. Born LA, Schwechheimer K, Maier H, Otto HF: Cytokeratin expression in normal salivary glands and in cystadenolymphomas demonstrated by monoclonal antibodies against selective cytokeratin polypeptides. Virchows Arch [A] 1987; 411:588–589.

17. Dardick I, Rippstein P, Skimming L, Boivin M, Dairkee SH: Immunohistochemistry and ultrastructure of myoepithelium and modified myoepithelium of the ducts of human major salivary glands: histogenetic implications for salivary gland tumors. Oral Surg Oral Med Oral Pathol 1987; 64:703–715.

18. Dardick I, Parks WR, Little J, Brown DL: Characterization of cytoskeletal proteins in basal cells of human parotid salivary gland ducts. Virchows Arch [A] 1988; 412:525–532.

19. Jacoby F, Leeson CR: The post-natal development of the rat submaxillary gland. J Anat 1959; 93:201–216.

20. Cutler LS, Chaudhry AP: Cytodifferentiation of acinar cells of the rat submandibular gland. Dev Biol 1974; 41:31–41.

21. Batsakis JG, Brannon RB, Sciubba JJ: Monomorphic adenomas of major salivary glands: a histologic study of 96 tumours. Clin Otolaryngol 1981; 6:129–143.

22. Daley TD, Dardick I: An unusual parotid tumor with histogenetic implications for salivary gland neoplasms. Oral Surg Oral Med Oral Pathol 1983; 55:374–381.

23. Batsakis JG, Kraemer B, Sciubba J: The pathology of head and neck tumors: the myoepithelial cell and its participation in salivary gland neoplasia, part 17. Head Neck Surg 1983; 5:222–233.

24. Batsakis JG, Pinkston GR, Luna MA, Byers RM, Sciubba JJ, Tillery GW: Adenocarcinomas of the oral cavity: a clinicopathologic study of terminal duct carcinoma. J Laryngol Otol 1983; 97:825–835.

25. Donath K, Seifert G, Lentrodt J: The embryonal carcinoma of the parotid gland: a rare example of an embryonal tumor. Virchows Arch [A] 1984; 403:425–440.

26. Dardick I, van Nostrand AWP: Myoepithelial cells in salivary gland tumors—revisited. Head Neck Surg 1985; 7:395–408.

27. Dardick I, van Nostrand AWP: Morphogenesis of salivary gland tumors: a prerequisite to improving classification. Pathol Annu 1987; 22(pt. 1):1–53.

28. Yaku Y: Ultrastructural studies on the development of human fetal salivary glands. Arch Histol Jpn 1983; 46, 677–690.

29. Friedman M, Hall JW: Radiation-induced squamous-cell metaplasia and hyperplasia of the normal mucous glands of the oral cavity. Radiology 1950; 55:848–851.

30. Tamarin A: Submaxillary gland recovery from obstruction: I. Overall changes and electron microscopic alterations of granular duct cells. J Ultrastruct Res 1971; 34:276–287.

31. Tamarin A: Submaxillary gland recovery from obstruction: II. Electron microscopic alterations in acinar cells. J Ultrastruct Res 1971; 34:288–302.

32. Tandler B: Ultrastructure of chronically inflamed human salivary glands. Arch Pathol Lab Med 1977; 101:425–431.

33. Harrison JD, Garrett JR: Histological effects of ductal ligation of salivary glands of the cat. J Pathol 1976; 118:245–254.

34. Harrison JD, Garrett JR: The effects of ductal ligation on the parenchyma of salivary glands of cat studied by enzyme histochemical methods. Histochem J 1976; 8:35–44.

35. Dardick I, Jeans MTD, Sinnott NM, Wittkuhn JF, Kahn HJ, Baumal R: Salivary gland components involved in the formation of squamous metaplasia. Am J Pathol 1985; 119:33–43.

36. Caselitz J, Osborn M, Wustrow J, Seifert G, Weber K: Immunohistochemical investigations on the epimyoepithelial islands in lymphoepithelial lesions: use of monoclonal keratin antibodies. Lab Invest 1986; 55:427–432.

37. Dardick I, van Nostrand AWP, Rippstein P, Skimming L, Hoppe D, Dairkee SH: Characterization of epimyoepithelial islands in benign lymphoepithelial lesions of major salivary gland: an immunohistochemical and ultrastructural study. Head Neck Surg 1988; 10:168–178.

38. Matthews TW, Dardick I: Morphological alterations of salivary gland parenchyma in chronic sialadenitis. J Otolaryngol 1988; 17:385–393.

39. Barka T: Induced cell proliferation: the effect of isoproterenol. Exp Cell Res 1965; 37:662–679.

40. Schneyer CA: β-Adrenergic effects of autonomic agents on mitosis and hypertrophy in rat parotid gland. Proc Soc Exp Biol Med 1969; 131:71–75.

41. Chang WWL: Cell population changes during acinus formation in the postnatal rat submandibular gland. Anat Rec 1974; 178:187–202.

42. Boshnell JL, Pennington C: Histological observations on the effects of isoproterenol on regenerating submandibular glands of the rat. Cell Tissue Res 1980; 213:411–416.

43. Klein RM: Acinar cell proliferation in the parotid and submandibular salivary glands of the neonatal rat. Cell Tissue Kinet 1982; 15:187–195.

44. Sharawy M, O'dell NL: Regeneration of submandibular salivary gland autografted in the rat tongue. Anat Rec 1981; 201:499–511.

45. Dardick I, van Nostrand AWP, Phillips MJ: Histogenesis of salivary gland pleomorphic adenoma (mixed tumor) with an evaluation of the role of the myoepithelial cell. Hum Pathol 1982; 13:62–75.

46. Schneyer CA, Humphreys-Beher M: Effects of epidermal growth factor and nerve growth factor on isoproterenol–induced DNA synthesis in rat parotid and pancreas following removal of the submandibular-sublingual glands. J Oral Pathol 1988; 17:250–256.

47. Ferguson DJP: Ultrastructural characterization of the proliferative (stem?) cells within the parenchyma of the normal "resting" breast. Virchows Arch [A] 1985; 407:379–385.

48. Joshi K, Smith JA, Perusinghe N, Monaghan P: Cell proliferation in the human mammary epithelium: Differential contribution by epithelial and myoepithelial cells. Am J Pathol 1986; 124:199–206.

49. Serratosa J, Domingo J, Enrich C, Bachs O: Nuclear growth and chromatin relaxation-condensation cycle in hepatocytes during the proliferative activation of rat liver. Virchows Arch [B] 1988; 55:57–64.

50. Sigler RE, Newkirk C, McDowell EM: Histogenesis and morphogenesis of epidermoid metaplasia in hamster tracheal organ explant culture. Virchows Arch [B] 1988; 55:47–55.

51. Dardick I, van Nostrand AWP: Recent contributions of electron microscopy to salivary gland pathology. In Motta PM, Riva A (eds.): Ultrastructure of the Extraparietal Glands of the Digestive Tract. Norwell, MA, Klüwer Academic Publishers, 1989; 75–98.

52. Dardick I, Kahn HJ, van Nostrand AWP, Baumal R: Salivary gland monomorphic adenoma: Ultrastructural, immunoperoxidase and histogenetic aspects. Am J Pathol 1984; 115:334–348.

53. Chaudhry AP, Cutler LS, Leifer C, Satchidanand S, Labay G, Yamane G: Histogenesis of acinic cell carcinoma of the major and minor salivary glands: An ultrastructural study. J Pathol 1986; 148:307–320.

54. Dardick I, George D, Jeans MTD, Wittkuhn JF, Skimming L, Rippstein P, van Nostrand AWP: Ultrastructural morphology and cellular differentiation in acinic cell carcinoma. Oral Surg Oral Med Oral Pathol 1987; 63:325–334.

55. Dardick I, Daya D, Hardie J, van Nostrand AWP: Mucoepidermoid carcinoma: Ultrastructural and histogenetic aspects. J Oral Pathol 1984; 13:342–358.

56. Nikai H, El-Bardaie AM, Takata T, Ogawa I, Ijuhin N: Histologic evaluation of myoepithelial participation in salivary gland tumors. Int J Oral Maxillofac Surg 1986; 15:597–605.

57. Dardick I, Hardie J, Thomas MJ, van Nostrand AWP: Ultrastructural contributions to the study of morphological differentiation in malignant mixed (pleomorphic) tumors of salivary gland. Head Neck Surg 1989; 11:5–21.

58. Dardick I, Claude A, Parks WR, Hoppe D, Stinson J, Burns BF, Little J, Brown DL, Dairkee SH: Warthin's tumor: An ultrastructural and immunohistochemical study of basilar epithelium. Ultrastruct Pathol 1988; 12:419–432.

59. Dardick I, van Nostrand AWP, Jeans MTD, Rippstein P, Edwards V: Pleomorphic adenoma: I. Ultrastructural organization of "epithelial" regions. Hum Pathol 1983; 14:780–797.

60. Dardick I, van Nostrand AWP, Jeans MTD, Rippstein P, Edwards V: Pleomorphic adenoma: II. Ultrastructural organization of "stromal" regions. Hum Pathol 1983; 14:798–809.

61. Erlandson RA, Cardon-Cardo C, Higgins PJ: Histogenesis of benign pleomorphic adenoma (mixed tumor) of the major salivary glands: an ultrastructural and immunohistochemical study. Am J Surg Pathol 1984; 8:803–820.

62. Hoshino M, Yamamoto I: Ultrastructure of adenoid cystic carcinoma. Cancer 1970; 25:186–198.

63. Nochomovitz LE, Kahn LB: Adenoid cystic carcinoma of the salivary gland and its histologic variants: A clinicopathologic study of thirty cases. Oral Surg Oral Med Oral Pathol 1977; 44:394–404.

64. Orenstein JM, Dardick I, van Nostrand AWP: Ultrastructural similarities of adenoid cystic carcinoma and pleomorphic adenoma. Histopathology 1985; 9:623–638.

65. Donath K, Seifert G, Schmitz R: Zur Diagnose und Ultrastruktur des Tubularen Speichelgangcarcinoms: Epithelial-myoepitheliales Schalstuckcarcinom. Virchows Arch [A] 1972; 356:16–31.

66. Corio RL, Sciubba JJ, Brannon RB, Batsakis JG: Epithelial-myoepithelial carcinoma of intercalated duct origin. Oral Surg Oral Med Oral Pathol 1982; 53:280–287.

67. Daley TD, Wysocki GP, Smout MS, Slinger RP: Epithelial-myoepithelial carcinoma of salivary glands. Oral Surg Oral Med Oral Pathol 1984; 57:512–519.

68. Luna MA, Ordonez NG, Mackay B, Batsakis JG, Guillamondegui O: Salivary epithelial-myoepithelial carcinomas of intercalated ducts: A clinical, electron microscopic, and immunocytochemical study. Oral Surg Oral Med Oral Pathol 1985; 59:482–490.

69. Chaudhry AP, Satchidanand S, Peer R, Cutler LS: Myoepithelial cell adenoma of the parotid gland: A light and ultrastructural study. Cancer 1982; 49:288–293.

70. Dardick I, van Nostrand AWP: Polymorphous low-grade adenocarcinoma: A case report with ultrastructural findings. Oral Surg Oral Med Oral Pathol 1988; 66:459–465.

71. Sciubba JJ, Brannon RB: Myoepithelioma of salivary glands: Report of 23 cases. Cancer 1982; 49:562–572.

72. Dardick I, Thomas MJ, van Nostrand AWP: Myoepithelioma—new concepts of histology and classification: A light and electron microscopic study. Ultrastruct Pathol 1989; 13:187–224.

73. Barnes L, Appel BN, Perez H, El-Attar AM: Myoepitheliomas of the head and neck: case report and review. J Surg Oncol 1985; 28:21–28.

74. Dardick I, Cavell S, Boivin M, Hoppe D, Parks

WR, Stinson J, Yamada S, Burns BF: Salivary gland myoepithelioma variants: Histological, ultrastructural, and immunohistochemical features. Virchows Arch [A] 1989; 416:25–42.

75. Mori M, Ninomiya T, Okada Y, Tsukitani: Myoepitheliomas and myoepithelial adenomas of salivary gland origin: Immunohistochemical evaluation of filament proteins, S-100 and glial fibrillary acidic proteins, neuron-specific enolase, and lactoferrin. Pathol Res Pract 1989; 184:168–178.

76. Mori M, Tsukitani K, Ninomiya T, Okada Y: Various expressions of modified myoepithelial cells in salivary pleomorphic adenoma. Pathol Res Pract 1987; 182:632–646.

77. Zarbo RJ, Hatfield JS, Trojanowski JQ, Crissman JD, Regezi JA, Maisel H, Batsakis JG: Immunoreactive glial fibrillary acidic protein in normal and neoplastic salivary glands: A combined immunohistochemical and immunoblot study. Surg Pathol 1988; 1:55–63.

78. Achtstatter T, Moll R, Anderson A, Kuhn C, Pilz S, Schwechheimer K, Franke WW: Expression of glial filament protein (GFP) in nerve sheaths and nonneural cells reexamined using monoclonal antibodies, with special emphasis on the co-expression of GFP and cytokeratins in epithelial cells of human salivary gland and pleomorphic adenoma. Differentiation 1986; 31:206–227.

79. Burns BR, Dardick I, Parks WR: Intermediate filament expression in normal parotid glands and pleomorphic adenoma. Virchows Arch [A] 1988; 413:103–112.

80. Yamada K, Shinohara H, Takai Y, Mori M: Monoclonal antibody-detected vimentin distribution in pleomorphic adenoma of salivary glands. J Oral Pathol 1988; 17:348–353.

81. Caselitz J, Löning T, Staquet MJ, Seifert G, Thivolet J: Immunocytochemical demonstration of filamentous structures in the parotid gland: Occurrence of keratin and actin in normal and tumoral parotid gland with special respect to the myoepithelial cells. J Cancer Res Clin Oncol 1981; 100:59–68.

82. Takeuchi J, Sobue M, Yoshida M, Sato E: Glycosaminoglycan-synthetic activity of pleomorphic adenoma, adenoid cystic carcinoma and nonneoplastic tubuloacinar cells of the salivary gland. Cancer 1978; 42:202–208.

83. Takeuchi J, Sobue M, Yoshida M, Esaki T, Katoh Y: Pleomorphic adenoma of the salivary gland with special reference to histochemical and electron microscopic studies and biochemical analysis of glycosaminoglycans in vivo and in vitro. Cancer 1975; 36:1771–1789.

84. Lam RMY: An electron microscopic histochemical study of the histogenesis of major salivary gland pleomorphic adenoma. Ultrastruct Pathol 1985; 8:207–223.

85. Toida M, Takeuchi J, Hara K, Sobue M, Tsukidate K, Goto K, Nakashima N: Histochemical studies of intercellular components of salivary gland tumors with special reference to glycosaminoglycan, laminin and vascular elements. Virchows Arch [A] 1984; 403:15–26.

86. Caselitz J, Schmitt P, Seifert G, Wustrow J, Schuppan D: Basal membrane associated substances in human salivary glands and salivary gland tumours. Pathol Res Pract 1988; 183:386–394.

87. Dardick I, Daley TD, van Nostrand AWP: Basal cell adenoma with myoepithelial cell-derived "stroma": a new major salivary gland tumor entity. Head Neck Surg 1986; 8:257–267.

88. Bernfield MR, Banerjee SD, Cohn RH: Dependence of salivary epithelial morphology and branching morphogenesis upon acid mucopolysaccharide-protein (proteoglycan) at the epithelial surface. J Cell Biol 1972; 52:674–689.

89. Banerjee SD, Cohn RH, Bernfield MR: Basal lamina of embryonic salivary epithelia: production by the epithelium and role in maintaining lobular morphology. J Cell Biol 1977; 73:445–463.

90. Ellis GL, Corio RL: Acinic cell adenocarcinoma: a clinicopathologic analysis of 294 cases. Cancer 1983; 52:542–549.

91. Mackay B, Ordóñez NG, Batsakis JG: Pleomorphic adenoma of parotid with myoepithelial cell predominance. Ultrastruct Pathol 1988; 12:461–468.

92. Hamper K, Schmitz-Watjen W, Mausch H-E, Caselitz J, Seifert G: Multiple expression of tissue markers in mucoepidermoid carcinomas and acinic cell carcinomas of the salivary glands. Virchows Arch [A] 1989; 414:407–413.

93. Gardner DG, Daley TD: The use of the terms monomorphic adenoma, basal cell adenoma and canalicular adenoma as applied to salivary gland tumors. Oral Surg Oral Med Oral Pathol 1981; 56:608–615.

94. Dardick I, van Nostrand AWP: Recent contributions of electron microscopy to salivary gland pathology. In Motta PM, Riva A (eds.): Ultrastructure of the Extraparietal Glands of the Digestive Tract. Norwell, MA, Kluwer Academic Publishers, 1989; 75–98.

95. Dairkee SH, Blayney C, Smith HS, Hackett AJ: Monoclonal antibody that identifies human myoepithelium. Proc Natl Acad Sci USA 1985; 82:7409–7413.

96. Dairkee SH, Blayney-Moore CM, Smith HS, Hackett AJ: Concurrent expression of basal and luminal epithelial markers in cultures of normal human breast analyzed using monoclonal antibodies. Differentiation 1986; 32:93–100.

97. Luna MA, Mackay B, Gomez-Araujo J: Myoepithelioma of the palate. Cancer 1973; 32:1429–1435.

98. Min BH, Miller AS, Leifer C, Putong PB: Basal cell adenoma of the parotid gland. Arch Otolaryngol 1974; 99:88–93.

99. Jao W, Keh PC, Swerdlow MA: Ultrastructure of the basal cell adenoma of the parotid gland. Cancer 1976; 37:1322–1333.

100. Suzuki J: Basal cell adenoma with acinic differentiation. Acta Pathol Jpn 1982; 32:1085–1092.

101. Hsu S-M, Raine L: Warthin's tumor—Epithelial cell differences. Am J Clin Pathol 1982; 77:78–81.

102. Palmer RM. Epithelial-myoepithelial carcinoma: An immunocytochemical study. Oral Surg Oral Med Oral Pathol 1985; 59:511–515.

103. Nicolatou O, Harwick RD, Putong P: Ultrastructural characterization of intermediate cells of mucoepidermoid carcinoma of parotid. Oral Surg Oral Med Oral Pathol 1979; 48:324–336.

104. Chen S-Y: Ultrastructure of mucoepidermoid carcinoma in minor salivary glands. Oral Surg Oral Med Oral Pathol 1979; 47:247–255.

105. Chomette G, Auriol M, Tereau Y, Vaillant JM: Les

tumeurs mucoepidermoides des glandes salivaires accessoires: Dénombrement. Etude clinicopathologique, histoenzymologique et ultrastructurale. Ann Pathol (Paris) 1982; 2:29–40.

106. Chaudhry AP, Cutler LS, Liefer C, Labay G, Satchidanand S, Yamane GM: Ultrastructural study of the histogenesis of salivary gland mucoepidermoid carcinoma. J Oral Pathol Med 1989; 18:400–409.

107. Hübner G, Kleinsasser O, Klein HJ: Zur Feinstruktur der Speichelgangcarcinome: Ein Beitrag zur Rolle der Myoepithelzellen in Speicheldrüsengeschwulsten. Virchows Arch [A] 1979; 346:1–14.

108. Smith JA, Warhol MJ, Brodsky GL: An immunohistochemical study of a carcinoma of the parotid gland exhibiting both ductal and acinic cell differentiation. Oral Surg Oral Med Oral Pathol 1983; 55:267–273.

109. Nagao K, Matsuzaki O, Saiga H, Sugano I, Kaneko T, Katoh T, Kitamura T, Shigematsu H, Maruyama N: Histopathologic studies on adenocarcinoma of parotid gland. Acta Pathol Jpn 1986; 36:337–347.

8

CLASSIFICATION OF SALIVARY GLAND NEOPLASMS

Gary L. Ellis and Paul L. Auclair

Classification involves the systematic categorization of tumors on the basis of designated characteristics for the purpose of predicting potential biologic behavior so that appropriate therapeutic modalities can be used. Although classification is particularly important for malignant neoplasms, it is advantageous to specifically classify benign tumors as well. Subtle variations in therapy may exist for different benign neoplasms, but more significantly, the ability to specifically classify a neoplasm instills confidence in its predicted biologic behavior and the selection of treatment.

The classification scheme for salivary gland neoplasms is not static. Indeed, it is a dynamic, evolving process that undergoes continuous refinement as research and experience increase our understanding of these diseases and the differences among them. Nor has there been a single, universally used classification system for salivary gland tumors. At the time of preparation of this text, the World Health Organization is in the process of revising its well-known classification of salivary gland neoplasms; Gary L. Ellis, one of the authors of this chapter as well as of this book, is on the committee that is formulating this revision. It appears that our classification system is similar to what will be the World Health Organization's revised system. The classification system that we currently use at the Armed Forces Institute of Pathology (AFIP) is given in Table 8–1. It is what we have termed a "morphologic working classification," and it segregates neoplastic entities by type and by predicted biologic behavior. Unquestionably, like all classifications of neoplasms, this classification system will undergo modification, just as it has in the past. In the future, some of the histogenetic and morphogenetic concepts and features described in Chapter 7 will undoubtedly

have a significant influence on the classification of salivary gland tumors. The developing information on oncogene expression, gene rearrangements, cytogenetic abnormalities, morphometry, flow cytophotometry, and other cellular and molecular parameters will also influence classification; however, histomorphology will probably continue as the foundation on which modifications in classification are made.

Tables 8–2 to 8–7 present several of the best-known and widely used tumor classification schemes that have been formulated during the past 35 years.[1–6] These provide not only a historical perspective on terminology and classification but also a regional perspective, since both American[1, 5] and European[2, 4, 6] authors are represented. The classification by Foote and Frazell[1] (Table 8–2) and that by Thackray and Lucas[4] (Table 8–5) have often been referred to by pathologists and others as the "AFIP classification" because they were published as part of the AFIP Fascicle series. However, we stress that these classifications were not authored by AFIP pathologists, were not based on the case materials at the AFIP, and do not necessarily represent the classification scheme used by pathologists at the AFIP. We hope this comment helps avoid confusion of our classification with those that have appeared or may appear in the Fascicles, which have typically been authored by individuals selected from outside the AFIP.

Despite the changes in terminology and the addition and deletion of some neoplastic entities from one classification system to the next, there is a core of neoplasms that has remained fairly consistent over time, including mixed tumor (pleomorphic adenoma), Warthin's tumor (papillary cystadenoma lymphomatosum, adenolymphoma),

Table 8–1. AFIP Morphologic Classification of Salivary Gland Neoplasms
by Ellis and Auclair, 1990

Primary Epithelial Neoplasms
Benign
  Mixed tumor (pleomorphic adenoma)
  Papillary cystadenoma lymphomatosum
    (Warthin's tumor)
  Oncocytoma
  Cystadenoma
  Basal cell adenoma
  Canalicular adenoma
  Ductal papillomas
    Sialadenoma papilliferum
    Inverted ductal papilloma
    Intraductal papilloma
  Myoepithelioma
  Sebaceous adenomas
    Sebaceous adenoma
    Sebaceous lymphadenoma
  Adenoma, not otherwise specified
Malignant
  Low-grade
    Mucoepidermoid carcinoma, low-grade
    Acinic cell adenocarcinoma
    Polymorphous low-grade adenocarcinoma
      (terminal duct carcinoma)
    Basal cell adenocarcinoma
    Adenocarcinoma, not otherwise specified,
      low-grade
    Metastasizing mixed tumor
  Intermediate-grade
    Mucoepidermoid carcinoma, intermediate-
      grade
    Adenoid cystic carcinoma, cribriform-
      tubular
    Epithelial-myoepithelial carcinoma
    Adenocarcinoma, not otherwise specified,
      intermediate-grade
    Clear cell carcinoma
    Cystadenocarcinoma
      Papillary
      Nonpapillary
    Sebaceous carcinomas
      Sebaceous carcinoma
      Sebaceous lymphadenocarcinoma
    Mucinous adenocarcinoma

High-grade
  Mucoepidermoid carcinoma, high-grade
  Adenoid cystic carcinoma, solid
  Malignant mixed tumor
    Carcinoma ex mixed tumor
    Carcinosarcoma
  Adenocarcinoma, not otherwise specified, high-
    grade
  Squamous cell carcinoma
  Undifferentiated carcinoma
    Small cell carcinoma
    Lymphoepithelial carcinoma (malignant
      lymphoepithelial lesion)
    Others
  Oncocytic carcinoma
  Adenosquamous carcinoma
  Salivary duct carcinoma
  Myoepithelial carcinoma
Nonepithelial Neoplasms of the Major Salivary Glands
Benign mesenchymal
  Hemangioma
  Schwannoma
  Neurofibroma
  Lipoma
  Others
Sarcomas
  Hemangiopericytoma
  Malignant schwannoma
  Fibrosarcoma
  Malignant fibrous histiocytoma
  Rhabdomyosarcoma
  Others
Lymphomas
  Non-Hodgkin's lymphoma
  Hodgkin's disease
Metastatic Neoplasms
Malignant melanoma
Squamous cell carcinoma
Renal cell carcinoma
Thyroid carcinoma
Others

Table 8–2. The Classification of Salivary Gland Neoplasms by Foote and Frazell, 1954*

Benign
    Mixed tumor
    Papillary cystadenomata lymphomatosa
    Oxyphil adenoma
    Sebaceous cell adenoma
    Benign lymphoepithelial lesion
    Unclassified
Malignant
    Malignant mixed tumor
    Mucoepidermoid tumor, low-grade and high-grade
    Squamous cell carcinoma
    Adenocarcinoma
        Adenoid cystic
        Trabecular or solid
        Anaplastic
        Mucous cell
        Pseudoadamantine
        Acinic cell
    Unclassified

*From Foote FW Jr, Frazell EL: Tumors of the Major Salivary Glands, Section IV, Fascicle 11, 1st series. Atlas of Tumor Pathology. Washington DC, Armed Forces Institute of Pathology, 1954; 8.

oncocytoma (oxyphil adenoma), mucoepidermoid tumor, acinic cell tumor, adenoid cystic carcinoma, adenocarcinoma, squamous cell (epidermoid) carcinoma, and carcinoma ex mixed tumor. Nevertheless, a few comments about terminology are necessary. We consider arguments for the preferability of either the term *mixed tumor* or the term *pleomorphic adenoma* to be unproductive; both terms are equally acceptable and universally recognized for what they represent. We have traditionally used the term *mixed tumor*. We do prefer the term *papillary cystadenoma lymphomatosum* to the term *adenolymphoma* because we think any implication that this tumor is associated with or related to lymphoma, a term which is accepted as meaning a malignant neoplasm of lymphocytes, is misleading. Perhaps the eponym *Warthin's tumor* is a good compromise and a term that seems to be universally recognized. Of course, *oxyphil cell adenoma* and *oncocytoma* are synonymous terms. We now consider all mucoepidermoid and acinic cell neoplasms to have at least some malignant potential and unequivocally prefer the terms *mucoepidermoid carcinoma* and *acinic cell adenocarcinoma* over mucoepidermoid *tumor* and acinic cell *tumor*, respectively, which have been used to indicate equivocation on biologic behavior or the inclusion of both benign and malignant variants.

Monomorphic adenoma is a term that has been widely used and, we believe, somewhat abused. There seems to be confusion or at least a lack of agreement about its exact connotation. It appears that the term was first used by Thackray and Sobin[3] in the World Health Organization classification (Table 8–4). In that classification and in the subsequent classifications of Thackray and

Lucas[4] (Table 8–5) and Seifert and colleagues[6] (Table 8–7), the term monomorphic adenoma is used to encompass *all* salivary gland adenomas other than mixed tumors (pleomorphic adenomas). On the other hand, Batsakis[5] and Shafer and colleagues[7] are more restrictive in their use of the term. Batsakis[5] (Table 8–6) excluded Warthin's tumor, oncocytoma, sebaceous adenoma, sebaceous lymphadenoma, and ductal papillomas as well as mixed tumor, whereas Shafer and

Table 8–3. The Classification of Salivary Gland Neoplasms by Evans and Cruickshank, 1970*

Epithelial tumors
    Benign
        Mixed tumor
        Adenolymphoma
        Mucoepidermoid tumor
        Acinic cell adenoma
        Solid adenoma
        Tubular solid adenoma
        Basal cell adenoma
        Oncocytoma
        Clear cell adenoma
        Sebaceous adenoma
        Sebaceous lymphoma
        Intraduct papilloma
        Mucinous cyst
    Malignant
        Carcinoma ex mixed tumor
        Malignant mixed tumor
        Mucoepidermoid tumor
        Acinic cell carcinoma
        Adenocystic carcinoma
        Malignant basal cell tumor
        Adenocarcinoma
        Sebaceous carcinoma
        Intraduct carcinoma
        Undifferentiated carcinoma
            Spindle cell
            Spheroidal
            Trabecular
        Squamous cell carcinoma
        Papillary carcinoma
        Adenoacanthoma
        Malignant oncocytoma
        Salivary duct carcinoma
    Connective tissue tumors
        Hemangioma
        Lymphangioma
        Lipoma
        Fibrosarcoma
        Chondrosarcoma
    Miscellaneous tumors
        Malignant lymphoma
        Melanoma
        Neuroblastoma
        Myelomatosis
        Branchial cyst
        Neurilemoma
        Neurofibroma
        Embryoma
    Metastatic tumors

*From Evans RW, Cruickshank AH: Epithelial Tumours of the Salivary Glands. Philadelphia, WB Saunders Co, 1970; 19.

Table 8–4. The Classification of
Salivary Gland Neoplasms by
the World Health Organization, 1972*

Epithelial tumors
  Adenomas
    Pleomorphic adenoma
    Monomorphic adenoma
      Adenolymphoma
      Oxyphilic adenoma
      Other
  Mucoepidermoid tumor
  Acinic cell tumor
  Carcinomas
    Adenoid cystic carcinoma
    Adenocarcinoma
    Epidermoid carcinoma
    Undifferentiated carcinoma
    Carcinoma in pleomorphic adenoma
Nonepithelial tumors
Unclassified tumors
Allied conditions
  Benign lymphoepithelial lesion
  Sialosis
  Oncocytosis

*From Thackray AC, Sobin LH: Histological Typing of Salivary Gland Tumours. Geneva, World Health Organization, 1972.

and should be recognized separately from basal cell adenoma (see Chapter 12).

The term *malignant mixed tumor (malignant pleomorphic adenoma)* has frequently been used to identify an adenocarcinoma that has arisen in a preexisting mixed tumor. Although it is certainly the most common type of malignant mixed tumor, this neoplasm is more appropriately called *carcinoma ex mixed tumor* because two other rare tumors, *carcinosarcoma* and *metastasizing mixed tumor,* may also be rightly considered malignant mixed tumors. See Chapter 20 for a thorough discussion.

As evident from Tables 8–1 to 8–7, the classification by Foote and Frazell[1] in 1954 (Table 8–2) was limited compared with the scopes of the subsequent classifications compiled by Evans and Cruickshank[2] (Table 8–3), Batsakis[5] (Table 8–6), and ourselves (Table 8–1). The World Health Organization classification (Table 8–4) in 1972 was also quite brief, but it was probably intended to satisfy the classification requirements for the majority of salivary gland neoplasms seen in an average general surgical pathology service at that time. In the context of current understanding of salivary gland tumors, the limitations and inadequacies of the World Health Organization's system have been realized, and we believe the revised

colleagues[7] seem to confine the use of the term to only basal cell adenoma and canalicular adenoma. Although these various investigators have differing parameters for monomorphic adenoma, they all exclude mixed tumor from this category and include a heterogeneous group of adenomas with varying histomorphology, incidence, and site predilection. Because a diagnosis of monomorphic adenoma will result in appropriate therapy in most cases, regardless of the specific type of adenoma, we have no quarrel with those pathologists who find it expedient to use that term, but we believe it is best to be as specific as possible. For example, we have found that some pathologists, including ourselves in the past, have used the term monomorphic adenoma for those occasional adenomas that defy specific classification into one of our defined categories of adenoma. Unfortunately, this group of monomorphic adenomas then combines specifically classifiable and unclassified adenomas in a conglomeration that seems to defeat the purpose of classification. Therefore, we have adopted a classification system for adenomas that categorizes currently unclassifiable adenomas as *adenoma, not otherwise specified,* and attempts to avoid the confusing term *monomorphic adenoma.*

Because we have mentioned canalicular adenoma and basal cell adenoma, we should state that there is some controversy about whether or not canalicular adenoma is an entity distinct from basal cell adenoma. We believe that canalicular adenoma has distinct clinicopathologic features

Table 8–5. The Classification of Salivary Gland Neoplasms by Thackray and Lucas, 1974*

Adenomas
  Pleomorphic adenoma
  Monomorphic adenoma
    Adenolymphoma
    Oxyphilic adenoma
    Tubular adenoma
    Clear cell adenoma
    Basal cell adenoma
    Trabecular adenoma
    Sebaceous adenoma
    Sebaceous lymphadenoma
Mucoepidermoid tumor
Acinic cell tumor
Carcinomas
  Adenoid cystic carcinoma
  Adenocarcinoma
  Epidermoid carcinoma
  Undifferentiated carcinoma
  Carcinoma in pleomorphic adenoma
  Malignant lymphoepithelial lesion
Connective tissue and other tumors
  Benign
    Hemangioma
    Lymphangioma
    Lipoma
    Neurinoma
  Sarcoma
  Lymphoma
Metastatic tumors

*From Thackray AC, Lucas RB: Tumors of the Major Salivary Glands. Fascicle 10, 2nd Series, Atlas of Tumor Pathology. Washington, DC, Armed Forces Institute of Pathology, 1974.

Table 8–6. The Classification of
Epithelial Salivary Gland Neoplasms
by Batsakis, 1979*

Benign
  Mixed tumor
  Papillary cystadenoma lymphomatosum (Warthin's tumor)
  Oncocytoma
  Monomorphic tumors
    Basal cell adenoma
    Glycogen-rich adenoma (?)
    Clear cell adenoma
    Membranous adenoma
    Myoepithelioma
  Sebaceous tumors
    Adenoma
    Lymphadenoma
  Papillary ductal adenoma (papilloma)
  Benign lymphoepithelial lesion
  Unclassified
Malignant
  Carcinoma ex pleomorphic adenoma
  Malignant mixed tumor
  Mucoepidermoid carcinoma; low-grade, intermediate-grade, and high-grade
  Adenoid cystic carcinoma
  Acinous cell carcinoma
  Adenocarcinoma
    Mucus-producing adenopapillary and nonpapillary carcinoma
    Salivary duct carcinoma
    Other
  Oncocytic carcinoma
  Clear cell carcinoma
  Squamous cell carcinoma
  Hybrid basal cell adenoma/adenoid cystic carcinoma
  Undifferentiated carcinoma
  Epithelial-myoepithelial carcinoma
  Miscellaneous
  Unclassified

*From Batsakis JG: Tumors of the Head and Neck: Clinical and Pathological Considerations, 2nd Ed. Baltimore, Williams & Wilkins, 1979; 9.

classification will be greatly expanded. The AFIP classification (Table 8–1) is fairly comprehensive and includes long-established and newly defined, but definitive, entities as well as a few tumors that have not been well defined in the literature.

Of the seven classification schemes presented (Tables 8–1 to 8–7), only those devised by Batsakis[5] (Table 8–6) and by ourselves include *myoepithelioma*. The argument can be made that myoepithelioma merely represents one extreme end of the spectrum of mixed tumor and that such tumors can be properly classified as mixed tumors. We do not disagree with this argument but base our justification of the segregation of myoepitheliomas on their distinctive histopathologic features, which are more easily confused with benign mesenchymal neoplasms than are the features of any other epithelial salivary gland neoplasm.

Epithelial-myoepithelial carcinoma and *salivary duct carcinoma* are two examples of uncommon salivary gland neoplasms that only recently have become clearly defined (see Chapters 24 and 27). In fact, Kleinsasser and colleagues[8] may be credited with one of the earliest descriptions of both of these tumors, but they described them as one entity under the term *salivary duct carcinoma*. It is only as additional reports of similar tumors have slowly accumulated in the literature that it has become apparent that there are two distinct histopathologic entities. The importance of segregating these two entities is punctuated by the fact that salivary duct carcinoma is a high-grade malignant tumor, whereas epithelial-myoepithelial carcinoma is an intermediate-grade tumor with a much better prognosis. It is also clear that several reports of so-called *clear cell adenoma* actually represented what we now identify as *epithelial-myoepithelial carcinoma* (see Chapter 24 and the discussion of clear cell tumors in Chapter 22). We consider all clear cell neoplasms of salivary glands to be malignant, except for the clear cell variant of oncocytoma (see Chapter 13). Therefore, although several of the previous classification schemes for salivary gland tumors[2, 4–6] (Tables 8–3 and 8–5 through 8–7) included clear cell adenoma, our classification system (Table 8–1) does not.

Another entity that does not appear in any of the previous classification systems is *polymorphous low-grade adenocarcinoma* (see Chapter 23). Our

Table 8–7. The Classification of
Salivary Gland Neoplasms
by Seifert and Colleagues, 1986*

Adenomas
  Pleomorphic adenoma
  Monomorphic adenoma
    Cystadenolymphoma
    Duct adenoma
    Basal cell adenoma
    Oncocytoma
    Sebaceous adenoma
    Clear cell adenoma
    Other
Malignant epithelial tumors
  Acinic cell tumor
  Mucoepidermoid tumor
  Carcinoma
    Adenoid cystic carcinoma
    Adenocarcinoma
    Squamous cell carcinoma
    Carcinoma ex pleomorphic adenoma
    Duct carcinoma
    Undifferentiated carcinoma
    Other
Nonepithelial tumors
Metastatic tumors

*From Seifert G, Miehlke A, Haubrich J, Chilla R: Diseases of the Salivary Glands: Pathology-Diagnosis-Treatment-Facial Nerve Surgery. Stuttgart, Georg Thieme Verlag, 1986; 171.

experience indicates that, since its definitive segregation from the heterogeneous group of adenocarcinomas, not otherwise specified, in 1983, this neoplasm is one of the more common malignant neoplasms of minor salivary glands. The identification of this tumor epitomizes both the evolutionary process and the purpose of classification. As a low-grade adenocarcinoma, its biologic potential and treatment are significantly different from those for adenocarcinoma, not otherwise specified, which is a neoplasm that is commonly considered to be a high-grade malignancy. The terminology for this neoplasm is still somewhat unsettled, as the terms *polymorphous low-grade adenocarcinoma, lobular carcinoma,* and *terminal duct carcinoma* have all been used synonymously. A majority seem to favor the term *polymorphous low-grade adenocarcinoma,* which is our preference as well.

REFERENCES

1. Foote FW Jr, Frazell EL: Tumors of the Major Salivary Glands, Section IV, Fascicle 11, Atlas of Tumor Pathology. Washington, DC, Armed Forces Institute of Pathology, 1954; 8.
2. Evans RW, Cruickshank AH: Epithelial Tumours of the Salivary Glands. Philadelphia, WB Saunders Co, 1970; 19.
3. Thackray AC, Sobin LH: Histological Typing of Salivary Gland Tumours. Geneva, World Health Organization, 1972.
4. Thackray AC, Lucas RB: Tumors of the Major Salivary Glands, Fascicle 10, 2nd Series. Atlas of Tumor Pathology. Washington, DC, Armed Forces Institute of Pathology, 1974.
5. Batsakis JG: Tumors of the Head and Neck: Clinical and Pathological Considerations, 2nd Ed. Baltimore, Williams & Wilkins, 1979; 9.
6. Seifert G, Miehlke A, Haubrich J, Chilla R: Diseases of the Salivary Glands: Pathology-Diagnosis-Treatment-Facial Nerve Surgery. Stuttgart, Georg Thieme Verlag, 1986; 171.
7. Shafer WG, Hine MK, Levy BM: A Textbook of Oral Pathology, 4th Ed. Philadelphia, WB Saunders Co, 1983; 235–237.
8. Kleinsasser O, Klein HJ, Hubner G: Speichelgangcarcinom: Ein den Milchgangcarcinomen der Brustdruse analoge Gruppe von Speicheldrusentumoren. Arch Klin Exp Ohre Nasen Kehlkopfheilkd 1968; 192:100–115.

Chapter

9

SALIVARY GLAND NEOPLASMS: GENERAL CONSIDERATIONS

Paul L. Auclair, Gary L. Ellis, Douglas R. Gnepp,
Bruce M. Wenig, and Christine G. Janney

Salivary gland tumors may arise from the parotid, submandibular, and sublingual glands; the minor glands throughout the oral mucosa and pharynx; the seromucous glands of the nasal passages, sinuses, and larynx; and ectopic salivary gland tissue. Although discussion of salivary gland tumors is usually limited to tumors that take origin from the epithelial parenchyma, primary nonparenchymal tumors represent a significant minority of the tumors arising in the major glands. Therefore, although most of our attention is devoted to epithelial tumors, mesenchymal neoplasms are also included in our discussion. Furthermore, in our experience, the frequency of metastatic disease in the parotid glands necessitates careful consideration of the possibility of this disease; thus data concerning metastases to the major glands are presented.

Before presentation of data, a few comments are needed regarding the nature of the cases accumulated by the Armed Forces Institute of Pathology (AFIP) that form much of the basis of this text. We recognize that in some respects the experience of the AFIP with salivary gland tumors is unique. For instance, the ratio of inflammatory to neoplastic salivary gland lesions in the AFIP files is low compared to the ratios reported by most surgical pathology laboratories. Obviously, consultations for inflammatory lesions are not sought as often as for neoplasms. It could also be suggested that many so-called "classic" examples of salivary gland tumors are less likely to be referred to the AFIP for consultation than are those that are atypical or less common; in other words, second opinions may be more likely to be sought for bizarre, one-of-a-kind cases. However, there are several reasons that lead us to consider

this effect as minimal. Only rarely are cases received for consultation from large "cancer treatment centers." Most cases are received from small- and medium-sized laboratories, in which all types of salivary gland tumors are considered relatively unusual. Lack of extensive experience often leads pathologists to seek second opinions on typical, more common tumors. Furthermore, our experience regarding the proportion of different salivary gland tumor types, in general, parallels that found in the few large, previously published series. In most instances, the proportion of specific histologic types and the clinical parameters, such as patient's age, sex, and site of the neoplasms, in the AFIP files closely reflect the experience of other investigators in the United States. The number of cases in the registry of salivary gland pathology at the AFIP exceeds that in any previously published series; this allows even less common tumors to be clinicopathologically characterized and correlated, which is often not possible in smaller series.

The cases in the AFIP registry have been accessioned from both military and civilian pathologists. The cases were accessioned during the last 45 years, and 61 per cent of all the cases in which the source is known were received from civilian institutions. During those 45 years, there have been many changes in the nomenclature, classification, and interpretation of salivary gland tumors. Undoubtedly, if we reviewed every case in the AFIP files, some would be reclassified. However, about 52 per cent of the cases have been accessioned since 1970, and we believe that the classification of the vast majority reflects contemporary knowledge and biologic concepts.

One last note concludes the introductory comments. The fascicle, *Tumors of the Major Salivary Glands*, written by Thackray and Lucas,[1] is often cited as reflecting the AFIP experience. The reader should be aware that the AFIP's affiliation with that monograph was limited to its publication. There is no connection between the monograph's contents and our experience with salivary gland tumors, either in the past or as presented in this text.

INCIDENCE OF SALIVARY GLAND NEOPLASMS

Because of the rarity of tumors of the salivary glands, they are often included as "miscellaneous" or "other" head and neck tumors in epidemiologic surveys of neoplasia. Nevertheless, although data on the incidence of benign tumors are frequently not available, cancer registries provide substantial data regarding the incidence of malignant tumors. However, as noted by Waterhouse and coworkers,[2] malignancy in some registries may be based on clinical parameters rather than on cytologic features; thus comparison of incidence rates must be performed with caution.

As shown in Table 9–1, the annual incidence of salivary gland tumors varies around the world from approximately 0.4 to 13.5 cases per 100,000 people.[3–16] As noted in the table, some of these

figures concern only parotid tumors, only tumors in the major glands, or only malignant tumors; one study included all tumors except Warthin's tumor. Evans and Cruickshank[9] estimated that from 1944 to 1956 the annual incidence of salivary gland tumors, excluding Warthin's tumor, in 2.8 million people living in the United Kingdom was 1.1 cases per 100,000 people; a later study[10] of the United Kingdom population demonstrated a higher annual incidence of 2.4 cases per 100,000 people. Furthermore, this later study was limited to parotid tumors, and the investigators felt their figure was an underestimation, because, although they could eliminate false-positive cases, they could not identify parotid tumors mistakenly classified as non-neoplastic disease. In their study of the people of eastern Scotland, Lennox and coworkers[11] showed that the annual incidence of all tumors of the major salivary glands was 4.2 per 100,000 people. They noted that numerous errors occurred in the reporting of the incidence of these tumors, but they too suggested that the errors were more likely to indicate too low an incidence than too high an incidence. The Danish Cancer Registry has recorded annual incidences per 100,000 people of 0.6 malignant salivary gland tumors in males and 0.4 in females in the years from 1973 to 1980.[13] From 1958 to 1962, the rates in men and women had been 1.2 and 1.3 cases, respectively, but steadily declined thereafter. Poulsen and colleagues[14] studied a population residing

Table 9–1. Incidence of Salivary Gland Tumors Around the World

Investigator(s) (Year Reported)	Geographic Location of Study	Annual Incidence (Number of Cases per 100,000 People)
Wallace and colleagues (1963)[5]	Canada (Eskimos)	13.5
Davies and colleagues (1964)[6]	Uganda	0.7
Loke (1967)[7]	Malaysia	1.0
Doll and colleagues (1970)[3]	Israel (western immigrants)	3.6
	South Africa (whites)	3.4
Evans and Cruickshank (1970)[9]	United Kingdom	1.1*
Lennox and colleagues (1978)[11]	Scotland	4.2†
Gunn and Parrott (1988)[10]	United Kingdom	2.4‡
Thomas and colleagues (1980)[8]	Malawi, Africa	0.4
Takeichi and colleagues (1983)[47]	Hiroshima City, Japan (non-exposed population)	0.6
Poulsen and colleagues (1987)[14]	Denmark (Funen county)	5.8‡
Dorn and Cutler (1959)[15]	United States	2.0¶
White females		2.1¶
White males		2.1¶
Nonwhite females		2.6¶
Nonwhite males		2.5¶
National Cancer Institute (1989)[16]	United States	
Both sexes, blacks and whites		0.9¶
Black females		0.7¶
White females		0.8¶
All females		0.8¶
Black males		0.8¶
White males		1.2¶
All males		1.2¶

*Excluded Warthin's tumor
†Major glands only
‡Parotid only
¶Malignant only

in one county in Denmark, and over a 5-year period, they found the yearly incidences per 100,000 people for malignant, benign, and all salivary gland tumors to be 0.7, 5.1, and 5.8 cases, respectively.

Historically, the one noteworthy exception to the otherwise relatively low incidence of salivary gland tumors among any population involves the Inuit living in the western and central Canadian Arctic.[17, 18] In the time period from 1950 to 1966, salivary gland tumors, predominantly lymphoepithelial carcinoma, accounted for 25 per cent of all cancers affecting this population. So prevalent were these tumors that they were coined "eskimomas." The mortality rate resulting from these tumors was nearly 100 and 400 times greater among Inuit men and women, respectively, than the rate among all Canadian men and women. However, although the rate of salivary gland carcinoma remained relatively high among these people after 1966, its relative frequency declined dramatically as cancers at other sites increased.[18]

In the United States, data on salivary gland tumors are generally limited to the incidence of salivary gland carcinoma. In 1959, Dorn and Cutler[15] reported slightly higher rates of carcinoma in nonwhites than in whites. Recent data (May, 1989) from the Surveillance, Epidemiology, and End Results (SEER) registries of the National Cancer Institute[16] show the age-adjusted incidence of salivary gland cancer from 1982 to 1986 in all races and both sexes to be 0.9 cases per 100,000 people. Incidences categorized by sex and race in the United States are shown in Table 9–1. Because most large studies in the United States have shown that malignant tumors comprise between 35 and 40 per cent of all salivary gland tumors, we estimate that the annual incidence of both benign and malignant salivary gland tumors in the United States is between 2.2 and 2.5 cases per 100,000 people. Recently Bouquot and colleagues[19] studied the changing incidence of salivary gland tumors in the population of Rochester, Minnesota during the period from 1935 to 1984. The average annual incidences per 100,000 people were 4.9 cases, 1.6 cases, and 6.5 cases for adenomas, carcinomas, and all salivary gland tumors, respectively. The carcinoma incidence rate decreased over the 49-year period from 3.2 to 0.9 cases per 100,000 people, whereas the adenoma incidence rate increased from 3.2 to 10.4 cases per 100,000 people. Age-specific incidence rates for adenomas showed a biphasic pattern with peaks in young adults and patients in their seventh and eighth decades of life. However, incidence rates for adenocarcinomas steadily increased with age and peaked in the seventh and eighth decades.

Frazell, one of the first investigators[20] to study large numbers of salivary gland tumors, determined that after excluding skin tumors major salivary gland tumors accounted for 5 per cent of all tumors seen in the Head and Neck Service of Memorial Hospital for Cancer and Allied Diseases, New York. Spiro and coworkers[21, 22] later reported from the same treatment center that salivary gland tumors accounted for about 1 percent of all admissions and about 6.5 percent of admissions for all head and neck tumors. Leegard and Lindeman[23] have stated that salivary gland tumors constitute about 2 percent of all neoplasms of the head and neck.

Ethnicity and geographic location of a population apparently have an effect on the frequency of occurrence of salivary gland tumors. Loke[7] studied the population of Malaysia, which was composed of three main racial groups, and found that of tumors at all sites, the proportion of salivary gland tumors was 4.1 percent among Malays, 2.3 percent among Chinese, and 1.7 percent among Indians. One survey[24] has shown that the incidence among several different ethnic groups was also influenced by their city of residence. For example, Japanese, Chinese, and whites (of European ancestry) all had higher age-adjusted incidence rates of salivary gland tumors if they lived in San Francisco rather than in Osaka, Hong Kong, or Los Angeles, respectively.

CLINICAL FINDINGS

At the time of the preparation of this chapter there were 13,749 benign and malignant epithelial salivary gland tumors in the files of the AFIP. In addition to these cases, there were 291 benign and malignant nonlymphoid mesenchymal tumors, 455 Hodgkin's and non-Hodgkin's malignant lymphomas, 490 metastatic tumors, and 85 cases that could not be further classified either histogenetically or by biologic potential. Thus, primary epithelial tumors constituted 91 percent of 15,070 neoplasms in the salivary glands. The breakdown of the cases by category and site of involvement is shown in Table 9–2.

Of the 13,749 epithelial salivary gland tumors, 63.2 percent were benign, and 36.8 percent were malignant. Comparison of these figures with those from other large series of cases from the Memorial Sloan-Kettering Cancer Center,[22] the Radiumhemmet and Karolinska Sjukhuset,[25] the Salivary Gland Register at the Pathology Institute of the University of Hamburg,[26] and the British Salivary Gland Panel[27] is shown in Table 9–3. There are probably several explanations for the observed differences in these series, including the nature of the cases normally referred to the reporting center, whether or not all tumors of the oral cavity were included, and possibly the geographic location of the patients. We have noted that the differences seem most closely related to the proportion of tumors reported that occurred in the minor salivary glands (see Table 9–3). More than 20 percent of all reported cases of tumors at the

Table 9–2. Distribution of All Salivary Gland Tumors, Including Metastases to the Major Glands, in the AFIP Registry by Category and Site of Involvement

Diagnosis	Major Glands				Minor Glands											Total
	Parotid	Sub-mandibular	Sub-lingual	Neck (NOS)*	Upper Lip	Lower Lip	Lip (NOS)*	Palate	Tongue	Cheek	Retro-molar	Floor of Mouth	Tonsil/Oro-pharynx	Other	Not Stated	
Benign epithelial	5,566	725	14	139	320	49	149	786	25	206	6	12	65	103	531	8,696
Malignant epithelial	2,656	510	33	38	93	74	31	692	150	210	52	90	46	196	182	5,053
Benign mesenchymal	174	27	1	—	—	—	—	—	—	—	—	—	—	—	4	206
Malignant mesenchymal	69	15	1	—	—	—	—	—	—	—	—	—	—	—	—	85
Lymphomas	340	101	1	—	—	—	—	—	—	—	—	—	—	—	13	455
Metastatic disease	400	71	—	—	—	—	—	—	—	—	—	—	—	—	19	490
Uncertain histogenesis	20	4	—	—	—	—	—	—	—	4	—	—	—	—	1	29
Uncertain biologic potential	37	7	—	—	—	—	1	4	—	5	—	—	—	1	1	56
Total	9,262	1,460	50	177	413	123	181	1,482	175	425	58	102	111	300	751	15,070

*NOS = not otherwise specified

Table 9–3. Proportions of Benign and Malignant Epithelial Salivary Gland Tumors in the AFIP Registry Compared With Those Reported in Several Previously Published Series

Series	Number of Cases	Percentage of Benign Tumors	Percentage of Malignant Tumors	Percentage of Minor Glands
Armed Forces Institute of Pathology	13,749	63.2	36.8	23.2
Memorial Sloan-Kettering Cancer Center[22]	2,807	54.5	45.5	21.6
Pathology Institute of the University of Hamburg[26]	2,579	74.3	25.7	9.0
Radiumhemmet and Karolinska Sjukhuset[25]	2,513	79.0	21.0	7.4*
British Salivary Gland Panel[27]	2,410	78.2	21.8	14.0

*Minor glands limited to those occurring in the palate

AFIP and Memorial Hospital occurred in the minor glands, and cases from both facilities predominantly involved patients from the United States. This figure of greater than 20 percent was considerably higher than those reported by institutions involving patients from West Germany, the United Kingdom, and Sweden.

Table 9–4 shows the total number of primary epithelial tumors in the AFIP registry occurring at specified sites and the proportions of benign tumors, of malignant tumors, and of all tumors that occurred at those sites. Although 69 percent of all benign tumors occurred in the parotid gland, a considerably smaller proportion (55 percent) of all malignant tumors occurred at that site. Conversely, the reported proportions of all malignant tumors occurring in the submandibular and sublingual glands and in all minor gland sites except the upper lip were greater than the corresponding proportions of all benign tumors occurring at these sites. About three fourths of all epithelial tumors occurred in the major glands (parotid 63.9 percent, submandibular 9.6 percent, sublingual 0.3 percent) and one fourth of all tumors arose from the minor glands. Nearly 12 percent of all tumors, 10 percent of benign tumors, and 14 percent of malignant tumors occurred in the palate.

Based on this experience, for every 100 parotid tumors there are about 40 minor gland tumors, 15 submandibular tumors, and less than 1 sublingual gland tumor. The distribution reported in 1968 by Thackray[28] in patients from the United Kingdom included 100 parotid tumors, 10 minor gland tumors, 10 submandibular gland tumors, and 1 sublingual gland tumor; this distribution varies most noticeably from the AFIP distribution in regard to minor gland tumors. However, differences in site distribution among different countries have long been recognized, and some large treatment centers may be less likely than others to receive intraoral tumors. As noted in Table 9–3, the frequency of tumors in minor glands in the four series (including AFIP data) that included all minor gland tumors[22, 26, 27] varied from 9.0 percent to a high frequency of 23.2 percent (AFIP cases). Similarly, the proportion of parotid gland tumors has varied from 75 percent in England[27] to 53 percent in Uganda.[6] Most recent large series show that the frequency of submandibular tumors varies from about 7.0[25] percent to 19.4 percent.[6]

Table 9–5 shows the separate numbers of benign and malignant tumors occurring in the major and minor glands and, at each specific site, the proportion that were benign and the proportion that were malignant. About one third of major gland tumors were malignant, but nearly one half of those occurring in the minor glands were malignant. The sites with the highest proportion of malignant tumors were the sublingual gland (70.2 percent), the tongue (85.7 percent), the floor of the mouth (88.2 percent), and the retromolar area (89.7 percent).

Of those patients with known occupational status (military/veteran or civilian), 39 percent were military personnel or veterans and 61 percent were civilian. There was a preponderance of males among all cases, and this was attributed to the greater number of males among military patients. As shown by Table 9–6, when only the civilian patients were considered, an approximately 3:2 predominance of cases involving female patients was seen (61 percent females, 39 percent males) for tumors occurring in all glands. Among patients with parotid and submandibular gland tumors, females accounted for a somewhat higher percentage of patients with benign tumors, and males accounted for more of those with malignant tumors. In the minor glands, these differences were not evident.

The difference in the average age between civilian and military patients for all tumors was only 1.6 years. Table 9–7 shows the mean ages of patients for benign and malignant tumors according to the sex of the patients and the site of occurrence. The ages of patients of all sites averaged 46.1 years for benign tumors and 47.1 years for malignant tumors. The median ages for benign and malignant tumors were 48 and 50 years, respectively. These latter figures, from the AFIP material, are similar to those reported from Sloan-Kettering Memorial Hospital Cancer Center,[22] in which the median ages for benign and malignant tumors were 46 and 54 years, respectively. However, our figures show median ages for civilian female and male patients with malignant tumors of 49 and 52 years, respectively, which are substantially lower than the comparable ages of 61 years in females and 64 years in males that were reported in the SEER registries by the National Cancer Institute.[16] Figure 9–1 compares age distribution data of the AFIP carcinoma cases with those of the cases from the SEER registries (from 1973 to 1977).[29] Although the two lines are close to parallel, the SEER data show a shift toward an older patient population. However, the SEER data included only 915 cases and were limited to major salivary gland carcinoma.

Although males with malignant tumors were, on average, 5.3 years older than males with benign tumors (49.4 years versus 44.1 years; see Table 9–7), there was a difference of only 1.1 years between the average age of females with malignant tumors and that of females with benign tumors (47.7 versus 46.6 years). The average age of women experiencing development of malignant tumors of the parotid and sublingual glands was lower than that for those experiencing development of benign tumors, but malignant submandibular tumors in both sexes occurred at least 6.6 years later than benign tumors. Little difference was seen between the average ages of patients with tumors of the major and minor glands, although there were differences between the two types at specific sites. The individual sites of neoplastic growth with the greatest average age differences

Table 9–4. Number of Benign and Malignant Primary Epithelial Tumors From the AFIP Registry Occurring at Specified Sites and the Percentage That Number Represents of Either All Benign, All Malignant, or Total of Benign and Malignant Epithelial Tumors From Among a Total of 12,859*

| | Major Glands | | | Minor Glands | | | | | | | | | | |
Diagnosis	Parotid	Sub-mandibular	Sub-lingual	Upper Lip	Lower Lip	Lip, NOS†	Palate	Tongue	Cheek	Retro-molar	Floor of Mouth	Tonsil/ Oro-pharynx	Other	Total
Benign	5,566	725	14	320	49	149	786	25	206	6	12	65	103	8,026
(Percentage of benign)	(69.0)	(9.0)	(0.2)	(4.0)	(0.6)	(1.9)	(9.8)	(0.3)	(2.6)	(0.1)	(0.2)	(0.8)	(1.3)	(100.0)
Malignant	2,656	510	33	93	74	31	692	150	210	52	90	46	196	4,833
(Percentage of malignant)	(55.0)	(10.6)	(0.3)	(1.9)	(1.5)	(0.6)	(14.3)	(3.1)	(4.3)	(1.0)	(1.9)	(0.9)	(4.1)	(100.0)
Total tumors at site	8,222	1,235	47	413	123	180	1,478	175	416	58	102	111	299	12,859
(Percentage of all cases)	(63.9)	(9.6)	(0.3)	(3.2)	(1.0)	(1.4)	(11.5)	(1.4)	(3.2)	(0.5)	(0.8)	(0.9)	(2.3)	(100.0)

*For example, 69 percent of benign tumors, 55 percent of malignant tumors, and 63.9 percent of all tumors occurred in the parotid glands
†NOS = not otherwise specified

Table 9–5. Total Number of Major and Minor Primary Epithelial Salivary Gland Tumors in the AFIP Files and Percentage of Those Cases Occurring at Selected Sites That Were Benign or Malignant

| | Major Glands | | | | Minor Glands | | | | | | | |
	All (Number [%])	Parotid (%)	Sub-mandibular (%)	Sub-lingual (%)	Upper Lip (%)	Lower Lip (%)	Palate (%)	Tongue (%)	Cheek (%)	Retro-molar (%)	Floor of Mouth (%)	Tonsil/ Oropharynx (%)
Benign tumors	(6,305 [66.3])	67.7	58.7	29.8	77.5	39.8	53.2	14.3	49.5	10.3	11.8	58.6
Malignant tumors	(3,199 [33.7])	32.3	41.3	70.2	22.5	60.2	46.8	85.7	50.5	89.7	88.2	41.4

Table 9–6. Sex Distribution of 7,021 Civilian Patients With Benign or Malignant Epithelial Salivary Gland Tumors With Stated Site, and Percentage of Benign, Malignant, or All Tumors by Sex

| | Parotid Gland | | | Submandibular Gland | | | Sublingual Gland | | | Minor Glands | | | All Glands | | |
	Benign	Malignant	Total	Benign	Malignant	Total	Benign	Malignant	Total	Benign	Malignant	Total	Benign	Malignant	Total
Number of tumors	2,568	1,668	4,236	309	294	603	7	21	28	978	1,176	2,154	3,862	3,159	7,021
Males (percentage)	36	43	39	32	42	37	29	33	32	39	38	38	37	41	39
Females (percentage)	64	57	61	68	58	63	71	67	68	61	62	62	63	59	61

Table 9–7. Average Age in Years of Patients With Benign and Malignant
Epithelial Salivary Gland Tumors by Site and Sex

Site	Average Age Males			Average Age Females			Average Age Both Sexes		
	Benign	*Malignant*	*Both*	*Benign*	*Malignant*	*Both*	*Benign*	*Malignant*	*Both*
Major Glands									
All major glands	43.8	48.9	45.5	46.1	46.1	46.1	44.8	47.7	45.8
Parotid gland	44.4	48.3	45.6	46.5	45.3	46.0	45.2	47.0	45.8
Submandibular gland	39.1	51.3	44.5	43.5	50.1	46.5	41.0	50.8	45.4
Sublingual gland	41.4	55.9	52.4	53.3	47.8	49.5	47.9	52.1	51.0
Minor Glands									
All minor glands	44.1	49.4	46.1	46.6	47.7	47.1	45.2	48.6	46.5
Lip, NOS*	36.0	42.9	37.5	45.6	46.5	45.9	39.6	44.7	40.8
Upper lip	49.9	50.9	50.1	56.6	46.0	55.3	52.7	51.5	52.5
Lower lip	49.4	50.5	50.1	54.0	53.1	54.0	51.6	51.8	52.0
Palate, NOS*	42.9	46.7	44.6	45.3	46.5	46.0	44.0	46.5	45.3
Hard palate	42.6	45.3	43.9	42.5	54.0	45.4	42.7	47.3	44.8
Soft palate	45.8	50.3	47.9	50.8	49.0	49.1	48.2	49.1	48.6
Tongue	41.8	58.2	55.6	45.3	56.6	55.5	43.7	57.4	55.6
Cheek	47.5	47.2	47.2	52.1	51.6	51.8	49.4	49.6	49.4
Retromolar area	20.5	49.1	46.1	60.0	50.3	51.7	46.8	49.3	49.0
Floor of mouth	53.0	62.5	61.5	46.0	57.1	56.2	47.2	60.4	59.0
Tonsil/oropharyngeal area	45.9	55.3	49.9	53.1	53.8	54.1	50.1	54.6	52.0
Total Major and Minor Glands	44.1	49.4	46.1	46.6	47.7	47.1	46.1	47.1	46.5

*NOS = not otherwise specified

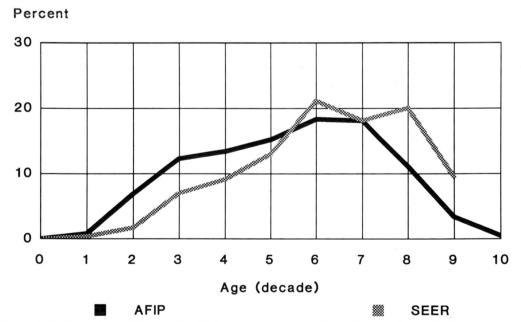

Figure 9–1. Comparison of the age distribution among patients with malignant salivary gland tumors as reported by the AFIP with the distribution reported by the SEER study.

between patients with benign and malignant tumors were the tongue (13.7 years) and the floor of mouth (13.2 years). Interestingly, malignant tumors of the upper lip in females occurred, on average, 10.6 years before their benign counterparts.

Figure 9–2 shows the age distribution of patients with benign and malignant tumors and demonstrates a peak in incidence among patients in the third decade of life for benign tumors, whereas the frequency of malignant tumors rises steadily among patients until their sixth decade of life. The distribution of incidence among patients by age in decades according to the histologic type of tumor is shown in Figure 9–3. According to this distribution, the incidence of mixed tumors peaks at an earlier patient age than that for other benign tumors. Similarly, among malignant tumors mucoepidermoid carcinoma and acinic cell adenocarcinoma peak among patients of relatively young age.

The number of cases of each histologic type of tumor occurring in specific sites and the percentage of that tumor type of all tumors occurring at that site are shown in Table 9–8. Slightly more than 79 percent of benign and 50 percent of all tumors were mixed tumors. These figures are very similar to those reported in three of the large studies that were previously cited,[22, 26, 27] but they differ from Eneroth's study.[25] Among AFIP cases mucoepidermoid carcinomas accounted for one third of all malignant tumors and were followed in decreasing order of frequency by acinic cell adenocarcinoma; adenocarcinoma, not otherwise specified (NOS); and adenoid cystic carcinoma. Acinic cell adenocarcinomas account for 10.3 per-

cent of all tumors in the buccal mucosa but only 1.4 percent of those occurring in the palate. Adenoid cystic carcinomas account for only 2 percent of parotid tumors, but they account for 8.3 percent of palatal tumors and 17.1 percent of tumors occurring in the tongue.

Of the 13,749 cases, the race of the patient was stated in 6,784 cases. The distribution by race for the most common tumors is shown in Table 9–9. Of all patients, 85.4 percent were white and 9.9 percent were black. Warthin's tumors were notable for their rarity among blacks (2.9 percent), but benign mixed tumors and adenocarcinomas, NOS, appeared to be disproportionately more common among black patients than among white patients. Spitz and Batsakis[57] have noted that, among salivary gland carcinomas, mucoepidermoid carcinomas and carcinomas ex mixed tumor were relatively more frequently diagnosed in black patients; however, our data show that, in addition to these two tumors, adenocarcinoma, NOS, and adenoid cystic carcinoma all account for a similar proportion of tumors occurring among blacks. The greatest proportion of tumors occurring among patients of Asian extraction were mixed tumors and cystadenomas.

ETIOLOGY

Viruses

In general, little is known about the cause of salivary gland tumors. One frequently investigated etiologic relationship concerns the association of

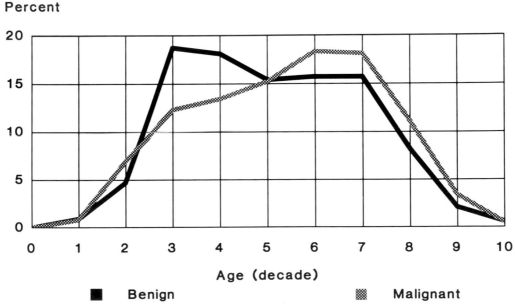

Figure 9–2. Comparison of the distribution by age of 13,263 patients with benign or malignant epithelial salivary gland tumors reported in the salivary gland registry of the AFIP.

SALIVARY GLAND NEOPLASMS: GENERAL CONSIDERATIONS

Figure 9–3. Age distribution by decade of patients with the most common types of benign and malignant salivary gland tumors in the AFIP files. (Note: NOS = not otherwise specified.)

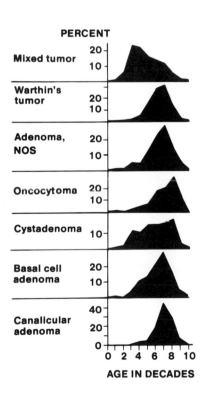

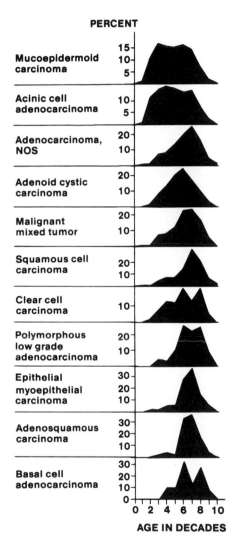

Table 9–8. Distribution of 13,749 Benign and Malignant Primary Epithelial Salivary Gland Tumors From the AFIP Registry by Histologic Type and Site and the Percentage (Shown in Parentheses) of All Tumors Occurring at Each Site

Diagnosis	Major Glands			Minor Glands												Total, All Sites
	Parotid	Sub-mandibular	Sublingual	Neck (NOS)	Upper Lip	Lower Lip	Lip, NOS*	Palate	Tongue	Cheek	Retro-molar	Floor of Mouth	Tonsil/Oropharyngeal	Minor/Other	Not Stated	
Benign																
Mixed tumor	4,359 (53.0)	657 (53.3)	10 (21.3)	89 (50.0)	147 (35.6)	20 (16.3)	130 (71.8)	711 (48.2)	16 (9.1)	126 (30.3)	3 (5.2)	7 (6.9)	38 (33.9)	79 (26.3)	488 (68.4)	6,880
Warthin's tumor	630 (7.7)	16 (1.3)	0 (0)	33 (18.5)	0 (0)	0 (0)	2 (1.1)	2 (<1.0)	0 (0)	2 (<1.0)	0 (0)	0 (0)	10 (8.9)	4 (1.3)	23 (3.2)	722
Adenoma, NOS*	170 (2.1)	10 (1.0)	2 (4.3)	4 (2.3)	54 (13.1)	9 (7.3)	8 (4.4)	23 (1.6)	2 (1.1)	27 (6.5)	0 (0)	2 (2.0)	3 (0)	6 (2.0)	9 (1.3)	329
Oncocytoma	156 (1.9)	18 (1.5)	0 (0)	6 (3.4)	0 (0)	1 (<1.0)	0 (0)	4 (<1.0)	0 (<1.0)	4 (<1.0)	0 (0)	0 (0)	3 (2.7)	1 (<1.0)	6 (<1.0)	200
Cystadenoma	112 (1.4)	13 (1.1)	1 (2.1)	1 (<1.0)	10 (2.4)	8 (6.5)	3 (1.7)	14 (<1.0)	0 (0)	16 (3.9)	2 (3.5)	1 (<1.0)	11 (9.8)	1 (<1.0)	3 (<1.0)	196
Basal cell adenoma	117 (1.4)	7 (1.0)	0 (0)	4 (2.3)	12 (2.9)	0 (0)	1 (<1.0)	6 (<1.0)	0 (0)	8 (1.9)	0 (0)	0 (<1.0)	0 (0)	3 (1.0)	1 (<1.0)	160
Canalicular adenoma	1 (<1.0)	0 (0)	0 (0)	1 (<1.0)	89 (21.6)	3 (2.5)	4 (2.2)	4 (<1.0)	0 (0)	15 (3.6)	0 (0)	0 (0)	0 (0)	4 (1.3)	0 (0)	121
Myoepithelioma	7 (<1.0)	4 (<1.0)	0 (0)	1 (<1.0)	3 (1.0)	0 (0)	0 (0)	9 (<1.0)	5 (2.9)	2 (<1.0)	0 (0)	1 (<1.0)	0 (0)	1 (<1.0)	0 (0)	33
Intraductal and inverted ductal papillomas	2 (<1.0)	0 (0)	0 (0)	0 (0)	5 (1.2)	8 (6.5)	1 (<1.0)	6 (1.0)	1 (<1.0)	5 (1.2)	0 (0)	0 (0)	0 (0)	1 (<1.0)	1 (<1.0)	30
Sialadenoma papilliferum	2 (<1.0)	0 (0)	1 (2.1)	0 (0)	0 (0)	0 (0)	0 (0)	7 (<1.0)	0 (0)	1 (<1.0)	1 (1.7)	0 (0)	0 (0)	3 (1.0)	0 (0)	15
Sebaceous adenomas	10 (<1.0)	0 (0)	0 (0)	0 (0)	0 (0)	0 (0)	0 (0)	0 (0)	0 (0)	0 (0)	0 (0)	0 (0)	0 (0)	0 (0)	0 (0)	10
Total	5,566 (67.7)	725 (58.8)	14 (29.8)	139 (78.5)	320 (77.5)	49 (39.8)	149 (82.8)	786 (53.2)	25 (14.3)	206 (49.5)	6 (10.3)	12 (11.8)	65 (58.5)	103 (34.4)	531 (74.5)	8,696
Malignant																
Mucoepidermoid carcinoma	791 (9.6)	112 (9.1)	17 (36.2)	5 (2.8)	12 (2.9)	37 (30.1)	9 (5.0)	305 (20.7)	58 (33.1)	93 (22.4)	40 (69)	51 (50)	11 (9.8)	106 (35.3)	54 (7.5)	1,701
Acinic cell adenocarcinoma	706 (8.6)	33 (2.7)	2 (4.3)	12 (6.7)	24 (5.8)	8 (6.5)	6 (3.3)	21 (1.4)	5 (2.9)	43 (10.3)	2 (3.5)	1 (<1.0)	1 (<1.0)	5 (1.7)	17 (2.4)	886
Adenocarcinoma, NOS	419 (5.1)	97 (7.9)	4 (8.5)	2 (1.1)	18 (4.4)	14 (11.4)	10 (5.5)	123 (8.3)	29 (16.6)	24 (5.8)	4 (6.9)	7 (6.9)	7 (6.3)	39 (13.0)	62 (8.7)	859
Adenoid cystic carcinoma	161 (2.0)	144 (11.7)	7 (14.9)	6 (3.4)	18 (4.4)	4 (3.3)	3 (1.6)	123 (8.3)	30 (17.1)	23 (5.5)	5 (8.6)	14 (13.7)	8 (7.1)	30 (10)	24 (3.4)	600
Malignant mixed tumor	210 (2.5)	43 (3.5)	1 (2.1)	6 (3.4)	6 (1.5)	0 (0)	0 (0)	36 (2.4)	4 (2.3)	4 (<1.0)	0 (0)	0 (0)	4 (3.6)	3 (1.0)	9 (1.3)	326

Squamous cell carcinoma	169 (2.1)	42 (3.4)	1 (2.1)	1 (<1.0)	0 (0)	0 (0)	0 (0)	0 (0)	0 (0)	0 (0)	0 (0)	0 (0)	0 (0)	0 (0)	11 (1.5)	224
Clear cell carcinoma	26 (<1.0)	10 (1.0)	0 (0)	2 (1.1)	0 (0)	8 (6.5)	2 (1.1)	20 (1.4)	4 (2.3)	3 (<1.0)	0 (0)	4 (3.9)	5 (4.5)	5 (1.7)	3 (<1.0)	92
Polymorphous low-grade adenocarcinoma	0 (0)	0 (0)	0 (0)	1 (<1.0)	12 (2.9)	1 (<1.0)	1 (<1.0)	44 (3.0)	1 (<1.0)	12 (2.9)	0 (0)	0 (0)	1 (<1.0)	2 (1.8)	0 (0)	75
Epithelial-myoepithelial carcinoma	43 (1.0)	7 (1.0)	0 (0)	0 (0)	0 (0)	0 (0)	0 (0)	3 (<1.0)	2 (1.1)	1 (<1.0)	0 (0)	0 (0)	0 (0)	2 (<1.0)	0 (0)	58
Adenosquamous carcinoma	0 (0)	0 (0)	0 (0)	0 (0)	0 (0)	2 (1.6)	0 (0)	11 (<1.0)	16 (9.1)	2 (<1.0)	1 (1.7)	12 (11.7)	8 (6.3)	4 (1.3)	1 (<1.0)	57
Basal cell adenocarcinoma	39 (<1.0)	4 (<1.0)	0 (0)	0 (0)	0 (0)	0 (0)	0 (0)	0 (0)	0 (0)	0 (0)	0 (0)	0 (0)	0 (0)	0 (0)	0 (0)	43
Oncocytic carcinoma	19 (<1.0)	3 (<1.0)	0 (0)	2 (1.1)	0 (0)	0 (0)	0 (0)	1 (<1.0)	0 (0)	1 (<1.0)	0 (0)	0 (0)	0 (0)	0 (0)	0 (0)	26
Cystadeno-carcinoma	14 (<1.0)	4 (<1.0)	1 (2.1)	0 (0)	2 (<1.0)	0 (0)	0 (0)	3 (0.20)	0 (0)	1 (0.24)	0 (0)	0 (0)	0 (0)	0 (0)	0 (0)	25
Undifferentiated carcinoma	14 (<1.0)	3 (<1.0)	0 (0)	1 (<1.0)	0 (0)	0 (0)	0 (0)	2 (<1.0)	1 (<1.0)	0 (0)	0 (0)	1 (<1.0)	1 (<1.0)	0 (0)	0 (0)	23
Small cell carcinoma	16 (<1.0)	1 (<1.0)	0 (0)	0 (0)	0 (0)	0 (0)	0 (0)	0 (0)	0 (0)	2 (<1.0)	0 (0)	0 (0)	0 (0)	0 (0)	1 (<1.0)	20
Lymphoepithelial carcinoma	11 (<1.0)	2 (<1.0)	0 (0)	0 (0)	0 (0)	0 (0)	0 (0)	0 (0)	0 (0)	0 (0)	0 (0)	0 (0)	0 (0)	0 (0)	0 (0)	13
Sebaceous carcinoma	10 (<1.0)	0 (0)	0 (0)	0 (0)	0 (0)	0 (0)	0 (0)	0 (0)	0 (0)	0 (0)	0 (0)	0 (0)	0 (0)	0 (0)	0 (0)	10
Carcinosarcoma	6 (<1.0)	2 (<1.0)	0 (0)	0 (0)	0 (0)	0 (0)	0 (0)	0 (0)	0 (0)	0 (0)	0 (0)	0 (0)	0 (0)	0 (0)	0 (0)	8
Salivary duct carcinoma	2 (<1.0)	0 (0)	0 (0)	0 (0)	0 (0)	0 (0)	0 (0)	0 (0)	0 (0)	1 (<1.0)	0 (0)	0 (0)	0 (0)	0 (0)	0 (0)	3
Malignant myoepithelioma	0 (0)	1 (<1.0)	0 (0)	0 (0)	1 (<1.0)	0 (0)	0 (0)	0 (0)	0 (0)	0 (0)	0 (0)	0 (0)	0 (0)	0 (0)	0 (0)	2
Mucinous adenocarcinoma	0 (0)	2 (<1.0)	0 (0)	0 (0)	0 (0)	0 (0)	0 (0)	0 (0)	0 (0)	0 (0)	0 (0)	0 (0)	0 (0)	0 (0)	0 (0)	2
Total	2,656 (32.3)	510 (41.2)	33 (70.2)	38 (21.5)	93 (22.5)	74 (60.2)	31 (17.2)	692 (46.8)	150 (85.7)	210 (50.5)	52 (89.7)	90 (88.2)	46 (42.3)	196 (65.6)	182 (26.1)	5,053
Total, Benign and Malignant	8,222	1,235	47	177	413	123	180	1,478	175	416	58	102	111	299	713	13,749

*NOS = not otherwise specified

Table 9–9. Distribution of Benign and Malignant Tumors by Race

Tumor	Total Number Race Stated	Percent White	Percent Black	Percent Asian	Percent Indian, Malayan
Benign					
Mixed tumor	3,262	83.3	10.7	4.8	
Warthin's tumor	384	95.8	2.9	0.5	
Adenoma, NOS*	151	87.4	7.9	5.3	
Basal cell adenoma	84	89.3	7.1	2.4	
Canalicular adenoma	57	91.2	7.0	0	
Cystadenoma	114	92.1	5.3	1.8	
Total	4,147	85.2	9.5	4.1	1.2
Malignant					
Mucoepidermoid carcinoma	1,028	84.7	11.1	3.3	
Acinic cell carcinoma	501	90.0	7.8	1.6	
Adenocarcinoma, NOS*	446	82.7	14.3	2.9	
Adenoid cystic carcinoma	372	84.4	11.0	2.2	
Malignant mixed tumor	189	83.1	11.1	3.7	
Squamous cell carcinoma	126	87.3	5.6	2.4	
Total	2,666	85.7	10.5	2.7	1.1
Total Benign and Malignant	6,784	85.4	9.9	3.6	1.2

*NOS = not otherwise specified

the Epstein-Barr virus, and possibly autoimmunity, with the form of salivary gland carcinoma often referred to as malignant lymphoepithelial lesion.[30–33] This type of tumor is extremely rare among people who are not of Asian extraction.[34] Although it has been shown that the incidence of infectious mononucleosis is low in Eskimo children from Greenland, by the age of 3 years, 100 percent of them have primary infection with Epstein-Barr virus.[35] Merrick and colleagues[36] believe this indicates that environmental factors in Greenland enhance humoral immunity to Epstein-Barr virus. The virus is normally present in the pharynx and salivary glands of this population; therefore the inter-relationships of immunity, environmental factors, and the genetic constitution of the host may all play a role in the malignant transformation of salivary gland epithelial cells. One study has demonstrated the presence of DNA from the Epstein-Barr virus in an adenocarcinoma of the parotid gland in a Finnish child.[37] Additionally, some possibly influential environmental factors relate to the Eskimo's lifestyle.[17] These include the additional chewing and salivation required to work leather and the consumption of raw frozen meat and fish.

Other viruses suspected as possible etiologic factors include polyoma virus, cytomegalovirus, type C particles similar to those associated with murine leukemia, type B particles similar to those associated with murine breast tumors,[38] and human papilloma virus types 16 and 18.[39] Salivary gland tumors can be induced in a high percentage of several strains of mice[40, 41] by injection of polyoma virus on the first day of birth. A markedly lower percentage of animals develop tumors if injection of the virus occurs after the first day, which suggests a relationship to the development of the immune system. Furthermore, injection of

virus is not age-related in athymic mice, again suggesting synergism with the immune system.[42] Tumors develop after a latent period of 10 to 12 weeks following injection of the virus in these animals. As noted by Scully,[38] some spontaneous salivary gland adenocarcinomas in animals reveal the presence of viral particles. However, he also points out that few studies in humans have examined the role that viruses may play in the development of salivary gland tumors and that much work remains to be done.

Radiation

Substantial evidence exists for a relationship between exposure to ionizing radiation and the later development of salivary gland tumors. Much of the stimulus for the work done in this area has come from studies of the thyroid gland. It has been noted in some series that more than 70 percent of children and as many as 40 percent of adults with thyroid cancer have a history of previous head and neck irradiation.[43]

Long-term observation of about 82,000 Japanese people who were exposed to radiation generated by the atomic bombs dropped on Hiroshima and Nagasaki has demonstrated increased risks of development of salivary gland neoplasia.[44–47] These studies have shown relative risks of 3.5- and 11-fold for benign and malignant salivary gland tumors, respectively. Risk for the development of malignant salivary gland tumors was significantly greater in those patients who experienced greater exposure, that is, in those closest to the hypocenter. As has been observed for leukemia in this population, the increased incidence of malignant salivary gland tumors per 100,000 people was higher in the period from 12 to 16 years after exposure than before or after that interval, although it remained substantially elevated 26 years later.

The tumorigenic effects of therapeutic radiation to the head and neck on salivary gland tissue have also been assessed. Some of the most thorough work on this relationship involved patients observed at the Michael Reese Hospital in Chicago.[48–51] The mean annual incidence per 100,000 people was 48 cases in an early period but increased to 77 per 100,000 people later in the study. This compared with 0.6 cases per 100,000 people from a nonexposed control group. Compared with normal expectations, there was a 40-fold increased risk in the irradiated population for development of malignant tumors.

Other studies on this topic have shown a similarly strong association. In most cases, the purpose of the therapeutic radiation was for benign conditions, such as hypertrophied tonsils and adenoids, tinea capitis, an enlarged thymus or thyroid gland, keloids, postmastoidectomies, unexplained deafness, acne, or tuberculous lymphadenitis.[48, 52–58] Several cases have followed radiotherapy for carcinoma, radium implants, or ^{131}I for hyperthyroidism.[56, 57, 59, 60] Hoffman and coworkers[59] studied a limited number of patients who were treated for hyperthyroidism with radioiodine (^{131}I), and they observed an elevated risk of cancer in organs that concentrated iodine (salivary glands, digestive tract, kidney, and bladder). The relative risk in the salivary glands was increased 6.4-fold.

The minimum tumorigenic dose is difficult to estimate and remains controversial. In the thyroid, a dose in the range of 250 to 1,000 rad is thought to be damaging,[61] but histologic radiation changes are not evident in the thyroid at these doses. Because the thyroid may play an important role in the processing of lymphocytes, it has been speculated that radiation damage to the immune component of this gland may be more important than damage to the epithelium.[61] Similar to the thyroid, the parotid gland also has lesions in which lymphocytes play a major role (e.g., Sjögren's syndrome, benign lymphoepithelial lesion). The substantial lymphoid component of the parotid gland may be more susceptible to low-dose radiation damage than the parenchyma.

A dose of 483 rad measured 1 cm below the skin in the parotid gland appears to significantly increase the risk of tumor development.[48] In many cases, it is difficult to determine if the glands were exposed to the primary beam or to scattered rays. It appears that doses as low as 140 rad may increase the risk of developing a salivary gland tumor and that this risk increases with the dose.[53, 55, 62–65]

Patients with radiation-related salivary gland tumors experience a high rate of second tumors of the salivary, thyroid, and parathyroid glands. Hawkins and colleagues[66] determined that, among childhood cancer survivors with no known genetic predisposition to developing cancer, those exposed to radiation experienced a fourfold increased risk of developing a second primary tumor, usually in tissue within or on the edge of the irradiated field. Investigators in two other studies[64, 67] observed tumors of the thyroid, parathyroid, breast, skin, and lung occurring in irradiated fields of patients with salivary gland tumors.

In summary, currently available evidence strongly indicates that radiotherapy is harmful to the salivary glands and should not be used to treat benign conditions.[68] Furthermore, data suggest that excessive use of medical or dental diagnostic radiographs could play a role in tumor initiation. One study[69] has shown an association between the development of malignant parotid tumors and patients who had five or more full-mouth dental radiographic series before 1960. It was estimated that these patients received from 11 to 32 rad in each parotid gland during each series. Other studies have shown that subjects who had a cumulative dose of 50 rad or more from dental radiography had an excess of malignant parotid tumors.[70, 71] Modern techniques, equipment, and films have resulted in much lower exposures, but care must be taken to ensure that patients are exposed to minimal doses.

Occupation

Certain occupations have been reported to place people at increased risks for the development of salivary gland carcinomas; these include asbestos mining;[72] manufacturing of rubber products and the industries, such as shoe manufacturing, that use these rubber products;[73] plumbing (exposure to metals);[74] and woodworking in the automobile industry.[75]

Lifestyle

Although severe malnutrition, such as kwashiorkor,[6] causes enlargement of salivary glands, an increased incidence of salivary gland tumors has not been observed. Similarly, no association of salivary gland tumors with heavy smoking or heavy alcohol consumption could be demonstrated by Keller[76] or by Williams and Horm.[77]

Hormones

It has been suggested that endogenous hormones may have a role in the carcinogenesis of salivary gland tumors.[78] One study[79] found nearly 80 percent of normal salivary gland samples to be positive for estrogen receptors (defined as receptor protein content of greater than or equal to 1 fmol/mg of cytosol protein). Additionally, these same investigators found that four of eight salivary gland tumors in women had estrogen receptor levels that would be considered hormonally dependent in breast carcinoma (greater than 10 fmol/mg of cytosol protein). Other studies have demonstrated prolactin-binding activity in both normal and neoplastic salivary gland tissue.[80] Further investigation of the effects of hormones on normal and neoplastic tissue and of the possible role for antiestrogen therapy in the treatment of salivary gland tumors is needed.

SALIVARY GLAND NEOPLASMS IN CHILDREN

The AFIP experience with salivary gland tumors in children (defined as persons under the age of 17 years) is shown in Table 9–10. Children accounted for 4.5 percent of all patients. Because mesenchymal tumors constitute such a large proportion of tumors occurring in this age group, they are also included.

Mixed tumors, mucoepidermoid carcinomas, and acinic cell adenocarcinomas accounted for over 92 percent of all epithelial tumors and about 77 percent of all tumors in this age group. In our experience, and in nearly all previous studies, mucoepidermoid carcinoma has been the most common salivary gland malignancy in children.[81–87, 89] The benign and malignant epithelial tumors together accounted for approximately 85 percent of all tumors reported in this age group. Essentially equal numbers of benign and malignant epithelial tumors were seen (Table 9–10). These figures contrast with those for patients of all ages, in whom over 63 percent of all epithelial tumors were benign. The observation that malig-

Table 9–10. Number of Benign and Malignant Salivary Gland Tumors in Patients Under 17 Years of Age, Percentage of All Tumors Occurring in This Age Group, and Percentage of Each Arising in Patients of All Ages*

Tumor Type	Number of Cases	Percentage of All Tumors Occurring in This Age Group	Percentage† of All Similar Tumors Occurring in All Age Groups
Benign Epithelial			
Mixed tumor	193	39.1	3.9
Warthin's tumor	5	1.0	0.9
Canalicular adenoma	4	0.8	3.4
Adenoma, NOS‡	4	0.8	1.2
Myoepithelioma	2	0.4	6.3
Oncocytoma	1	0.2	0.6
Basal cell adenoma	1	0.2	0.6
Total benign	210	42.5	3.3
Malignant Epithelial			
Mucoepidermoid carcinoma	123	24.9	7.7
Acinic cell adenocarcinoma	65	13.2	7.6
Adenocarcinoma, NOS‡	13	2.6	1.8
Adenoid cystic carcinoma	6	1.2	1.0
Squamous cell carcinoma	2	0.4	1.2
Small cell carcinoma	1	0.2	1.1
Clear cell carcinoma	1	0.2	12.5
Carcinosarcoma	1	0.2	12.5
Total malignant	212	42.9	5.2
Benign Mesenchymal			
Hemangioma	40	8.1	78.4
Neurofibroma	7	1.4	28.0
Lymphangioma	5	1.0	41.7
Fibromatosis	5	1.0	45.5
Schwannoma	3	0.6	8.8
Lipoma	1	0.2	6.6
Total benign	61	12.3	35.6
Malignant Mesenchymal			
Sarcoma, NOS‡	4	0.8	44.4
Rhabdomyosarcoma	2	0.4	40.0
Fibrosarcoma	2	0.4	22.2
Malignant schwannoma	2	0.4	18.2
Alveolar soft part sarcoma	1	0.2	50.0
Total malignant	11	2.2	14.6
Total Benign and Malignant	494	100.0	4.5

*For example, 39.1 percent of all salivary gland tumors in patients under 17 years of age were mixed tumors, and 3.9 percent of mixed tumors in all age groups occurred in patients under 17 years of age
†Percent of patients with age stated
‡NOS = not otherwise specified

nant tumors are relatively more common than benign tumors in younger patients has been previously noted[84–88] and suggests that the pathogenesis of tumors in children may be different from that in adults. Whereas mixed tumors accounted for about 52 percent of all epithelial tumors in patients of all ages, they accounted for only 39.3 percent of tumors in children.

Over 14 percent of tumors in children were mesenchymal tumors. Over one half of all mesenchymal tumors occurring in the salivary glands occurred in children, although, as noted earlier, children represented only 4.5 percent of all patients. Hemangiomas were the predominant mesenchymal tumor in the AFIP registry, but some investigators have found them to be the most common of all salivary gland tumors in children. A previous AFIP study[89] of patients under the age of 15 years reported that hemangiomas and lymphangiomas together were second in frequency only to mixed tumors. In our current survey, the two vascular lesions (45 cases) not only were less common than mixed tumors but, together, were also less common than either mucoepidermoid or acinic cell carcinoma. The percentage of vascular tumors reported by others[85, 87, 90–92] exceeds that observed in the AFIP registry.

Figure 9–4 shows the age distribution from birth through 16 years of age of patients with epithelial tumors. Among patients between the ages of 8 and 12 years, both benign and malignant tumors simultaneously demonstrated an increased frequency, which initiated an irregular, but continuous, upward trend through each age category to the sixth decade of life (see Fig. 9–2).

SECOND PRIMARY NEOPLASMS FOLLOWING SALIVARY GLAND TUMORS

In 1968 Berg, Hutter, and Foote[93] reported that patients with known salivary gland cancers experienced an eightfold increased risk of developing second primary cancers in the breast. Berg and coworkers also noted that a greater than expected number of skin cancers developed in their patients but attributed this increase to radiation therapy. Since that time, many other investigators have tried to confirm that patients with primary salivary gland cancer are at increased risk of developing a second primary carcinoma of the breast or of other sites.[93–103] Moertel and Elveback[94] used a similar method in an attempt to validate the findings of Berg and associates[93] but found no association between neoplasms of the breast and salivary glands. They instead concluded that such studies often lacked an appropriate source of controls, which precluded accurate estimation of the expected tumor rate. Since this observation, investigators have chosen the cancer registries used for comparison more carefully.

In addition to the study done by Moertel and Elveback,[94] at least two other studies[101, 102] have been unable to confirm an increase in the frequency of breast carcinoma that is associated with salivary gland tumors, but several others[95, 97, 100] have shown an increased risk, although it is more modest than that reported by Berg and colleagues.[93] Some investigators have found increased frequencies of tumors at sites other than the breast. Table 9–11 shows the secondary sites

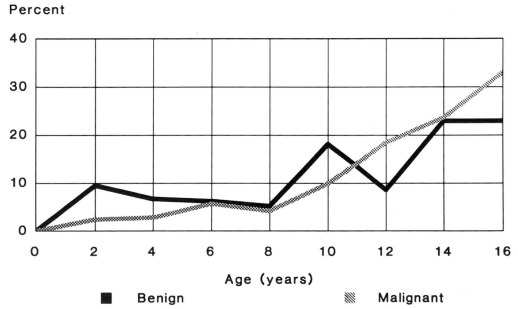

Figure 9–4. Comparison (in percentages) of the distribution by age of 210 patients with benign epithelial salivary gland tumors and 212 patients with malignant epithelial salivary gland tumors. All patients were younger than 17 years of age.

Table 9–11. Risk of Second Cancer in Patients Who Have Had a Previous Salivary Gland Tumor

Study	Total Number of Patients	Second Primary Site for Females (Relative Risk)	Second Primary Site for Males (Relative Risk)	Notes
Berg and colleagues[93]	396	Breast (7.8)	—	Malignant SGT* only
Moertel and Elveback[94]	297	Breast (1.0)	—	Malignant SGT* only
Dunn and colleagues[95]	349	Breast (2.0)	—	Major glands only
Newell and colleagues[96]	—	—	Prostate and lung (3.0)	Blacks; malignant SGT* only
Prior and Waterhouse[97]	925	Breast (2.3)	Prostate (4.2)	Benign and malignant SGT*
		Bronchus (6.5)	Skin (4.5)	
Biggar and colleagues[98]	782	Ovary (5.3)	Respiratory (2.8)	Malignant SGT* only
Abbey and colleagues[100]	372	Breast (4.8)	—	Benign and malignant SGT, all sites
Spitz and colleagues[102]	498	Breast (1.0)	Skin (2.5–4.3)	Whites; malignant SGT only
Johns and colleagues[103]	198	—	Major salivary glands (400)	Malignant SGT only
			Larynx (40.8)	
			Colon (14.0)	

*SGT = salivary gland tumor

reportedly at increased risk in females and males and the risks of developing tumors at those sites relative to the expected number of cases. Among female patients, the bronchial tree and ovaries have shown increased susceptibility to the development of second primaries. Among male patients, there is less concurrence, but the most frequent association appears to be with skin cancer, both prior to and subsequent to the diagnosis of salivary gland cancer,[97, 98, 102, 103] and increased numbers of second primaries of the salivary glands have been reported (see later).

In some regions of the United States more than others, patients with primary salivary gland tumors may be at increased risk for the development of primary tumors at other sites. However, the conflicting conclusions among the various studies diminish their value and clinical application.

MULTIPLE HISTOLOGICALLY DISTINCT SALIVARY GLAND NEOPLASMS

Multiple synchronous or metachronous salivary gland tumors are extremely unusual. In a review in 1989, Gnepp and coworkers[104] reported on 25 patients with synchronous, unilateral salivary gland tumors, 23 of which were from the files of the AFIP; they also reviewed the literature on both unilateral and bilateral synchronous and metachronous tumors.

These investigators found that the most common tumor to occur bilaterally, either synchronously or metachronously, was Warthin's tumor, and they noted that over 100 such cases had been reported. About one third as many mixed tumors

developed in a similar manner; most involved the parotid glands, but on occasion, they affected the parotid and submandibular glands or the major and minor glands. The next most common tumors to occur bilaterally were acinic cell adenocarcinoma and oncocytoma.

Gnepp and colleagues[104] found that Warthin's tumors were more often one among several distinctly separate, unilateral tumors than any other type. Most often, the second tumor focus, or in some cases the third, was another Warthin's tumor or a mixed tumor, although other benign and malignant tumor types were also recorded. The second most likely unilateral combination was mixed tumor with another mixed tumor, and this combination was followed in frequency by multiple foci of basal cell adenoma or oncocytoma.

Although occurrence of multiple tumors within salivary glands is uncommon, awareness of this possibility may help avoid an incorrect interpretation of malignancy. This is especially important in cases of basal cell adenomas or oncocytomas, where encapsulation may be absent.

CLINICAL STAGING OF SALIVARY GLAND CARCINOMAS

Much of the work of staging criteria for carcinoma of the major salivary glands was done at Memorial Hospital by Spiro and coworkers.[105, 106] A TN (tumors and nodes) staging system (TNM [tumors, nodes, and metastases] modification) was developed for tumors of the parotid or submandibular glands. Consideration was given to the size of the tumor, to its mobility, and to whether or not the facial nerve was intact. N0 and N1 designations were applied to the absence or presence of suspected cervical lymph node metastases.

In a comprehensive, retrospective, multicenter study that involved 861 patients, Levitt and colleagues[107] found that prognosis was principally related to the size of the primary tumor and that further prognostic accuracy could be achieved by additionally considering the presence or absence of local extension. Other variables that played a lesser role were the palpability of and suspected metastasis to the regional lymph nodes and the presence or absence of distant metastasis. Lymph nodes considered as regional included those within or immediately adjacent to the salivary glands and the deep cervical lymph nodes. Tumor involvement of nodes other than these were considered as distant metastases. Although no attempt was made to include the histopathologic grade in the staging system, it was noted that patients with undifferentiated carcinomas and poorly differentiated mucoepidermoid carcinomas had a poor prognosis, regardless of the size, extension, fixation, or consistency of the tumor.

These criteria were accepted with minor modifications by the American Joint Committee on Cancer in 1988[108] and are shown in Table 9–12. The staging system proposed by this committee uses four clinical variables: tumor size, local extension of the tumor, the palpability of and suspected metastasis to regional nodes, and the presence or

absence of distant metastases. It was determined that local extension was far less ominous in smaller tumors than in larger ones; thus the presence or absence of local extension was designated by a suffix within each T category. This change was reflected in the stage grouping in that T1 and T2 lesions with local extension were considered stage II rather than stage III as in the system proposed by Levitt and coworkers.[107]

Currently there are no staging systems that specifically address tumors of the intraoral minor salivary glands. However, Spiro and associates[109] have shown good prognostic correlation for mucoepidermoid carcinoma of these glands by staging according to criteria used for epidermoid carcinoma arising in the oral cavity, pharynx, larynx, or sinuses.

FROZEN SECTION DIAGNOSIS

The process of preparing histologic sections for microscopic examination from frozen diseased tissues was first introduced in Holland by de Reimer in 1818.[110–112] However, it was not until the invention and refinement of the cryostat during the 1940s and 1950s that the use of the intraoperative frozen section technique became generally accepted.[113]

Several recent reports question the accuracy of

Table 9–12. Staging System for Major Salivary Gland Carcinoma Proposed by the American Joint Committee on Cancer*

Primary Tumor (T)†				
TX	Primary tumor cannot be assessed			
T0	No evidence of primary tumor			
T1	Tumor 2 cm or less in greatest diameter			
T2	Tumor more than 2 cm but not more than 4 cm in greatest dimension			
T3	Tumor more than 4 cm but not more than 6 cm in greatest dimension			
T4	Tumor more than 6 cm in greatest dimension			
Regional Lymph Nodes (N)				
NX	Regional lymph nodes cannot be assessed			
N0	No regional lymph node metastasis			
N1	Metatasis in a single ipsilateral lymph node, 3 cm or less in greatest dimension			
N2	Metatasis in a single ipsilateral lymph node, more than 3 cm but not more than 6 cm in greatest dimension; or in multiple ipsilateral lymph nodes, none more than 6 cm in greatest dimension; or in bilateral or contralateral lymph nodes, none more than 6 cm in greatest dimension			
N2a	Metastasis in a single ipsilateral lymph node more than 3 cm but not more than 6 cm in greatest dimension			

N2b	Metastasis in multiple ipsilateral lymph nodes, none more than 6 cm in greatest dimension			
N2c	Metastasis in bilateral or contralateral lymph nodes, none more than 6 cm in greatest dimension			
N3	Metastasis in a lymph node more than 6 cm in greatest dimension			
Distant Metastasis (M)				
MX	Presence of distant metastasis cannot be assessed			
M0	No distant metastasis			
M1	Distant metastasis			
Stage Grouping				
Stage I	T1a	N0	M0	
	T2a	N0	M0	
Stage II	T1b	N0	M0	
	T2b	N0	M0	
	T3b	N0	M0	
Stage III	T3b	N0	M0	
	T4a	N0	M0	
	Any T (except T4b)	N1	M0	
Stage IV	T4b	Any N	M0	
	Any T	N2, N3	M0	
	Any T	Any N	M1	

*Table modified from Beahrs OH, Henson DE, Hutter RVP, Myers MT (eds.): Manual for Staging of Cancer, 3rd ed. Philadelphia, JB Lippincott, 1988; p. 52.

†All T categories are subdivided into (a) no local extension and (b) local extension. Local extension is clinical or macroscopic evidence of invasion of skin, soft tissues, bone, or nerve.

Table 9–13. Accuracy of Frozen Section Diagnosis of Salivary Gland Lesions

Reference	Number of Frozen Sections	False-Positive Diagnoses	False-Negative Diagnoses	Deferred Diagnoses
Pitts and colleagues (1958)[130]	19	1	1	0
Khoo (1965)[125]	12	0	0	0
Nakazawa and colleagues (1968)[114]	109	1	3	1
Elsner (1968)[124]	44	0	0	0
Funkhouser and colleagues (1979)[129]	23	0	0	0
Bauer (1970)[127]	31	0	2	3
Iri and colleagues (1977)[135]	6	0	2	0
Dehner and Rosai (1977)[121]	11	0	0	0
Miller and colleagues (1979)[116]	132	0	6	10
Dalal and colleagues (1979)[128]	22	0	1	1
Hillel and Fee (1983)[115]	75	0	4	7
Remsen and colleagues (1984)[126]	118	0	4	0
Wheelis and Yarington (1984)[118]	256	4	6	—
Dindzans and Van Nostrand (1984)[131]	110	0	3	2
Granick and colleagues (1985)[119]	462	8	12	0
Dankwa and Davies (1985)[122]	5	0	0	0
Cohen and colleagues (1986)[132]	21	0	1	1
Kaufman and colleagues (1986)[123]	3	0	0	0
Rigual and colleagues (1986)[133]	100	2	2	—
Layfield and colleagues (1987)[134]	38	0	4	2
Gnepp and colleagues (1987)[120]	301	2	4	7
Total from all references	1,898	18 (0.9%)	55 (2.9%)	34

frozen section diagnosis of salivary gland lesions, especially involving malignant neoplasms.[114–119] However, a recent study of 301 lesions, including 162 benign neoplasms, 72 malignant neoplasms, and 67 benign non-neoplastic masses, reported an accuracy rate of 98 percent, excluding deferred diagnoses.[120] This compares favorably with the published average accuracy rate, from 25 series, of 98.6 percent without deferred diagnoses for 45,698 frozen sections from other regions of the body.[113] However, the overall average accuracy rate in 21 series[114–116, 118–135] of 96.2 percent of salivary gland frozen section diagnoses, excluding deferred frozen sections (Table 9–13), is slightly less accurate. Furthermore, if salivary gland lesions are divided into benign and malignant

groups (Tables 9–14, 9–15), it becomes apparent that the accuracy rate is excellent for the benign group, which accounts for 78 percent of the frozen sections. However, in the malignant tumor group, the accuracy rates with and without deferred diagnoses are 77.1 and 85.7 percent, respectively (Table 9–15).

Fifty-seven percent of the false-positive diagnoses involved pleomorphic adenomas. The pathologist must be aware that it is not unusual for cellular areas in benign mixed tumors to contain tightly packed ductal cells, some of which may be rather atypical and have an active mitotic rate (Fig. 9–5). Care must be taken not to "overdiagnose" these latter areas as carcinoma. Slightly more than 20 percent of false-positive diagnoses

Table 9–14. Accuracy of Frozen Section Diagnosis of Benign Salivary Gland Lesions

Reference	Number of Frozen Sections	Erroneously Called Malignant	Deferred Diagnoses
Nakazawa and colleagues (1968)[114]	79	1	0
Elsner (1968)[124]	44	0	0
Funkhouser and colleagues (1970)[129]	21	0	0
Bauer (1974)[127]	24	0	0
Dehner and Rosai (1977)[121]	10	0	0
Miller and colleagues (1979)[116]	107	0	6
Hillel and Fee (1983)[115]	61	0	3
Remsen and colleagues (1984)[126]	99	0	0
Wheelis and Yarington (1984)[118]	204	4	—
Dindzans and Van Nostrand (1984)[131]	90	0	2
Granick and colleagues (1985)[119]	376	8	0
Cohen and colleagues (1986)[132]	19	0	0
Rigual and colleagues (1986)[133]	80	2	—
Gnepp and colleagues (1987)[120]	229	2	3
Total from all references	1,443	17 (1.2%)	14

Table 9–15. Accuracy of Frozen Section Diagnosis of Malignant Salivary Gland Lesions

Reference	Number of Frozen Sections	Erroneously Called Benign	Deferred Diagnoses
Nakazawa and colleagues (1968)[114]	20	3	1
Funkhouser and colleagues (1970)[129]	2	0	0
Bauer (1974)[127]	7	2	3
Iri and colleagues (1977)[135]	3	2	0
Dehner and Rosai (1977)[121]	1	0	0
Miller and colleagues (1979)[116]	25	6	4
Hillel and Fee (1983)[115]	14	4	4
Remsen and colleagues (1984)[126]	19	4	4
Wheelis and Yarington (1984)[118]	52	6	—
Dindzans and Van Nostrand (1984)[131]	20	3	0
Granick and colleagues (1985)[119]	86	12	0
Cohen and colleagues (1986)[132]	2	1	1
Rigual and colleagues (1986)[133]	20	2	—
Gnepp and colleagues (1987)[120]	72	4	4
Total from all references	343	49 (14.3%)	21

were associated with benign lymphoepithelial lesions or cysts causing confusion with lymphoma or mucoepidermoid carcinoma. Oncocytomas and a case of sarcoidosis also have caused difficulty.[120, 133]

Mucoepidermoid carcinoma was the tumor most commonly involved with a false-negative diagnosis (32 percent), whereas acinic cell carcinoma (18 percent), adenoid cystic carcinoma (16 percent), and malignant mixed tumor (16 percent) also

caused difficulty.[120, 131–133] Mucoepidermoid carcinomas must be differentiated from chronic sialadenitis and necrotizing sialometaplasia. Occasionally, in cases of chronic sialadenitis, one may find ectatic salivary ducts with mucinous metaplasia. The epithelial lining in these ducts appears similar to normal excretory duct epithelium except for an increased density of mucin-secreting cells; however, if the mucosa is focally thickened to more than three times that of normal mucosa and has

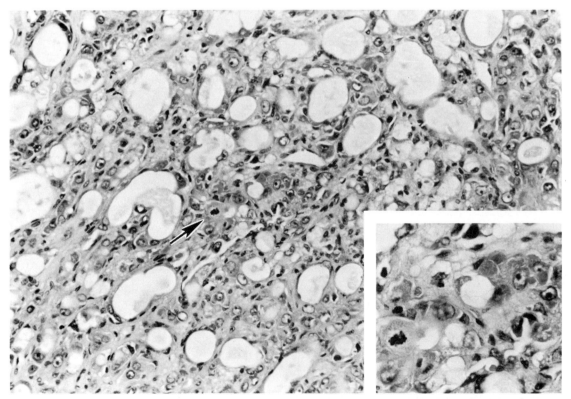

Figure 9–5. Portion of a mixed tumor demonstrating marked crowding of epithelial cells with focally prominent nucleoli and a rare mitotic figure (arrow) (× 100). *Inset,* detail of atypical but benign epithelium (× 200).

areas of mucinous and squamous differentiation, mucoepidermoid carcinoma is most likely the correct diagnosis.

Necrotizing sialometaplasia is a non-neoplastic, inflammatory, commonly ulcerating, and self-healing lesion of salivary glands (see Chapter 5). A history of previous trauma or surgery, usually within the past several weeks, is helpful in separating necrotizing sialometaplasia from squamous carcinoma that is growing down salivary excretory ducts. The need for this distinction is often a problem when freezing surgical margins of the palate, the larynx, the nasal cavity, or in the paranasal sinus regions. If diagnosis is in doubt, an additional piece of tissue should be obtained for frozen section examination. This usually will resolve the problem. One recent case of proliferative sialometaplasia was reported in which squamous sialometaplasia arising from ductal inclusions within an intraparotid lymph node simulated malignancy.[136] Necrotizing sialometaplasia is important in the differential diagnosis whenever frozen section diagnosis is performed on any mass or surgical margin that is obtained from areas where salivary or seromucinous glands are found.

Many of the false-negative errors are caused by poor sampling, by either the surgeon or the pathologist. Although sampling errors cannot be avoided completely, they can be minimized. It is preferable for the pathologist to receive the entire specimen, if surgically possible, and to select the area to freeze. The variable histologic appearance of many salivary gland tumors is well known, and inadequate sampling may lead to erroneous results. Carcinomas arising in a pleomorphic adenoma are often localized to one region and may only infiltrate focally. Also, acinic cell and mucoepidermoid carcinomas may present as cystic masses, diminishing suspicion of malignancy. The specimen should be carefully examined, and areas that appear necrotic, solid, or cystic should be separately sampled. Sections should always include the neoplasm, capsule, and adjacent soft tissues to evaluate as much of the tumor's interface with surrounding tissues as possible. Sections should never be limited to the middle of the tumor. Poorly defined borders that blend imperceptibly into adjacent soft tissues suggest malignancy. Sampling risks can be minimized only by careful examination of the entire specimen by the pathologist.

The histologic characteristics of the majority of tumors should not present diagnostic difficulty. It is the exceptional carcinoma, the unusual pleomorphic or monomorphic adenoma, and occasionally, a lymphoma that may cause diagnostic problems. It should also be remembered that pleomorphic and monomorphic adenomas often contain small areas resembling adenoid cystic carcinoma, especially when arising in minor salivary glands.[137] Also, lymph nodes are commonly found in periparotid and intraparotid locations or adjacent to the submandibular gland. Tumor may directly infiltrate these nodes, or the nodes may contain ectopic salivary gland tissue that occasionally may give rise to primary intranodal tumors. This is illustrated by the report of missed diagnoses of two intranodal acinic cell carcinomas and the seeding of a lymph node by a benign pleomorphic adenoma, which, at the time of its recurrence, caused a false-positive diagnosis.[120]

Oncocytomas may be misdiagnosed as acinic cell carcinomas, and acinic cell carcinomas may be "underdiagnosed" as oncocytomas. Oncocytoma nuclei are usually relatively small and centrally placed, whereas acinic cell carcinoma cells have larger, more pleomorphic nuclei often found at the cell periphery.[137] Also, areas of papillary and ductal differentiation may be found in acinic cell carcinomas but usually are not found in oncocytomas.

If the tumor is completely encapsulated and grossly uniform in appearance, and the initial frozen section reveals a classic histologic pattern, a specific diagnosis often can be rendered. If the tumor is multifocal, necrotic, or appears invasive, it should be carefully sampled with two or more frozen sections before a specific diagnosis is given. Recurrent mixed tumors, oncocytic lesions, dermal analogue tumors, and canalicular adenomas of the upper lip are benign neoplasms that may present as multinodular masses.[138, 139] In problematic cases, a specific histologic diagnosis is not always prudent. Furthermore, often the only information the surgeon needs to plan an operative approach is whether a tumor is benign or malignant. If there is any uncertainty or doubt, it is best to consult another pathologist, and if doubt still persists, the diagnosis should await permanent sections.

It is possible to accurately diagnose salivary gland neoplasms by examining frozen sections.[140] However, the literature does suggest caution when dealing with malignant tumors. Optimal accuracy is obtained by the pathologist who is aware of the gross and microscopic spectrum of salivary gland neoplasia, who examines specimens carefully for evidence of macroscopic variation, who does not hesitate to sample additional areas when faced with problematic and unusual microscopic patterns, and who places discretion above valor when microscopic findings indicate that deferral until permanent section is prudent. Finally, it is important to remember that a therapeutic decision should never be made on the basis of a frozen section diagnosis alone; it should always be made in conjunction with the clinical findings.

THE MERITS AND LIMITATIONS OF FINE-NEEDLE ASPIRATION IN THE DIAGNOSIS OF SALIVARY GLAND LESIONS

The role of fine-needle aspiration (FNA) has gained increasing acceptance in the diagnosis of abnormal masses in all body sites. The diagnostic accuracy of FNA, coupled with its cost containment and low associated morbidity rate, makes it an ideal preoperative procedure for assessing neoplastic lesions and directing subsequent therapy. From an anatomic standpoint, salivary gland lesions are easily accessible to needle aspiration. Despite a long history of use in the diagnosis of salivary gland neoplasms in Scandinavian countries[141-148] as well as in the United States,[149, 150] only later in its history did FNA gain support in the United States as a diagnostic procedure of choice in assessing salivary gland lesions. This emergence is based on numerous studies that demonstrate the high accuracy rate in needle aspiration diagnosis of salivary gland lesions.[151-158] The purpose of this review is to analyze the merits and pitfalls of needle aspiration in regard to salivary gland lesions.

An array of pathologic processes may cause enlargement of the salivary glands. These include non-neoplastic and neoplastic conditions. The overwhelming majority of major salivary gland neoplasms are benign, and nearly 80 percent of these are mixed tumors. As such, from a purely statistical viewpoint, a lesion of the parotid gland, in the appropriate clinical setting, is a mixed tumor until proved otherwise. However, salivary gland pathology is diverse, and despite good correlation between the clinical picture and the pathologic diagnosis, discrepancies can occur. Although malignancy may be obvious in some patients, most malignant salivary gland neoplasms are clinically indistinguishable from their benign counterparts.[22, 159] It would be an invaluable aid in planning definitive therapy to be able to establish a diagnosis employing a safe, quick, inexpensive, and accurate method. FNA offers such a technique; however, despite its practicality and increasing utility, it has deficiencies. The practicing pathologist must fully understand its limitations in diagnosis. According to most sources, the diagnostic accuracy with regard to benignancy versus malignancy is about 98 percent for benign salivary gland neoplasms, 93 percent for primary malignant salivary gland tumors, and 88 percent for metastatic tumors.[21] This starkly contrasts with a diagnostic accuracy of 31 percent reported prior to 1963.[155, 160] Experience and advances in the technique account for this increase in diagnostic accuracy, leading some to claim similar results for needle aspiration and for surgical biopsy.[160] A recent review of 3,615 cases from 13 series indicated false-positive and false-negative rates of 1.2 percent and 4.5 percent, respectively.[134] However, one should remember that the exact histologic diagnosis can be established in only about 75 percent of patients.[134, 187] Further, both false-positive and false-negative diagnoses are rare in the interpretation of FNA specimens of salivary gland lesions.[161] Virtually every conceivable lesion of major and minor salivary glands as well as lesions that arose in adjacent soft tissue,

overlying skin, or metastatic tumors to the salivary glands has been diagnosed by FNA.[141-148, 151-156, 160-191]

Among the many arguments cited in support of diagnosis of salivary gland lesions via FNA are cost containment,[153, 192] negligible associated morbidity and/or complications,[153, 160, 192, 193] rapidity in arriving at a diagnosis, high diagnostic accuracy,[151-158] and ability to use this procedure in determining patient management.[151, 156, 162, 183, 192] In addition, tumor implantation along the needle tract following aspiration biopsy, which is a complication that occurs at other body sites[194, 195] as well as in salivary glands with the use of large-bore needles for aspiration,[196] has not been reported with the use of smaller gauge needles.[160] Among the diagnostic limitations of aspirated material, in contrast to conventional biopsy material, are the limited histologic architectural features and the absence of the tumor-stroma interface, which are both of critical importance in the diagnosis of many salivary gland neoplasms. Although statistically FNA is a sensitive and specific technique, many diagnoses hinge on architectural features and evidence of the presence or absence of invasion. The status of invasion is considered by us and others to be one of the most important criteria in predicting biologic behavior.[143, 197] The small sample obtained by needle aspiration precludes the disclosure of these features to the pathologist. Examples illustrating these points include the difficulties in separating a benign mixed tumor from adenoid cystic carcinoma[141, 148, 183, 198] and polymorphous low-grade adenocarcinoma,[178, 184] variants of monomorphic adenoma from adenoid cystic carcinoma,[168, 173, 181, 182, 198, 199] basal cell adenoma from basal cell adenocarcinoma,[200] infectious or autoimmune sialadenitides from lymphomas,[134, 160] and benign mixed tumor from carcinoma arising in mixed tumor.[174] The last example highlights the potential pitfall of chance aspiration of a region with atypical cytologic features in an otherwise typical benign tumor (see Fig. 9–5). This has been the source of false-positive diagnoses in several reports.[143, 146, 148, 162] Conversely, carcinoma arising in benign mixed tumor can be missed in limited samples and yield false-negative results.[147, 199] Furthermore, bias based on the limited clinical history of benignancy or malignancy may lead to erroneous conclusions on the limited sampling of aspirated material. Therefore, as others point out,[149, 199] larger biopsies are preferred to aspirated samples when the biopsies can be obtained with limited difficulty.

As previously mentioned, many studies cite the high sensitivity and specificity of FNA in salivary gland lesions. However, Hajdu and Melamed[199] point out that "the diagnosis of cancer is simpler than its classification." The complexity and diversity of salivary gland lesions are such that limited sampling precludes an overall evaluation of a lesion that may be composed of multiple patterns and cellular components. Familiarity with the var-

Vienna, International Atomic Energy Agency, 1978; 71–81.

47. Takeichi N, Hirose F, Yamamoto H, Ezaki H, Fujikura T: Salivary gland tumors in atomic bomb survivors, Hiroshima, Japan: II. Pathologic study and supplementary epidemiologic observations. Cancer 1983; 52:377–385.

48. Schneider AB, Favus MJ, Stachura ME, Arnold MJ, Frohman LA: Salivary gland neoplasms as a late consequence of head and neck irradiation. Ann Intern Med 1977; 87:160–164.

49. Colman M, Kirsch M, Creditor M: Tumours associated with medical x-ray therapy exposure in childhood. *In* Late Biological Effects of Ionizing Radiation. Vienna, International Atomic Energy Agency, 1978; 71–81.

50. Shore-Freedman E, Abrahams C, Recant W, Schneider AB: Neurilemomas and salivary gland tumors of the head and neck following childhood irradiation. Cancer 1983; 51:2159–2163.

51. Schneider AB, Shore-Freedman E, Ryo UY, Bekerman C, Favus M, Pinsky S: Radiation-induced tumors of the head and neck following childhood irradiation: Prospective studies. Medicine 1985; 64:1–15.

52. Hempelmann LH: Neoplasms in youthful populations following x-ray treatment in infancy. Environ Res 1967; 1:338–358.

53. Modan B, Baidatz D, Mart H, Steinitz R, Levin SG: Radiation-induced head and neck tumours. Lancet 1974; 1:277–278.

54. Shore RE, Albert RE, Pasternack BS: Follow-up study of patients treated by x-ray epilation for tinea capitis: Resurvey of post-treatment illness and mortality experience. Arch Environ Health 1976; 31:17–24.

55. Hazen RW, Pifer JW, Toyooka ET, Livingood J, Hempelmann H: Neoplasms following irradiation of the head. Cancer Res 1966; 26:305–311.

56. Palmer JA, Mustard RA, Simpson WJ: Irradiation as an etiologic factor in tumours of the thyroid, parathyroid and salivary glands. Can J Surg 1980; 23:39–42.

57. Spitz MR, Batsakis JG: Major salivary gland carcinoma: Descriptive epidemiology and survival of 498 patients. Arch Otolaryngol 1984; 110:45–49.

58. Spitz MR, Tilley BC, Batsakis JG, Gibeau JM, Newell GR: Risk factors for major salivary gland carcinoma: A case comparison study. Cancer 1984; 54:1854–1859.

59. Hoffman DA, McConahey WM, Fraumeni JF, Kurland LT: Cancer incidence following treatment of hyperthyroidism. Int J Epidemiol 1982; 11:218–224.

60. Loy TS, McLauglin R, Odom LF, Dehner LP: Mucoepidermoid carcinoma of the parotid as a second malignant neoplasm in children. Cancer 1989; 64:2174–2177.

61. Katz AD: Thyroid and associated polyglandular neoplasms in patients who received head and neck irradiation during childhood. Head Neck Surg 1979; 1:417–422.

62. Katz AD, Preston-Martin S: Salivary gland tumors and previous radiotherapy to the head or neck: Report of a clinical series. Am J Surg 1984; 147:345–348.

63. Ju DMC: Salivary gland tumors occurring after radiation of the head and neck area. Am J Surg 1968; 116:518–523.

64. Sener SF, Scanlon EF: Irradiation induced salivary gland neoplasia. Ann Surg 1980; 191:304–306.

65. Maxon HR, Saenger EL, Buncher CR, Thomas SR, Kereiakes JG, Shafer ML, McLaughlin CA: Radiation-associated carcinoma of the salivary gland: A controlled study. Ann Otol 1981; 90:107–108.

66. Hawkins MM, Draper GJ, Kingston JE: Incidence of second primary tumours among childhood cancer survivors. Br J Cancer 1987; 56:339–347.

67. Swelstad JA, Scanlon EF, Ovledo MA, Hugo NE: Irradiation-induced polyglandular neoplasia of the head and neck. Am J Surg 1978; 135:820–824.

68. Watkin GT, Hobsley M: Should radiotherapy be used routinely in the management of benign parotid tumours. Br J Surg 1986; 73:601–603.

69. Preston-Martin S, Henderson BE, Bernstein L: Medical and dental x-rays as risk factors for recently diagnosed tumors of the head. NCI Monogr 1985; 69:175–179.

70. Preston-Martin S, Thomas DC, White SC, Cohen D: Prior exposure to medical and dental x-rays related to tumors of the parotid gland. J Natl Cancer Inst 1988; 80:943–949.

71. Preston-Martin S, White SC: Brain and salivary gland tumors related to prior dental radiography: Implications for current practice. JADA 1990; 120:151–158.

72. Graham S, Blanchet M, Rohrer T: Cancer in asbestos-mining and other areas of Quebec. J Natl Cancer Inst 1977; 59:1139–1145.

73. Mancuso TF, Brennan MJ: Epidemiological considerations of cancer of the gallbladder, bile ducts and salivary glands in the rubber industry. J Occup Med 1970; 12:333–341.

74. Milham S Jr: Cancer mortality patterns associated with exposure to metals. Ann NY Acad Sci 1976; 271:243–249.

75. Swanson GM, Belle SH: Cancer morbidity among woodworkers in the US automotive industry. J Occup Med 1982; 24:315–319.

76. Keller, AZ: Residence, age, race and related factors in the survival and associations with salivary tumors. J Epidemiol 1969; 90:269–277.

77. Williams RR, Horm JW: Association of cancer sites with tobacco and alcohol consumption and socioeconomic status of patients: Interview from the Third National Cancer Survey. J Natl Cancer Inst 1977; 58:525–547.

78. Armstrong B: Endocrine factors in human carcinogenesis. IARC Sci Publ 1982; 39:193–221.

79. Dimery IS, Jones LA, Verjan RP, Raymond AK, Goepfert H, Hong WH: Estrogen receptors in normal salivary gland and salivary gland carcinoma. Arch Otolaryngol Head Neck Surg 1987; 113:1082–1085.

80. Abbey LM, Witorsch RJ: Prolactin binding in minor salivary gland tumors. Oral Surg Oral Med Oral Pathol 1985; 60:44–49.

81. Seifert G, Okabe H, Caselitz J: Epithelial salivary gland tumors in children and adolescents. Analysis of 80 cases (Salivary Gland Register 1965–1984). ORL 1986; 48:137–149.

82. Dahlqvist Å, Östberg Y: Malignant salivary gland tumours in children. Acta Otolaryngol 1982; 94:175–179.

83. Catania VC, Bozzetti F, Santangelo A, Salvadori B: Parotid tumors in infants and children. Tumori 1977; 63:195–198.

84. Shikhani AH, Johns, ME: Tumors of the major salivary glands. Head Neck Surg 1988; 10:257–263.

85. Castro EB, Huvos AG, Strong EW, Foote F: Tumors of the major salivary glands in children. Cancer 1972; 29:312–317.

86. Baker SR, Malone B: Salivary gland malignancies in children. Cancer 1985; 55:1730–1736.

87. Lack EE, Upton MP: Histopathologic review of salivary gland tumors in childhood. Arch Otolaryngol Head Neck Surg 1988; 114:898–906.

88. Jaques DA, Krolls SO, Chambers RG: Parotid tumors in children. Am J Surg 1976; 132:469–471.

89. Krolls SO, Trodahl JN, Boyers RC: Salivary gland lesions in children. A survey of 430 cases. Cancer 1972; 30:459–469.

90. Chong GC, Beahrs OH, Chen MLC, Hayles AB: Management of parotid tumors in infants and children. Mayo Clin Proc 1975; 50:279–283.

91. Welch KJ, Trump DS: The salivary glands. *In* Ravitch MM, Welch KJ, Benson CD, Aberdeen E, Randolph JG (eds.): Pediatric Surgery, ed. 3. Chicago, Year Book Medical Publishers, Inc., 1979; 308–323.

92. Schuller DE, McCabe BF: The firm salivary mass in children. Laryngoscope 1977; 87:1891–1898.

93. Berg JW, Hutter RVP, Foote FW JR: The unique association between salivary gland cancer and breast cancer. JAMA 1968; 204:771–774.

94. Moertel CG, Elveback LR: The association between salivary gland cancer and breast cancer. JAMA 1969; 210:306–308.

95. Dunn JE, Bragg KU, Sautter C, Gardipee C: Breast cancer risk following a major salivary gland carcinoma. Cancer 1972; 29:1343–1346.

96. Newell GR, Krementz ET, Roberts JD: Multiple primary neoplasms in blacks compared to whites: II. Further cancers in patients with cancer of the buccal cavity and pharynx. J Natl Cancer Inst 1974; 52:639–642.

97. Prior P, Waterhouse JAH: Second primary cancer in patients with tumors of the salivary glands. Br J Cancer 1977; 36:362–368.

98. Biggar RJ, Curtis RE, Hoffman DA, Flannery JT: Second primary malignancies following salivary gland cancers. Br J Cancer 1983; 47:383–386.

99. Belson TP, Toohil RJ, Lehman RH, Chobanian SL, Grossman TW, Malin TC: Adenoid cystic carcinoma of the submaxillary gland. Laryngoscope 1982; 92:497–501.

100. Abbey LM, Schwab BH, Landau GC, Perkins ER: Incidence of second primary breast cancer among patients with a first primary salivary gland tumor. Cancer 1984; 54:1439–1442.

101. Schou G, Storm HH, Jensen OM: Second cancer following cancers of the buccal cavity and pharynx in Denmark, 1943–80. NCI Monogr 1985; 68:253–276.

102. Spitz MR, Newell GR, Gibeau JM, Byers RM, Batsakis JG: Multiple primary cancer risk in patients with major salivary gland carcinoma. Ann Otol Rhinol Laryngol 1985; 94:129–132.

103. Johns ME, Shikhani AH, Kashima HK, Matanoski GM: Multiple primary neoplasms in patients with salivary gland or thyroid gland tumors. Laryngoscope 1986; 96:718–721.

104. Gnepp DR, Schroeder W, Heffner D: Synchronous tumors arising in a single major salivary gland. Cancer 1989; 63:1219–1224.

105. Spiro RH, Huvos AG, Strong EW: Cancer of the parotid gland: A clinicopathologic study of 288 primary cases. Am J Surg 1975; 130:452–459.

106. Spiro RH, Hajdu SI, Strong EW: Tumors of the submaxillary gland. Am J Surg 1976; 132:463–468.

107. Levitt SH, McHugh RB, Gómez-Marin O, Hyams VJ, Soule EH, Strong EW, Sellers AH, Woods JE, Guillamondegui OM: Clinical staging system for cancer of the salivary gland: A retrospective study. Cancer 1981; 47:2712–2724.

108. Beahrs OH, Henson DE, Hutter RVP, Myers MH (eds.): Manual for Staging of Cancer, 3rd Ed. Philadelphia, JB Lippincott, 1988; 51–56.

109. Spiro RH, Huvos AG, Berk R, Strong EW: Mucoepidermoid carcinoma of salivary gland origin: A clinicopathologic study of 367 cases. Am J Surg 1978; 136:461–468.

110. Krumbhaar EB: Clio Medica. A Series of Primers on the History of Medicine: 19, Pathology. New York, PB Hoeber Inc., 1937; 171.

111. Long ER: A History of Pathology. Baltimore, Williams & Wilkins, 1928; 212.

112. French AJ, Lafler CJ: Frozen sections: Rapid tissue diagnosis. J Michigan Med Soc 1960; 59: 591–595.

113. Gnepp DR: Frozen sections. *In* Gnepp DR (ed.): Pathology of the Head and Neck. New York, Churchill Livingstone, 1988; 1–24.

114. Nakazawa H, Rosen P, Lane N, Lattes R: Frozen section experience in 3,000 cases: Accuracy, limitations and value in residency training. Am J Clin Pathol 1968; 49:41–51.

115. Hillel AD, Fee WE Jr: Evaluation of frozen section in parotid gland. Surgery 1983; 109:230–232.

116. Miller RH, Calcaterra TC, Paglia DE: Accuracy of frozen section diagnosis of parotid lesions. Ann Otol Rhinol Laryngol 1979; 88:573–576.

117. Conley JJ: Salivary Glands and the Facial Nerve. New York, Grune & Stratton, 1975; 85–88.

118. Wheelis RF, Yarington CT Jr: Tumors of the salivary glands: Comparison of frozen-section diagnosis with final pathologic diagnosis. Arch Otolaryngol 1984; 110:76–77.

119. Granick MS, Erickson ER, Hanna DC: Accuracy of frozen-section diagnosis in salivary gland lesions. Head Neck Surg 1985; 7:465–467.

120. Gnepp DR, Rader WR, Cramer SF, Cook LL, Sciubba J: Accuracy of frozen section diagnosis of the salivary gland. Otolaryngol Head Neck Surg 1987; 96:325–330.

121. Dehner LP, Rosai J: Frozen section examination in surgical pathology: A retrospective study of one year experience, comprising 778 cases. Minn Med 1977; 60:83–94.

122. Dankwa EK, Davies JD: Frozen section diagnosis: An audit. J Clin Pathol 1985; 38:1235–1240.

123. Kaufman Z, Lew S, Griffel B, Dinbar A: Frozen-section diagnosis in surgical pathology: A prospective analysis of 526 frozen sections. Cancer 1986; 57:377–379.

124. Elsner B: La biopsia por congelacion: Su valor asistencial y en la educacion medica del patologo. Pren Med Argent, 1968; 55:1741–1749.

125. Khoo TK: Frozen section service in the general hospital, Singapore. Singapore Med J 1965; 6:219–225.

126. Remsen KA, Lucente FE, Biller HF: Reliability of frozen section diagnosis in head and neck neoplasms. Laryngoscope 1984; 94:519–524.

127. Bauer WC. The use of frozen sections in otolaryngology. Otorhinolaryngology 1974; 78:88–97.
128. Dalal BI, Malik AK, Datta BN: Frozen section diagnosis: A review of 1051 cases. Indian J Cancer 1979; 16:59–65.
129. Funkhouser JW, Oosting M, Kelly M, Straughen WJ: Evaluation of frozen sections using the cryostat in a community hospital: Analysis of 3968 consecutive cases. Ohio State Med J 1970; 66:46–49.
130. Pitts HH, Sturdy JH, Coady CJ: Frozen sections II. Value in cases of suspected malignancy. Can Med Assoc J 1958; 79:110–113.
131. Dindzans LJ, Van Nostrand AWP: The accuracy of frozen section diagnosis of parotid lesions. J Otolaryngol 1984; 13:382–386.
132. Cohen MB, Ljung BE, Boles R: Salivary gland tumors. Fine-needle aspiration vs frozen-section diagnosis. Arch Otolaryngol Head Neck Surg 1986; 112:867–869.
133. Rigual RR, Milley P, Lore JM Jr, Kaufman S: Accuracy of frozen section diagnosis in salivary gland neoplasms. Head Neck Surg 1986; 8:442–446.
134. Layfield LJ, Tan P, Glasgow BJ: Fine-needle aspiration of salivary gland lesions: Comparison with frozen sections and histologic findings. Arch Pathol Lab Med 1987; 111:346–353.
135. Iri H, Mikata A, Takeuchi H, Kameya T: Frozen section diagnosis. Indication, limitation and diagnostic value. Rinsho Byori 1977; 25:499–509.
136. Goldman RL, Klein HZ: Proliferative sialometaplasia arising in an intraparotid lymph node. Am J Clin Pathol 1986; 86:116–119.
137. Perzin KH: Systematic approach to the pathologic diagnosis of salivary gland tumors. In Fenoglio CM, Wolff M (eds.): Progress in Surgical Pathology, Vol. 4. New York, Masson Publishing USA, Inc, 1982:137–179.
138. Batsakis JG, Brannon RB, Sciubba JJ: Monomorphic adenomas of major salivary glands: A histologic study of 96 tumors. Clin Otolaryngol 1981; 6:129–143.
139. Daley TD: The canalicular adenoma: Considerations on differential diagnosis and treatment. J Oral Maxillofac Surg 1984; 42:728–730.
140. Luna MA: Uses, abuses and pitfalls of frozen section diagnoses of diseases of the head and neck. In Barnes EL (ed.): Surgical Pathology of the Head and Neck. New York, Marcel Dekker Inc, 1985; 7–22.
141. Mavec P, Eneroth CM, Franzen S, Moberger G, Zajicek J: Aspiration biopsy of salivary gland tumours. I. Correlation of cytologic reports from 652 aspiration biopsies with clinical and histologic findings. Acta Otolaryngol (Stockh) 1964; 58:472–484.
142. Eneroth CM, Zajicek J: Aspiration biopsy of salivary gland tumors. II. Morphologic studies on smears and histologic sections from oncocytic tumors (45 cases of papillary cystadenoma lymphomatosum and 4 cases of oncocytoma). Acta Cytol 1965; 9:355–361.
143. Eneroth CM, Zajicek J: Aspiration biopsy of salivary gland tumors. III. Morphologic smears and histologic sections from 368 mixed tumors. Acta Cytol 1966; 10:440–454.
144. Eneroth CM, Franzen S, Zajicek J: Aspiration biopsy of salivary gland tumors: A critical review of 910 biopsies. Acta Cytol 1967; 11:470–472.

145. Eneroth CM, Franzen S, Zajicek J: Cytologic diagnosis of aspirate from 1,000 salivary gland tumors. Acta Otolaryngol Suppl (Stockh) 1967; 224:168–171.
146. Eneroth CM, Zajicek J: Aspiration biopsy of salivary gland tumors. IV. Morphologic studies on smears and histologic sections from 45 cases of adenoid cystic carcinoma. Acta Cytol 1969; 13:59–63.
147. Persson PS, Zettergren L: Cytologic diagnosis of salivary gland tumors by aspiration biopsy. Acta Cytol 1973; 17:351–354.
148. Lindberg LG, Akerman M: Aspiration cytology of salivary gland tumors. Diagnostic experience from six years of routine laboratory work. Laryngoscope 1976; 86:584–594.
149. Martin HE, Ellis EB: Biopsy by needle puncture and aspiration. Ann Surg 1930; 92:169–181.
150. Stewart FW: The diagnosis of tumors by aspiration. Am J Pathol 1933; 9:801–815.
151. Kolson H, Aslam P: Accuracy and value of needle biopsy of the parotid gland. Arch Otolaryngol 1968; 87:501–505.
152. Frable WJ, Frable MA: Thin-needle aspiration biopsy in the diagnosis of head and neck tumors. Laryngoscope 1974; 84:1069–1077.
153. Young JEM, Archibald SD, Shier KJ: Needle aspiration cytologic biopsy in head and neck masses. Am J Surg 1981; 142:484–489.
154. Sismanis A, Merriam JM, Kline TS, Davis K, Shapshay SM, Strong MS: Diagnosis of salivary gland tumors by fine needle aspiration biopsy. Head Neck Surg 1981; 3:482–489.
155. Qizilbash AH, Sianos J, Young JEM, Archibald SD: Fine needle aspiration biopsy cytology of major salivary glands. Acta Cytol 1985; 29:503–512.
156. O'Dwyer P, Farrar WB, James AG, Finkelmeier W, McCabe DP: Needle aspiration biopsy of major salivary gland tumors: Its value. Cancer 1986; 57:554–557.
157. Slack RWT, Croft CB, Crome LP: Fine needle cytology in the management of head and neck masses. Clin Otolaryngol 1985; 10:93–96.
158. Lau T, Balle VH, Bretlau P: Fine needle aspiration biopsy in salivary gland tumours. Clin Otolaryngol 1986; 11:75–77.
159. Dunn EJ, Kent T, Hines J, Cohn I: Parotid neoplasms: A report of 250 cases and review of the literature. Ann Surg 1976; 184:500–506.
160. Qizilbash AH, Young JEM: Salivary glands. In Qizilbash AH, Young JEM (eds.): Guides to Clinical Aspiration Biopsy Head and Neck. Tokyo, Igaku-Shoin, 1988; 15–116.
161. Kline TS, Merriam JM, Shapshay SM: Aspiration biopsy cytology of the salivary gland. Am J Clin Pathol 1981; 76:263–269.
162. Webb AJ: Cytologic diagnosis of salivary gland lesions in adults and pediatric surgical patients. Acta Cytol 1973; 17:51–58.
163. Malberger E: Aspiration cytology in the diagnosis of orofacial masses. Int J Oral Surg 1974; 3:137–143.
164. Woyke S, Olszewski W, Domagala W, Marzecki Z: Cytodiagnosis of acinic cell carcinoma: Ultrastructural study of material obtained by fine needle aspiration biopsy. Acta Cytol 1975; 19:110–116.
165. Zajicek J, Eneroth CM, Jakobsson P: Aspiration biopsy of salivary gland tumors. VI. Morphologic studies on smears and histologic sections from

mucoepidermoid carcinoma. Acta Cytol 1976; 20:35–41.

166. Frable WJ: Thin needle aspiration biopsy: A personal experience with 469 cases. Am J Clin Pathol 1976; 65:168–181.

167. Pellegrino SV: Malignant lymphoma and salivary obstruction. J Oral Maxillofac Surg 1978; 36:223–226.

168. Hood IC, Qizilbash AH, Salama SS, Alexopoulou I: Basal-cell adenoma of the parotid: Difficulty of differentiation from adenoid cystic carcinoma on aspiration biopsy. Acta Cytol 1983; 27:515–520.

169. Hood IC, Qizilbash AH, Salama SS, Young JEM, Archibald SD: Needle aspiration of sebaceous carcinoma. Acta Cytol 1984; 28:305–312.

170. Jayaram G: Cytology of hemangioendothelioma. Acta Cytol 1984; 28:153–156.

171. Balle VH, Greisen O: Neurilemmomas of the facial nerve presenting as parotid tumors. Ann Otol Rhinol Laryngol 1984; 93:70–72.

172. Yazdi HM, Hogg GR: Malignant lymphoepithelial lesion of the submandibular salivary gland. Am J Clin Pathol 1984; 82:344–348.

173. Layfield LJ: Fine needle aspiration cytology of a trabecular adenoma of the parotid gland. Acta Cytol 1985; 29:999–1002.

174. Geisinger KR, Reynolds GD, Vance RP, McGuirt WF: Adenoid cystic carcinoma arising in a pleomorphic adenoma of the parotid gland. Acta Cytol 1985; 29:522–526.

175. Gal R, Strauss M, Zohar Y, Kessler E: Salivary duct carcinoma of the parotid gland: Cytologic and histopathologic study. Acta Cytol 1985; 29:454–456.

176. Aufdemorte TB, Ramzy I, Holt GR, Thomas JR, Duncan DL: Focal adenomatoid hyperplasia of salivary glands: A differential diagnostic problem in fine needle aspiration biopsy. Acta Cytol 1985; 29:23–28.

177. Ebbs SR, Webb AJ: Adenolymphoma of the parotid: Aetiology, diagnosis and treatment. Br J Surg 1986; 73:627–630.

178. Frierson HF, Covell JL, Mills SE: Fine-needle aspiration cytology of terminal duct carcinoma of minor salivary gland. Diagn Cytopathol 1987; 3:159–162.

179. Austin MB, Frierson HF, Feldman PS: Oncocytoid adenocarcinoma of the parotid gland: Cytologic, histologic and ultrastructural findings. Acta Cytol 1987; 31:351–356.

180. Mair S, Phillips JI, Cohen R: Small cell undifferentiated carcinoma of the parotid gland: Cytologic, histologic, immunohistochemical and ultrastructural features of a neuroendocrine variant. Acta Cytol 1988; 33:164–168.

181. Hruban RH, Erozan YS, Zinreich SJ, Kashima HK: Fine-needle aspiration cytology of monomorphic adenomas. Am J Clin Pathol 1988; 90:46–51.

182. Stanley MW, Horwitz CA, Henry MJ, Burton LG, Lowhagen T: Basal-cell adenoma of the salivary gland: A benign adenoma that cytologically mimics adenoid cystic carcinoma. Diagn Cytopathol 1988; 4:342–346.

183. Bedrossian CWM, Martinez F, Silverberg AB: Fine needle aspiration. In Gnepp DR (ed.): Pathology of the Head and Neck. New York, Churchill Livingstone, 1988; 54–69.

184. Young JA: Fine needle aspiration cytology of salivary glands. Ear Nose Throat J 1989; 68:120–129.

185. Chan MKM, McGuire LJ: Fine needle aspiration cytodiagnosis of an unusual parotid mass. Acta Cytol 1989; 33:274–276.

186. Elliot JN, Oertel YC: Lymphoepithelial cysts of the salivary glands: Histologic and cytologic features. Am J Clin Pathol 1990; 93:39–43.

187. Rodriguez HP, Silver CE, Moisa II, Chacho MS: Fine-needle aspiration of parotid tumors. Am J Surg 1989; 158:342–344.

188. Currens HS, Sajjad SM, Lukeman JM: Aspiration cytology of oat cell carcinoma metastatic to the parotid gland. Acta Cytol 1982; 26:566–567.

189. Gattuso P, Castelli MJ, Shah PA, Kron T: Fine needle aspiration cytologic diagnosis of metastatic Merkel cell carcinoma in the parotid gland. Acta Cytol 1988; 32:576–578.

190. Powers CN, Raval P, Schmidt WA: Fine needle aspiration cytology of metastatic lymphoepithelioma: A case report. Acta Cytol 1989; 33:254–258.

191. Melnick SJ, Amazon K, Dembrow V: Metastatic renal cell carcinoma presenting as a parotid tumor: A case report with immunohistochemical findings and a review of the literature. Hum Pathol 1989; 20:195–197.

192. Frable MAS, Frable WJ: Fine-needle aspiration biopsy revisited. Laryngoscope 1981; 92:1414–1418.

193. McLoughlin MJ, Ho CS, Tao LC: Percutaneous needle aspiration biopsy. CMAJ 1978; 119:1324–1328.

194. Smith FP, Macdonald JS, Schein PS, Ornitz RD: Cutaneous seeding of pancreatic cancer by skinny-needle aspiration biopsy. Arch Intern Med 1980; 140:855.

195. Ferucci JT, Wittenberg J, Margolies MN, Carey RW: Malignant seeding of the tract after thin-needle aspiration biopsy. Radiology 1979; 130:345–346.

196. Yamaguchi KT, Strong MS, Shapshay SM, Soto E: Seeding of parotid carcinoma along Vim-Silverman needle tract. J Otolaryngol 1979; 8:49–52.

197. Eneroth CM, Zetterberg A: A cytochemical method of grading the malignancy of salivary gland tumours preoperatively. Acta Otolaryngol 1976; 81:489–495.

198. Orell SR, Nettle WJS: Fine needle aspiration biopsy of salivary gland tumours, problems and pitfalls. Pathology 1988; 20:332–337.

199. Hajdu SI, Melamed MR: Limitations of aspiration cytology in the diagnosis of primary neoplasms. Acta Cytol 1984; 28:337–345.

200. Ellis GL, Gnepp DR: Unusual salivary gland tumors. In Gnepp DR (ed.): Pathology of the Head and Neck. New York, Churchill Livingstone, 1988; 617–623.

201. Lininger JR, Corell JR, Feldman PS: The diagnosis of mucoepidermoid carcinoma of the salivary gland by fine needle aspiration. Acta Cytol 1981; 25:720–724.

202. Kern SB: Necrosis of a Warthin's tumor following fine needle aspiration. Acta Cytol 1988; 32:207–208.

203. Johns ME, Kaplan MJ: Malignant neoplasms. In Cummings CW, Fredrickson JM, Harker LA, Krause CJ, Schuller DE (eds.): Otolaryngology—Head and Neck Surgery. St. Louis, CV Mosby, 1986; 1035–1069.

204. McGahan JP, Walter JP, Bernstein L: Evaluation of the parotid gland: Comparison of sialography, non-contrast computed tomography, and CT sialography. Radiology 1984; 152:453–458.

205. Berg HM, Jacobs JB, Kaufman D, Reede DL: Correlation of fine needle aspiration biopsy and CT scanning of parotid masses. Laryngoscope 1986; 96:1357–1362.

206. Hannson LG, Johansen CC: CT sialography and conventional sialography in the investigation of parotid masses. Oral Surg Oral Med Oral Pathol 1987; 64:494–500.

207. Zbaren P, Ducommun JC: Diagnosis of salivary gland disease using ultrasound and sialography: A comparison. Clin Otolaryngol 1989; 14:189–187.

208. Johns ME, Goldsmith MM: Current management of salivary gland tumors. Oncology 1989; 3:85–91.

209. Sandberg AA, Turc-Carel C: The cytogenetics of solid tumors. Cancer 1987; 59:387–395.

210. Heim S, Mitelman F: Cancer Cytogenetics. New York, Alan R. Liss, Inc., 1987; 227–261.

211. Mark J, Dahlenfors R: Cytogenetical observations in 100 human benign pleomorphic adenomas: Specificity of the chromosomal aberrations and their relationship to sites of localized oncogenes. Anticancer Res 1986; 6:299–308.

212. Sandros J, Stenman G, Mark J: Cytogenetic and molecular observations in human and experimental salivary gland tumors. Cancer Genet Cytogenet 1990; 44:153–167.

213. Bullerdiek J, Takla G, Bartnitzke S, Brandt G, Chilla R, Haubrich J: Relationship of cytogenetic subtypes of salivary gland pleomorphic adeno-mas with patient age and histologic type. Cancer 1989; 64:876–880.

214. Mark J, Sandros J, Wedell B, Stenman G, Ekedahl C: Significance of the choice of tissue culture technique on the chromosomal patterns in human mixed salivary gland tumors. Cancer Genet Cytogenet 1988; 33:229–244.

215. Scappaticci S, Lo Curto F, Mira E: Karyotypic variation in benign pleomorphic adenoma of the parotid and in normal salivary glands. Acta Otolaryngol 1973; 76:221–228.

216. Mark J, Dahlenfors R, Ekedahl C, Stenman G: The mixed salivary gland tumor—a normally benign human neoplasm frequently showing specific chromosomal abnormalities. Cancer Genet Cytogenet 1980; 2:231–241.

217. Bullerdiek J, Chilla R, Haubrich J, Meyer K, Bartnitzke S: A causal relationship between chromosomal rearrangements and the genesis of salivary gland pleomorphic adenomas. ORL 1988; 245:244–249.

218. Tsukamoto AS, Grosschedl R, Guzman RC, Parslow T, Varmus HE: Expression of the int-1 gene in transgenic mice is associated with mammary gland hyperplasia and adenocarcinomas in male and female mice. Cell 1988; 55:619–625.

219. Bullerdiek J, Boschen C, Barnitzke S: Aberrations of chromosome 8 in mixed salivary gland tumors—cytogenetic findings on seven cases. Cancer Genet Cytogenet 1987; 24:205–212.

220. Sandros J, Mark J, Happonen RP, Stenman G: Specificity of 6q- markers and other recurrent deviations in human malignant salivary gland tumors. Anticancer Res 1988; 8:637–644.

10

MIXED TUMOR (PLEOMORPHIC ADENOMA) AND MYOEPITHELIOMA

Charles A. Waldron

TERMINOLOGY

The mixed tumor, or pleomorphic adenoma, is the most common neoplasm involving both the major and minor salivary glands. Both designations, *mixed tumor* and *pleomorphic adenoma*, are widely used today, and the choice of term is a matter of personal preference. The current literature suggests that use of the term *mixed tumor* is possibly more common in the United States, whereas pathologists in Europe, Canada, and Asia appear to favor the designation *pleomorphic adenoma*, which is used in the World Health Organization's classification system.[1] According to Foote and Frazell,[2] the term *mixed tumor* dates from Minssen's review in 1874, which is cited by Ahlbom.[3] Many years ago, mixed tumors of the salivary glands were believed to originate from cells of more than one germ layer, and their benign nature was questioned. They were designated by terms such as *branchioma, enclavoma, teratoma, myxochondrocarcinoma, cylindroma, myxochondrosarcoma,* and *chondromyxohemangioendotheliosarcoma.* There is now universal agreement that the salivary gland mixed tumor is entirely of epithelial origin.

It must be emphasized that current use of the term *mixed tumor* of salivary gland origin does not imply origin from cells of more than one germ layer; it is used simply as a descriptive term for a neoplasm that characteristically shows combined features of epithelioid and connective tissue–like growth. Use of the term *mixed tumor*, likewise, is not derived from the fact that the tumor is uniquely composed of both ductal and myoepithelial cells, because a number of currently recognized salivary gland tumors, such as adenoid cystic carcinoma, epithelial-myoepithelial carcinoma, and polymorphous low-grade adenocarcinoma, also show active myoepithelial cell participation. With evolving study and experience, a number of well-recognized tumors, such as adenoid cystic carcinoma (cylindroma), mucoepidermoid carcinoma, epithelial-myoepithelial carcinoma, and basal cell and canalicular adenomas, which were formerly included under the general term *mixed tumor,* have been recategorized as specific entities.

Apparently, the term *pleomorphic adenoma* was first suggested by Willis[4] and is an equally appropriate designation. This term avoids confusion with tumors that occur in other parts of the body that are composed of more than one type of tissue and are also called mixed tumors. However, the designation *mixed tumor* is the personal preference of the author and is used in this chapter.

Tumors composed primarily of myoepithelial cells are designated as *myoepithelioma* and are also discussed in this chapter. These tumors represent one extreme end of the histopathologic spectrum of mixed tumor, but, because of their monomorphous appearance, it is advantageous to identify them separately.

MIXED TUMOR

Clinical Features

There is universal agreement that the mixed tumor is the most common neoplasm of salivary gland origin. According to various studies,[5-10] mixed tumors account for about 60 to 70 percent of all parotid neoplasms, 40 to 60 percent of all submandibular tumors, and 40 to 70 percent of minor salivary gland tumors. The sublingual gland is seldom the site for salivary tumors, and mixed tumors in this location are exceedingly rare. Table 10–1 shows the site distribution of 6,880 mixed tumors in a total of 13,749 primary epithelial salivary gland tumors registered at the Armed Forces Institute of Pathology (AFIP). Table 10–2 shows the reported frequency of mixed tumors in various sites compiled from selected reports of large numbers of cases.[5–10] The lower frequency of mixed tumors in the report by Spiro[6] undoubtedly reflects the patient referral pattern to a major cancer treatment center.

Occasionally, mixed tumors may arise in unusual locations. A few examples have been found in the cheek, along Stensen's duct, arising in accessory parotid tissue that is separated from the body of the gland.[11] Mixed tumors may also develop in salivary gland tissue inclusions within lymph nodes in the neck. Although uncommon, salivary gland tumors of several histologic types may also occur within the mandible or maxilla. Mucoepidermoid carcinoma is the most common type to occur at either of these sites;[12, 13] however, examples of intrabony mixed tumors have been reported.[14] Mixed tumors are almost invariably solitary lesions, although a recent review cited 34 examples of synchronous or metachronous involvement of 2 or more major salivary glands with mixed tumors.[15] Mixed tumors may also be found in combination with other types of salivary gland tumors, most commonly Warthin's tumor.[16]

Table 10–1. Anatomic Distribution of 6,880 Cases of Mixed Tumors from the Salivary Gland Registry of the Armed Forces Institute of Pathology

Anatomic Site	Number of Cases	Percentage
Major Glands		
Parotid gland	4,359	63.4
Submandibular gland	657	9.5
Sublingual gland	10	0.1
Neck, NOS*	89	1.3
Minor Glands		
Palate (total)	711	10.3
Palate, NOS*	(483)	(7.0)
Hard palate	(118)	(1.7)
Soft palate	(110)	(1.6)
Lip (total)	297	4.3
Upper lip	(147)	(2.1)
Lower lip	(20)	(0.3)
Lip, NOS*	(130)	(1.9)
Tongue	16	0.2
Cheek	126	1.8
Floor of mouth	7	0.1
Tonsil/oropharynx	38	0.6
Retromolar area	3	—
Other	79	1.1
Not Stated	488	7.1
Total†	6,880	100

*NOS = not otherwise specified
†Does not include numbers in parentheses

Table 10–2. Frequency of Mixed Tumors in Various Anatomic Sites as Reported in Selected Reviews of Large Numbers of Salivary Gland Tumors[5–10]

Site	Number of Tumors	Percent Mixed Tumors (Range)
Parotid gland	5,379	66–77
Submandibular gland	594	45–60
Sublingual gland	7	0
Intraoral glands	1,833	19–53

Twenty-four cases of mixed tumor associated synchronously or metachronously with other salivary gland tumors are described in the files of the AFIP. The most common combination was mixed tumor and Warthin's tumor, but mucoepidermoid carcinoma, adenoid cystic carcinoma, and acinic cell carcinoma also have occurred in combination with mixed tumors.

Mixed tumors may develop in patients from a wide range of ages, but these tumors are most commonly diagnosed in patients between the ages of 30 and 50 years. The mean age for 4,911 mixed tumor patients of known age from the AFIP files was 41.2 years. Mixed tumors are uncommon in patients who are in the first 2 decades of life, although tumors may occur in very young children.[17, 18] In the AFIP series, 51 cases (1 percent of mixed tumors) were found in patients under 10 years of age, and 289 cases (5.9 percent) occurred in patients between 10 and 19 years of age (Fig. 10–1). The clinical behavior of mixed tumors in children is similar to that noted in adults.[17] Mixed tumors are generally stated to be somewhat more common in females, with male-to-female ratios ranging from 1:3 to 1:4. The AFIP data on 5,094 patients with stated gender showed a predominance of cases occurring in males (58.3 percent). Because 48 percent of these cases were received from military or Veterans Administration sources, this predominance of cases among males probably does not reflect the true sex distribution in the general population. Among the 3,031 cases of AFIP mixed tumors received from civilian sources, 65.7 percent occurred in females (female-to-male ratio of 1.9:1.0).

The usual clinical presentation is that of a painless, slowly growing, firm mass. In the parotid gland, this tumor most often presents in the lower pole of the superficial lobe as a mass over the angle of the mandible, below and in front of the ear. About 10 percent of parotid mixed tumors arise in the deeper portion of the gland. These may extend between the ascending ramus of the mandible and the stylomandibular ligament in a dumbbell shape into the parapharyngeal space. In such instances, the tumor presents as a mass in the tonsillar fossa, soft palate, or lateral pharynx.[19, 20]

In early development, parotid mixed tumors

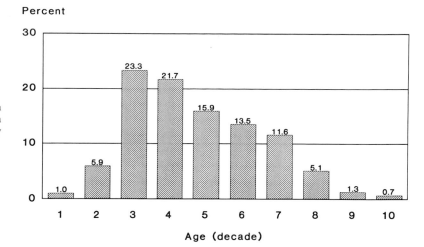

Figure 10–1. Age distribution by decade of 4,911 patients with mixed tumor as documented by the AFIP files.

are usually movable, but with continued growth, the tumor becomes more nodular and less movable. Recurrent mixed tumors of the parotid gland are usually multinodular and appear clinically as multiple small nodules that may seem fixed on palpation. Mixed tumors of the submandibular gland typically present as firm, discrete masses within the gland.

Although mixed tumors may arise in all sites where minor salivary gland tissue is present, the palate (54 percent), upper lip (18 percent), and buccal mucosa (11 percent) are the sites of most tumors occurring in the intraoral salivary glands.[8] These three sites were the location of 82.2 percent of all minor salivary gland tumors with specified locations included in the AFIP material. These minor gland tumors also clinically present as painless, slow-growing, submucosal masses. The covering mucosa is seldom ulcerated, unless it has been secondarily traumatized. Because the mucosa of the hard palate is tightly bound to the palatal bone, mixed tumors of the hard palate are not movable; however, those in other sites generally are mobile. Palatal mixed tumors usually are located laterally on the palate and seldom cross the midline, unless a neglected lesion grows to a large size. The majority of intraoral mixed tumors are less than 3.0 cm in diameter when they are excised, although rare examples of huge intraoral mixed tumors may be seen. Most intraoral mixed tumors are surfaced by normal-appearing oral mucosa. Larger lesions, however, frequently are covered by an erythematous-appearing mucosa, which is due to congestion of the capillary bed in the lamina propria of the intact covering mucosa.

Magnetic resonance imaging and computed tomography have been widely applied to the study of parotid tumors and may yield valuable information. Magnetic resonance imaging appears superior to computed tomography in demonstrating tumor margins and can show whether a deep-seated mass is multicentric or a single, markedly lobulated mass. Computed tomography is less ef-

fective in demonstrating tumor margins but shows calcifications that are sometimes present in mixed tumors.[21, 22]

Gross Pathology

Mixed tumors of the parotid and submandibular glands appear as well-circumscribed masses with smooth or bosselated surfaces. Tumors larger than 3.0 cm in diameter tend to exhibit increased surface bosselation. The tumor is usually surrounded by a fibrous capsule of varying thickness, and a clear demarcation between the tumor and the adjacent salivary gland tissue is present. A section of the mixed tumor is usually solid and white and may contain variable areas of firmer, somewhat translucent, bluish tissue that correspond to the cartilagelike material seen microscopically. Sections from mixed tumors that are predominantly myxoid demonstrate a soft, somewhat gelatinous tissue. Cystic degeneration in mixed tumors is relatively uncommon and is found most often in long-standing, large tumors (Fig. 10–2). Soft, hemorrhagic areas of infarction within the tumor may occasionally be found, particularly in large, long-standing mixed tumors. Infarcted or hemorrhagic areas may also be noted in tumors that have been subjected to preoperative fine-needle aspiration (FNA).

In contrast to the unifocal character of primary mixed tumors, recurrent lesions characteristically are multinodular.[23] Small to large discrete nodules of tumor may be present within the salivary gland parenchyma, in adjacent fat and connective tissue, or in the dermis along the scar line (Fig. 10–3). These nodules of recurrent tumor are frequently myxoid in nature. The multifocal nature of the recurrence is often the result of incomplete enucleation, which may leave small bosselated extensions of the tumor in the wound or may seed the wound bed by rupture of a mucoid mixed tumor during removal.

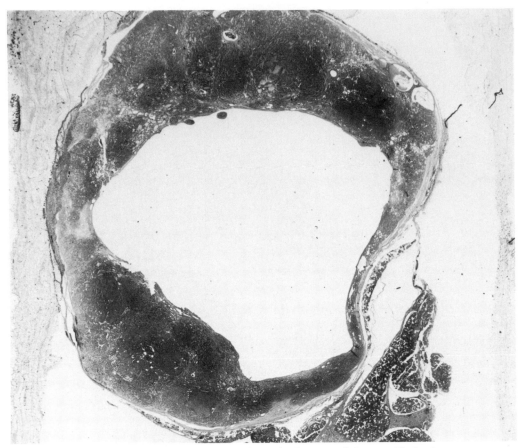

Figure 10–2. Central cystic area in a mixed tumor of the parotid gland.

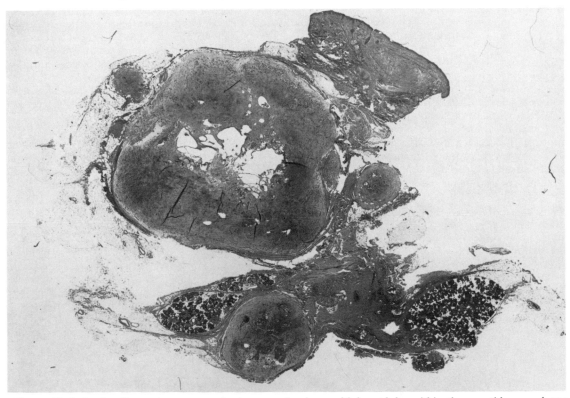

Figure 10–3. Section from a recurrent mixed tumor showing multiple nodules within the parotid parenchyma (bottom) and in the overlying dermis. A wedge of skin is present at the top of the photograph.

Minor salivary gland mixed tumors generally occur as well-circumscribed, smooth, firm masses, which appear whitish in sections. Because the majority of minor salivary gland mixed tumors are removed when they are less than 2.0 cm, the prominent surface bosselations noted in larger parotid mixed tumors are not seen frequently. A prominent fibrous capsule is not often apparent, but the tumor is clearly demarcated from the surrounding tissues. If the covering mucosa is included in the specimen, it will usually appear grossly normal, but it may be ulcerated if it has been secondarily traumatized. Because minor gland mixed tumors histologically contain less myxoid and chondroid material than their major gland counterparts, the gelatinous or cartilagelike areas are generally not as conspicuous on gross examination of the cut surface.

Microscopic Findings

Morphologic diversity is the hallmark of mixed tumors, and few other neoplasms manifest a wider morphologic spectrum. Considerable variation is often present within a single tumor, and it is relatively uncommon to encounter a mixed tumor with a homogenous histologic composition. All mixed tumors demonstrate combinations of gland-like epithelium and mesenchyma-like tissue, but the proportions of each vary widely. Some are predominantly myxoid with a scant epithelial-appearing component (Fig. 10–4). Other lesions are chiefly cellular, and the characteristic myxo-chondroid tissue is present only in limited areas (Fig. 10–5). Foote and Frazell[2] analyzed 250 mixed tumors and categorized them into the following four types: (1) principally myxoid (36 percent), (2) myxoid and cellular components present in about equal proportions (30 percent), (3) predominantly cellular (22 percent), and (4) extremely cellular (12 percent). Similar findings were reported by Seifert and colleagues,[24] who found that about 30 percent of mixed tumors of the parotid gland had a mucoid stroma that constituted 30 to 50 percent of the tumor mass, while in 55 percent of the tumors the mucoid stroma constituted 80 percent of the tumor. The remaining 15 percent of the tumors were cellular, and the stroma constituted less than 20 percent of the tumor.

The epithelial-appearing component of a mixed tumor may take the form of ducts, small cellular nests, solid sheets of cells, anastomosing cords, and foci of either keratinizing squamous cells or

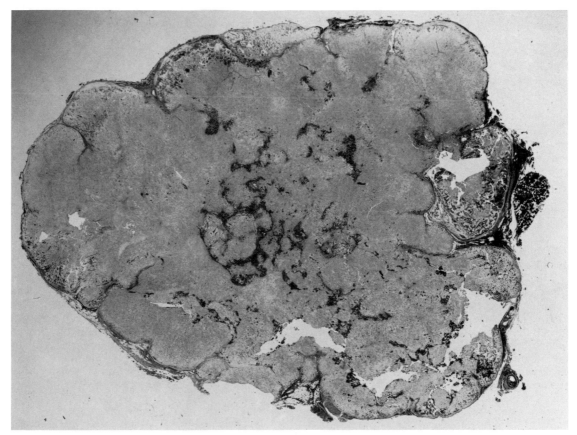

Figure 10–4. Section from a predominantly mucoid mixed tumor of the parotid gland containing only scant epithelial structures, which appear as the dark areas in the photograph.

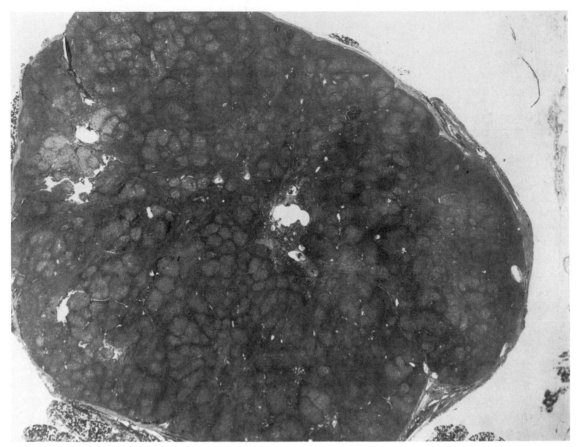

Figure 10–5. Section from a predominantly cellular mixed tumor of the parotid gland. Only small foci of mucoid and hyaline stroma are present.

spindle-shaped cells. The role of the myoepithelial cell has received considerable attention and has been studied extensively by immunohistochemical and ultrastructural methods. Studies indicate that myoepithelial cells constitute a major component of mixed tumors and that myoepithelium is responsible for development of the characteristic myxoid and chondroid stroma.[25–27]

Ductal structures present in mixed tumors resemble normal salivary gland intercalated ducts with lumina that are lined by a single layer of ductal epithelium surrounded by darker staining, angular myoepithelial cells. The ductal lumina frequently contain eosinophilic material that stains positive with periodic acid–Schiff stain (Fig. 10–6). In contrast to normal intercalated ducts, the myoepithelial cells in mixed tumors form thick "collars" around the ducts. Accumulation of basophilic mucoid material between the myoepithelial cells separates them into either small groups or narrow strands of cells. The cartilaginous areas that are often present in mixed tumors are the result of more extensive accumulation of mucoid material around individual myoepithelial cells. Vacuolar degeneration of the cell results in a cartilaginous appearance (Fig. 10–7). The carti-

lage in mixed tumors was formerly designated as pseudocartilage, but it cannot be differentiated from cartilage of mesenchymal derivation by routine microscopic examination. Eosinophilic hyaline material is also common in mixed tumors. This material may appear as foci within cellular masses or may form bands that separate the epithelial cells into either small nests or long strands of cells (Fig. 10–8). This hyaline material is believed to be basal lamina produced by the myoepithelial cells. Foci of squamous cells, sometimes with keratin pearl formation, are present in about 20 percent of mixed tumors. These usually form in solid cellular zones of presumed myoepithelial cells or in myxoid areas rather than in relation to preexisting ducts. Small squamous epithelium–lined cysts that contain keratin are frequently present (Fig. 10–9). The solid cellular areas in a mixed tumor may take the form of interlacing trabeculae or masses of loosely cohesive cells that form numerous tubular structures (Fig. 10–10). Some mixed tumors may show large areas composed almost entirely of plump, eosinophilic-staining, spindle-shaped cells that form anastomosing bands or fascicles. Nuclear palisading may be present, and the pattern may resemble that of a

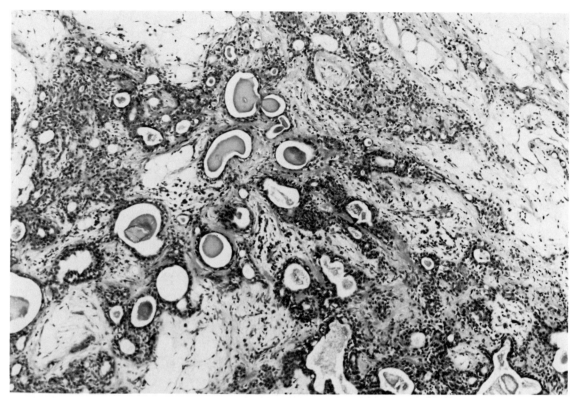

Figure 10–6. Ductal structures surrounded by myoepithelial cells in a mixed tumor. Many of the ducts contain eosinophilic material.

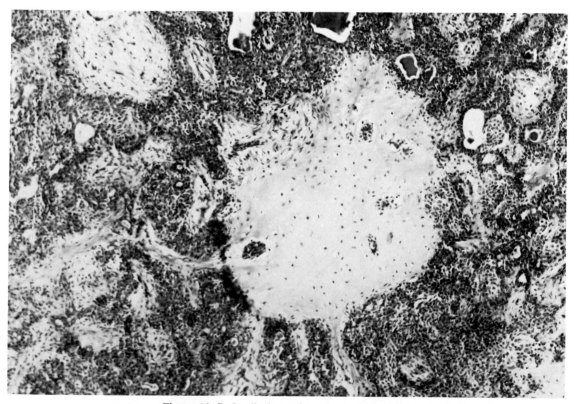

Figure 10–7. Cartilaginous focus in a mixed tumor.

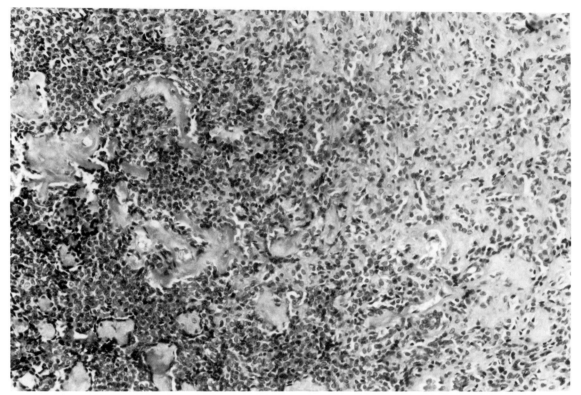

Figure 10–8. Hyaline stroma separating myoepithelial cells into narrow cords (right) or occurring between sheets of myoepithelial cells (left).

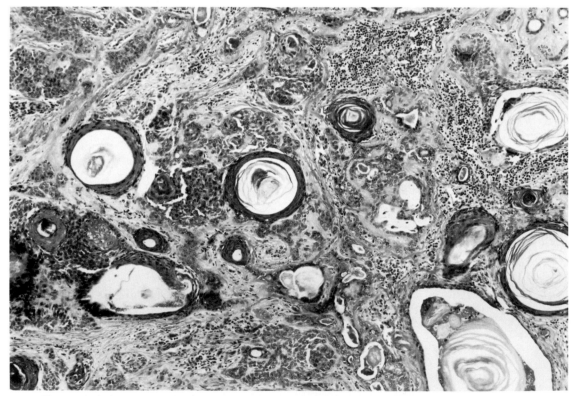

Figure 10–9. Squamous epithelial islands with formation of multiple squamous epithelium–lined cysts.

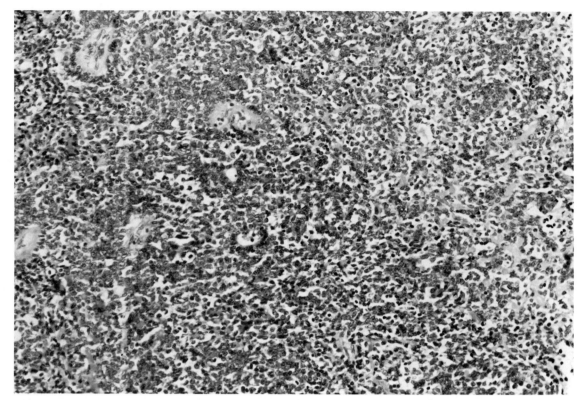

Figure 10–10. Cellular area in a mixed tumor showing sheets of loosely cohesive cells with formation of occasional tubular structures.

leiomyoma or schwannoma (Fig. 10–11). These cells, however, have been demonstrated to be of myoepithelial differentiation by immunohistochemical and ultrastructural studies.[28] Other mixed tumors may show diffuse masses of round cells with hyalinized eosinophilic cytoplasm and eccentric nuclei that resemble plasma cells. The myoepithelial derivation of these plasmacytoid cells has been established. This feature is somewhat more prominent in mixed tumors that arise in the minor salivary glands than in those arising in the major salivary glands (Fig. 10–12).[29, 30]

Epithelial islands with a cribriform structure are occasionally seen in otherwise typical mixed tumors (Fig. 10–13).[16] Although these islands closely resemble the histologic features of adenoid cystic carcinoma, their presence in a mixed tumor has no bearing on prognosis, and this feature must not lead to "overdiagnosis." Mucous goblet cells may also be found in association with squamous cells in mixed tumors, and isolated foci may resemble mucoepidermoid carcinoma (Fig. 10–14). However, this feature by itself, like that of cribriform areas that resemble adenoid cystic carcinoma, does not indicate malignancy and is of no prognostic significance. Other types of cells that may be encountered in mixed tumors include sebaceous cells in association with squamous elements and large, eosinophilic ductal epithelial cells that resemble oncocytes. In focal areas, these eo-

sinophilic ductal epithelial cells may even resemble an oncocytoma. Focal collections of adipose tissue are occasionally present in mixed tumors. Whether these are representative of preexisting fat that has been incorporated into the tumor or are the result of stromal metaplasia is not clear. Bone formation is also occasionally seen. This appears to result from stromal metaplasia rather than from ossification of preexisting chondroid stroma (Fig. 10–15).

Deposits of crystalline material may be located in mixed tumors of both the major and minor salivary glands. These may be found in isolated foci or may be extensively deposited throughout the tumor. Several types of crystalloids have been reported. In some instances, they are arranged in petal-shaped clusters of glossy, eosinophilic, structureless masses that surround a central core. These structures are refractile and have been designated as tyrosine-rich crystals. They stain positively with Millon's reagent. These tyrosine-rich crystals are found more often in black patients and have been observed in 21 percent of mixed tumors from black patients.[31] Other crystalloid materials appear as radially arranged, nonrefractile, needle-shaped structures. These do not stain histochemically for tyrosine and have been designated as collagen-rich crystalloids (Fig. 10–16).[32] Oxalate crystals have also been reported in mixed tumors.[33] These crystalloid structures do not ap-

Text continued on page 177

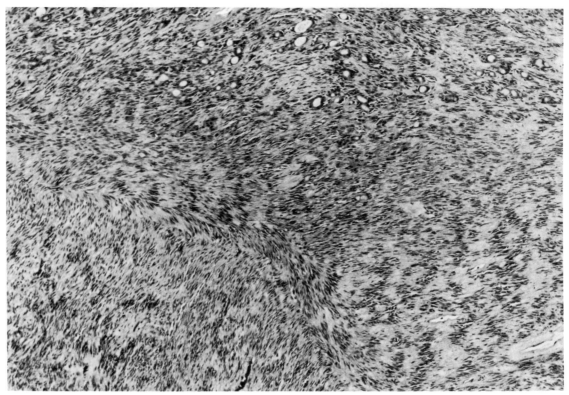

Figure 10–11. Mixed tumor with a prominent spindle-shaped myoepithelial cell component. Nuclear palisading in these areas resembles a neurilemoma. Epithelial ductal structures are present at the top of the photograph.

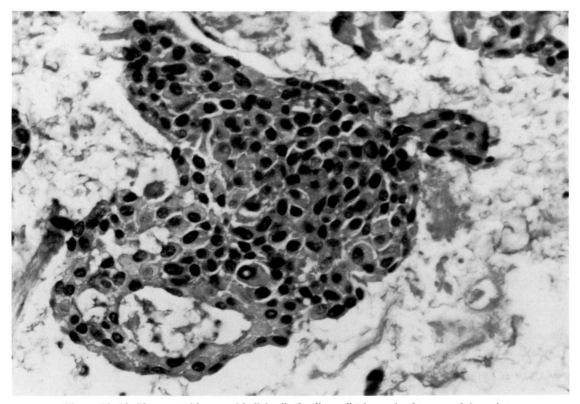

Figure 10–12. Plasmacytoid myoepithelial cells (hyaline cells) in a mixed tumor of the palate.

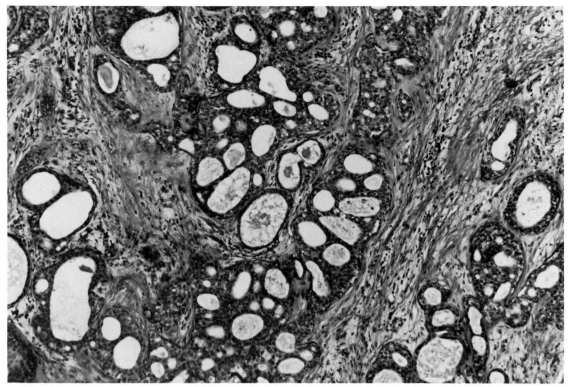

Figure 10–13. Focus of cells with a cribriform pattern present in an otherwise typical mixed tumor of the parotid gland.

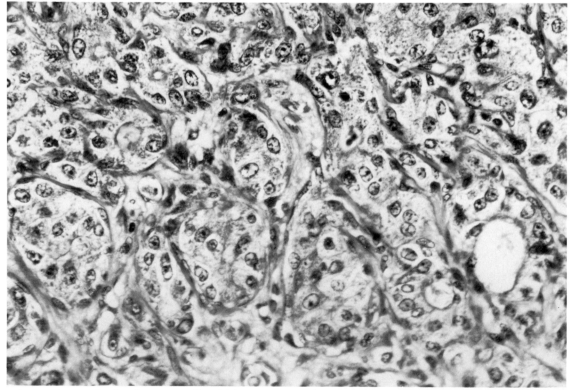

Figure 10–14. Islands of mucous cells, which were present in an otherwise typical mixed tumor of the parotid gland.

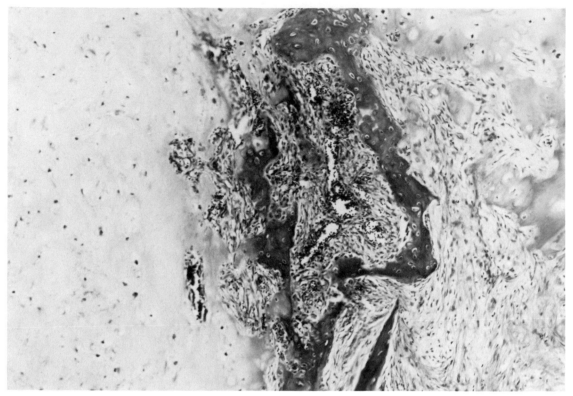

Figure 10–15. Bone formation adjacent to a chondroid focus in a parotid mixed tumor.

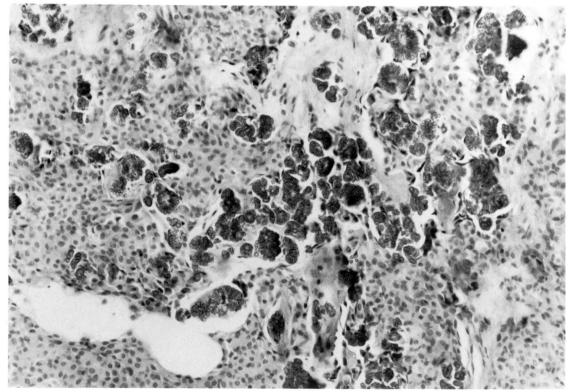

Figure 10–16. Collagen-rich crystalloids in a mixed tumor of the palate. These structures did not stain for tyrosine but showed a positive result when staining for collagen by the van Gieson method.

pear to be related to the age of the patient or to duration of the tumor and apparently have no bearing on behavior or prognosis.

Mixed tumors arising in the oral and pharyngeal minor salivary glands show the same histologic features as those of their major gland counterparts. However, minor salivary gland mixed tumors tend to be more cellular with fewer myxoid and chondroid components. Although they are well circumscribed, they frequently do not have well-defined capsules. This absence of a capsule must not be interpreted as infiltration into adjacent salivary gland acini and connective tissue, which occurs in adenocarcinomas. The tumors may closely approximate the overlying mucosal epithelium, but they do not invade it (Fig. 10–17). Ulceration of the surface mucosa is very uncommon, even in large tumors, unless they have been traumatized.

Immunohistochemistry and Ultrastructure

Immunohistochemical methods have been extensively applied to the study of mixed tumors in recent years.[34–37] Although immunohistochemical analyses are not necessary or useful for the routine diagnosis of the vast majority of mixed tumors encountered in medical and dental practice, these studies have provided considerable information about the histogenesis of these tumors, especially the role of the myoepithelial cell. Myoepithelial cells are difficult to identify by routine light microscopy. In normal salivary gland tissue, myoepithelial cells adjacent to acini have a stellate or basketlike morphology, and those adjacent to intercalated ducts are spindle-shaped. Immunohistochemistry has been very useful in the diagnosis of some variants of mixed tumors, particularly those with a predominance of spindle or plasmacytoid myoepithelial cells. The myoepithelial nature of these cells may be suggested with the use of appropriate immunohistochemical stains. Myoepithelial cells in mixed tumors have been shown to be immunoreactive for keratin, S-100 protein, glial fibrillary acidic protein, actin, and vimentin by the immunoperoxidase method on formalin-fixed and paraffinized tissue.[9, 38] Ductal epithelial cells and solid cellular nests with a tubular structure in these tumors have been strongly immunoreactive for cytokeratin and moderately reactive for antiepithelial membrane and carcinoembryonic antigens.[39]

Ultrastructural studies have also been widely employed in the study of mixed tumors. Ultrastructural identification of desmosomes, cytoplasmic actin microfilaments, and remnants of basal lamina may be used to help confirm the myoepithelial origin of both spindle and plasmacytoid cells present in mixed tumors.[27, 34, 40]

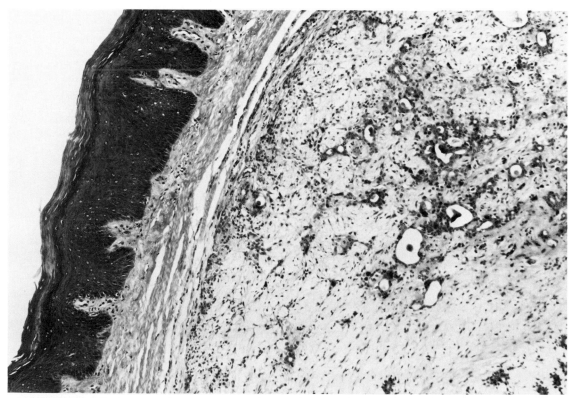

Figure 10–17. Mixed tumor of the palate. A well-defined capsule is not present. The tumor is proximal to the surface epithelium, but it does not invade into it.

Behavior and Treatment

With adequate surgical excision, the prognosis for a patient with mixed tumor is excellent. Adequate initial surgical removal is almost always curative. Based on a review of 52 separate studies with adequate follow-up data comprising 804 cases of mixed tumor, Hickman and colleagues[41] found a 5-year recurrence-free rate of 96.6 percent and a 10-year recurrence-free rate of 93.7 percent. Formerly, mixed tumors of the parotid were often treated by local enucleation procedures that were undoubtedly responsible for the frequency of local recurrence.[42] Today, parotid tumors are almost always treated by superficial or total parotidectomy with preservation of the facial nerve. When this surgical approach is used initially, the incidence of recurrence approaches zero.[43, 44] Submandibular mixed tumors are generally treated by total excision of the gland. Minor salivary gland tumors are best treated by total excision that includes a rim of surrounding tissue. Recurrence after such procedures is rare. Even with less than "optimal" surgical margins, recurrence of minor gland mixed tumors seldom develops. Open biopsy of suspected salivary gland tumors of the parotid and submandibular glands is not recommended because of the risk of seeding the wound and the subsequent multinodular recurrence. Because clinical differentiation between benign and malignant minor salivary gland tumors is usually difficult, if not impossible, and because intraoral biopsy is a minor surgical procedure, incisional biopsy of larger minor gland tumors, particularly those on the palate, is often performed to determine the nature of the tumor and to plan the extent of the surgery required. It is important for the surgeon to include a portion of adjacent normal tissue so that the tumor interface can be evaluated. The biopsy incision line through the covering mucosa should be included in the subsequent surgical excision specimen.

Fine-needle aspiration has been extensively used in Europe for the preoperative evaluation of salivary gland tumors,[45] but it has been slower to gain acceptance in the United States.[46] Several recent reports have shown that FNA has been up to 93 percent accurate in detecting the presence of a neoplasm when a parotid mass was subjected to aspiration.[46, 47] In experienced hands, the accuracy of FNA diagnosis for benign salivary gland tumors is claimed to be greater than 90 percent, but this method is less accurate for malignant tumors.[47] The high percentage of false-negative FNA biopsies for malignant salivary gland tumors makes this method unreliable if used alone. The accuracy of FNA diagnosis appears to be quite similar to that of frozen-section diagnosis when they are compared to the final pathologic diagnosis (see Chapter 9).[48] Benign salivary gland tumors have been reported to be correctly diagnosed by frozen section in 96 percent of instances, whereas the

accuracy rate for malignant tumors dropped to 86 percent, excluding deferred diagnoses.[49] One major cancer center reports a waning enthusiasm for FNA in recent years, because treatment decisions were not significantly influenced by FNA results even when the correct pathologic diagnosis was obtained.[6]

Radiation therapy is not widely used as an adjunct in treatment of mixed tumors, although some centers have employed this method.[50]

Mixed tumors of salivary glands are one of the few benign neoplasms that can undergo malignant transformation. The likelihood of malignant change in mixed tumor increases with the duration of the tumor and with the age of the patient. Carcinoma ex mixed tumor is discussed in Chapter 20.

Differential Diagnosis

The typical mixed tumor that contains both epithelial and myxochondroid mesenchyma-like areas seldom, if ever, presents a problem in differential diagnosis. However, the microscopic appearance of a chondroid syringoma (mixed tumor) of the skin is essentially identical to that of some mixed tumors of salivary gland origin. A small, deep-seated, dermal tumor overlying the parotid gland or in the dermis of the upper lip may be difficult or impossible to differentiate from a mixed tumor arising from salivary gland tissue, unless adjacent salivary tissue is included in the specimen.

Mixed tumors that show a predominantly epithelial structure and almost complete absence of the characteristic myxochondroid structure may be difficult to differentiate from monomorphic salivary gland adenomas. Even experienced pathologists may disagree on interpretation of a given case. If the epithelial pattern in such a lesion is similar to that seen in more typical mixed tumors and if there is some evidence of spindle or plasmacytoid differentiation, the diagnosis of mixed tumor is appropriate even in the absence of any appreciable areas of myxochondroid tissue (Fig. 10–18). In any event, the distinction between mixed tumor and a type of monomorphic adenoma in such cases is more academic than practical because the treatment and prognosis for both are similar. Mixed tumors consisting predominantly of myxoid or chondroid mesenchyma-like tissue may not demonstrate convincing epithelial elements on a given section. These lesions may be confused with some type of mesenchymal neoplasm such as myxoma, myxoid lipoma, or myxoid neurofibroma. Study of sections from multiple blocks may be necessary to detect small areas of typical epithelial structures that will confirm the diagnosis of mixed tumor (Fig. 10–19). Immunohistochemical analysis in such cases may also confirm the myoepithelial character of the mesenchyma-like cells.

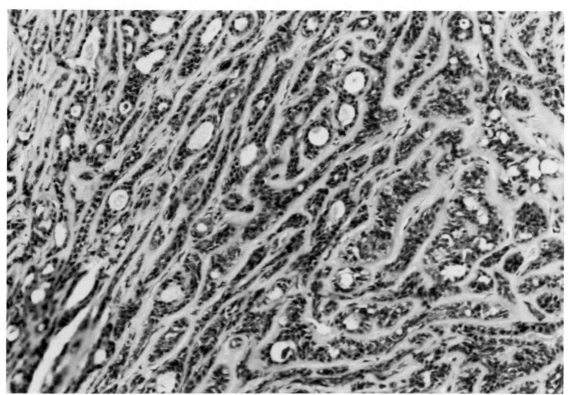

Figure 10–18. Parotid cellular mixed tumor, which contained only isolated foci of myxoid stroma. A number of experienced pathologists favored a diagnosis of basal cell adenoma for this lesion, whereas others diagnosed it as a mixed tumor.

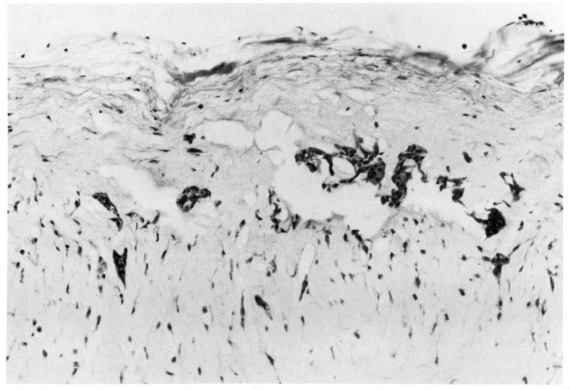

Figure 10–19. A largely myxoid mixed tumor of the parotid gland, which shows only small epithelial islands at the periphery of the tumor.

A major concern in differential diagnosis relates to the evaluation of possible malignant transformation in a mixed tumor. Nodules of tumor may be present within the salivary parenchyma outside the apparent capsule of a mixed tumor. This feature, by itself, is not indicative of invasion or malignant change. Serial sections almost invariably demonstrate that these apparently detached nodules represent bulging bosselated extensions of the main tumor mass that are connected to the tumor in another tissue plane (Fig. 10–20).[51] Similarly, benign mixed tumors may occasionally show small foci of capsular penetration by islands of tumor. In an otherwise histologically benign mixed tumor, this feature is not of concern (Fig. 10–21). In some tumors, a definite fibrous capsule may not be present for significant areas around the periphery, and the tumor tissue will be immediately adjacent to the salivary gland parenchyma. Care must be taken to distinguish the pushing border in these cases from malignant invasion.

Mixed tumors may contain variable-sized foci of epithelial cells that demonstrate nuclear hyperchromatism or other cytologic features suggestive of malignancy. If careful study of sections from multiple blocks fails to demonstrate convincing evidence of invasion into the surrounding salivary gland parenchyma or fibrofatty tissue, the lesion is best considered a benign mixed tumor.[52]

These changes are sometimes referred to as *intracapsular carcinoma* or *carcinoma-in-situ* (Fig. 10–22). If the surgical excision has been adequate, the prognosis is probably the same as in other mixed tumors that do not show these features. Atypical epithelial cells may also be present adjacent to areas of infarction or ischemia in mixed tumors; this feature alone, likewise, is not indicative of malignant change (Fig. 10–23). Mixed tumors showing extensive stromal hyalinization and fibrosis with or without areas of infarction or ischemic change should be carefully examined in multiple blocks to look for the presence of frank carcinomatous change in other areas. As already stated, foci of cribriform structures that resemble adenoid cystic carcinoma or focal areas of intermingled epidermoid and mucous cells that resemble mucoepidermoid carcinoma may be present in a mixed tumor; such areas are not indicative of malignant change.[16]

A problem in differential diagnosis may be encountered in markedly cellular mixed tumors, where distinction between benign mixed tumor and some form of adenocarcinoma may be very difficult. These cellular lesions are sometimes designated as "cellular" or "atypical" mixed tumors.

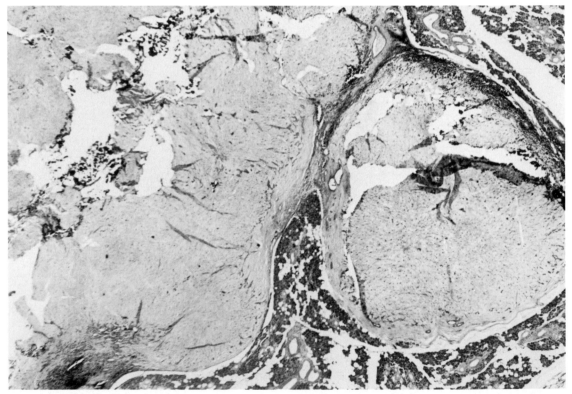

Figure 10–20. A small, bosselated nodule of mixed tumor, which is largely surrounded by parotid parenchyma (right) and appears separated from the main tumor (left). Deeper sections showed that the nodule was attached to the main tumor.

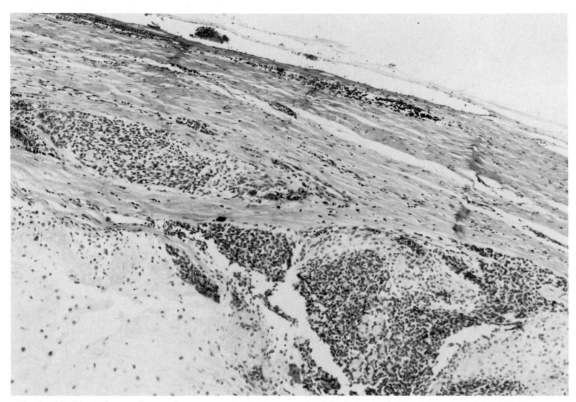

Figure 10–21. A focus of capsular penetration by tumor cells in a mixed tumor of the parotid gland. The tumor was otherwise histologically benign and capsular penetration was found in only isolated areas.

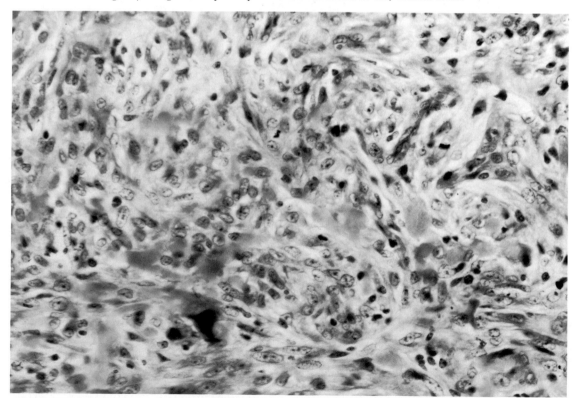

Figure 10–22. Mixed tumor of the parotid gland, showing areas of atypical epithelial cells with numerous mitoses. Sections from multiple blocks showed no evidence of invasion through the capsule. These features may be considered as "intracapsular carcinoma" or carcinoma-in-situ.

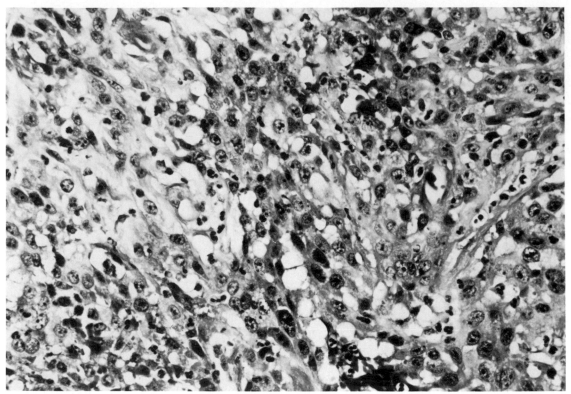

Figure 10–23. Focus of cellular atypia adjacent to an area of infarction in a mixed tumor of the parotid gland. A fine-needle aspiration had been performed prior to surgical removal of the tumor. The tumor was otherwise a typical benign mixed tumor.

A marked increase in mitotic activity (1 to 5 mitotic figures per high-power field) has been claimed to indicate aggressive behavior and metastatic potential.[53] A fragmented, cellular mixed tumor specimen, most often the result of careless surgical or tissue processing techniques, may be difficult, if not impossible, to differentiate from adenocarcinoma. Good tissue specimens can solve many problems in diagnosis and can prevent equivocal or incorrect interpretations.

MYOEPITHELIOMA

Tumors composed entirely or almost exclusively of myoepithelial cells are uncommon, accounting for less than 1 percent of all salivary gland tumors. The term *myoepithelioma* was apparently first used in 1943 by Sheldon,[54] who reported that 3 of 54 cases of so-called mixed salivary gland tumors were primarily composed of basket (myoepithelial) cells. The taxonomy of these lesions is somewhat controversial. Some investigators prefer to classify these tumors as a separate type of monomorphic adenoma of the salivary gland and designate them as myoepithelioma.[55, 56] We and other pathologists use the designation of myoepithelioma but acknowledge that these adenomas represent one end of the spectrum of mixed tumor.[26, 28, 57] Since

occasional ductal elements may be present in an otherwise predominantly myoepithelial tumor, the designation of *myoepithelioma* as opposed to *mixed tumor with myoepithelial predominance* is largely a matter of personal preference. Barnes and associates[58] suggest that such a tumor is best designated as *mixed tumor with a high content of myoepithelial cells* if one or more ductal structures are noted in every $220 \times$ magnification field or if more than one small cluster of ducts is present within the tumor.

Clinical Features

A review in 1985 by Barnes and associates[58] noted 40 previously reported cases to which the authors added one new case. Twenty-one (51 percent) of the myoepitheliomas were located in the parotid gland, 11 (27 percent) were found on the palate, and 5 (12 percent) were located in the submandibular gland. Two cases were present in the lip and cheek, and the gingiva and retromolar area accounted for one case each. A review of 33 cases of myoepithelioma from the files of the AFIP showed that 21 percent were located in the parotid gland, 12 percent involved the submandibular gland, and 67 percent arose in the minor salivary glands, with slightly over half of these being located on the palate. The age and sex distribution of myoepitheliomas is similar to that of mixed tumors. There are no distinctive clinical features, and, similar to most other salivary gland tumors, myoepitheliomas present as asymptomatic, slowly growing masses.

Gross and Microscopic Features

Macroscopically, myoepitheliomas appear as well-circumscribed, frequently encapsulated tumors that show no features distinct from mixed tumors except for the absence of grossly myxoid or chondroid areas. Parotid myoepitheliomas are usually encapsulated, whereas those arising in the minor salivary glands may not demonstrate a capsule. Microscopically, they show three morphologic patterns. The *spindle cell* pattern is the most common and consists of a proliferation of spindle-shaped cells with eosinophilic cytoplasm. These may be arranged in diffuse sheets or interlacing fasicles (Fig. 10–24). Little intercellular fibrous stroma or ground substance is present. The *plasmacytoid* pattern shows groups of round cells with eccentric nuclei and eosinophilic, often hyaline-appearing cytoplasm. Some authors have referred to these cells as hyaline cells.[29, 30] These may be present in sheets of closely packed cells or in groups of cells separated by a loose, myxoid

stroma (Fig. 10–25). The third and least common pattern shows a combination of plasmacytoid and spindle-shaped cells. The spindle-cell pattern is most common in parotid tumors, whereas the plasmacytoid pattern is more commonly seen in palatal tumors. The uncommon myoepitheliomas of the tongue tend to show a myxoid pattern. Lesions designated as myoepithelioma do not contain the characteristic myxochondroid stroma of the mixed tumor.

Immunohistochemistry and Ultrastructure

Neoplastic myoepithelial cells show immunoreactivity for cytokeratin, S-100 protein, glial fibrillary acidic protein, vimentin, and actin. Ultrastructurally, myoepithelial cells demonstrate desmosomes, cytoplasmic microfilaments, and basal lamina.

Behavior and Treatment

Treatment of myoepitheliomas is similar to that of mixed tumors and consists of complete surgical removal. Most myoepitheliomas pursue a benign course with minimal tendency for recurrence. A few examples of malignant myoepithelioma have

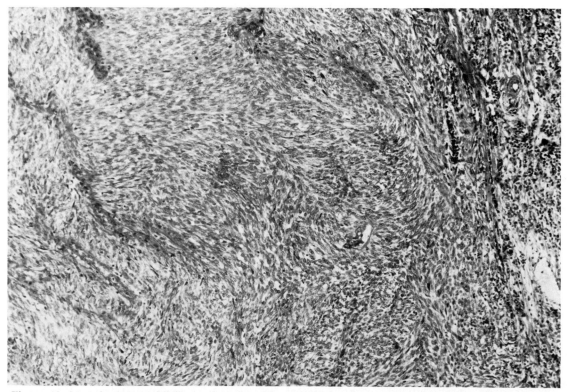

Figure 10–24. Palatal myoepithelioma, demonstrating interlacing fascicles of spindle-shaped cells. No epithelial ductal structures were seen in this tumor.

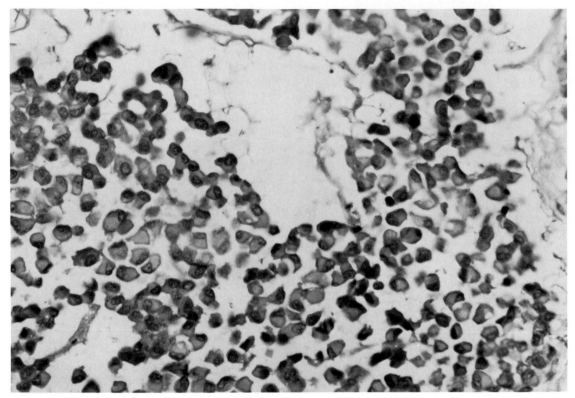

Figure 10–25. Plasmacytoid (hyaline) myoepithelial cells in a myoepithelioma of the parotid gland.

been reported.[39, 59] According to several investigators,[39, 59] there is some indication that the behavior of spindle-cell myoepitheliomas is correlated with the degree of cellular differentiation. Well-differentiated lesions behave in a benign fashion, whereas less-differentiated tumors with a myoepithelial nature that may be uncertain as visualized by light microscopy tend to behave in an aggressive or malignant manner. Plasmacytoid myoepitheliomas tend to follow a benign course.

Differential Diagnosis

The rarity of myoepitheliomas and the varied phenotypic expression of myoepithelial cells may cause problems in diagnosis. Sciubba and Brannon[28] noted that 7 of the 23 cases accessioned at the AFIP at the time of their study were initially mistaken for a malignant epithelial or mesenchymal lesion. Tumors consisting predominantly of spindle-shaped myoepithelial cells may be difficult to differentiate from mesenchymal lesions, such as fibrous histiocytoma, leiomyoma, or schwannoma. Use of immunohistochemical methods to demonstrate positive staining for immunoreactive cytokeratin, S-100 protein, and glial fibrillary acidic protein helps to confirm the myoepithelial nature of the tumor. Similarly, a mixed tumor composed predominantly or entirely of plasma-

cytoid myoepithelial cells might be confused with a plasmacytoma. In such cases, immunohistochemical or ultrastructural studies may be used to confirm the diagnosis. Immunohistochemical or electron-microscopic studies may be necessary to establish the correct diagnosis.

REFERENCES

1. Thackray AC, Sobin LH: Histologic Typing of Salivary Gland Tumors. Geneva, World Health Organization, 1973.
2. Foote FW Jr, Frazell EL: Tumors of the Major Salivary Glands. Atlas of Tumor Pathology, Section IV, Fascicle 11, 1st Series. Washington DC, Armed Forces Institute of Pathology, 1954.
3. Ahlbom HE: Mucous and salivary gland tumors: Clinical study with special reference to radiotherapy based on 254 cases treated at the Radiumhemmet, Stockholm. Acta Radiol 1935; 23(Suppl):1–452.
4. Willis RA: Pathology of Tumors. St. Louis, CV Mosby Co, 1948; 321.
5. Eveson JW, Cawson RA: Salivary gland tumors: A review of 2410 cases with particular reference to histologic types, site, age and sex distribution. J Pathol 1985; 146:51–58.
6. Spiro RH: Salivary neoplasms: Overview of a 35 year experience with 2,807 patients. Head Neck Surg 1986; 8:177–184.
7. Eneroth CM: Salivary gland tumors in the parotid

gland, submandibular gland and the palate region. Cancer 1971; 27:1415–18.

8. Waldron CA, El-Mofty S, Gnepp DR: Tumors of the intraoral minor salivary glands: A demographic and histologic study of 426 cases. Oral Surg Oral Med Oral Pathol 1988; 66:323–333.

9. Regezi JA, Lloyd RV, Zarbo RJ, McClatchey KD: Minor salivary gland tumors: A histologic and immunochemical study. Cancer 1985; 55:108–115.

10. Da Quan M, Guang-Yan Y: Tumors of the minor salivary glands: A clinicopathologic study of 243 cases. Acta Otol 1987; 103:325–331.

11. Frommer J: The human accessory parotid gland: Its incidence, nature and significance. Oral Surg Oral Med Oral Pathol 1977; 43:671–676.

12. Browand BC, Waldron CA: Central mucoepidermoid tumors of the jaws: Report of nine cases and review of the literature. Oral Surg Oral Med Oral Pathol 1975; 40:631–643.

13. Gingell JC, Beckerman T, Levy BA, Snider LA: Central mucoepidermoid carcinoma: Review of the literature and report of a case associated with an apical periodontal cyst. Oral Surg Oral Med Oral Pathol 1984; 57:436–440.

14. Miller AS, Winnick M: Salivary gland inclusion in the anterior mandible: Report of a case with a review of the literature on aberrant salivary gland tissue and neoplasms. Oral Surg Oral Med Oral Pathol 1971; 31:790–797.

15. Gnepp DR, Schroeder W, Heffner D: Synchronous tumors arising in a single major salivary gland. Cancer 1989; 63:1219–1224.

16. Thackray AC, Lucas RB: Tumors of the Major Salivary Glands. Atlas of Tumor Pathology, Second Series, Fascicle 10. Washington DC, Armed Forces Institute of Pathology, 1974.

17. Malone B, Barker SR: Benign pleomorphic adenomas in children. Ann Otol Rhin Larygol 1984; 93:210–214.

18. Krolls SO, Trodahl JN, Boyers RC: Salivary gland lesions in children: A survey of 430 cases. Cancer 1972; 30:459–469.

19. Goodwin WJ Jr, Chandler JR: Transoral excision of lateral pharyngeal space tumors presenting intraorally. Laryngoscope 1988; 98:266–269.

20. Nigro MF, Spiro RH: Deep lobe parotid tumors. Am J Surg 1977; 134:523–527.

21. Som PM, Shugar JMA, Sacher M, Stollman AL, Biller HF: Benign and malignant pleomorphic adenomas: CT and MR studies. J Comp Asst Tomog 1988; 12:65–69.

22. Mirich DR, McArdle CB, Kulkarni MV: Benign pleomorphic adenomas of the salivary glands: Surface coil MR imaging versus CT. J Comp Asst Tomog 1987; 11:620–623.

23. Batsakis JG: Recurrent mixed tumors. Ann Otol Rhinol Laryngol 1986; 95:543–544.

24. Siefert G, Miehlke A, Haubrich J, Chilla R: Diseases of the Salivary Glands. Diagnosis, Pathology, Treatment, Facial Nerve Surgery. Stuttgart, Georg Thieme Verlag, 1980; 184.

25. Dardick I, van Nostrand AWP: Myoepithelial cells in salivary gland tumors-revisited. Head Neck Surg 1985; 7:395–408.

26. Batsakis JG, Kraemer B, Sciubba J: The pathology of head and neck tumors: the myoepithelial cell and its participation in salivary gland neoplasia. Head Neck Surg 1983; 5:222–233.

27. Dardick I, van Nostrand AWP, Phillips MJ: Histogenesis of salivary gland pleomorphic adenoma (mixed tumor) with evaluation of the role of the myoepithelial cell. Hum Pathol 1982; 13:62–75.

28. Sciubba JJ, Brannon R: Myoepithelioma of salivary glands: Report of 23 cases. Cancer 1982; 47:562–572.

29. Lomax-Smith JD, Azzopardi JG: The hyaline cell: A distinctive feature of "mixed" salivary tumors. Histopathology 1978; 2:77–92.

30. Buchner A, David R, Hansen LS: "Hyaline" cells in pleomorphic adenomas of salivary gland origin. Oral Surg Oral Med Oral Pathol 1981; 52:506–512.

31. Thomas K, Hutt MS: Tyrosine crystals in salivary gland tumors. J Clin Pathol 1981; 34:1003–1005.

32. Campbell WG Jr, Priest RE, Weathers DR: Characterization of two types of crystalloids in pleomorphic adenomas of minor salivary glands: A light microscopic, electron microscopic and histochemical study. Am J Pathol 1985; 118:194–202.

33. Dyke PL, Hajdu SI, Strong EW, Erlandson RA, Fleisher M: Mixed tumor of parotid containing oxylate crystals. Arch Pathol 1971; 91:89–92.

34. Erlandson RA, Cardon-Cardo C, Higgins PJ: Histogenesis of benign pleomorphic adenoma (mixed tumor) of the major salivary glands: An ultrastructural and immunohistochemical study. Am J Surg Pathol 1984; 8:803–820.

35. Mori M, Tsukitani K, Minomiya T, Okada Y: Various expressions of modified myoepithelial cells in pleomorphic adenoma: Immunohistochemical studies. Pathol Res Pract 1987; 182:632–646.

36. Tsukitani K, Kobayashi K, Murase N, Sumitomo S, Mitani H, Mori M: Characterization of cells in salivary gland lesions by immunohistochemical identification of carcinoembryonic antigens. Oral Surg Oral Med Oral Pathol 1985; 59:595–599.

37. Sato M, Hayashi Y, Yoshida H, Yanagawa T, Yura Y, Nitta T: Search for specific markers of neoplastic epithelial duct and myoepithelial cell lines established from human salivary gland and characterization of their growth in vitro. Cancer 1984; 54:2959–2967.

38. Stead RH, Qizilbach AH, Kontozoglu T, Daya AD, Riddill RH: An immunohistochemical study of pleomorphic adenomas of the salivary gland: Glial fibrillary acidic protein-like immunoreactivity identifies a major myoepithelial component. Hum Pathol 1988; 19:32–40.

39. Singh R, Cawson RA: Malignant myoepithelial carcinoma (myoepithelioma) arising in a pleomorphic adenoma of the parotid gland: An immunohistochemical study and review of the literature. Oral Surg Oral Med Oral Pathol 1988; 66:65–70.

40. Dardick I: A role for electron microscopy in salivary gland neoplasms. Ultrastruct Pathol 1985; 9:151–161.

41. Hickman RE, Cawson RA, Duffy SW: The prognosis of specific types of salivary gland tumors. Cancer 1984; 54:1620–1654.

42. Krolls SO, Boyers RC: Mixed tumors of salivary glands. Long term follow-up. Cancer 1972; 30:276–281.

43. Martis C: Parotid benign tumors: Comments on treatment of 263 cases. Int J Oral Surg 1983; 12:211–220.

44. Maran AG, Machenzie IJ, Stanley RE: Recurrent

pleomorphic adenomas of the parotid gland. Arch Otolaryngol Head Neck Surg 1984; 110:167–171.

45. Eneroth C-M, Franzen S, Zajicek J: Cytologic aspirates from 1000 salivary gland tumors. Acta Otolaryngol 1967; 224:168–172.

46. O'Dwyer P, Farrar WB, James AG, Finkelmeir W, McCabe DP: Needle aspiration biopsy of major salivary gland tumors: Its value. Cancer 1986; 57:554–557.

47. Cohen MB, Ljung BM, Boles R: Salivary gland tumors: Fine needle aspiration vs frozen section diagnosis. Arch Otolaryngol Head Neck Surg 1986; 112:867–869.

48. Wheelis RF, Yarington CT Jr: Tumors of the salivary glands. Comparison of frozen-section diagnosis with final pathologic diagnosis. Arch Otolaryngol 1984; 110:76–77.

49. Gnepp DR, Rader WR, Cramer SF, Cook LL, Sciubba JJ: Accuracy of frozen section diagnosis of the salivary gland. Otolaryngol Head Neck Surg 1987; 96:325–330.

50. Dawson AK, Orr JA: Long-term results of local excision and radiotherapy in pleomorphic adenoma of the parotid. Int J Radiat Oncol Biol Phys. 1985; 11:451–455.

51. Eneroth C-M: Histologic and clinical aspects of parotid tumors. Acta Otolaryngol 1964; 191:1–99.

52. LiVolsi VA, Perzin KH: Malignant mixed tumors arising in salivary gland. I. Carcinomas arising in mixed tumors: A clinicopathologic study. Cancer 1977; 39:2209–2230.

53. Ryan RE Jr, Desanto LW, Weiland LH, DeVine KD, Beahrs OH: Cellular mixed tumors of the salivary glands. Arch Otolaryngol 1978; 104:451–453.

54. Sheldon WH: So-called mixed tumors of salivary glands. Arch Pathol 1943; 35:1–20.

55. Chaudhry AP, Satchidanad S, Peer R, Cutler LS: Myoepithelial adenoma of the parotid gland: A light and ultrastructural study. Cancer 1982; 49:288–293.

56. Toto PD, Hsu D-J: Product definition in a case of myoepithelioma. Oral Surg Oral Med Oral Pathol 1986; 62:169–174.

57. Batsakis JG: Myoepithelioma. Ann Otol Rhinol Laryngol 1985; 94:523–524.

58. Barnes L, Appel BN, Perez H, El-Attar AM: Myoepithelioma of the head and neck: Case report and review. J Surg Oncol 1985; 28:21–28.

59. Crissman JD, Wirman JA, Harris A: Malignant myoepithelioma of the parotid gland. Cancer 1977; 40:3042–3049.

11

PAPILLARY CYSTADENOMA LYMPHOMATOSUM (WARTHIN'S TUMOR)

Gary R. Warnock

Papillary cystadenoma lymphomatosum (PCL) is a benign neoplastic process characterized by histologic and clinical features that are so distinctive that they render this tumor one of the most readily identifiable salivary gland lesions. Papillary cystadenoma lymphomatosum was first described by Hildebrad[1] in 1895 as a form of congenital cyst of the neck. In 1910, Albrecht and Arzt[2] recorded two cases as papillary cystadenoma of lymphoid stroma and considered the lesions to be pharyngeal endodermal anlagen. The first cases in the English language literature were reported by Nicholson[3] in 1923 as adenomas of heterotopic salivary glands. Two additional cases, which were the first recorded in the United States, were reported in 1929 by Warthin,[4] who coined the present name *papillary cystadenoma lymphomatosum.*

The nomenclature for this tumor has long been a point of confusion, precipitated by different opinions in regard to the tumor's histogenesis. Chaudhry and Gorlin[5] reviewed the world literature in 1958 and cited 23 synonyms for the neoplasm. The most frequently used synonyms in the English language literature include *cystic papillary adenoma,*[3] *papillary cystadenoma lymphomatosum,*[4] *branchial cysts of the parotid,*[6] *branchiogenic adenoma,*[7] *oncokocytoma,*[8] *adenolymphoma,*[9] *lymphoglandular cystome,*[10] and *Warthin's tumor.*[11] *Papillary cystadenoma lymphomatosum* is now generally held to be the most appropriate name because it is fully descriptive and unlikely to be misinterpreted. Other terms that are frequently encountered are *Warthin's tumor* and *adenolymphoma. Warthin's tumor* was first applied by Martin and Ehrlich[11] in respect to Warthin, who published the first American cases; this term is widely held as synonymous with PCL by pathologists and clinicians alike. *Adenolymphoma,*

although descriptive, overstates the importance of the lymphoid component, and the uninformed may even infer it to signify a malignant condition. Thus, the use of *adenolymphoma* should be discouraged. Carmichael and coworkers[12] reviewed the first large series, which involved 26 cases. Among the many additional series, the largest series were those reported by Orloff[13] and by Chaudhry and Gorlin[5] The registry of salivary gland pathology at the Armed Forces Institute of Pathology (AFIP) contains 722 cases of PCL.

CLINICAL FEATURES

The majority of PCLs occur in the parotid area, and most estimates of incidence have included both ectopic sites and malignant variants. The cited incidence has varied from 2 to 15 percent of parotid gland tumors.[14, 15] In Warthin's[4] description, the tumor represented only 2 cases of 700 reviewed, whereas later reviews by Orloff[13] reported an incidence of 2 to 6 percent of all parotid tumors and 1.6 to 4.2 percent of all salivary gland neoplasms. The generally accepted range of occurrence in parotid gland is held to be 5 to 6 percent, which has been supported by Chaudhry and Gorlin[5] and Thackray and Lucas[16] at 5.0 and 6.5 percent, respectively.

Among the 13,749 primary epithelial salivary gland tumors in the files of the AFIP, the 722 cases of PCL have an incidence of 5.3 percent. This incidence is in concurrence with previously reported large series. Of the 699 cases with specific sites identified, 633 (95 percent) involved the parotid gland. When considering only benign parotid tumors, the incidence is 11.9 percent. PCL is almost exclusively a parotid lesion, and occurrence at any other site should be considered ectopic. Numerous unusual sites have been reported, including the submandibular gland,[17, 18] palate,[19-21] lower lip,[20, 22] buccal mucosa,[20, 23] tonsil,[24, 25] larynx,[26] and maxillary sinus.[27] Review of the documented cases at unusual sites substantiates the occurrence of histologically acceptable cases; however, as several authors have noted, the tumors often appear as papillary cystadenomas with poorly developed lymphoid components. When considering a diagnosis of PCL in a site other than the parotid gland, strict histologic criteria, including both epithelial and lymphoid features, should be employed to avert an inappropriate diagnosis. Sites other than the parotid gland that are recorded in the AFIP files include submandibular gland (16 cases), tonsil (10 cases), lip (2 cases), palate (2 cases), buccal mucosa (2 cases), mandible (2 cases), oral cavity (2 cases), and pharynx (1 case). Evans and Cruikshank[28] attributed development of some ectopic tumors to extensions of the parotid gland lying subjacent to the submandibular gland. With this possibility in mind, the AFIP's submandibular cases were reviewed. Of the 12 cases reviewed, none unequivocally arose in the submandibular gland.

Papillary cystadenoma lymphomatosum has long been considered as a tumor of the elderly and is seen only sporadically before the third decade.[11, 29] In documented cases, patients' ages have ranged from 30 months to 92 years, and most patients are in the fifth and sixth decades of life.[30] In Chaudhry and Gorlin's[5] review of 242 cases, the mean age was 55.6 years. Previous findings are substantiated by data in the AFIP series, which show an average age of 57.3 years and a range from 1 to 90 years. Some investigators have noted an earlier development of lesions in females;[11] the AFIP series shows a mean age of 55.8 years for females and 57.6 years for males.

The majority (76.7 percent) occurred in patients between the ages of 40 and 70 years (Fig. 11–1).

Historically, few salivary gland tumors have shown as distinctive a sex predilection as PCL. The typically cited ratio of men to women is 5 to 1, and ratios as high as 10 to 1 have been reported.[5, 11, 16] Of interest are studies by Kennedy[31] and Lamelas and colleagues[32] in which the male predominance is refuted. Of the 606 cases from the AFIP series in which sex was specified, 506 involved men. In the military population, the male-to-female ratio was heavily predominated by males at 40 to 1. In contrast, the civilian data show a male-to-female ratio of 1.2 to 1.0 (106 men versus 91 women). These data agree with the investigations by Kennedy[31] and by Lamelas and colleagues.[32]

Racial statistics indicate that PCL occurs primarily among whites. Occasional tumors have been reported in Orientals, East Indians, Egyptians, and African blacks.[5] In the AFIP cases, 95.8 percent of the patients were white; blacks represented 3 percent; and there were scattered cases among Malaysians, Mongolians, and Native Americans.

Unique to PCL is its frequency of occurring bilaterally, ranging from 5 to 14 percent.[29, 33] Most bilateral PCLs do not occur simultaneously but are metachronous. Six simultaneously bilateral cases have been reported.[34-38] Numerous authors have purported PCL to be a multicentric or multifocal disease, which is proposed as the explanation for bilaterality.[39, 40] The multifocal concept may account for the large number of synchronous tumors and has been documented by studies of serially sectioned tumors with multifocality as high as 80 percent.[41, 42] Other benign and malignant tumors have been associated with PCL in the same gland with unusually high frequency.[43-45] Gnepp and colleagues[46] in an excellent review of synchronous tumors of major salivary glands documented cases of monomorphic adenoma, mixed tumor,

Percent

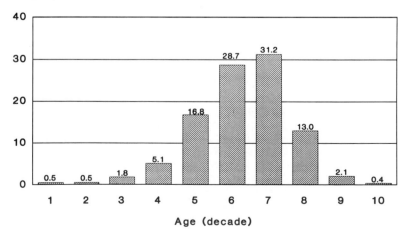

Figure 11–1. Age distribution by decade of 571 patients with PCLs in the AFIP registry of salivary gland disease.

acinic cell adenocarcinoma, oncocytoma, basal cell adenoma, ductal adenocarcinoma, and adenoid cystic carcinoma associated with PCL. They found that PCL is the most frequent synchronous tumor, which is probably attributable to its multifocality.

Sialography is not useful in differentiating PCL from other salivary gland tumors, but scintigraphy may be helpful. Radiosialography is based on the extraction of iodine from peritubular capillaries and secretion into the ductal lumina of normal glands as well as accumulation in tumors.[47] Gates and Work[48] cited the advantages of technetium-99m pertechnetate over ^{131}I and selenomethionine in radiosialography. In PCL, there is increased uptake of technetium-99m pertechnetate that presents as a smooth-margined, radiopositive "hot" nodule.[49] Ishikawa and Ishii[50] noted a unique propensity for PCL to retain radionuclide in the core of the tumor. This scintigraphic picture of the "hot" nodule is in contrast to that of space-occupying "cold" nodules that are indicative of mixed tumors, nonfunctioning malignant tumors, and most metastatic tumors except thyroid lesions. In addition to PCL, other lesions that accumulate technetium-99m pertechnetate are oncocytoma, sialadenitis, lymphangioma, and parotid cyst. Uptake of ^{123}I by PCL has been seen incidentally while a thyroid scan was being performed.[51] Positive scintigraphy with ^{123}I could indicate PCL, but the possibility of ectopic thyroid tissue or metastatic thyroid tumor must also be considered.[52] When a presumptive diagnosis is required before surgery, radioscintigraphy is an appropriate diagnostic study.

Similar to other parotid salivary gland tumors, PCL is usually a solitary, nodular, slowly enlarging swelling. Superficially located PCLs may cause facial asymmetry. Typically, PCL is located in the inferior pole of the parotid, next to the angle of the mandible, and it is usually 2 to 3 cm in size at the time of diagnosis. The tumor may also develop in lymph nodes in the superficial and medial portions of the parotid gland. They vary from moderately firm to fluctuant on palpation and are asymptomatic. Fewer than 10 percent of patients present with pain, pressure, or rapid increase in tumor size.[15] The average duration is approximately 36 months, but at clinical presentation lesions have been present for as long as 3 decades.[5] When the tumor is located inferior to and outside the parotid gland, the clinical impression may be branchial cleft cyst, chronic lymphadenitis, lymphoma, or tuberculosis.[53]

FINE-NEEDLE ASPIRATION

Fine-needle aspiration for cytologic diagnosis (see Chapter 9) is applicable to PCL.[54] PCL has positive correlation between histologic and cytologic diagnosis in 61 to 83 percent of cases.[55, 56] Aspiration biopsy typically produces cystic fluid that may contain tiny, visible tissue fragments. A smear from PCL consists of cystic fluid, lymphocytes, and clumps of oncocytic epithelial cells (Fig. 11–2). The lymphocytic component is evenly scattered throughout the fluid background of the cyst, which is amorphous with some cellular debris or mucoid material.[57] Atypical epithelial features are likely to correspond to PCL tumors that exhibit cystic degeneration, necrosis, or squamous metaplasia.[58] Because oncocytes with irregular nuclei, clumped chromatin, and loss of granular cytoplasm may be seen in aspirates of benign PCLs, differentiation from carcinoma may be extremely difficult and injudicious on a cytologic aspirate.

GROSS PATHOLOGIC FEATURES

The surgical specimen is usually a spheric or oval mass that is covered by a thin, tough capsule, which is usually intact. The tumor has a smooth, red-gray, lobulated surface. The typical PCL measures about 3 cm in diameter, and few tumors that are smaller than 2 cm or larger than 6 cm are removed. Tumor consistency varies from fluctuant in specimens with a single large cystic space (Fig. 11–3) to firm and rubbery in more solid tumors with small or few cysts (Fig. 11–4). The features of the tumor's cut surface are nearly pathognomonic, varying with the number and the size of the cysts.[29] Rarely, a single cyst will form, but usually, multiple cysts ranging in diameter from a few millimeters to a centimeter are seen. The cystic compartments contain fluid of variable viscosity that may be clear, serous, mucoid, brown-tinged (chocolate), or semisolid caseous material. The linings of the cyst appear shaggy and irregular with multiple intricate papillae that extend from the cyst wall. The solid portions of the tumor are gray-white and correspond to the lymphoid component. Within the solid areas, numerous tiny white nodules can be seen after scraping the surface; these nodules represent lymphoid follicles. Papillary cystadenoma lymphomatosum can usually be diagnosed grossly; however, tumors with liquefaction may lead to an inappropriate diagnosis of tuberculous lymphadenitis or branchial cleft cyst.[15]

MICROSCOPIC FEATURES

The combination of lymphoid matrix and papillations of eosinophilic epithelial cells forming cystic spaces presents a distinct and pathognomonic histopathologic picture (Fig. 11–5). The epithelial cells are arranged in two cell layers of uniform rows. Tall columnar cells approximate the cystic space (Fig. 11–6). The columnar cells contain darkly stained, pyknotic nuclei that are centrally placed near the luminal space. An inner cell layer is composed of cuboidal and polygonal

Text continued on page 192

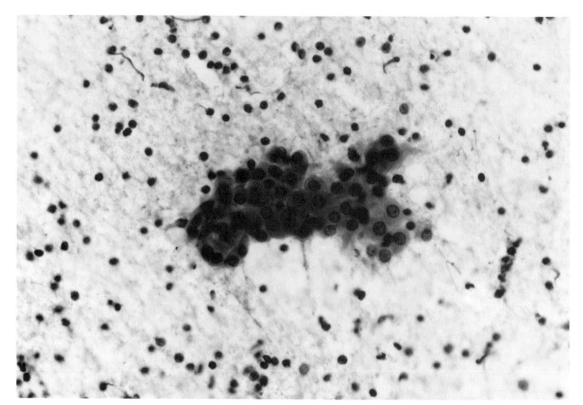

Figure 11–2. Cytologic aspiration of PCL shows cuboidal oncocytes with a background of scattered lymphocytes (× 300).

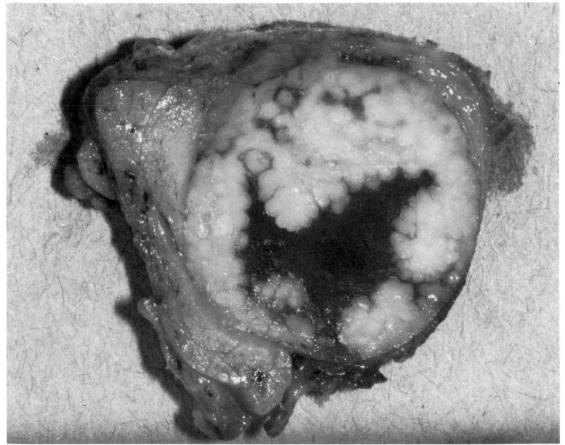

Figure 11–3. Transected PCL exhibits a solitary cyst surrounded by solid, white, homogenous tissue representing the lymphoid component.

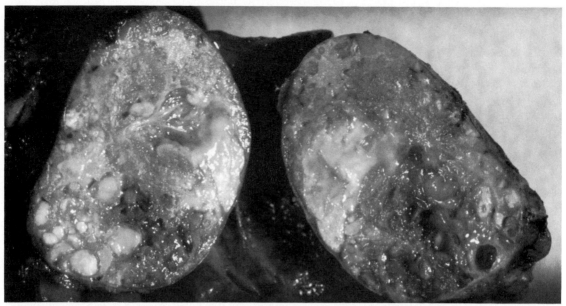

Figure 11–4. Transected PCL shows a multicystic pattern with multiple white nodules throughout, which correspond to the lymphoid component.

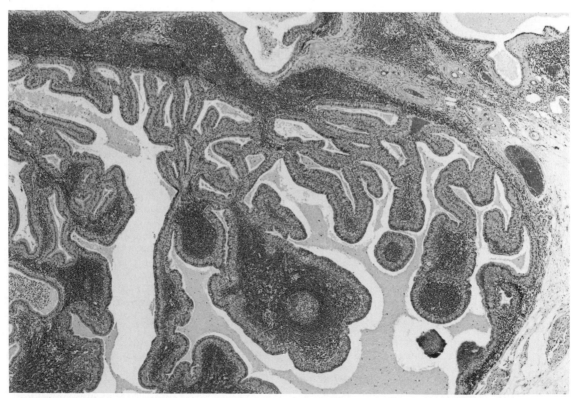

Figure 11–5. PCL shows cystic spaces partially filled with homogenous fluid circumscribed by double rows of oncocytes bordered by lymphoid tissue ($\times$ 30).

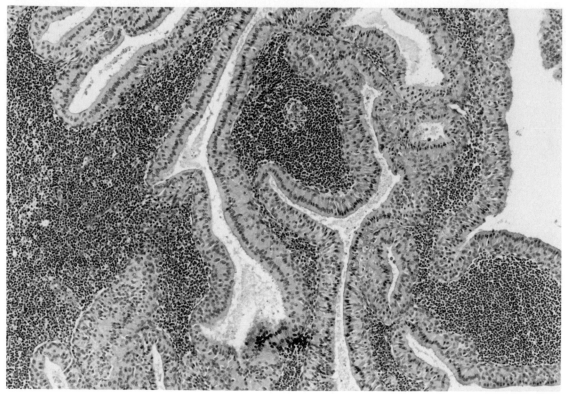

Figure 11–6. Papillary cystadenoma lymphomatosum with regimented rows of oncocytes in two cell layers and with accompanying lymphoid stroma (× 75).

cells that contain nuclei with prominent nucleoli (Fig. 11–7). The cytoplasm of both cell layers is finely granular and distinctly eosinophilic. Staining intensity varies according to the density of mitochondria, which are demonstrable with phosphotungstic acid–hematoxylin stain. The epithelial papillations project into cystic spaces that are often filled with homogenous eosinophilic granular material that stains with periodic acid–Schiff stain. Luminal lining cells are rarely ciliated but often have a "fuzzy" luminal surface (Fig. 11–7), which is attributed to the presence of microvilli. The epithelial cells are separated from the lymphoid stroma by a thin basement membrane. The lymphoid component appears reactive with germinal centers and occasional sinusoids and subcapsular spaces, but the amount of lymphoid stroma is variable and may be only a scanty lymphocytic infiltrate. Because at least four cases of lymphoma developing in PCL have been reported, the benign polymorphous character of the stroma should be histologically confirmed.

The most frequent histologic variations in PCL are oncocytosis, squamous metaplasia, mucous cell prosoplasia, and, rarely, inclusions of sebaceous glands.[59] Oncocytosis is characterized by sheets and nests of disorganized oncocytic cells that show loss of papillary formation (Fig. 11–8). Focal oncocytosis within the tumor mass should not be construed as a separate neoplasm or as a malig-

nant degeneration. PCL frequently shows focal areas of squamous metaplasia, presenting as a flattened, luminal surface with loss of regimented columnar cells (Fig. 11–9). Because mucous cells are normally found in salivary gland tissue, including the parotid gland ducts, the presence of mucous cells interdigitated between epithelial cells of PCL is not unusual (Fig. 11–10). When associated with inflammation, PCL may show spontaneous necrosis and squamous metaplasia (Fig. 11–11). In areas of metaplasia, the squamous cells have uniform bland cytologic features. If cytologic atypia is encountered (Fig. 11–12), the possibility of malignant transformation should be considered. A diagnosis of malignancy, however, requires evidence of stromal invasion (Fig. 11–13) or metastasis. Malignant transformation of the epithelial component of PCL has been reported in 14 cases, 2 of which were bilateral.[60, 61] Malignant tumors arising in PCLs include squamous cell carcinoma,[62–66] undifferentiated carcinoma,[67–69] adenocarcinoma,[70–72] and mucoepidermoid carcinoma.[73] The existence of malignant tumors has often been controversial as a result of scanty histologic documentation, lack of metastasis, and patients with concomitant malignant lesions. However, convincing cases have been presented by De la Pava and colleagues,[63] Kessler and colleagues,[67] Ruebner and Bramhall,[70] and Gadient and Kalfayan.[73] Three cases of malignant lymphoma have
Text continued on page 196

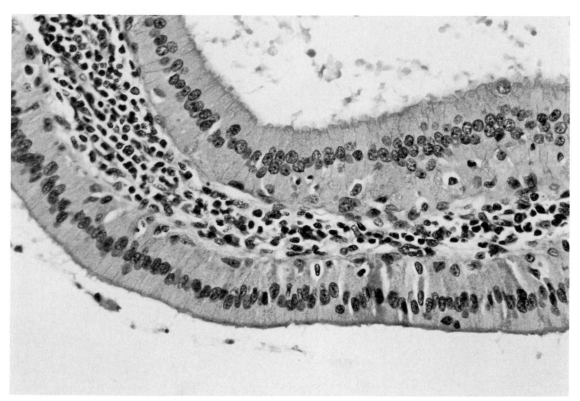

Figure 11–7. Oncocytic cells in papillary cystadenoma lymphomatosum include scattered cuboidal basal cells and columnar luminal cells with pseudociliated appearance (× 150).

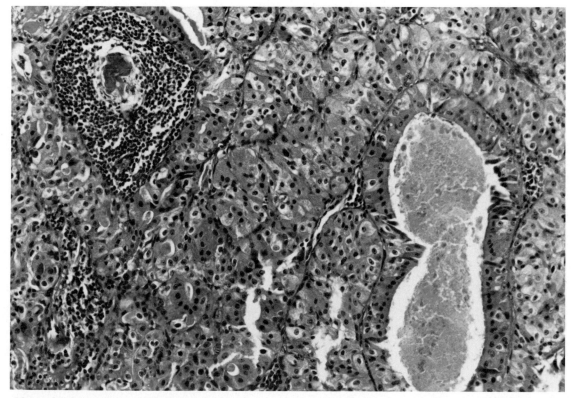

Figure 11–8. Papillary cystadenoma lymphomatosum is shown with focal oncocytosis that presents as back-to-back oncocytes with loss of papillary pattern (× 75).

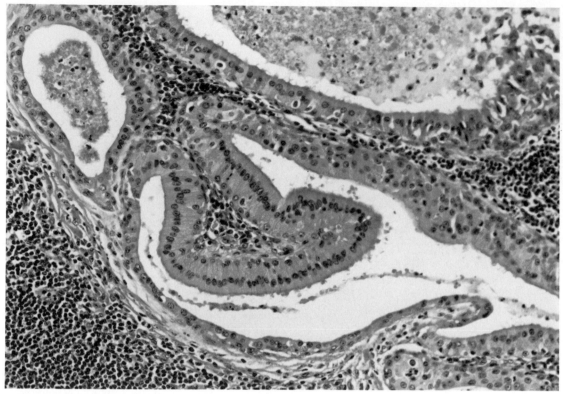

Figure 11–9. Papillary cystadenoma lymphomatosum has luminal oncocytes that exhibit focal metaplasia and partial loss of a regimented pattern (× 150).

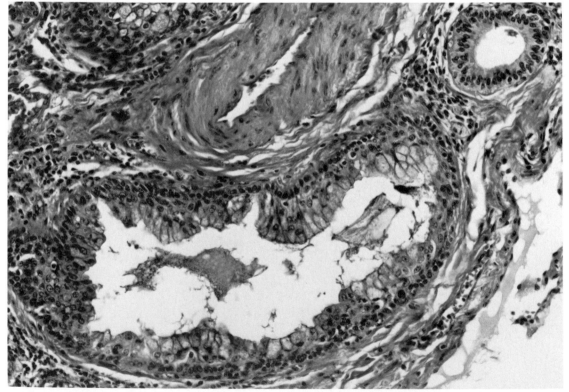

Figure 11–10. Papillary cystadenoma lymphomatosum shows focal mucous prosoplasia and goblet cell formation (× 150).

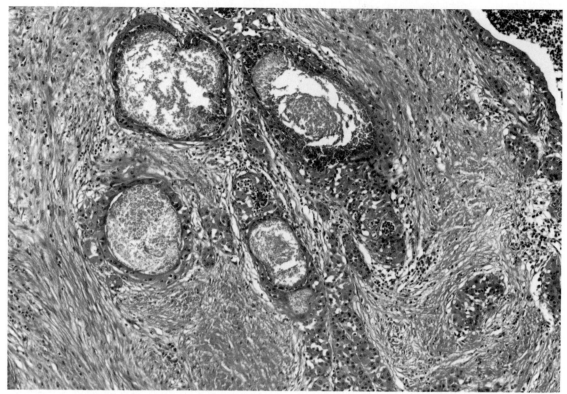

Figure 11–11. Marked squamous metaplasia and focal necrosis associated with secondary inflammation (× 75).

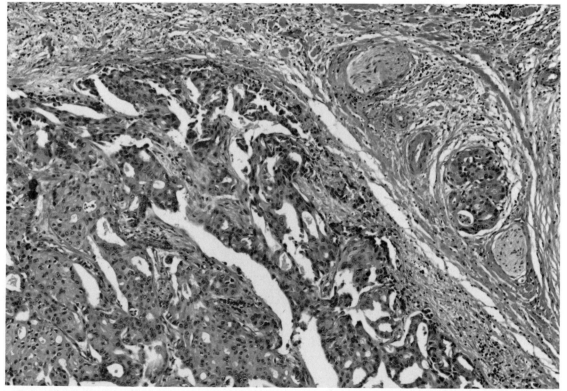

Figure 11–12. Malignant transformation of PCL shows focus of tumor with marked cytologic atypia associated with neural and vascular structures (× 150).

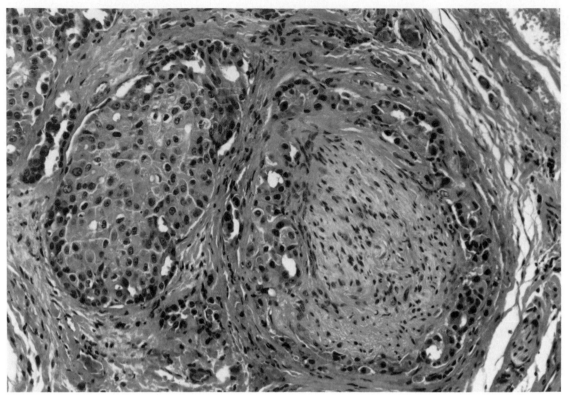

Figure 11–13. Malignant oncocytic component of PCL surrounds nerve bundles and invades adjacent stroma (× 150).

also been reported with PCL; however, the authors indicated that the pathogenesis was debatable and dissemination from another ectopic primary site should be considered.[74, 75] The AFIP files contain six documented cases of malignant transformation in PCL; squamous cell carcinoma (two cases), undifferentiated carcinoma (one case), adenocarcinoma (one case), mucoepidermoid carcinoma (one case), and lymphoma (one case). The AFIP data for malignant PCLs approximate a frequency of 1 percent. Because of the rarity of malignant PCL, caution is advised before establishing the diagnosis, and metastasis from another tumor site should first be ruled out.

Histochemical studies have little value in the diagnosis of PCL and are primarily for research interest. Lymphocyte marker studies have shown a predominance of T lymphocytes, which is consistent with normal lymph node tissue.[76, 77] Hsu and colleagues[78] reported that 80 percent of plasma cells in a PCL were IgA-producing plasma cells, whereas in the study by Korsrud and Brandtzaeg,[79] lymphoid markers were consistent with a reactive lesion, showing IgG (48.6 percent), IgA (38.5 percent), IgM (8.9 percent), IgD (3.3 percent), and IgE (0.7 percent). Immunohistochemical studies of luminal epithelial cells demonstrate reactivity for IgA and peanut agglutinin in the basal cell layer.[80] Korsrud and Brandtzaeg[79] also demonstrated IgA secretory component and carcinoembryonic antigen in the epithelial cells.

Zarbo and coworkers'[81] series on S-100 protein in salivary gland tumors provided negative results for the oncocytic tumors, including PCL.

DIFFERENTIAL DIAGNOSIS

The pathognomonic histology of PCL allows little latitude for confusion in the differential diagnosis. Papillary cystadenoma bears some resemblance to PCL. The amount and organization of lymphoid stroma necessary to separate the PCL from papillary cystadenoma vary among observers; however, most would agree that some organization of the lymphocytic component is required to render a diagnosis of PCL. Lesions with sparse, unorganized lymphocytic infiltrates that surround an oncocytic cyst lining are probably more appropriately diagnosed as papillary cystadenoma with chronic inflammation. When metaplasia involves squamous and mucous cells, small nests and sheets may emulate a mucoepidermoid carcinoma. Although mucoepidermoid carcinomas have arisen in PCL,[73, 74] the possibility is remote, and the diagnosis should be rendered with trepidation. Diagnosis of malignant transformation in PCL should always be done with caution and with the realization that oncocytosis, squamous metaplasia with necrosis, and mucous prosoplasia are seen in the benign PCL. It should also be remembered that several other benign and malignant salivary gland tumors, including sebaceous lymphadenoma, acinic cell carcinoma, and mucoepidermoid carcinoma, may have a prominent lymphoid component.

ULTRASTRUCTURAL FEATURES

The oncocytic cells of PCL have been of great interest to electron microscopists. As with most oncocytic neoplasms, the primary ultrastructural feature is an increased amount of mitochondria.[82-84] Most of the epithelial cells show prominent mitochondria throughout the cytoplasm, and those cells adjacent to the cystic lumina show densely packed mitochondria. In contrast, normal striated ducts of parotid do not have packed mitochondria in the apical portion but do share other ultrastructural features. The mitochondria range from normal size to three times larger with pleomorphic forms. The cristae of the aberrant mitochondria are increased in length and number and form closely packed lamellar sheaves (Fig. 11–14). Cristae may produce rouleaux or spheric concentric rings, or they may be arranged haphazardly in villous forms.[85] Crystalloids have been

described in the pyramidal cells and appear as rectangular prisms. Tonofilaments are infrequently seen but, when present, are found in tumors displaying significant metaplasia. Electron microscopy confirms the presence of true cilia in PCL, which is not entirely unexpected because cilia can be seen in normal parotid gland striated ducts. The apical surfaces of the epithelial cells frequently exhibit microvilli (Fig. 11–15). Kim and coinvestigators[86] documented the presence of membrane-bound granules in the apical area of degenerating columnar cells that were interpreted as lysosomes. The lysosomal granules were shown to contain acid phosphatase by cytochemical studies and were theorized to be related to a lytic process.

TREATMENT AND PROGNOSIS

The established treatment for PCL is surgical removal.[87, 88] Because most PCLs are superficially located in the parotid, the tumor is easily removed with minimal loss of glandular function and with preservation of the facial nerve. The principal debate regarding treatment usually concerns the amount of normal tissue removal required to

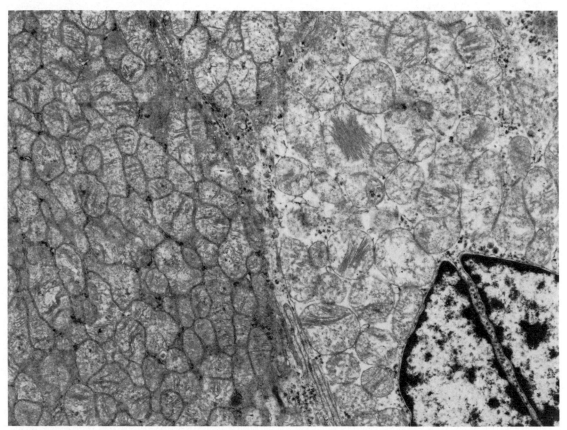

Figure 11–14. Electron micrograph of epithelium in PCL shows closely packed, enlarged, and irregular mitochondria ($\times$ 12,000).

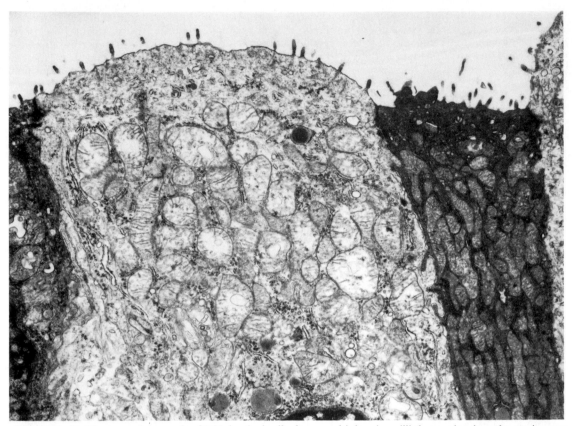

Figure 11–15. Electron micrograph of PCL luminal cells shows multiple microvilli that project into the cystic space at the top (× 10,000).

attain minimal recurrence rates. Two theories of surgical treatment are (1) tumor enucleation with resection of a minimal amount of surrounding tissue, and (2) a somewhat more aggressive superficial parotidectomy. Enucleation may be sufficient treatment for PCL. However, other tumors require more aggressive therapy, and it is difficult to be certain of tumor type at the time of surgery. In addition, although frozen section diagnosis can easily identify PCL, violation of the capsule is associated with a higher recurrence rate.[89] Shugar and colleagues[40] have proposed that minimal therapy should involve superficial parotidectomy because numerous investigations have documented the multifocality of PCL. Radiation therapy reduces tumor mass but does not eradicate the tumor and is not recommended. A judicious treatment approach is dictated by tumor location and accessibility and by a desire to attain minimal recurrence rates.

Recurrence rates for PCL are difficult to assess accurately because of the multifocal nature of the lesion. It can be assumed that a portion of lesions described as recurrent are actually multicentric lesions. Foote and Frazell[29] in an early follow-up study of PCL found 6 recurrences among 49 tumors, resulting in a 12 percent recurrence rate. Later studies by Beahrs[89] and Thackray and Lucas[16] reported rates of 9 percent (3 of 33) and

11.7 percent (2 of 17), respectively. The largest series reporting recurrence rates were by Chaudhry and Gorlin[5] and Orloff,[13] who found substantially lower recurrence rates of 6.7 and 5.5 percent, respectively.

PATHOGENESIS

The pathogenesis of PCL has long been controversial in regard to the origin of both the epithelium and the lymphoid stroma. As mentioned previously, Hildebrad[1] in his original description of the tumor ascribed the lesion to a variant of lateral cervical cyst and remnants of the branchial pouches. Soon after this description, Albrecht and Arzt[2] proposed heterotopic salivary rests in parotid lymph nodes as the origin, which is a position held by numerous authors.[90–93] In Warthin's[4] introduction of the lesion in the American literature, he suggested that PCL arose from heterotopic pharyngeal endoderm. Hevenor and Clark[94] supported Warthin and specified ectopic eustachian tube endoderm as the tissue of origin. Other theories of histogenesis have included orbital inclusions, heterotopic oncocytes, sebaceous glands, hypertrophic lymph node endothelium, and thymic anlage.[5, 16, 95]

Thompson and Bryant[96] conducted an embryology-based study of PCL and described parotid ductal epithelium in lymph nodes in the immediate vicinity of the parotid gland. They also described tumors with typical epithelial elements that showed no evidence of normal lymph node architecture, and they suggested a second theory that involved neoplastic proliferation of parotid ductal epithelium and concomitant secondary formation of lymphoid tissue. Subsequently Bernier and Bhaskar[97] documented cases in which the lymphoid tissue appeared to be true lymph nodes with subcapsular spaces and medullary sinusoids. Histochemical investigation by Azzopardi and Smith[98] indicated that PCL most likely arose from salivary ducts in lymphoid stroma. The theory of enclaved parotid epithelium in a lymph node was proved by Azzopardi and Hou,[99] who demonstrated two cases of PCL in association with lymph nodes containing salivary gland inclusions with two incipient PCL tumors. Although evidence has been presented that supports the enclaved ductal epithelium theory, other theories regarding the lymphoid stroma cannot be entirely discarded. These are the concepts concerning the secondary neoplastic proliferation and the accompanying inflammatory process.[100, 101] A high frequency of bilateral occurrence and the absence of lymph node architecture support a reactive pathogenesis.

Allergro[102] has proposed hypersensitivity as the main cause, suggesting a cascade of events as follows: oxyphilic metaplasia of striated ducts; papillary formations with secretion; cyst formation; infiltration of the basement membrane by basophils and histiocytes that eventuates in a complete delayed hypersensitivity reaction; and formation of the lymphoid stroma. This theory is supported by an immunohistochemical investigation that indicates a distribution of IgA and IgG that is similar to that seen with autoimmune thyroiditis and the presence of Langerhans's cells.[103] Other studies have not supported the delayed hypersensitivity theory but, rather, confirmed that the lymphoid elements are similar to polyclonal tonsillar tissue that produces all immunoglobulins with the exception of IgE.[104] It appears that a reactive histogenesis cannot be entirely ruled out (particularly in those lesions with poorly developed lymphoid elements). However, the theory involving development from heterotopic tissue in a lymph node has stood the test of time and continues to be the most substantiated pathogenesis.

REFERENCES

1. Hildebrad O: Veber angeborne epitheliale Cysten und Fisteln des Halse. Arch F Klin Chir 1895; 49:167–192.
2. Albrecht H, Arzt L: Beitrage zur frage der gewebsrerirrung gapillare cystadenome lymphdrusen. Frankfurt Ztsch F Path 1910; 4:47–69.
3. Nicholson GW: Studies in tumor formation. Guy's Hosp Rep 1923; 73:37.
4. Warthin AS: Papillary cystadenoma lymphomatosum: A rare teratoid of the parotid region. J Cancer Res 1929; 14:116–125.
5. Chaudhry AD, Gorlin RJ: Papillary cystadenoma lymphomatosum. Am J Surg 1958; 95:923–931.
6. Cunningham WF: Branchial cysts of the parotid gland. Ann Surg 1929; 90:114–117.
7. Handford JM: Branchiogenic adenoma of the neck. Ann Surg 1931; 94:461–464.
8. Jaffe RH: Adenolymphoma (onkocytoma) of parotid gland. Am J Cancer 1932; 16:1415–1423.
9. Hall EM: Adenolymphoma (orbital inclusion adenoma) of the parotid gland. Arch Pathol 1935; 19:756–757.
10. Norrish RE: An unusual tumor of the neck. Br J Surg 1935; 23:188–190.
11. Martin H, Ehrlich HE: Papillary cystadenoma lymphomatosum (Warthin's tumor) of the parotid gland. Surg Gynecol Obstet 1944; 79:611–623.
12. Carmichael R, Davie TB, Stewart MJ: Adenolymphoma of the salivary glands. J Pathol Bacteriol 1935; 40:601–615.
13. Orloff MJ: Collective review: Benign epitheliolymphoid lesions of parotid gland, papillary cystadenoma lymphomatosum and Mikulicz's disease. Surg Gynecol Obstet 1956; 103:521–541.
14. Batsakis JG: Tumors of the Head and Neck: Clinical and Pathologic Considerations, 2nd Ed. Baltimore, Williams & Wilkins, 1979; 54–56.
15. Seifert G, Miehlke A, Haubrich, J, Chilla R: Diseases of the Salivary Glands. Stuttgart, Georg Thieme Verlag, 1986; 195–213.
16. Thackray AC, Lucas RB: Tumors of the Major Salivary Glands: Atlas of Tumor Pathology, 2nd Series, Fascicle 10. Washington, DC, Armed Forces Institute of Pathology, 1974; 40–53.
17. Smith AG, Broadbent TR, Zavaleta AA: Tumors of oral mucous glands. Cancer 1954; 7:224–233.
18. Kurreja HK, Jain HK: Adenolymphoma of submandibular salivary gland. J Laryngol Otol 1972; 85:1201–1203.
19. Fantasia JE, Miller AS: Papillary cystadenoma lymphomatosum arising in minor salivary gland. Oral Surg Oral Med Oral Pathol 1981; 52:411–416.
20. Baden E, Pierce M, Selmon AJ, Roberts TW, Doyle JL: Intra-oral papillary cystadenoma lymphomatosum. J Oral Surg 1976; 34:533–541.
21. Hendrick JW: Papillary cystadenoma lymphomatosum of the palate. Arch Otolarynol 1964: 79:31–33.
22. Akin RK, Kreller AJ, Walters PJ: Papillary cystadenoma of the lower lip. Oral Surg Oral Med Oral Pathol 1973; 31:858–869.
23. Hart MN, Andrews JL: Papillary cystadenoma lymphomatosum arising in the oral cavity. Oral Surg Oral Med Oral Pathol 1968; 26:588–591.
24. Singh RS: Adenolymphoma presenting as pharyngeal tumour. J Laryngol Otol 1966; 80:199–203.
25. Fahmy S: Adenolymphoma of the tonsillar fossa. J Laryngol 1973; 87:675–679.
26. Foulsham CK, Snyder GG, Carpenter RJ: Papillary cystadenoma lymphomatosum of the larynx. Otolaryngol Head Neck Surg 1981; 89:960–964.
27. Sruthers AM, Williams H, Parkhill EM: Papillary cystadenoma of the maxillary paranasal sinus (atypical Warthin's tumor). Arch Otolaryngol 1954; 59:241–244.

28. Evans RW, Cruickshank AH: Epithelial Tumours of the Salivary Glands. Philadelphia, WB Saunders Co, 1970; 37–57.

29. Foote FW, Frazell EI: Tumors of the major salivary glands. Cancer 1953; 6:1065–1133.

30. Peel RL, Gnepp DR: Diseases of salivary glands. *In* Barnes L (ed.): Surgical Pathology of the Head and Neck. New York, Marcel Dekker Inc, 1985; 565–569.

31. Kennedy TL: Warthin's tumor: A review indicating no male predominance. Laryngoscope 1983; 93:889–891.

32. Lamelas J, Terry JH, Alfonso AE: Warthin's tumor: Multicentricity and increasing incidence in women. Am J Surg 1987; 154:347–351.

33. Eveson JW, Cawson RA: Warthin's tumor (cystadenolymphoma) of salivary glands: A clinicopathologic investigation of 278 cases. Oral Surg Oral Med Oral Pathol 1986; 61:256–262.

34. Hales B, Hansen JE: Bilateral simultaneous Warthin's tumor in a woman. South Med J 1977; 70:257–258.

35. Kurzer A, Villegas LF: Bilateral simultaneous Warthin's tumors in women. Plast Reconstr Surg 1986; 78:87–90.

36. Kavka SJ: Bilateral simultaneous Warthin's tumors. Arch Otolaryngol 1970; 91:302–303.

37. Akira I, Kawasaki T, Nakajima T: Bilateral Warthin's tumor: Report of case and review of the Japanese literature. J Oral Surg 1981; 39:362–366.

38. Tveteras K, Kristensen S: Warthin's tumour with bilateral synchronous presentation: Survey of the literature and a new case. J Laryngol Otol 1986; 100: 487–491.

39. Beck LD, Maguda TA: Papillary cystadenoma lymphomatosum (Warthin's tumor): A multicentric benign tumor. Laryngoscope 1967; 77:1840–1847.

40. Shugar JM, Som PM, Biller HF: Warthin's tumor, a multifocal disease. Ann Otol Rhinol Laryngol 1982; 91:246–249.

41. Patey DH, Thackray AC: The treatment of parotid tumors in the light of a pathologic study of parotid material. Br J Surg 1958; 45:477–487.

42. Turnbull AD, Frazell EL: Multiple tumors of the major salivary glands. Am J Surg 1969; 118:787–788.

43. Lumerman H, Freedman P, Caracciolo P, Remigio PS: Synchronous malignant mucoepidermoid tumor of the parotid gland and Warthin's tumor in adjacent lymph node. Oral Surg Oral Med Oral Pathol 1975; 39:954–958.

44. Astacio JN: Papillary cystadenoma lymphomatosum associated with pleomorphic adenoma of the parotid gland. Oral Surg Oral Med Oral Pathol 1974; 38:91–95.

45. Chait GE, Snell GED, van Nostrand AWP: Multiple tumors of parotid gland. J Otolaryngol 1979; 8:435–438.

46. Gnepp DR, Schroeder W, Heffner D: Synchronous tumors arising in a single major salivary gland. Cancer 1989; 63:1219–1224.

47. Gates GA: Sialography and scanning of salivary glands. Otolaryngol Clin North Am 1970; 10:379–390.

48. Gates GA, Work WP: Radioisotopes scanning of the salivary glands: A preliminary report. Laryngoscope 1967; 77:861–875.

49. Stebner FC, Eyler WR, Dusault LA, Block MA: Identification of Warthin's tumor by scanning of salivary glands. Am J Surg 1968; 116:513–517.

50. Ishikawa H, Ishii Y: Evaluation of salivary gland scintigraphy was evaluated in 32 histologically proven cases. J Oral Maxillofac Surg 1984; 42:429–434.

51. Burt RW: Accumulation of ^{123}I in Warthin's tumor. Clin Nucl Med 1978; 3:155–156.

52. Moinuddin M, Rockett JF: Warthin's tumor and I-123 scan. J Nucl Med 1980; 21:898–899.

53. Shaw HJ, Friedman I: Bilateral adenolymphoma of the parotid salivary gland associated with tuberculosis. Br J Surg 1959; 46:500–505.

54. Mavec P, Eneroth CM, Frazen S, Moberger G, Zajicck J: Aspiration biopsy of salivary gland tumors: Correlation of cytologic findings from 652 aspiration biopsies with clinical and histologic observations. Acta Otolaryngol 1964; 58:471–484.

55. Bottles K, Lowhagen T, Miller TR: Mast cells in the aspiration cytology differential diagnosis of adenolymphoma. Acta Cytol 1985; 29:513–515.

56. Kline TS, Merriam JM, Shapshay SM: Aspiration biopsy cytology of the salivary gland. Am J Clin Pathol 1981; 76:263–269.

57. Eneroth CM, Zajicek L: Aspiration biopsy of salivary gland tumors. II. Morphologic studies on smears and histologic sections from oncocytic tumors. Acta Cytol 1965; 9:355–361.

58. Person PS, Zettergren L: Cytologic diagnosis of salivary gland tumors by aspiration biopsy. Acta Cytol 1973; 17:351–354.

59. Meza-Chavez L: Sebaceous glands in normal and neoplastic parotid glands: Possible significance of sebaceous glands in respect to the origin of tumors of the salivary gland. Am J Pathol 1949; 25:627–645.

60. Dieter A: Bilateral carcinoma of parotid, one cancer arising in a Warthin's tumor. Am J Clin Pathol 1974; 61:270–274.

61. Tanaka N, Chen WC: A case of bilateral papillary cystadenoma lymphomatosum. (Warthin's tumor) of the parotid complicated with mucoepidermoid. Gann 1953; 44:229–231.

62. McClatchy KD, Appelblat NH, Langin JL: Carcinoma in papillary cystadenoma lymphomatosum (Warthin's tumor). Laryngoscope 1982; 92:98–99.

63. De la Pava S, Knutson GH, Mukhtar F, Pickren JW: Squamous cell carcinoma arising in Warthin's tumor of the parotid gland. Cancer 1965; 18:790–794.

64. Dajanov I, Sneff EM, Dclerme AN: Squamous cell carcinoma arising in Warthin's tumor of the parotid gland. Oral Surg Oral Med Oral Pathol 1983; 55:286–290.

65. Little JW, Rickles NH: Malignant papillary cystadenoma lymphomatosum. Cancer 1965; 18: 851–856.

66. Baker M, Yuzon D, Baker BH: Squamous cell carcinoma arising in benign adenolymphoma (Warthin's tumor) of the parotid gland. J Surg Oncol 1980; 15:7–10.

67. Kessler E, Koznizky LL, Schindel J: Malignant Warthin's tumor. Oral Surg Oral Med Oral Pathol 1977; 43:111–115.

68. Moosavi H, Ryan CK, Schwartz S, Connelly JA: Malignant adenolymphoma. Hum Pathol 1980; 11:80–83.

69. Brown L, Aparicio SP: Malignant Warthin's tumor:

An ultrastructural study. J Clin Pathol 1984; 37:170–175.

70. Ruebner B, Bramhall JL: Malignant papillary cystadenoma lymphomatosum. Arch Pathol 1960; 69:110–117.

71. Dobrossy L, Ronay P, Molnar L: Malignant papillary cystadenoma lymphomatosum. Oncology 1972; 26:457–465.

72. Nakashima NK: Malignant papillary cystadenoma lymphomatosum. Virchows Arch [A] 1983; 399:207–219.

73. Gadient SE, Kalfayan B: Mucoepidermoid carcinoma arising within a Warthin's tumor. Oral Surg Oral Med Oral Pathol 1975; 40:391–398.

74. Banik S, Howell JS, Wright DH: Non-Hodgkin's lymphoma arising in adenolymphoma—A report of two cases. J Pathol 1985; 146:167–177.

75. Miller R, Yanagihara ET, Aaron AD, Lukes RJ: Malignant lymphoma in a Warthin's tumor. Cancer 1982; 50:2948–2950.

76. Diamond LW, Braylan RC: Cell surface markers on lymphoid cells from Warthin's tumors. Cancer 1979; 44:508–583.

77. Howard DR, Bagley C, Batsakis JG: Warthin's tumor: A functional immunologic study of the lymphoid cell component. Am J Otolaryngol 1982; 3:15–19.

78. Hsu S, Hsu P, Nayak RN: Warthin's tumor: An immunohistochemical study of its lymphoid stroma. Hum Pathol 1981; 12:251–257.

79. Korsrud FR, Brandtzaeg P: Immunohistochemical characterization of cellular immunoglobulins and epithelial marker antigens in Warthin's tumor. Hum Pathol 1983; 15:361–367.

80. Hsu S, Raine L: Warthin's tumor, epithelial cell differences. Am J Clin Pathol 1981; 77:78–82.

81. Zarbo RJ, Regezi JA, Batsakis JG: S-100 protein in salivary gland tumors: An immunohistochemical study of 129 cases. Head Neck Surg 1986; 8:268–275.

82. Tandler B: Warthin's tumor. Arch Otolaryngol 1966; 84:68–76.

83. McGarvan MH: The ultrastructure of papillary cystadenoma lymphomatosum of the parotid. Virchows Arch [A] 1965; 338:195–202.

84. Balogh K, Roth SI: Histochemical and electron microscopic studies of eosinophilic granular cells (oncocytes) in tumors of the parotid gland. Lab Invest 1965; 44:310–320.

85. Tandler B, Shipkey FH: Ultrastructure of Warthin's tumor. J Ultrastruc Mol Struct Res 1964; 11:292–305.

86. Kim S, Weatherbee L, Nasjleti GE: Lysosomes in the epithelial component of Warthin's tumor. Arch Pathol 1973; 95:56–62.

87. Eneroth CM, Hamburger CA: Principles of treatment of different types of parotid tumors. Laryngoscope 1974; 84:1732–1740.

88. Woods JE: Parotidectomy versus limited resection for benign parotid masses. Am J Surg 1985; 149:749–750.

89. Beahrs OH: Surgical management of parotid lesions. Arch Surg 1960; 80:890–903.

90. Harris PN: Adenocystoma lymphomatosum of the salivary glands. Am J Pathol 1937; 13:81–87.

91. Smith JF: Classification of major gland lesions. Arch Otolaryngol 1964; 80:322–349.

92. Plaut JA: Adenolymphoma of the parotid gland. Ann Surg 1942; 116:43–53.

93. Lloyd OC: Salivary adenoma and adenolymphoma. J Pathol 1946; 58:699–710.

94. Hevenor EP, Clark CE: Adenolymphoma (papillary cystadenoma lymphomatosum). Surg Gynecol Obstet 1950; 90:746–751.

95. Kaissel CL, Stout AP: "Orbital inclusions" cysts and cystadenoma of parotid salivary glands. Arch Surg 1933; 24:485–499.

96. Thompson AS, Bryant HC: Histogenesis of papillary cystadenoma lymphomatosum (Warthin's tumor) of the parotid salivary gland. Am J Pathol 1950; 26:807–849.

97. Bernier JL, Bhaskar SN: Lymphoepithelial lesions of the salivary glands. Cancer 1958; 11:1156–1178.

98. Azzopardi JG, Smith OD: Salivary gland tumors and their mucins. J Pathol 1959; 77:131–140.

99. Azzopardi JG, Hou LT: The genesis of adenolymphoma. J Pathol 1964; 88:213–218.

100. Bauer WH, Bauer JD: Classification of glandular tumors of salivary glands. Arch Pathol 1953; 55:328–346.

101. Hicks JD: The histogenesis of adenolymphoma of the salivary glands. J Pathol 1953; 65:169–174.

102. Allegro SR: Warthin's tumor: A hypersensitivity disease. Hum Pathol 1971; 2:403–420.

103. Foulsham CK, Johnson GS, Snyder GG, Carpenter RJ, Shafi NQ: Immunohistopathology of papillary cystadenoma lymphomatosum (Warthin's tumor). Ann Clin Lab Sci 1984; 14:47–63.

104. Korsrud FR, Brandtzaeg P: Immunohistochemical studies on epithelium and lymphoid components of Warthin's tumor. Acta Otolaryngol (Suppl) 1979; 360:221–224.

Chapter

12

CANALICULAR ADENOMA AND BASAL CELL ADENOMA

Frank J. Kratochvil

The nomenclature for the salivary gland neoplasms known as canalicular adenoma and basal cell adenoma has historically been inconsistent and confusing. Although histogenetic and pathogenetic similarities exist between these two adenomas, we believe clinicopathologic differences are sufficient to identify them as separate and distinct entities. In 1926, Schutz[1] reported a case of "adenoma" of the parotid gland, which included a description and photomicrographs that suggested that this lesion may represent a basal cell adenoma. Eggers[2] illustrated two examples of what was called "adenoma" of the palate, one of which was consistent with a canalicular adenoma. McFarland,[3] in writing about "histopathologic prognosis," reviewed the histology and follow-up of 304 cases of "mixed tumors" and reported a group he classified as "simple canalicular tumors." Limited information precludes definitive retrospective diagnosis, but the photomicrograph of one lesion is highly suggestive of a canalicular adenoma. Although Bauer and Bauer[4] used the term *canalicular adenoma* in 1953, Bhaskar and Weinmann[5] were the first to use the term to describe this neoplasm as we now identify it in minor salivary glands. They noted a propensity for these lesions to develop in the upper lip.

Kleinsasser and Klein[6] were the first to suggest using the term *basal cell adenoma* for a group of salivary gland tumors and to describe characteristic microscopic features. They proposed that basal cell adenoma be recognized as an entity that is separate from mixed tumors. Evans and Cruickshank[7] also recognized these lesions as separate entities and devoted a chapter in their text to basal cell adenoma. However, among the basal cell adenomas in their series, apparently two canalicular adenomas of the upper lip were included. Following this report, it became clear that various investigators disagreed in regard to the appropriate terminology for these two groups of tumors.

In 1970, Rauch and colleagues[8] classified benign salivary gland neoplasms into two broad categories: monomorphic adenoma and pleomorphic adenoma. They noted that monomorphic adenomas could be classified according to growth patterns but that distinct separation failed in some areas. In 1972, in the World Health Organization's *Histological Typing of Salivary Gland Tumors*, Thackray and Sobin[9] supported the same broad use of the term *monomorphic adenoma*. They recognized the well-established terms *adenolymphoma*, or *papillary cystadenoma lymphomatosum*, and *oxyphilic adenoma*, or *oncocytoma*, as distinct entities encompassed by this broad category. In addition, they suggested a third category that they called *other types of monomorphic adenoma*, which consisted of tumors that were not as well defined. They noted that the so-called "basal cell adenoma" came under the third category (*other types*). Thackray and Lucas[10] later embraced this classification. In 1972, Eneroth and coworkers[11] supported the same general classification system and the use of the term *monomorphic adenoma* as presented by Thackray and Sobin.

Although some authors have used the terms *monomorphic adenoma, basal cell adenoma,* and *canalicular adenoma* synonymously, others have used them individually to imply specific diagnoses.[12–21] Furthermore, in 1981, Batsakis and Brannon[22] described the "dermal analogue tumor" and concluded that this lesion was the salivary gland counterpart of the dermal eccrine cylindroma. They noted that these neoplasms contained prominent extracellular hyaline material and that they had formerly been classified as basal cell adenomas.

In 1982, Nagao and colleagues[23] reported the microscopic features of 40 basal cell adenomas and classified them histologically into four subtypes: basal cell, tubular, trabecular, and papillary. In 1983, Gardner and Daley[24] reviewed the literature in an attempt to clarify the use of the terms *monomorphic adenoma, basal cell adenoma,* and *canalicular adenoma.* They recommended that *monomorphic adenoma* be used as a general term for any benign salivary gland neoplasm that is not a pleomorphic adenoma. According to these investigators, basal cell adenoma was a distinct entity within the monomorphic adenoma group that exhibited a number of histologic subtypes that included the following: solid, trabecular, tubular, and membranous. Canalicular adenoma was considered a separate entity that was distinct from basal cell adenoma. In a later paper, Daley and colleagues[25] reported five cases of canalicular adenoma and eight cases of basal cell adenoma and observed that the clinical, histologic, histochemical, and ultrastructural features of these two neoplasms are distinctly different. They stated that although the biologic behavior of these neoplasms is similar, they are separate entities. Others have used these terms similarly.[12, 26-30]

In this chapter, use of the term *monomorphic adenoma* is not recommended. In my opinion, it is an ambiguous term that detracts from the terms used for adenomas that have relatively specific clinical and histopathologic features. Comparison of the clinical features of 160 cases classified as basal cell adenoma and 121 cases classified as canalicular adenoma in the AFIP registry of salivary gland pathology supports the view that they represent different neoplastic entities.[31] Furthermore, these adenomas have distinctive histologic features.

CANALICULAR ADENOMA

Clinical Features

The files of the AFIP contain 121 cases of canalicular adenoma. The average age among patients with canalicular adenoma is 65 years with a range of 34 to 88 years. All of the patients have been at least in their fourth decade of life, and there is a dramatic peak in the adenoma's occurrence in the seventh decade (Fig. 12–1). The average age of patients with canalicular adenomas (64.6 years) is older than that for basal cell adenomas (57.7 years), and the range in patients' ages is narrower. Other authors have reported a patient age range of 33 to 87 years, and an average age of 60 to 67 years.[17, 20, 25, 28, 32]

The sex of the patient was reported for 118 patients. When the few military patients are excluded, there is a definite female predominance of 1.7 to 1.0. Surprisingly, in 1973, Nelson and Jacoway[28] found a male predominance (55 percent). This finding may be the result of a significant number of military patients in their study. Regezi and colleagues[32] found a nearly equal sex distribution of 11 females and 12 males in their study. Other investigators have reported female prevalences that ranged from 1.2 to 1.8 females for each male.[17, 20, 25]

Information on patients' race is available for only a limited number of patients (57 cases); however, among these patients, 91 percent were white, 7.0 percent were blacks, and 2 percent were Native American. Although the numbers are relatively small, they do suggest a possible propensity for canalicular adenoma to develop among whites. Blacks make up 12 percent of the American population but only 7 percent of the population of patients with canalicular adenoma in this series. Other investigators have also stated that canalic-

Figure 12–1. Graph depicts distribution by age in decades of 119 patients with canalicular adenoma who are listed in the AFIP salivary gland registry.

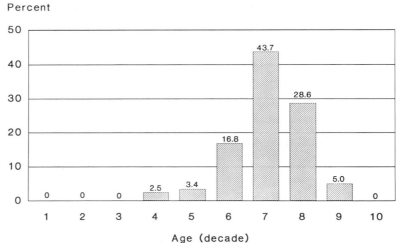

Percent

Age (decade)

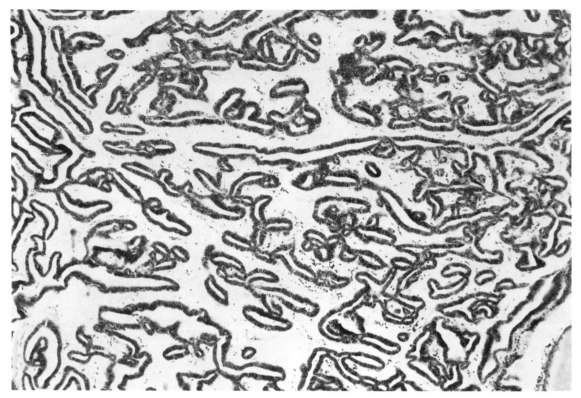

Figure 12–4. Canalicular adenoma showing single rows of cells that are arranged in parallel lines, which form long lumina that have a "canalicular" appearance (× 75).

It is not unusual for large cystic spaces to be present (Fig. 12–5). Multiple, smaller cystic dilatations can give the neoplasm a microcystic appearance, and larger cysts may result in a prominent cystic presentation, both microscopically and grossly. When cystic, the tumors may have papillary projections into the lumina (Fig. 12–6). These projections are covered by the same columnar or cuboidal cells that make up the body of the neoplasm. In areas where papillary projections are present, psammoma bodies may be seen (Fig. 12–7). The presence of psammoma bodies has been mentioned by others.[19, 20] Occasionally, mucous cells or oncocytic cells may be seen (Fig. 12–8). Mintz and coworkers[20] reported the presence of mucous cells in 8 of 21 cases in their series.

It is not unusual to find focal areas of the tumors that are composed of groups of more rounded cells. This appearance, in many cases, results from a tangential plane of section, which produces an "on face" presentation of the normal columnar cells and gives them a more basaloid appearance (Fig. 12–9). In rare cases, more solid cellular proliferations are evident, which result in tumors that show features of both canalicular and basal cell adenomas (Fig. 12–10).

The remarkable features of the stroma of canalicular adenoma are the sparse fibrillarity, the lack of cellularity, and the prominent vascularity (Figs. 12–2 to 12–4). The stroma contains few fibroblasts and minimal to moderate collagen. In many areas of sections stained with hematoxylin and eosin, the stroma has an edematous, lightly basophilic appearance with a few scattered inflammatory cells. The relatively acellular stroma stains with mucicarmine, alcian blue, and periodic acid–Schiff, with and without diastase predigestion. The material within the smaller ducts and canals also reacts with these stains. The prominent vascularity is striking (Fig. 12–11). The loose fibrous connective tissue stroma contains numerous delicate, endothelium-lined vascular spaces, some of which appear engorged with blood. Hemosiderin deposition is often seen in association with the vascularity. This product of the breakdown of blood can be seen in foci of macrophages or as finely granular pigment found apparently within epithelial cells. This apparent epithelial cell pigmentation resembles melanin, but iron stains confirm its true nature.

For the most part, lesions of significant size are well circumscribed and appear to be surrounded by a thin fibrous capsule (Fig. 12–12). As noted, a significant number of canalicular adenomas are multifocal. In these cases, the larger foci are usually encapsulated, but the scattered smaller foci are often unencapsulated and appear as nidi of proliferation within the salivary gland parenchyma (Fig. 12–13). It is important to avoid interpreting these small foci as a feature of malignancy.

Text continued on page 211

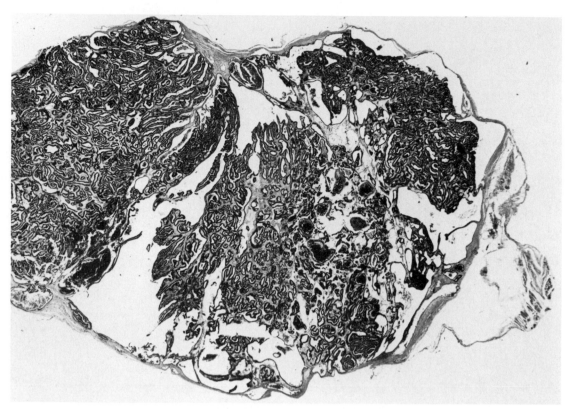

Figure 12–5. Canalicular adenoma exhibits a cystic pattern and a thin connective tissue capsule (× 15).

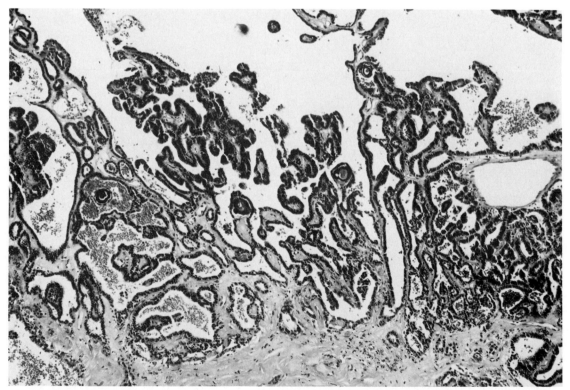

Figure 12–6. Canalicular adenoma with a cystic pattern exhibits papillary projections surfaced by columnar or cuboidal cells (× 75).

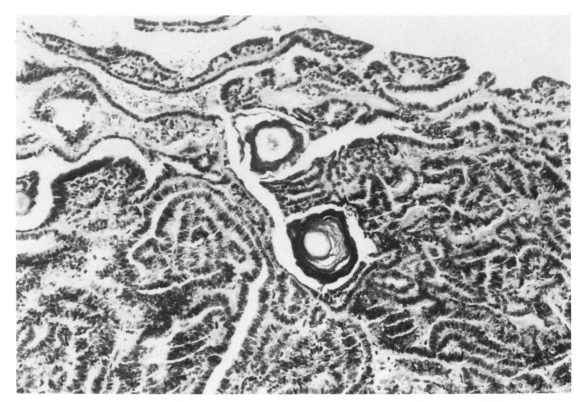

Figure 12–7. Canalicular adenoma with psammoma bodies in a papillary area (× 150).

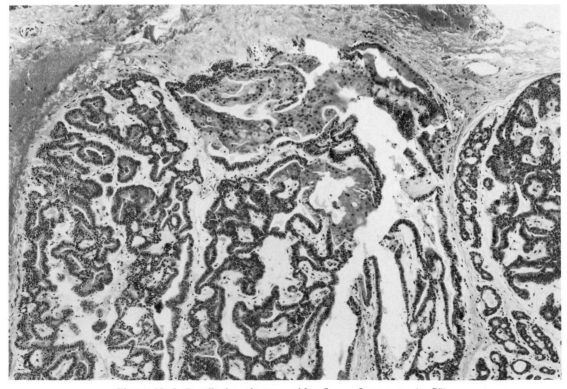

Figure 12–8. Canalicular adenoma with a focus of oncocytes (× 75).

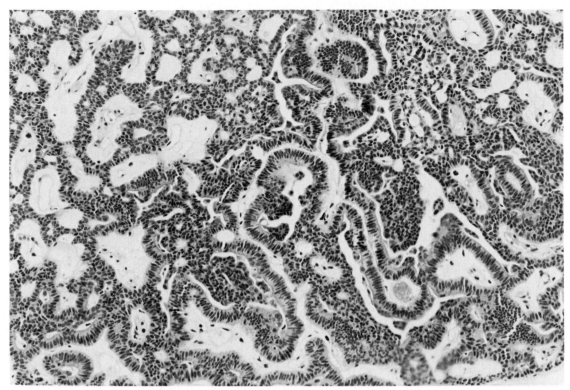

Figure 12–9. Canalicular adenoma in which "on face" plane of section of columnar cells produces the appearance of a "hybrid neoplasm" that has features of canalicular and basal cell adenomas (× 150).

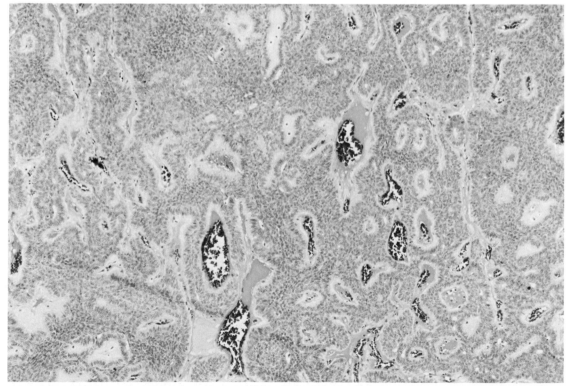

Figure 12–10. Minor salivary gland neoplasm exhibits a limited, hypocellular, vascular stroma; columnar peripheral cells that are typical of canalicular adenoma; and solid proliferation of smaller cells more reminiscent of basal cell adenoma (× 75).

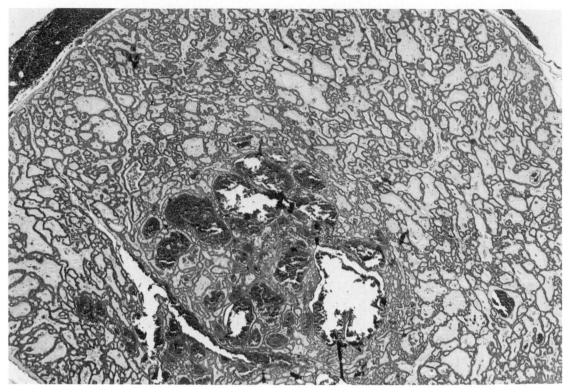

Figure 12–11. Canalicular adenoma tissue demonstrates prominent vascularity ($\times$ 30).

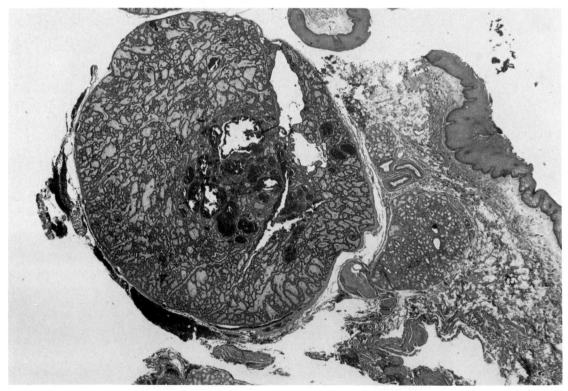

Figure 12–12. Large circumscribed nodule of canalicular adenoma has a thin capsule and prominent vascularity ($\times$ 15).

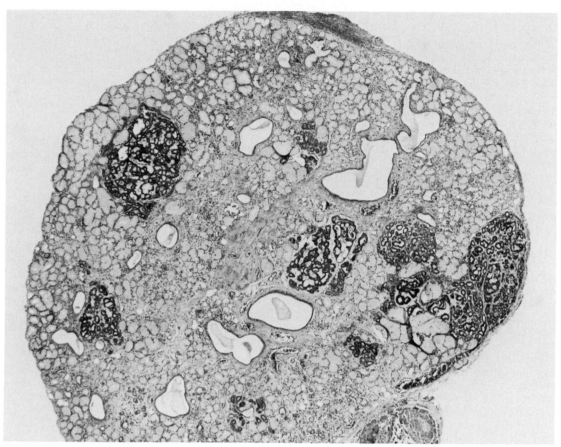

Figure 12–13. Canalicular adenoma of the upper lip demonstrates multifocal proliferation within minor salivary gland tissue (× 10).

Ultrastructural Features

Reports on the ultrastructural features of canalicular adenomas vary. Chen and Miller[29] noted two rows of interdigitating cells, one of tall columnar cells positioned toward the lumen and another of conical cells that are in contact with the stromal connective tissue. Guccion and Redman[33] reported that the cells were arranged in a single layer around the lumen. The nuclei are described as ovoid with generally small but prominent nucleoli.[29, 33] The nuclei contain abundant euchromatin and slightly patchy chromatin condensation.

The supportive connective tissue exhibits small numbers of collagen fibrils and few fibroblasts in a large amount of mucoid material.[29]

Investigators have noted that although the epithelial cells in canalicular adenomas exhibit desmosomes, they tend to be small and relatively few in number.[25, 29] Daley and colleagues[25] found that canalicular adenomas had fewer tonofilaments than basal cell adenomas. Chen and Miller[29] pointed out that the basement membrane did not show any obvious hemidesmosomes in their case of canalicular adenoma.

Some intracellular microfilaments are present in canalicular adenoma and range from 4 to 7 nm in diameter, and occasionally they are densely packed or are present in tangled clusters.[25, 34] Guccion and Redman[33] did not find any tumor cells that resembled myoepithelial cells, but they did see some oval to fusiform cells adjacent to the tumor capsule that contained microfilaments with focal densities.

As opposed to the prominent reduplicated basement membrane seen in many basal cell adenomas, the basement membrane in canalicular adenomas tends to be single but somewhat thickened.[25, 29] Guccion and Redman[33] reported reduplication of the basal lamina in a few focal areas but noted that many capillaries in the adjacent stroma had moderate to marked replication of their basal lamina. Mair and Stalsberg[34] described frequent reduplication of basal laminae, although their transmission electron micrographs showed minimal reduplication in comparison with that of basal cell adenomas.

A moderately developed Golgi complex, prominent rough endoplasmic reticulum, mitochondria, and clusters of glycogen granules are also noted.[29] Some investigators[29, 34] have reported the presence of secretory granules, although Guccion and Redman[33] did not observe them. In addition, microvilli have been reported.[34]

Immunohistochemical Findings

Zarbo and coworkers[39] reported that the epithelium in canalicular adenomas showed significant S-100 protein immunoreactivity but nonreactive stromal cells. Other salivary gland neoplasms with S-100 protein immunoreactivity that was limited to the epithelium were their so-called salivary duct adenoma and membranous type of basal cell adenoma. This contrasts with benign mixed tumors and the trabeculotubular form of basal cell adenoma, which tend to show S-100 protein immunoreactivity in mesenchymal-like tissue.

Differential Diagnosis

The clinical differential diagnosis of a swelling in the upper lip has been reviewed by Daley.[38] It includes sialolith, mucus extravasation phenomenon, mucus retention cyst, and salivary gland neoplasms, notably mixed tumor. In our experience, about 36 percent of all upper lip salivary gland tumors are mixed tumors, and about 22 percent are canalicular adenomas (see Table 9–8). However, canalicular adenomas generally affect older patients.

We agree with various investigators who have stated that the microscopic differential diagnosis for canalicular adenoma, depending on the site of involvement, may include ameloblastoma,[35] cutaneous basal cell carcinoma,[35] adenoid cystic carcinoma,[17, 19, 20, 32] and mixed tumor.[19, 20] In the upper lip, the presence of ameloblastoma would require extension from the anterior maxilla, whereas basal cell carcinoma is not a consideration for intraoral tumors. Nelson and Jacoway[28] noted that four of the canalicular adenomas in their series were initially diagnosed as adenoid basal cell carcinoma, two as papillary cystadenocarcinoma, and one as papillary adenocarcinoma.

Distinction from adenoid cystic carcinoma may sometimes be difficult. Both are composed of morphologically bland basaloid cells that form numerous ductlike structures. Fantasia and Neville[17] pointed out that two important distinguishing features are (1) circumscription of canalicular adenoma compared with the invasive pattern of adenoid cystic carcinoma and (2) the lack of vascularity in the cribriform areas of adenoid cystic carcinoma in contrast to the numerous endothelium-lined channels in the adenomas. These criteria are generally true, although not absolute. Several authors[20, 32] have noted that the incorrect diagnosis of canalicular adenoma as adenoid cystic carcinoma could result in "overtreatment." For this reason, I concur with Mintz and colleagues[20] who stressed that limited or fragmented biopsy specimens should be interpreted with caution and that an invasive pattern and irregular cytologic features should be viewed with suspicion of malignancy. They and others[32, 38] also noted that the

multifocal nature of some of these lesions might be misconstrued as malignancy.

Prognosis and Treatment

Recurrence of canalicular adenomas after surgical treatment is unusual.[13, 17, 19, 20, 28, 34] Two of three patients who had recurrences had previously had lesions that were multifocal in nature.[25, 32] Mair and Stalsberg[34] wondered why more canalicular adenomas did not recur despite their multifocal nature.

Various surgical procedures, including surgical excision, enucleation, or limited extracapsular excision, have been used without tumor recurrence.[13, 19, 20] However, Klein and Goldman[35] cautioned that canalicular adenomas should not be treated by enucleation because complete excision of a tumor that was previously only enucleated revealed residual tumor. Mintz and colleagues[20] and Daley[38] recommend that clinically benign neoplasms of the upper lip should be treated as though they were mixed tumors, i.e., excision with a cuff of apparently uninvolved tissue.

BASAL CELL ADENOMA

Clinical Features

There are 160 basal cell adenomas in the AFIP salivary gland registry. They constitute 1.8 percent of all benign primary epithelial salivary gland tumors in these files. As will be discussed, on the basis of their morphologic appearance, basal cell adenomas may be divided into the following four subtypes: solid, trabecular, tubular, and membranous. Other investigators[6, 10, 23] have found that basal cell adenomas represented 1.8 to 7.5 percent of their salivary gland tumors.

The average age of patients is 57.7 years, and the age range is from 0.1 to 93 years. These figures are in agreement with those reported by others.[25, 41] The patient age distribution by decade was more evenly spread between the third through the ninth decades of life than that for canalicular adenomas; however, similar to that for canalicular adenomas, the peak incidence of basal cell adenoma occurred in the sixth decade of life (Fig. 12–14).

Three publications[7, 10, 23] have pointed out that basal cell adenomas tend to occur in an older patient population than does the mixed tumor; this agrees with our experience (see Fig. 9–3).

Of the 130 civilian patients in the AFIP registry, 66.2 percent are female. Other investigators[6, 10, 23] have also reported an increased frequency of basal cell adenomas in females. Daley and coworkers[25] however, reported an equal distribution between males and females, and Luna and colleagues,[40] in

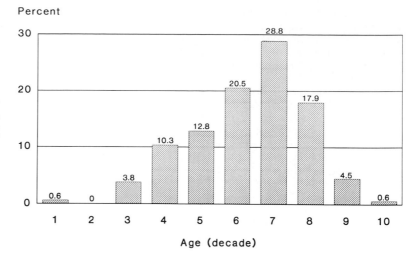

Figure 12–14. Distribution by decade of the ages of 156 patients with basal cell adenoma who were included in the AFIP registry of salivary gland disease.

their review of membranous basal cell adenomas, found that over 90 percent occurred in males.

Among the AFIP patients with basal cell adenoma whose race is known, 90 percent are white and 7 percent are black. This series represents the largest series reported and does suggest a possible propensity for basal cell adenoma to develop in whites. Blacks make up 12 percent of the American population but only 7.1 percent of the population of patients with basal cell adenoma in the AFIP series. However, in another series, 11 of 17 patients whose race was known were white, and 6 were black.[25]

The most common site for basal cell adenoma is the parotid gland, with 73.1 percent occurring in this location (Table 12–1). These findings demonstrate that this adenoma has a significant predilection for major glands, especially the parotid. Four lesions in this series that were listed as occurring in the neck most likely were parotid tumors or submandibular tumors. There are, however, reports[18, 40] of these lesions occurring in lymph nodes. If the neoplasms listed as occurring in the neck are counted among the major gland tumors, then over 80 percent of basal cell adenomas occur in major glands, which may be compared with 1.7 percent of canalicular adenomas. Many other investigators[6, 7, 10, 18, 23, 25, 41, 42] also report a marked preference for basal cell adenomas to occur in the parotid gland.

Basal cell adenomas are clinically indistinguishable from mixed tumors. They tend to occur in the superficial portion of the parotid, are freely movable, and show no predisposition for either the right or the left side.[7, 10, 18, 25, 41, 42] Their greatest dimension is usually less than 3.0 cm, and the surgeon may mistake them for hyperplastic lymph nodes because of their encapsulation and color.[41] Jao and colleagues[43] reported two cases of painful membranous basal cell adenoma. One was hard and immobile, whereas the other was firm but freely movable.

As first pointed out in 1976 by Crumpler and

associates,[16] some basal cell adenomas histologically resemble eccrine cylindroma. In 1977, Headington and colleagues[44] reported a patient who had a basal cell adenoma of the parotid gland and multiple dermal cylindromas and trichoepitheliomas. They pointed out that the histologic features of the salivary gland tumor and the skin tumors were remarkably similar and demonstrated the presence of prominent hyaline membrane. They suggested the term *membranous adenoma* for the salivary gland lesion, and they noted that the synchronous occurrence of morphologically similar tumors at different sites may result from a single pleotropic gene that acts on ontogenetically similar stem cells.

There have been other reports of the membranous form of basal cell adenoma associated with dermal appendage tumors, such as dermal cylindromas or trichoepitheliomas.[18, 45–49] Batsakis and coworkers[18, 22] suggested the term *dermal analogue tumor* for these salivary gland membranous basal cell adenomas because of their histologic similarity to the cutaneous lesions and their occurrence in individuals who have multiple cutaneous lesions.

A number of investigators[45–49] have noted the genetic component of this salivary gland/skin tumor diathesis with as many as four generations of patients affected, some with multiple bilateral salivary gland tumors. The reported incidence of skin tumors in patients with membranous basal cell adenoma is between 25 and 37 percent.[18, 40] It has been suggested[48] that individuals with salivary basal cell adenomas should be screened for skin lesions. There have been two recorded cases of individuals with the salivary gland/skin tumor diathesis who have developed salivary gland malignancies.[46, 49]

Pathologic Features

Grossly, basal cell adenomas have been described as round or ovoid, well-circumscribed or with a smooth-surfaced capsule, and with a soft to moderately firm consistency.[7, 10, 27, 42, 46, 50] Their appearance has been described by several authors as similar to that of an enlarged lymph node.[14, 27] Membranous basal cell adenomas, especially in individuals with the salivary gland/skin tumor diathesis, may consist of multiple nodules.[46]

Basal cell adenomas tend to be under 3.0 cm in diameter with a range of 1.2 to 8.0 cm.[7, 14, 16, 46] The cut surface often has a homogenous, solid appearance that may be interrupted by cysts of varying sizes that are filled with brown/red mucinous material or blood.[7, 9, 16, 50] The color of the cut surface can vary, depending on the tissue fixation, but it tends to be uniform and varies from gray-white to pink-red or brown.[7, 9, 14, 27, 42, 46, 50]

As noted by Ellis and Gnepp[51] and as mentioned previously in this chapter, basal cell adenomas may be divided on the basis of their morphologic pattern into four subtypes: solid, trabecular, tubular, and membranous. Despite these different histologic growth patterns, there are basic underlying histologic features that facilitate their diagnosis. The cells that make up the neoplasms are, for the most part, uniform and regular from tumor to tumor. These basaloid cells have two morphologic forms that are intermixed. One is a small cell with scant cytoplasm and a round, deeply basophilic nucleus. The other is a larger cell with amphophilic to eosinophilic cytoplasm and a nucleus that is more ovoid and paler staining than

that of the smaller cells. The larger, pale cells generally predominate with the smaller, darker cells often located in the peripheral portions of the epithelial tumor nests, cords, or islands (Fig. 12–15). Often, the nuclei have a slightly irregular outline and may have a grooved appearance. One or two chromatin condensations may be seen, or the nuclei may have small eosinophilic nucleoli. Rarely mitosis may be seen.

In addition to the relatively regular cellular population, there are two other consistent features that help in their recognition. One feature is a sharp demarcation between the neoplastic epithelial cells and the surrounding connective tissue. The second feature is the palisading of peripheral cuboidal or slightly columnar cells that accentuates the epithelioconnective tissue interface (Fig. 12–16).

The most common type of basal cell adenoma is the solid variant. It consists of islands and cords of neoplastic epithelial cells that have a broad, rounded, lobular pattern. The hyperchromatic peripheral layer of cells often demonstrates palisading (Fig. 12–17). These peripheral palisaded cells are either cuboidal or columnar.

The epithelial cells that make up the inner portions of the tumor islands often appear to have a directional orientation that tends to parallel the basilar cells. In some tumors, these inner cells have a tendency to produce scattered whorled eddies. On occasion, these eddies may mature into

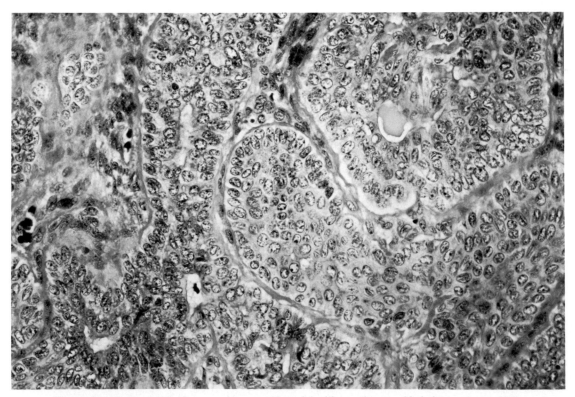

Figure 12–15. Basal cell adenoma shows ovoid nuclei with regular, speckled chromatin (× 360).

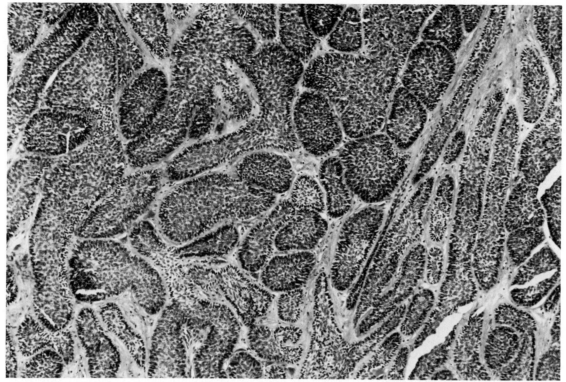

Figure 12–16. Basal cell adenoma shows sharp demarcation between islands of neoplastic epithelial cells with peripheral palisading and the connective tissue (× 75).

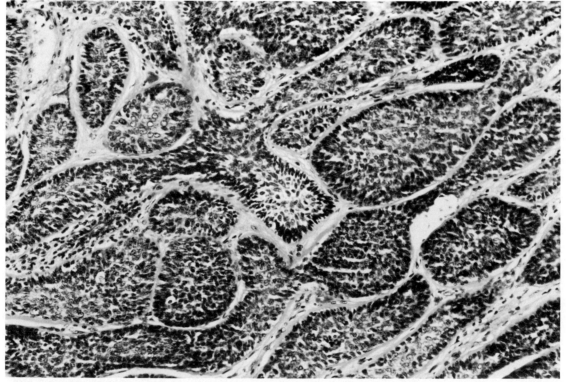

Figure 12–17. Solid variant of basal cell adenoma is composed of islands of tumor with a hyperchromatic, palisaded, peripheral layer of cells (× 150).

squamous cells and may produce keratin to give the appearance of small keratin cysts, or "keratin pearls" (Fig. 12–18). Ductlike structures are not prominent in this pattern, and the tumor nests do not have the thick eosinophilic basement membrane that is seen in the membranous basal cell adenoma.

The trabecular histologic subtype has the same cytologic features as the solid form, but the epithelial islands are narrower and cordlike and form interconnecting tonguelike islands with rounded borders (Fig. 12–19). These strands of epithelium may be only two cells thick in some areas. In areas where the trabeculae of epithelium are thicker, the morphologic character more closely resembles the solid pattern.

The tubular pattern exhibits multiple small, round, ductlike structures (Fig. 12–20). On many occasions, this pattern may be seen in conjunction with the trabecular pattern to form a trabeculotubular composite (Fig. 12–21). Focally, this pattern often has the appearance of richly epithelial areas seen in mixed tumors. Some investigators have suggested that some of these basal cell adenomas exhibit ultrastructural and immunohistochemical characteristics of mixed tumors.[39, 52]

The membranous basal cell adenoma has an interesting and distinct microscopic picture that is quite similar to that of the dermal cylindroma. At low magnification, the pattern is very similar to that of the solid variant of basal cell adenoma with the exception that it is usually multilobular and is encapsulated in only about one half of the cases. The epithelial islands are arranged in large lobules that appear to mold to the shape of other lobules so as to fit closely together in a "jigsaw puzzle" pattern. Although the cells are regular in pattern, the peripheral palisaded cells have a darker, more compact appearance, whereas the more central cells have the appearance of being slightly larger, with lighter nuclei. The distinctive feature of membranous basal cell adenomas is the thick, eosinophilic hyaline layer that surrounds the epithelial islands and separates them from one another (Fig. 12–22). This hyaline material stains positive for periodic acid–Schiff stain (Fig. 12–23) and has been shown by electron microscopy to represent a reduplicated basement membrane. Similar material is often seen within the epithelial islands and appears as hyaline droplets. These interepithelial droplets are often associated with, or surrounded by, slightly darker and smaller epithelial cells (Fig. 12–24). In some instances, the hyaline droplets coalesce and produce large irregular eosinophilic masses.

Batsakis and coworkers[18] separate the membranous adenoma from other basal cell adenomas because of its distinctive microscopic features, its higher incidence of recurrence, and its association with genetically predisposed turban tumors. However, although these differences are important, the morphologic overlap among basal cell ade-

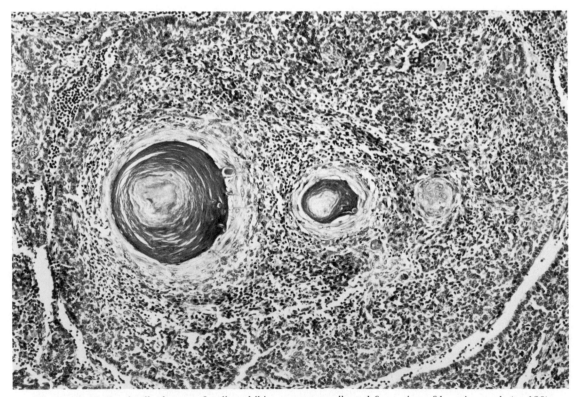

Figure 12–18. Basal cell adenoma focally exhibits squamous cells and formation of keratin pearls (× 120).

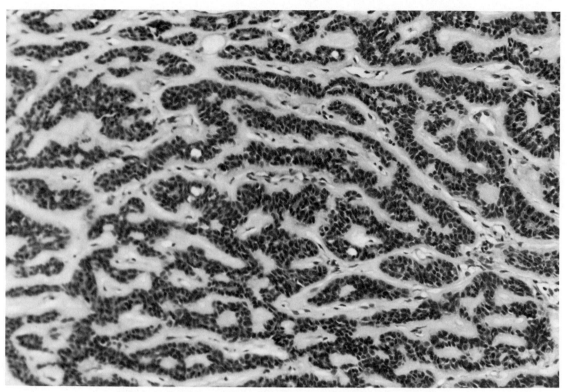

Figure 12–19. Basal cell adenoma has a trabecular pattern (× 150).

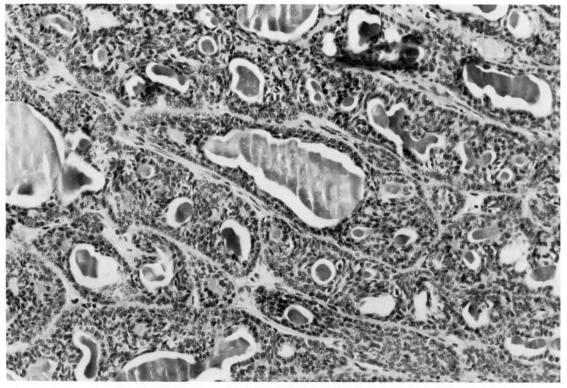

Figure 12–20. Basal cell adenoma illustrates tubular pattern (× 150).

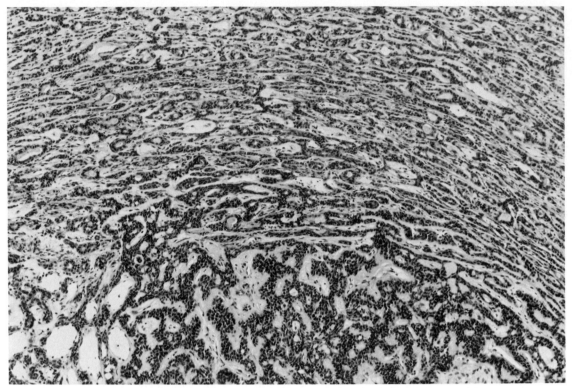

Figure 12–21. Basal cell adenoma demonstrates trabeculotubular pattern (× 75).

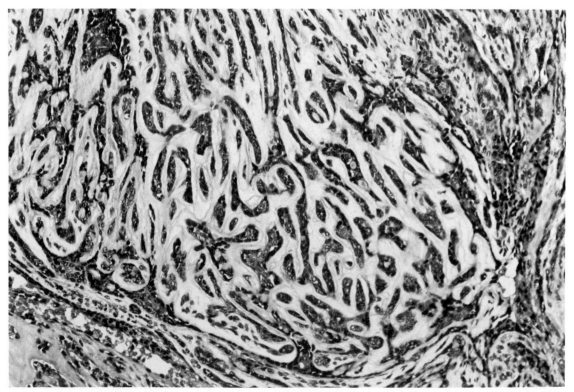

Figure 12–22. Membranous basal cell adenoma has a thick, eosinophilic hyaline layer that surrounds and separates the epithelial islands (× 150).

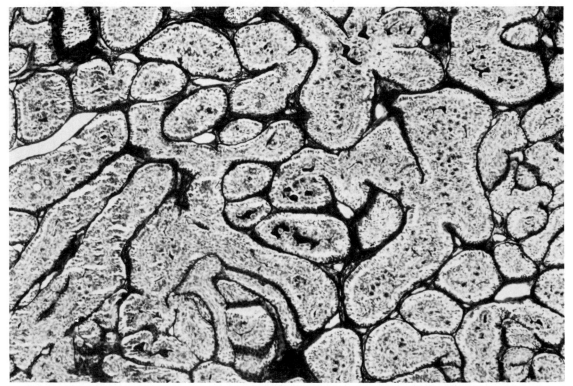

Figure 12–23. Membranous basal cell adenoma demonstrates positive staining of the hyaline layer with periodic acid–Schiff stain (× 99).

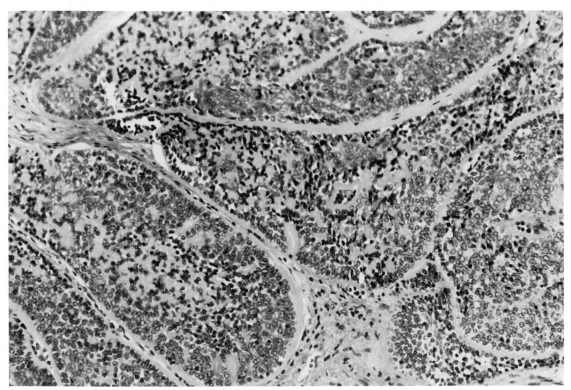

Figure 12–24. Membranous basal cell adenoma with a hyaline layer surrounding epithelial islands contains interepithelial hyaline droplets (× 150).

noma subtypes is indisputable and suggests a common pathogenesis. Furthermore, focal areas with more than one of the microscopic patterns are seen in some tumors.

Ultrastructural Findings

There have been varying ultrastructural findings reported for basal cell adenomas. Although some authors[40, 52] have observed similarities between basal cell adenomas, mixed tumors, and adenoid cystic carcinomas, others[53] have stated that electron microscopy is useful in distinguishing the more differentiated basal cell adenoma from the less differentiated adenoid cystic carcinoma.

Some difference of opinion concerns the diversity of the cell population that makes up the epithelial clusters or nests. Some investigators support the existence of a single cell type.[23, 50, 54–56] Others report that they can distinguish from two to five different cell types, including secretory cells, intermediate cells, myoepithelial cells, and luminal cells.[43, 45, 52, 57]

The presence and contribution of myoepithelial cells in basal cell adenoma has been a controversial topic in ultrastructural evaluation of these tumors. Several investigators[43, 45, 50, 53–56, 58] have pointed out that myoepithelial cells are absent or are an insignificant component in these neoplasms; however, others[23, 52, 57] have reported their presence. Dardick and coworkers[52] feel that the presence of outer epithelial and stromal myoepithelial cells in the trabeculotubular form of basal cell adenoma may suggest that this form of neoplasm may actually represent a cellular form of mixed tumor or a hybrid form of basal cell adenoma and myoepithelioma.

Probably the most distinctive ultrastructural characteristic of the basal cell adenoma is the presence of reduplicated, multilayered, basal laminae. This reduplicated basal lamina surrounds the epithelial cell clusters. Several authors have mentioned marked cytoplasmic invagination of the basement membrane material that closely approximates the nucleolus.[43, 53, 59]

Many investigators[23, 43, 50, 53–56] have pointed out the numerous desmosomes and conspicuous tonofilaments in basal cell adenomas. Microfilaments have been reported as numerous,[58] variable,[23] and occasional.[43] The cells have been described as having few organelles,[54, 55, 58] but others have noted numerous parallel arrays of rough endoplasmic reticulum[43] and prominent surface microvilli.[45, 53, 56] Another feature that has been reported by some investigators,[23, 43, 45, 50, 56, 57] but not by others,[54, 55] is the presence of secretory granules.

Immunohistochemical Findings

Hara and colleagues[60] reported that S-100b protein-positive cells were seldom seen in basal cell adenomas that were stained by the peroxidase-antiperoxidase method. On this basis, they suggested that myoepithelial cells are not a component of these neoplasms. Dardick and colleagues[52] performed immunohistochemical stains on six trabeculotubular basal cell adenomas. In addition to the staining of the basal cells of the tumor clusters for S-100 protein, their most surprising finding was the moderate to strong staining of the stromal regions by antibodies to S-100 protein. This was not seen in two cases of canalicular adenoma and basal cell adenoma that were used as controls. Dardick and colleagues suggested that this is a unique form of neoplasm that displays tricellular differentiation and may represent a hybrid of basal cell adenoma and myoepithelioma or a cellular pleomorphic adenoma. Similar findings and conclusions were reported by Zarbo and associates[39] after staining three trabeculotubular adenomas. It is possible that results from future studies may eventually indicate an advantage to separating the trabeculotubular subtype from the other basal cell adenomas.

Fine-Needle Aspiration

The cytologic distinction of basal cell adenoma from adenoid cystic carcinoma by fine-needle aspiration is difficult. Layfield[61] has noted that both adenoid cystic carcinoma and basal cell adenoma contain hyaline globules, which stain red-blue with May-Grünwald-Giemsa stain, surrounded by neoplastic cells. He noted that the hyaline globules had a slightly bluer color in basal cell adenoma and a redder color in adenoid cystic carcinoma. Also, minimally greater nuclear atypia may be seen in adenoid cystic carcinoma. Aspirates from pleomorphic adenomas can be distinguished from basal cell adenomas by the cytologic heterogeneity of the cell types seen in pleomorphic adenomas; the cells in pleomorphic adenomas may display a spindle cell population in addition to polygonal cells. In addition, aspirates of pleomorphic adenomas often contain a myxoid or chondroid substance.

Differential Diagnosis

The clinical differential diagnosis for a movable, asymptomatic swelling in the parotid area could include any benign salivary gland neoplasm, especially mixed tumor. Other considerations include an enlarged lymph node or a lesion of the skin, such as an epidermal inclusion cyst.

Microscopically, basal cell adenomas might be misinterpreted as ameloblastoma because of the palisaded nature of the peripheral layer of cells.[7, 14, 27, 62] This distinction could be especially problematic for lesions that occur in the hard palate, which fortunately are uncommon. Examination of radiographs for alveolar bone involvement can be helpful in making this distinction. Likewise, if basal cell adenoma occurs adjacent to or encroaches on the dermis, it may be misinterpreted as cutaneous basal cell carcinoma.[7, 27, 62] In cases where tumors are enucleated with no surrounding normal tissue, this distinction may be impossible.

Mixed tumor often is a consideration in the differential diagnosis for basal cell adenomas.[7, 10, 16, 27, 58, 63] Important distinguishing features include the absence of histologically recognizable myoepithelial cells and the sharp demarcation between the epithelium and stroma in basal cell adenomas. The stroma of basal cell adenomas tends to be scanty, and there is an absence of myxoid or chondroid elements. The thickened basement membrane of membranous basal cell adenoma must not be interpreted as the hyalinized mesenchyme-like element that is seen in mixed tumors. The hyalinized material in membranous basal cell adenoma is relatively acellular, as opposed to the myxochondroid tissue of the mixed tumor. In the absence of areas that present a more recognizable solid pattern, the possibility of a "cellular" mixed tumor or an inadequately sampled mixed tumor should be entertained.

The most difficult differential consideration is adenoid cystic carcinoma. An important distinguishing feature is that adenoid cystic carcinoma has an invasive appearance, both on gross examination and in a histologic comparison with the circumscription or encapsulation of basal cell adenoma (Fig. 12–25). The presence of multiple peripheral nests of basaloid cells that vary in size are unusual for basal cell adenoma and should alert the pathologist to the possibility of adenoid cystic carcinoma. The presence of two cell types with palisaded peripheral cells supports a diagnosis of basal cell adenoma. The membranous basal cell adenoma, because of its regular cellular features and hyaline production, also may be confused microscopically with adenoid cystic carcinoma. The three important features pointed out by Ellis and Gnepp[64] that help distinguish membranous adenoma from adenoid cystic carcinoma are the whorled eddies of epithelial cells that are not seen in adenoid cystic carcinoma, the haphazard arrangement of the hyaline material that is seen in the membranous adenoma, and the absence of parenchymal and perineural invasion by basal cell adenoma.

Prognosis and Treatment

Recurrence of basal cell adenomas after surgical treatment is unusual.[16, 18, 20, 23, 30, 62] Nagao and colleagues[23] reported no recurrences in a series of 40 cases and stated that basal cell adenomas may have a better prognosis than mixed tumors. How-

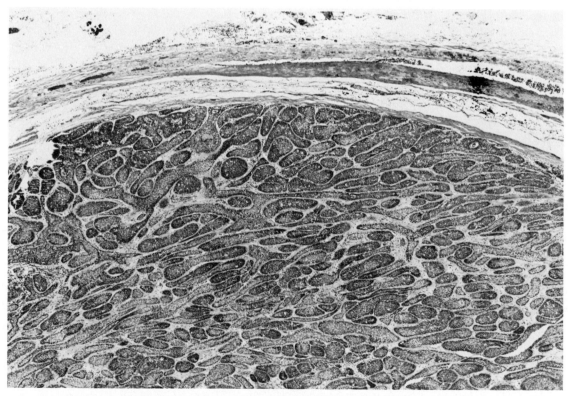

Figure 12–25. Basal cell adenoma shows circumscription and encapsulation (× 30).

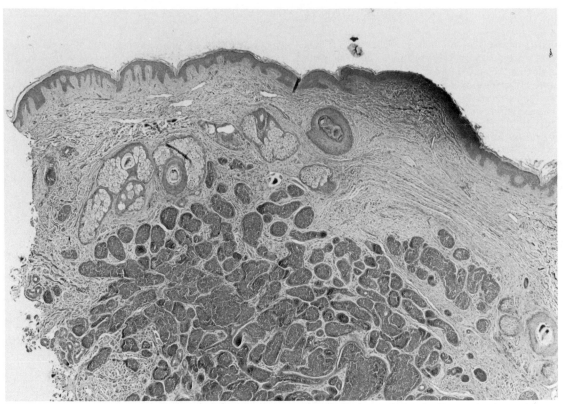

Figure 12–26. Cutaneous cylindroma demonstrates microscopic similarity to tissue of salivary gland membranous basal cell adenoma. Patient had a salivary gland skin tumor diathesis (× 30).

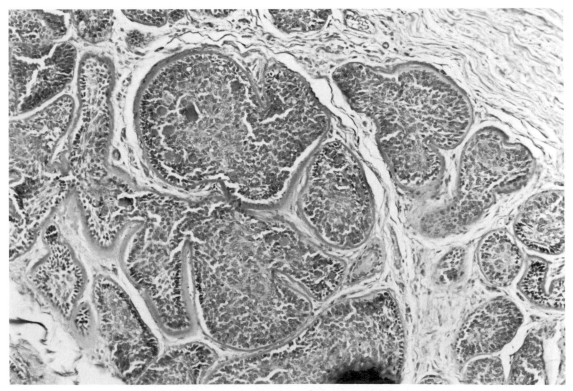

Figure 12–27. Cutaneous cylindroma shows a hyaline layer that surrounds islands of epithelial cells with palisaded peripheral cells (× 150).

ever, there are reports of recurrences, including a palatal tumor that recurred 4 years after surgery, probably as a result of incomplete primary excision.[30, 62] Membranous basal cell adenomas are the type that are most commonly associated with recurrence.[18, 22, 25, 46, 47, 49] The recurrence rate has been reported as 25 and 37 percent, and it has been observed that this rate was similar to that for the cutaneous cylindromas.[18, 22] A number of investigators have noted that these cases are often associated with the salivary gland/skin tumor diathesis (Figs. 12–26 and 12–27) and may be related to the multifocal nature of these neoplasms, rather than to true recurrences.[18, 22, 46, 49]

Excision may be adequate treatment, and recurrence should not be expected.[7, 10, 14, 23] Thackray and Lucas[10] recommended an operation similar to what would be appropriate for mixed tumor and speculated that incomplete removal or tumor implantation in the wound would result in recurrence.

An unusual finding is malignant transformation in basal cell adenoma. So-called "hybrid tumors" that consist of basal cell adenoma and adenoid cystic carcinoma have been reported.[7, 14] Malignant change has also been reported in basal cell adenomas associated with membranous basal cell adenoma or the salivary gland/skin tumor diathesis.[46, 49, 65, 66] However, most malignant basaloid tumors of the salivary glands arise de novo (see Chapter 26).

REFERENCES

1. Schutz CB: Adenoma of the salivary gland. Am J Pathol 1926; 2:153–157.
2. Eggers HE: Mixed tumors of the palate. Arch Pathol 1928; 6:378–395.
3. McFarland J: The histopathologic prognosis of salivary gland mixed tumors. Am J Med Sci 1942; 203:502–519.
4. Bauer WH, Bauer JD: Classification of glandular tumors of salivary glands: Study of one hundred forty-three cases. Arch Pathol 1953; 55:328–346.
5. Bhaskar SN, Weinmann JP: Tumors of the minor salivary glands. Oral Surg Oral Med Oral Pathol 1955; 8:1278–1297.
6. Kleinsasser O, Klein HJ: Basalzelladenome der Speicheldrusen. Arch Klin Exp Ohren Nasen Kehlkopfheilkd 1967; 189:302–316.
7. Evans RW, Cruickshank AH: Epithelial Tumours of the Salivary Glands. Philadelphia, WB Saunders Co, 1970; 58–76.
8. Rauch S, Seifert G, Gorlin RJ: Diseases of the salivary glands, tumors. In Gorlin RJ, Goldman HM, (eds.): Thoma's Oral Pathology. 6th Ed. St. Louis, CV Mosby Co, 1970; 1003–1006.
9. Thackray AC, Sobin LH: Histological Typing of Salivary Gland Tumours. Geneva, World Health Organization, 1972; 20–22.
10. Thackray AC, Lucas RB: Tumors of major salivary glands, Atlas of Tumor Pathology, Series II, Fascicle 10. Washington, DC, Armed Forces Institute of Pathology, 1974; 59–68.
11. Eneroth CM, Hiertman L, Moberger G: Salivary gland adenomas of the palate. Acta Otolaryngol 1972; 73:305–315.
12. McL.Davis W, McL.Davis W: Canalicular adenoma: Report of case. J Oral Surg 1971; 29:500–502.
13. Christ TF, Crocker D: Basal cell adenoma of minor salivary gland origin. Cancer 1972; 30:214–219.
14. Bernacki EG, Batsakis JG, Johns ME: Basal cell adenoma: Distinctive tumor of salivary glands. Arch Otolaryngol 1974; 99:84–87.
15. Seifert G, Donath K: Classification of the pathohistology of diseases of the salivary glands: Review of 2,600 cases in the salivary gland register. Beitr Pathol 1976; 159:1–32.
16. Crumpler C, Scharfenberg JC, Reed RJ: Monomorphic adenomas of salivary glands: Trabecular-tubular, canalicular, and basaloid variants. Cancer 1976; 38:193–200.
17. Fantasia JE, Neville BW: Basal cell adenomas of the minor salivary glands. Oral Surg Oral Med Oral Pathol 1980; 50:433–440.
18. Batsakis JG, Brannon RB, Sciubba JJ: Monomorphic adenomas of major salivary glands: A histologic study of 96 tumours. Clin Otolaryngol 1981; 6:129–143.
19. Levine J, Krutchkoff DJ, Eisenberg E: Monomorphic adenoma of minor salivary glands: A reappraisal and report of nine new cases. J Oral Surgery 1981; 39:101–107.
20. Mintz GA, Abrams AM, Melrose RJ: Monomorphic adenomas of the major and minor salivary glands: Report of twenty-one cases and review of the literature. Oral Surg Oral Med Oral Pathol 1982; 53:375–386.
21. Waldron CA, El Mofty SK, Gnepp DR: Tumors of the intraoral minor salivary glands: A demographic and histologic study of 426 cases. Oral Surg Oral Med Oral Pathol 1988; 66:323–333.
22. Batsakis JG, Brannon RB: Dermal analogue tumors of major salivary glands. J Laryngol Otol 1981; 95:155–164.
23. Nagao K, Matsuzaki O, Saiga H, Sugano I, Sigematsu H, Kaneko T, Katoh T, Kitamura T: Histopathologic studies of basal cell adenoma of the parotid gland. Cancer 1982; 50:736–745.
24. Gardner DG, Daley TD: The use of the terms monomorphic adenoma, basal cell adenoma, and canalicular adenoma as applied to salivary gland tumors. Oral Surg Oral Med Oral Pathol 1983; 56:608–615.
25. Daley TD, Gardner DG, Smout MS: Canalicular adenoma: Not a basal cell adenoma. Oral Surg Oral Med Oral Pathol 1984; 57:181–188.
26. Eversole LR: Histogenic classification of salivary tumors. Arch Pathol 1971; 92:433–443.
27. Batsakis JG: Basal cell adenoma of the parotid gland. Cancer 1972; 29:226–230.
28. Nelson JF, Jacoway JR: Monomorphic adenoma (canalicular type): Report of 29 cases. Cancer 1973; 31:1511–1513.
29. Chen SY, Miller AS: Canalicular adenoma of the upper lip: An electron microscopic study. Cancer 1980; 46:552–556.
30. Pogrel MA: The intraoral basal cell adenoma. J Craniomaxillofac Surg 1987; 15:372–375.
31. Kratochvil FJ, Auclair PL, Ellis GL: Clinical Features of 160 cases of basal cell adenoma and 121 cases of canalicular adenoma. Oral Surg Oral Med Oral Pathol 1990; 70:605.

32. Regezi JA, Lloyd RV, Zarbo RJ, McClatchey KD: Minor salivary gland tumors: A histologic and immunohistochemical study. Cancer 1985; 55:108–115.

33. Guccion JG, Redman RS: Canalicular adenoma of the buccal mucosa: An ultrastructural and histochemical study. Oral Surg Oral Med Oral Pathol 1986; 61:173–178.

34. Mair IW, Stalsberg H: Basal cell adenomatosis of minor salivary glands of the upper lip. Arch Otorhinolaryngol 1988; 245:191–195.

35. Klein HZ, Goldman RL: Basal cell adenoma involving the lip. Arch Pathol 1973; 95:94–96.

36. Strychalski J: Basal cell adenoma of intraoral minor salivary gland origin. J Oral Surg 1974; 32:595–600.

37. Hruban RH, Erozan YS, Zinreich SJ, Kashima HK: Fine needle aspiration cytology of monomorphic adenomas. Am J Clin Pathol 1988; 90:46–51.

38. Daley TD: The canalicular adenoma: Considerations on differential diagnosis and treatment. J Oral Maxillofac Surg 1984; 42:728–730.

39. Zarbo RJ, Regezi JA, Batsakis JG: S100 protein in salivary gland tumors: An immunohistochemical study of 129 cases. Head Neck Surg 1986; 8:268–275.

40. Luna MA, Tortoledo ME, Allen M: Salivary dermal analogue tumors arising in lymph nodes. Cancer 1987; 59:1165–1169.

41. Batsakis JG: Tumors of the Head and Neck. Clinical and Pathologic Considerations, 2nd Ed. Baltimore, Williams & Wilkins Co, 1979; 50–53.

42. Walter P, Prevot M, Ludwig L: Ademes a cellules basales des glandes salivaires: Analyse de 7 observations et de la litterature etude comparative avec les cylindromes. Ann Anat Pathol (Paris) 1977; 22:233–250.

43. Jao W, Keh P, Swerdlow MA: Ultrastructure of the basal cell adenoma of the parotid gland. Cancer 1976; 37:1322–1333.

44. Headington JT, Bataskis JG, Beals TF, Campbell TE, Simmons JL, Stone WD: Membranous basal cell adenoma of parotid gland, dermal cylindromas, and trichoepitheliomas: Comparative histochemistry and ultrastructure. Cancer 1977; 39:2460–2469.

45. Zarbo RJ, Ricci A, Kowalczyk PD, Cartun RW, Knibbs DR: Intranasal dermal analogue tumor (membranous basal cell adenoma): Ultrastructure and immunohistochemistry. Arch Otolaryngol 1985; 111:333–337.

46. Reingold IM, Keasbey LE, Graham JH: Multicentric dermal type cylindromas of the parotid glands in a patient with florid turban tumor. Cancer 1977; 40:1702–1710.

47. Herbst EV, Utz W: Multifocal dermal type basal cell adenomas of parotid glands with coexisting dermal cylindromas. Virchows Arch [A] 1984; 95–102.

48. Ferrandiz C, Campo E, Baumann E: Dermal cylindromas (turban tumour) and eccrine spiradenomas in a patient with membranous basal cell adenoma of the parotid gland. J Cutan Pathol 1985; 12:72–79.

49. Hyma BA, Scheithauer BW, Weiland LH, Irons GB: Membranous basal cell adenoma of the parotid gland: Malignant transformation in a patient with multiple dermal cylindromas. Arch Pathol Lab Med 1988; 112:209–211.

50. Luna MA, Mackay B: Basal cell adenoma of the parotid gland: Case report with ultrastructural observations. Cancer 1976; 37:1615–1621.

51. Ellis GL, Gnepp DR: Unusual salivary gland tumors. In Gnepp DR (ed.): Pathology of the Head and Neck. New York, Churchill Livingstone Inc, 1988; 587.

52. Dardick I, Daley TD, van Nostrand AW: Basal cell adenoma with myoepithelial cell derived "stroma": A new major salivary gland tumor entity. Head Neck Surg 1986; 257–267.

53. Le Charpentier Y, Chomette G, Auriol M, Karkouche B, Lamas G: Adenome a celluler basaler de la parotide: A propos d'un cas avec etude ultrastructurale. Ann Pathol 1986; 6:228–232.

54. Klima M, Wolfe K, Johnson PE: Basal cell tumors of the parotid. Arch Otolaryngol 1978; 104:111–116.

55. Youngberg G, Sambasiva R: Ultrastructural features of monomorphic adenoma of the parotid gland. Oral Surg Oral Med Oral Pathol 1979; 47:458–461.

56. Chaudhry AP, Cutler LS, Satchidanand S, Labay G, Raj MS, Lin CC: Monomorphic adenomas of the parotid glands: Their ultrastructure and histogenesis. Cancer 1983; 52:112–120.

57. Dardick I, Kahn HJ, van Nostrand AWP, Baumal R: Salivary gland monomorphic adenoma: Ultrastructural, immunoperoxidase, and histogenetic aspects. Am J Pathol 1984; 115:334–348.

58. Hubner G, Kleinsasser O, Klein HJ: Zur feinstruktur der basalzelladenome der speicheldrusen. Virchows Arch [A] 1971; 353:333–346.

59. Min BH, Miller AS, Leifer C, Putong PB: Basal cell adenoma of the parotid gland. Arch Otolaryngol 1974; 99:88–93.

60. Hara K, Ito M, Takeuchi J, Iijima S, Endo T, Hidaka H: Distribution of S100 protein in normal salivary glands and salivary gland tumors. Virchows Arch [A] 1983; 401:237–249.

61. Layfield LJ: Fine needle aspiration cytology of a trabecular adenoma of the parotid gland. Acta Cytol 1985; 29:999–1002.

62. Pogrel MA: Tumors of the salivary glands: a histological and clinical review. Br J Oral Surg 1979; 17:47–56.

63. Kozlovskii OM: Bazal'nokletochnye adenomy sliunnykh zhelez. Arkh Patol 1975; 37:60–64.

64. Ellis GL, Gnepp DR: Unusual salivary gland tumors. In Gnepp DR (ed.): Pathology of the Head and Neck. New York, Churchill Livingstone Inc, 1988; 586–592.

65. Chen KT: Carcinoma arising in monomorphic adenoma of the salivary gland. Am J Otolaryngol. 1985; 6:39–41.

66. Luna MA, Batsakis JG, Tortoledo ME, DelJunco GW: Carcinomas ex monomorphic adenoma of salivary glands. J Laryngol Otol 1989; 103:756–759.

13

ONCOCYTOMA*

Robert K. Goode

An oncocytoma is a tumor characterized by large epithelial cells (oncocytes) that contain a brightly eosinophilic, granular cytoplasm. The oncocyte, which is derived from the Greek word *onkousthai*, meaning swollen or enlarged, was initially described in 1897 by Schaffer,[1] who observed this tumor in ductal and acinar elements of salivary glands in the tongue, pharynx, and esophagus. Zimmermann[2] also noted that histopathologic phenomenon in the sublingual gland; he referred to these cells as "pyknocytes" because of their condensed nuclear chromatin or pyknotic nuclei. Jaffe[3] first used the term *oncocytoma*, although differently from its present connotation, to describe what we currently consider to be papillary cystadenoma lymphomatosum (Warthin's tumor). The first case report of oncocytoma, although not referred to as such, was by McFarland[4] in 1927. In 1931, Hamperl[5] first applied the term *onkocyte* to cells that make up what we now consider to be oncocytoma. He reported that these large cells were usually observed in the tissue of the salivary glands of individuals who were in their sixth decade of life or older as well as in the tissues of the kidney and of the thyroid, parathyroid, pituitary, and adrenal glands and in the tumors affecting each of these organs.[6, 7] Oncocytes have also been observed in the liver, pancreas, fallopian tubes, testes, stomach, and bronchi.[8] Ackerman,[9] in 1934, advocated discontinuation of Jaffe's application of the term *oncocytoma* to papillary cystadenoma lymphomatosum, pointing out that the histopathologic distinction of a prominent lymphocytic component in the latter entity warranted such a separation. There are numerous other names that have been advocated for oncocytoma. Meza-Chavez[10] proposed the term *oxyphilic granular cell adenoma* in 1949, and Eneroth[11] considered

that term synonymous with *oncocytoma*. Other investigators who reported cases as *oxyphilic granular cell adenoma* included Boley and Robinson,[12] Codington,[13] Lane,[14] Chaudhry and Gorlin,[15] and Smoler.[16] Buxton and coworkers[17] favored *acidophilic granular cell tumor* as being more descriptive of the histopathologic features observed. Stump[18] preferred *oncocytic adenoma*, whereas Schafer and colleagues[19] expanded the former to *oncocytic cell adenoma*. Although we agree that many of these alternative terms are descriptively accurate, we prefer the term *oncocytoma*, which we use throughout this chapter.

PATHOGENESIS

Several theories have been advanced regarding the pathogenesis of oncocytoma, but an unequivocal determination of the pathogenesis for this lesion has not yet been established. Schaffer[1] believed the oncocyte was the result of a degenerative phenomenon in salivary gland parenchymal cells. Hamperl[5, 6, 20] initially considered the oncocyte to be a "peculiar degeneration" that was irreversible with age; however, in 1962, he expanded his position to suggest that the oncocyte could be seen in a variety of pathologic conditions.[21] Hamperl[21] suggested that individual cells or aggregates of cells either could undergo permanent modification into oncocytes as a metaplastic process or could proliferate as a hyperplastic or neoplastic process. Meza-Chavez[10] supported this proposition and postulated that oncocytoma could evolve from a hyperplastic state. The observation of malignant transformation of previously benign oncocytic lesions and the existence of de novo oncocytic adenocarcinoma would seem to endorse the existence of a benign neoplastic process.

In contrast, Blanck and coinvestigators[22] proposed that oncocytoma is not a neoplasm but

---

*All material in this chapter is in the public domain, with the exception of any borrowed figures or tables.

Table 13–1. Comparison of the Incidence of Oncocytomas in Several Series of Salivary Gland Tumors

Author	Total Number of Cases	Number of Oncocytomas	Percentage
Buxton and colleagues[17]	280	3	1.0
Foote and Frazell[8]	877	1	0.1
Kirklin and colleagues[29]	909	4	0.4
Blanck and colleagues[22]	1,678	13	0.8
Tandler and colleagues[25]	1,578	12	0.7
Eneroth[11]	1,019	7	0.6
Chaudhry and colleagues[30]	1,414	2	0.1
AFIP	13,749	200	1.4*

*Percentage of all benign and malignant epithelial salivary gland tumors included in this series.

rather—based on its multinodular nature and bilateral occurrence in 5 of their 13 cases—is a nodular hyperplasia.

Numerous ultrastructural studies of oncocytoma have demonstrated vastly increased numbers of mitochondria within the cytoplasm of the oncocyte, and histochemical studies have compared concentrations of oxidative enzymes of the oncocyte to those of normal salivary gland acinar and ductal cells.[23–28] Although there are some morphologic similarities between the oncocyte and the intercalated duct reserve cell at the ultrastructural level, a definitive conclusion on the cell of origin remains speculative. Some of these studies can be interpreted to suggest that the salivary gland oncocyte may be an adaptive or compensatory hyperplastic cell that occurs secondary to an undetermined somatic mutation rather than a purely degenerative process.

INCIDENCE

There have been several studies with significant numbers of cases that indicate that the oncocytoma is indeed an uncommon neoplasm.[8, 11, 17, 22, 25, 29, 30] These reports place the incidence of oncocytoma among all salivary gland tumors at approximately 1 percent (Table 13–1). At this time, there are 13,749 primary epithelial salivary gland tumors in the salivary gland registry of the Armed Forces Institute of Pathology (AFIP). Only 200 oncocytomas are in that compilation (1.4 percent). Oncocytomas make up 2.3 percent of benign epithelial salivary gland tumors and are, in my experience, among the least common types of benign salivary gland tumors.

CLINICAL FEATURES

Although oncocytomas have occasionally been reported in patients in the first decade of life,[31, 32] this is considered to be an exception from the usual presentation. Data from large series, as reflected in Table 13–2, indicate oncocytoma is predominantly observed in the older adult population with distribution over the sixth, seventh, and eighth decades of life.[11, 14, 15, 21, 33] The age distribution of patients with oncocytomas reviewed at the AFIP (Fig. 13–1) ratifies that which has previously been reported. Approximately 85 percent of the cases registered at the AFIP occur in patients who fall within the sixth through ninth decades of life. The highest percentage (31.3 percent) of AFIP cases was observed in patients in the 9th decade. The average patient age among all AFIP cases is 64.1 years. Males demonstrate an average age of occurrence of 61.9 years, whereas females tend to present at a slightly older 66.9 years. This conforms to Hastrup and colleagues'[34] findings in which the average age of occurrence for males was lower than that for females, 59 years versus 64 years, respectively.

The scientific literature does not address a racial predilection for oncocytoma, and no conclusion regarding racial preference for oncocytoma can be made based on the AFIP experience. Of 200 AFIP cases, 88 (44 percent) reported race of the patient; based on this limited information, it was ascertained that 80 patients (90.9 percent) were white, 6 patients (6.8 percent) were black, and 2 patients (2.3 percent) were Asian.

Conflicting reports about the gender predilection of oncocytoma are observed in the scientific literature. Evans and Cruickshank,[35] in their classic monograph on epithelial salivary gland tumors, reported a predominant occurrence in females. This conclusion was supported by Eneroth,[11] Hamperl,[21] and a review of previously reported cases by Chaudhry and Gorlin[15] in 1958. In contrast, in 1962, Lane's[14] evaluation of previously

Table 13–2. Average Ages of Patients with Oncocytoma Reported in Various Series

Author	Average Age of Occurrence (Years)
Eneroth[11]	64.0
Lane[14]	70.4
Chaudhry and colleagues[15]	62.8
Hamperl[21]	60.0
Gray and colleagues[33]	64.8
AFIP	64.1

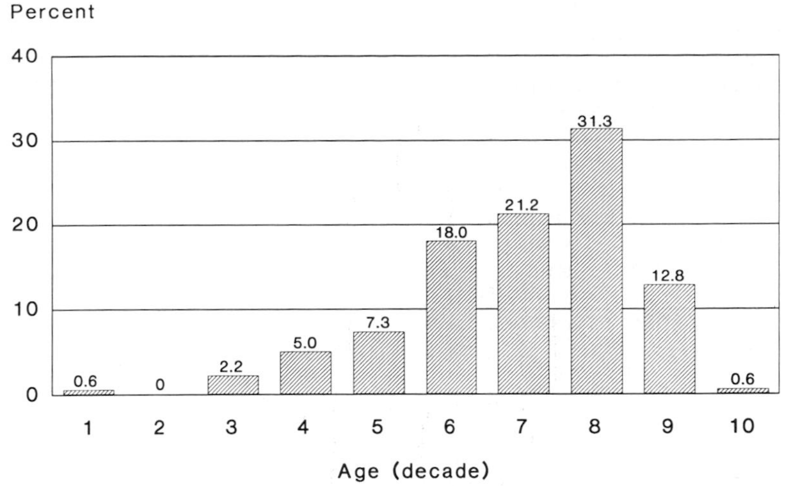

Percent

Figure 13–1. Graph showing distribution by age of 200 patients with oncocytoma in the AFIP registry of salivary gland pathology.

reported cases found a nearly equal male-to-female ratio. Gray and coworkers'[33] report of 10 oncocytomas supports Lane's findings.

Initial analysis of the AFIP experience with oncocytoma would seem to support a slight male predilection. When the 178 cases from both military/veteran and civilian sources that stated gender were analyzed, 96 cases (54 percent) occurred in males, and 82 cases (46 percent) occurred in females. However, a significant bias was noted, because all 25 cases of oncocytoma submitted from military/veteran sources were males. When 153 oncocytomas submitted to the AFIP from civilian institutions were analyzed, 82 tumors (53.6 percent) occurred in females, and 71 tumors (46.4 percent) occurred in males.

Review of published case reports indicates oncocytoma is predominantly a tumor of the major salivary glands. In the major glands, the vast majority of oncocytomas are seen in the parotid gland, although occurrence in the submandibular gland has been reported.[36, 37] Several studies report the occurrence of bilateral oncocytomas of the parotid glands.[12, 22, 38]

Fewer than 20 cases of oncocytomas are reported in minor salivary glands. Published data suggest that the palatal mucosa is the most common location, followed in frequency by the buccal mucosa and the tongue.[30–33, 39–45]

The AFIP experience regarding location of oncocytoma confirms previous reports. Of the 200 tumors reported, 156 (78.0 percent) were in the parotid gland. The submandibular gland was found to be the site of an additional 18 cases (9.0 percent), and no cases were observed in the sublingual gland. The remaining 26 cases were distributed over a variety of sites (Table 13–3). The palate, buccal mucosa, and pharynx were the most common locations. The seven cases listed as occurring in the neck and mandible most likely represent tumors that developed in the parotid or submandibular glands.

The oncocytoma is clinically indistinguishable from other benign tumors of the major salivary glands. It most frequently presents as an indolent, single, often multilobulated, firm, solid mass in the superficial lobe of the parotid gland. It has often been described as "shelling out" with blunt dissection during surgery. Oncocytoma may also be located in the deep lobe of the parotid gland and may be insinuated between branches of the facial nerve. In most instances, oncocytoma does not evoke pain or paresthesia unless branches of the facial nerve are compromised. Tumor size varies with duration of the lesion, but it generally does not exceed 4.0 cm. The tumor is usually freely movable on palpation. Intraoral oncocytomas fail to demonstrate any distinguishing clinical symptoms that would permit differentiation from other benign or malignant minor salivary gland tumors. Oncocytoma of minor salivary gland origin may become secondarily ulcerated by trauma to the overlying mucosa.

The use of certain imaging techniques can be valuable in the clinical discrimination of oncocytoma from certain other salivary gland lesions. Grove and Di Chiro[46] first performed scintigraphy

Table 13–3. Anatomic Distribution of 200 Cases of Oncocytoma in the AFIP Registry

Anatomic Site	Number	Percent
Parotid gland	156	78.0
Submandibular gland	18	9.0
Lower lip	1	0.5
Palate	2	1.0
Soft palate	2	1.0
Pharynx	3	1.5
Tongue	1	0.5
Buccal mucosa	4	2.0
Neck	6	3.0
Mandible	1	0.5
Site not stated	6	3.0

studies with technetium-99m pertechnetate on various salivary gland lesions in 1968. Their findings were amplified by others, who demonstrated that oncocytoma and papillary cystadenoma lymphomatosum (Warthin's tumor) were the only salivary gland neoplasms to exhibit an increased uptake and accumulation of pertechnetate anion.[47–51] Resultant "hot" radionucleotide scans of salivary gland lesions were interpreted as indicative of benign oncocytic "functioning" tumors. However, further study now suggests that "hot" radionucleotide scans of salivary gland lesions may not be limited to benign oncocytic salivary gland tumors.[52] Noyek and coinvestigators[52] reported a malignant parotid gland tumor that on scintigraphy mimicked the findings that were previously considered consistent only with oncocytoma and papillary cystadenoma lymphomatosum.

GROSS FINDINGS

The external surface of the tumor is smooth and may be multinodular or lobulated. The cut surface is a white-gray with focal areas of red-brown hemorrhage reported. The tumor is generally homogenous in consistency and demonstrates distinct intersecting fibrous connective tissue septa within the tumor mass.

An oncocytoma from the minor glands is usually a solid tumor that may occasionally exhibit a focal cystic component. It is covered by an unremarkable oral mucosa, unless secondarily ulcerated. The tumor is well defined; however, complete encapsulation is not necessarily observed. In the hard palate, pressure resorption of the underlying bone by the tumor without evidence of intrabony invasion may be observed.

MICROSCOPIC FINDINGS

Oncocytoma is a well-circumscribed tumor (Fig. 13–2) that is composed of oncocytes arranged in solid sheets (Fig. 13–3) or in nests and cords, which form alveolar or organoid patterns (Fig. 13–4). Some of these structures may have small central lumina. A mild, chronic inflammatory cell infiltrate may be present.

The oncocyte is a large, well-defined, polyhedral or round cell that is characterized by brightly eosinophilic cytoplasm with prominent granular-

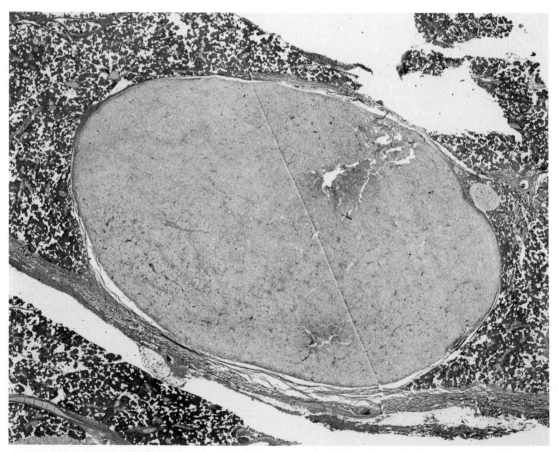

Figure 13–2. Well-circumscribed oncocytoma exhibits sharply demarcated interface between tumor capsule and parenchyma of parotid gland (× 4).

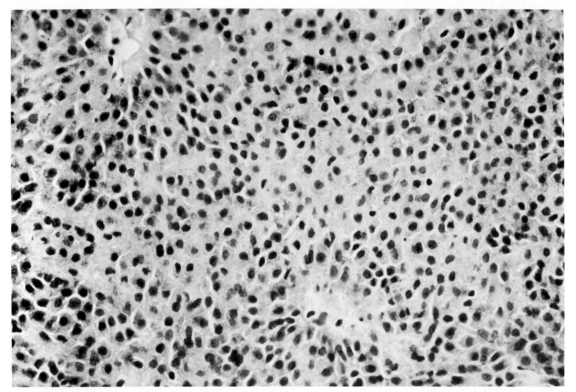

Figure 13–3. Solid pattern demonstrates round and polyhedral oncocytic cells with relatively large, centrally located nuclei. Note loss of cohesion of cells (× 300).

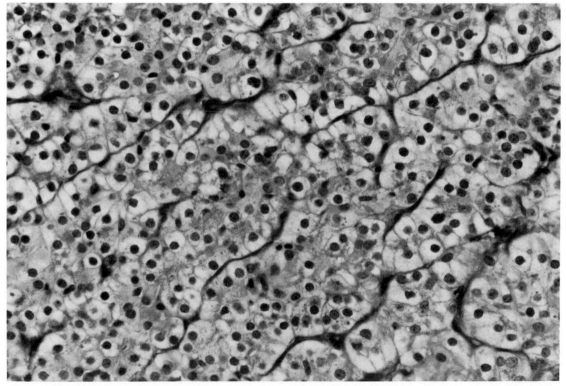

Figure 13–4. Alveolar pattern is delineated by clusters of oncocytic cells that are supported by thin, fibrous, connective tissue septa and small blood vessels. Note oncocytes have clear cytoplasm that is interspersed with typical oncocytes, which demonstrate cytoplasmic granularity (× 300).

ity. The intensity of eosinophilic staining is proportional to the degree of cytoplasmic granularity. Individual oncocytes appear closely adherent and have distinct cellular boundaries unless the tissue has been poorly preserved, in which case acantholysis may be noted (Figs. 13–5 and 13–6). Cells with clear cytoplasm may be seen scattered focally throughout the tumor, or occasionally, as solid masses. Groups of oncocytes are supported by numerous, thin, fibrous connective tissue septa that contain small endothelium-lined vascular spaces (Figs. 13–7 and 13–8). A centrally located nucleus may be small and hyperchromatic or large and vesiculated with prominent nucleoli (Fig. 13–9). Few mitoses are observed.

Some degree of increased cellular atypia, nuclear hyperchromatism, and pleomorphism is accepted as compatible with benignancy in oncocytoma. These atypical histopathologic features might be considered more ominous if observed in other salivary gland tumors; however, in the absence of concomitant infiltration, these features should not serve as a basis for a malignant interpretation. The histopathologic criteria for malignant transformation of oncocytoma are included in Chapter 27 with the discussion of oncocytic carcinoma.

Although observation of bright pink cytoplasmic granularity during examination of slides stained with hematoxylin and eosin is often sufficient to convince the pathologist that an accurate interpretation of oncocytoma can be rendered, special and immunohistochemical stains may prove to be valuable in confirming the diagnosis. Special stains may be particularly dependent on correct tissue preservation and proper handling by the surgeon and laboratory histotechnologist. If unexpected results are observed with special stains, the diagnosis of oncocytoma can be confirmed or excluded with electron microscopic evaluation.

As noted by Azzopardi and Smith,[53] oncocytomas demonstrate a positive reaction for glycogen if stained by periodic acid–Schiff reagent before and after digestion with diastase. Staining procedures for acid mucopolysaccharide with alcian blue and mucicarmine stains produce a negative result.

The cytoplasmic granularity observed in oncocytoma results from the packing of the cytoplasmic volume with mitochondria. One of the procedures most helpful in identifying this organelle, in our experience, is examination of the phosphotungstic acid hematoxylin stain (PTAH). Cytoplasmic granules seen at the light microscopic level stain a deep blue color with PTAH. Less reliable than PTAH, Bensley's aniline-acid fuchsin on frozen tissue stains the cytoplasmic granules of oncocytoma red. Oncocytoma also demonstrates a strong Luxol-

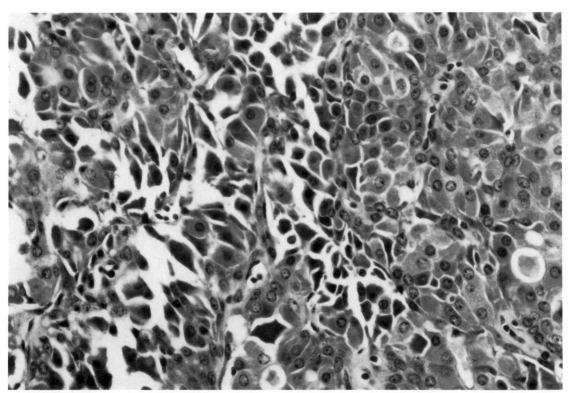

Figure 13–5. Oncocytoma demonstrates an area of syncytial arrangement of oncocytes with little pleomorphism (right) with transition to area of acantholytic oncocytes. Note variable cytoplasmic granularity, pleomorphism, nuclear hyperchromatism, and foci reminiscent of ducts (× 300).

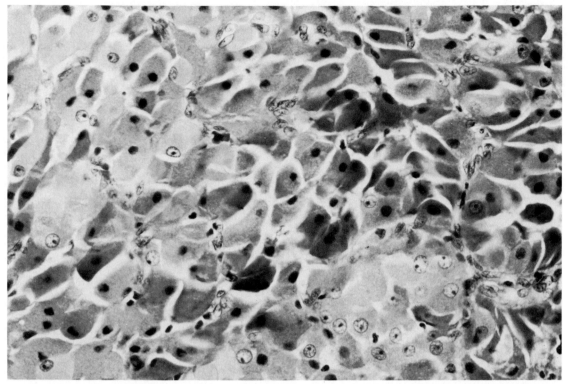

Figure 13–6. This oncocytoma is composed of large oncocytes with most cells exhibiting prominent, eosinophilic cytoplasmic granularity and small, dark nuclei (× 300).

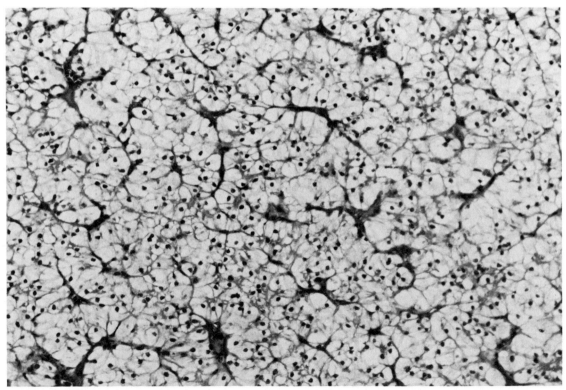

Figure 13–7. Clear cell oncocytoma has an alveolar pattern of oncocytes, which are separated by thin fibrous septa (× 150).

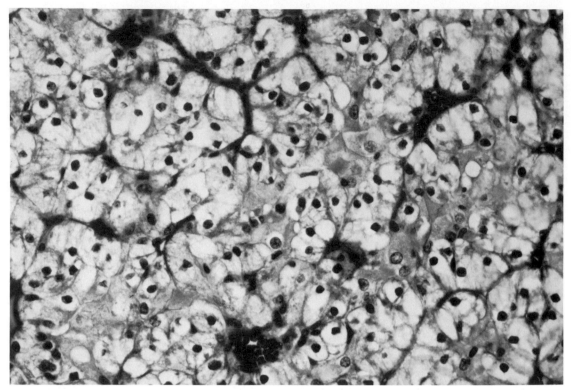

Figure 13–8. Clear cell oncocytoma is composed of oncocytes with granular cytoplasm that are interspersed between aggregated cells with clear cytoplasm (× 300).

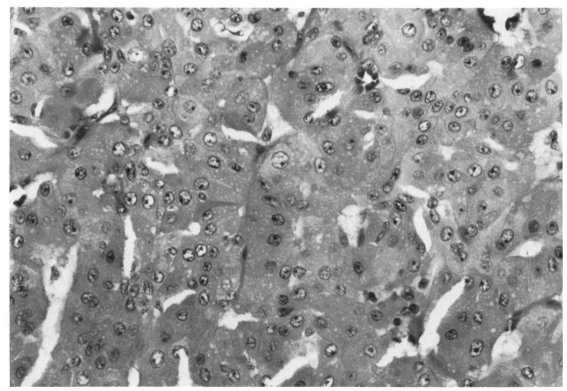

Figure 13–9. Oncocytes arranged in organoid pattern have large, vesicular nuclei with prominent nucleoli (× 300).

fast-blue reaction and reacts metachromatically with thionin and cresyl violet stains.

Limited immunohistochemical studies conducted at the AFIP indicate the oncocyte stains positively for cytokeratin and negatively for S-100 protein and muscle-specific actin. The last two observations are often used to identify myoepithelial differentiation. Immunohistochemical studies of oncocytic cells by Hara and colleagues[54] and Takahashi and coworkers[55] are in agreement with our findings.

Previous reports by some investigators have noted observation of cells with clear cytoplasm interspersed among what proved to be typical oncocytes.[15, 22, 33, 56, 57] Ellis[58] reported ten cases of "clear cell" oncocytoma, which he distinguished from other clear cell salivary gland tumors that were considered to be of low-grade malignant potential. Light microscopic demonstration of typical granular cytoplasm in some cells, PTAH staining, and electron microscopic observation of mitochondria confirm the oncocytic nature of the tumor. The clear cytoplasm that predominates in this variant of oncocytoma is believed to be caused by accumulation of glycogen and by artifactual change.

DIFFERENTIAL DIAGNOSIS

Christopherson[59] inappropriately reported an oncocytoma as a tumor exhibiting chondroid matrix within its stroma. Pulitzer and Reitmeyer[60] correctly recognized this histopathologic feature as more compatible with oncocytic pleomorphic adenoma. The light microscopic differential diagnosis for oncocytoma might reasonably include benign mixed tumor as well as mucoepidermoid carcinoma with oncocytic features, acinic cell carcinoma, low-grade clear cell carcinoma of salivary gland origin, and metastatic carcinoma of the adrenal and thyroid glands, the liver, and the kidney. Observation of keratin pearl formation; osseous, myxoid, or chondroid metaplasia; or spindle or plasmacytoid myoepithelial cell differentiation in tumors that also exhibit oncocytic histomorphology should be considered oncocytoid pleomorphic adenomas. Positive PTAH staining for mitochondria and the absence of intracytoplasmic sialomucin, as determined by special staining procedures, can be useful in differentiating oncocytomas from some well-differentiated mucoepidermoid carcinomas. Unlike acinic cell adenocarcinoma, oncocytoma lacks well-differentiated acinar cells and contains glycogen. Oncocytomas and oncocytosis with prominent clear cells may be confused with the parenchymal infiltration observed in low-grade, clear cell carcinoma. Recognition of typical oncocytes, lack of a stromal reaction, and absence of parenchymal destruction by invasion favor interpretation as oncocytoma. Similarly, oncocytomas with clear cells bear a resemblance to certain metastatic tumors. Immunohistochemical studies for thyroglobulin may be useful in excluding thyroid origin. Similar procedures to identify alpha-fetoprotein and hepatitis B antigens, as well as special stains for bile, may prove useful in differentiating oncocytomas from metastatic hepatic carcinoma. At the light microscopic level, it may not always be possible to unequivocally distinguish metastatic renal cell carcinoma from salivary gland oncocytoma. Clinical evaluation of the patient for a primary tumor in the kidney is worthy of consideration in such cases.

Cytoplasmic granularity at the light microscopic level may result from the presence of secretory granules, lysosomes, endoplasmic reticulum, or mitochondrial organelles. Diagnostic confirmation of oncocytoma may require electron microscopic examination when the PTAH reaction is equivocal.

ULTRASTRUCTURAL FEATURES

The ultrastructural characteristic that *defines* the oncocyte is a cytoplasmic volume packed with mitochondria to the exclusion of most other organelles (Fig. 13–10). One quantitative study of oncocytes estimates that mitochondria constitute approximately 60 percent of the total cell volume. The nucleus fills an additional 20 percent of the total cell volume, leaving 20 percent for all other organelles.[61] Sun and coworkers[62] described two types of oncocytic cells: the typical oncocyte with relatively uniform mitochondria and a condensed oncocyte characterized by fused and degenerating mitochondria. Balough and Roth[24] described oncocytic cell mitochondria that varied in size and shape from 0.2-by-5.0-micrometer filamentous forms to 3.0-micrometer, swollen, spherical forms with long, interdigitating cristae and varying degrees of pleomorphism (Fig. 13–11).

Ultrastructural features that identify the oncocyte as an epithelial cell include the basement membrane and the desmosomal attachments. Occasional tonofilaments are seen in association with cell attachments. The microvilli that extend into a narrow lumen and the few secretory granules help identify the oncocyte as a glandular cell.

Although mitochondria occupy the majority of the cytoplasmic space, other organelles can be observed in oncocytes, including free ribosomes, endoplasmic reticulum, Golgi apparatus, lysosomes, and glycogen. Myofibrillar structures were observed in the cytoplasm of myoepithelial type oncocytic cells in an oncocytoma reported by Askew and colleagues.[63]

The oncocyte nucleus contains evenly distributed chromatin and one or more nucleoli. It may also exhibit an irregular nuclear membrane.

Johns and colleagues[27] and Lee and Roth[64] have compared the ultrastructural differences between oncocytoma and oncocytic adenocarcinoma. In

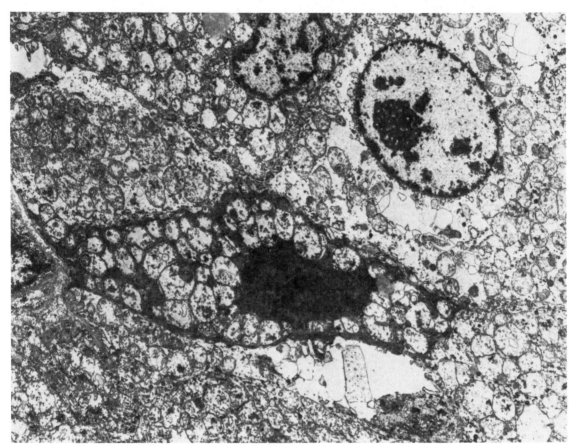

Figure 13–10. Electron micrograph of oncocytoma exhibits cytoplasm that is predominantly filled with swollen mitochondria, a round nucleus with condensed chromatin at the nuclear membrane, and a prominent nucleolus (× 12,800).

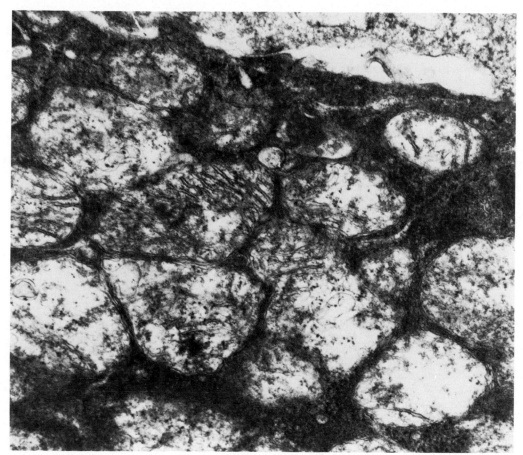

Figure 13–11. Electron micrograph of oncocytoma shows enlarged mitochondria with linear cristae (× 29,575).

benign oncocytoma, the intercellular space is less prominent, with glycogen, myofilaments, and basal lamina observed; this contrasts with oncocytic adenocarcinoma, which lacks these features. However, Johns and colleagues[27] state that the basic ultrastructural similarity between benign and malignant oncocytes precludes absolute determination of biologic behavior. This evaluation is properly based on the histopathologic features that are seen at the light microscopic level and the clinical behavior of the neoplasm.

CLINICAL BEHAVIOR AND TREATMENT

Review of selected published reports[10, 11, 15, 43, 45] indicates that oncocytomas in the major and minor salivary glands can be expected to demonstrate a low rate of recurrence after complete surgical removal. Persistent tumor occurring after incomplete removal is the primary cause of recurrent lesions, as suggested by Chaudhry and Gorlin.[15] Gray and coinvestigators'[33] study of 10 oncocytomas reported a 20 percent recurrence rate but

did not indicate the treatment rendered. Their review of the literature summarized four cases of locally aggressive, benign oncocytomas of minor salivary gland origin (palate or nasal mucosa). Batsakis[65] considered all solid oncocytomas arising from glands of the upper respiratory tract (nasal cavity and paranasal sinuses) to be low-grade malignant neoplasms. Chau and Radden[44] recognized a need for further study of the behavior of solid oncocytomas in the minor salivary glands. Damm and colleagues[45] reviewed the literature regarding oncocytoma of minor salivary glands and reported a case of oncocytoma in the buccal mucosa. They determined that a solid oncocytoma of a minor salivary gland displays no evidence of aggressive behavior. Consequently, minor salivary gland oncocytomas should be separated from those of the upper respiratory tract.

Malignant transformation of a previously benign oncocytoma has been reported.[11, 66] In one case, transformation was marked by rapid growth after an indolent period of 19 years.[11] Another case was preceded by multiple surgical attempts to extirpate recurrent oncocytoma; therefore, oncocytomas that demonstrate a sudden increase in size or multiple recurrences should be viewed with increased suspicion.

Surgery is the most common and accepted treatment for oncocytoma. Although most parotid gland oncocytomas are encapsulated and located rather superficially, partial parotidectomy with facial nerve preservation, whenever possible, is the preferred method of treatment. This method ensures complete tumor removal and should reduce the likelihood of recurrent disease. Curettage or simple enucleation of the tumor is to be avoided. If the facial nerve must be sacrificed, microneurosurgical repair attempts are worthy of consideration. In addition to facial nerve paralysis, another complication of parotid gland surgery is auriculotemporal syndrome or gustatory sweating.

Complete glandectomy is recommended for oncocytoma in the submandibular gland. Oncocytoma of minor salivary gland origin can be treated by local excision that includes a margin of tumor-free tissue.

Radiation therapy in the treatment of oncocytoma has been considered unfavorable by McFarland,[4] Lane,[14] and Chaudhry and Gorlin.[15] McFarland's[4] case of oncocytoma recurred following radiation therapy. Lane[14] as well as Chaudhry and Gorlin[15] found radiation therapy to have little efficacy. Blanck and coworkers[22] reported that radiation therapy was employed in 10 of 13 patients with oncocytoma. Four patients experienced recurrence (30 percent). Kosuda and coworkers[67] reported a recurrent oncocytoma treated by administration of radioisotope ^{131}I that resulted in a reduction in tumor size.

REFERENCES

1. Schaffer J: Beitrage zur Histologie Menischlicher Organe. IV. Zunge. V. Mundhohle-Schlundkopf. VI. Oesophagus VII. Cardia. Sitzungsber. d. Kais. Akad. d. Wissensch., Math. naturwiss. Classe, Abth. III 1897; 106:353–357.
2. Zimmermann KW: Die Speicheldrusen der Mundhohle und die Bauchspeicheldruse. In Von Mollendorff W: Handbuch der Mikroskopischen Anatomie der Menschen. Berlin, Julius Springer, 1927; 5:128.
3. Jaffe RH: Adenolymphoma (onkocytoma) of the parotid gland. Am J Cancer 1932; 16:1414–1423.
4. McFarland J: Adenoma of salivary glands with a report of a possible case. Am J Med Sci 1927; 174:362–378.
5. Hamperl H: Onkocyten und Geschwulste der Speicheldrusen. Virchows Arch [A] 1931; 282:724–736.
6. Hamperl H: Über das Vorkommen von Onkocyten in verschiedenen Organen und ihren Geschwulsten. Virchows Arch [A] 1936; 298:327–375.
7. Hamperl H: Onkocytes and the so-called Hürthle cell tumor. Arch Pathol Lab Med 1950; 49:563–567.
8. Foote FW Jr, Frazell EL: Tumors of the Major Salivary Glands. Atlas of Tumor Pathology, Section 4, Part 11, 1st Series. Washington, DC, Armed Forces Institute of Pathology, 1954; 137–139.
9. Ackerman LV: Oncocytoma of the parotid gland. Arch Pathol Lab Med 1943; 36:508–511.
10. Meza-Chavez L: Oxyphilic granular cell adenoma of the parotid gland (oncocytoma): Report of five cases and study of the oxyphilic granular cells (oncocytes) in normal parotid glands. Am J Pathol 1949; 25:523–537.
11. Eneroth CW: Oncocytoma of major salivary glands. J Laryngol Otol 1965; 79:1064–1072.
12. Boley JO, Robinson DW: Bilateral oxyphilic granular cell adenoma of the parotid. Arch Pathol Lab Med 1954; 58:564–567.
13. Codington JB: Oxyphilic granular cell adenoma of the parotid gland. Am J Surg 1959; 97:333–335.
14. Lane SL: Oxyphilic granular cell adenoma (oncocytoma) of the parotid. Plast Reconstr Surg 1962; 30:88–94.
15. Chaudhry AP, Gorlin RJ: Oxyphilic granular cell adenoma (oncocytoma). Oral Surg Oral Med Oral Pathol 1958; 11:897–905.
16. Smoler J: Oxyphilic granular cell adenoma of the parotid gland. Arch Otolaryngol Head Neck Surg 1968; 87:540–542.
17. Buxton RW, Maxwell JH, French AJ: Surgical treatment of epithelial tumors of the parotid gland. Surg Gynecol Obstet 1953; 97:401–441.
18. Stump DJ: Oncocytic adenoma of the salivary glands. Arch Pathol Lab Med 1949; 48:287.
19. Schafer EL, Gruet M, Jackson AS: Oncocytic cell adenoma of the parotid gland. Am J Surg 1956; 91:272–278.
20. Hamperl H: Beitrage zur normalen und pathologischen histologie menischilicher speicheldrusen. Zeitschrift Mikropischanatomische Forschung (Leipzig) 1931; 27:1–22.
21. Hamperl H: Benign and malignant oncocytoma. Cancer 1962; 15:1019–1027.
22. Blanck C, Eneroth CM, Jakobsson PA: Oncocytoma of the parotid gland: Neoplasm or nodular hyperplasia. Cancer 1970; 24:919–925.
23. Roth SI, Olsen E, Hansen LS: The eosinophilic cells of the parathyroid (oxyphil cells), salivary (oncocytes) and thyroid (Hurthle cell) glands, light and electron microscopic observations. Lab Invest 1962; 11:933–941.
24. Balough K, Roth SI: Histochemical and electron microscopic studies of eosinophilic granular cells (oncocytes) in tumors of the parotid gland. Lab Invest 1965; 14:310–320.
25. Tandler B, Hutter R, Erlandson R: Ultrastructure of oncocytoma of the parotid gland. Lab Invest 1970; 23:567–580.
26. Koboyaski H, Hosino M, Tauchi H: Ultrastructural study of cytochrome oxidase in oncocytoma. Nagoya J Med Sci 1972; 34:25–32.
27. Johns ME, Regezi JA, Batsakis JG: Oncocytic neoplasms of salivary glands: An ultrastructural study. Laryngoscope 1977; 87:862–871.
28. Fischer R: Uber den histochemischen Nachweis oxydativer enzyme in Oncocyten verschidener Organe. Virchow Arch [A] 1961; 334:445–452.
29. Kirklin JW, McDonald JR, Harrington SW, New GB: Parotid tumors: Histopathology, clinical behavior, and end results. Surg Gynecol Obstet 1951; 92:721–733.

30. Chaudhry AP, Vickers RA, Gorlin RJ: Intraoral minor salivary gland tumors: An analysis of 1414 cases. Oral Surg Oral Med Oral Pathol 1961; 14:1194–1226.
31. Das S, Sengupta P, Chatterjee SK, Sarkar SK: Oncocytoma of tongue in a child. J Pediatr Surg 1976; 11:113–114.
32. Zipermam HH, Capers TH: Oxyphil cell adenoma of the tongue. US Armed Forces Med J 1955; 6:1039–1042.
33. Gray SR, Cornog JL, Seo IS: Oncocytic neoplasms of salivary glands: A report of 15 cases including two malignant oncocytomas. Cancer 1976; 38:1306–1317.
34. Hastrup N, Bretlau P, Kroudahl A, Melchiors H: Oncocytomas of the salivary glands. J Laryngol Otol 1982; 96:1027–1032.
35. Evans RW, Cruickshank AH: Epithelial Tumours of the Major Salivary Glands. Philadelphia, WB Saunders Co, 1970; 27–37.
36. Dibble PA, Sanford DM: Submaxillary oncocytoma. Arch Otolaryngol 1961; 74:81–83.
37. Batsakis JG, Martz DG: Oxyphilic cell tumor of the submaxillary gland. US Armed Forces Med J 1960; 11:1383–1386.
38. Deutsch E, Eilon A, Zelig S, Ariel I: Synchronous bilateral oncocytoma of the parotid glands. ORL Otorhinolaryngol Relat Spec 1984; 46:66–68.
39. Cohen MA, Batsakis JG: Oncocytic tumors (oncocytomas) of minor salivary glands. Arch Otolaryngol Head Neck Surg 1968; 88:71–73.
40. Jalisi M: Oncocytoma of the accessory salivary glands. J Laryngol Otol 1968; 82:257–259.
41. Bergman F: Tumors of the minor salivary glands: A report of 46 cases. Cancer 1969; 23:538–543.
42. Crocker DJ, Cavalaris CJ, Finch R: Intraoral minor salivary gland tumors: Report of 38 cases. Oral Surg Oral Med Oral Pathol 1970; 29:60–68.
43. Pogrel MA: Tumours of the salivary glands: A histological and clinical review. Br J Oral Surg 1979; 17:47–56.
44. Chau MNY, Radden BG: Intraoral benign solid oncocytoma. Int J Oral Maxillofac Surg 1986; 15:503–506.
45. Damm DD, White DK, Geissler RH, Drummond JF, Henry BB: Benign solid oncocytoma of intraoral minor salivary glands. Oral Surg Oral Med Oral Pathol 1989; 67:84–86.
46. Grove AS Jr, Di Chiro G: Salivary gland scanning with technetium 99m pertechnetate. Am J Roentgen 1968; 102:109–116.
47. Ausband JR, Kittrell BJ, Cowan RJ: Radioisotope scanning for parotid oncocytoma. Arch Otolaryngol Head Neck Surg 1971; 93:628–629.
48. Lunia S, Chodos RB, Lunia C, Chandramouly BS: Oxyphilic adenoma of the parotid gland: Identification with 99mTc-pertechnetate. Radiology 1978; 128:690.
49. Noyek AM, Greyson ND, Cooter N, Shapiro BJ: Radionucleotide salivary gland imaging of maxillary sinus oncocytoma. J Otolaryngol Otol 1982; 1:17–22.
50. Kosuda S, Gokan T, Tamura K, Kubo A: Radionucleotide imaging for parotid oncocytoma. Clin Nucl Med 1987; 12:150–151.
51. Higashi T, Murahashi H, Ikuta H, Mori Y, Watanabe Y: Identification of Warthin's tumor with technetium-99m pertechnetate. Clin Nucl Med 1987; 12:796–800.
52. Noyek AM, Greyson ND, Fernandes BJ, Chapnik JS: Radionucleotide salivary scan imaging of a "functioning" malignant parotid tumor (mucus-producing papillary adenocarcinoma). J Otolaryngol 1982; 11:83–85.
53. Azzopardi JG, Smith OD: Salivary gland tumors and their mucins. J Pathol 1959; 77:131–140.
54. Hara K, Ito M, Takeuchi J, Iijima S, Endo T, Hidaka H: Distribution of S-100 protein in normal salivary glands and salivary gland tumors. Virchows Arch [A] 1983; 401:237–249.
55. Takahashi H, Tsuda N, Tezuka F, Okabe H: An immunohistochemical investigation of S-100 protein in the epithelial component of Warthin's tumor. Oral Surg Oral Med Oral Pathol 1986; 62:57–62.
56. Corridan M: Glycogen-rich clear-cell adenoma of the parotid gland. J Pathol 1956; 72:623–626.
57. Goldman RL, Klein H: Glycogen-rich adenoma of the parotid gland: An uncommon benign clear-cell tumor resembling certain clear-cell carcinomas of salivary origin. Cancer 1972; 30:749–754.
58. Ellis GL: "Clear cell" oncocytoma of salivary gland. Hum Pathol 1988; 19:862–867.
59. Christopherson WM: Oncocytoma of the parotid gland. Arch Pathol 1949; 48:96–98.
60. Pulitzer DR, Reitmeyer WJ: Oncocytic pleomorphic adenoma of the parotid gland. J Surg Oncol 1987; 34:198–201.
61. Carls B, Domeij S, Helander HF: A quantitative ultrastructural study of a parotid oncocytoma. Arch Pathol Lab Med 1979; 103:471–474.
62. Sun CN, White HJ, Thompson BW: Oncocytoma (mitochondrioma) of the parotid gland: An electron microscopical study. Arch Pathol Lab Med 1975; 99:208–214.
63. Askew JB, Bentinck DC, Jensen AB, Fechner RE: Epithelial and myoepithelial oncocytes: Ultrastructural study of a salivary gland oncocytoma. Arch Otolaryngol Head Neck Surg 1971; 93:46–54.
64. Lee SC, Roth LL: Malignant oncocytoma of the parotid gland: A light and electron microscopic study. Cancer 1976; 37:1607–1614.
65. Batsakis JG: Tumors of the Head and Neck: Clinical and Pathologic Considerations, 2nd Ed. Baltimore, Williams & Wilkins, 1979; 57–62.
66. Goode RK, Corio RL: Oncocytic adenocarcinoma of salivary glands. Oral Surg Oral Med Oral Pathol 1988; 65:61–66.
67. Kosuda S, Ishikawa M, Tamura K, Kubo A, Hashimoto S: Iodine-131 therapy for parotid oncocytoma. J Nucl Med 1988; 29:1126–1129.

14

DUCTAL PAPILLOMAS

Gary L. Ellis and Paul L. Auclair

It is not unusual for salivary gland tumors to have a papillary configuration that is either the principal morphologic pattern or foci among other morphologic forms. The papillary cystadenoma lymphomatosum, or Warthin's tumor, is the most common papillary tumor; however, cystadenoma, acinic cell adenocarcinoma, polymorphous low-grade adenocarcinoma, mucoepidermoid carcinoma, and cystadenocarcinoma can certainly have foci with a papillary conformation. On the other hand, besides Warthin's tumor, benign papillary tumors of the salivary glands are quite rare. In many published surveys of salivary gland neoplasms, benign papillomatous tumors are not specifically identified or categorized.[1–10] In some of these tumor analyses, it may be presumed that salivary gland papillomas are included in categories such as "other adenomas" or "monomorphic adenomas," but it is more likely that this group of tumors is often ignored or unrecognized.

Chaudhry and coworkers[11] identified 4 tumors among 189 minor salivary gland tumors that they had classified as intraductal papillary hyperplasia. Seifert and colleagues[12] apparently included sialadenoma papilliferum, intraductal papilloma, and inverted ductal papilloma within a broad category of monomorphic adenomas that they called ductal adenoma. Neville and colleagues[13] found one intraductal papilloma among 103 labial salivary gland tumors. In an analysis of 426 minor salivary gland tumors, Waldron and coinvestigators[14] categorized 5 tumors as sialadenoma papilliferum and 4 tumors as unicystic cystadenomas, whereas Regezi and colleagues[15] found 2 sialadenoma papilliferums and 4 inverted ductal papillomas among 229 minor salivary gland tumors. Chau and Radden[16] listed a single papillary cystadenoma within their survey of 98 intraoral salivary gland neoplasms.

Although benign papillary tumors of the salivary gland, other than Warthin's tumors, are relatively rare, there are three types with unique histopathologic features that allow these types to be easily identified and classified. These three types of papillary tumors are *sialadenoma papilliferum, inverted ductal papilloma,* and *intraductal papilloma.* The anatomic sites of occurrence of the salivary duct papillomas in the Armed Forces Institute of Pathology (AFIP) registry of salivary gland pathology are given in Table 14–1.

SIALADENOMA PAPILLIFERUM

Abrams and Finck[17] first described sialadenoma papilliferum in 1969 when they reported two cases. They chose the term *sialadenoma papilliferum* because of the histologic similarity of this type of salivary gland tumor to the syringocystadenoma papilliferum of skin adnexal origin.[18] Including these two originally reported cases, to date, we have found 26 acceptable cases reported in the English language literature.[19–35] These include the first two cases in a study by Whittaker and Turner[22] that were categorized as oncocytic adenomatous hyperplasia. We have also included the case reported as "intraductal papilloma" by Castigliano and Gold[19] many years before Abrams and Finck[17] defined the term *sialadenoma papilliferum;* by our evaluation, this tumor is more appropriately classified as sialadenoma papilliferum than as intraductal papilloma. We have not accepted the case of sialadenoma papilliferum of the parotid gland reported by Grushka and colleagues[36] because it lacked surface exophytic growth, which we consider requisite for the diagnosis. Nor have we included the case reported by Chan and colleagues[37] because it was described clinically as a nodule and because the micrographs and the microscopic description did not indicate the exophytic papillary features of sialadenoma papilliferum. Solomon and colleagues[38] reported a palatal lesion with features suggestive of sialadenoma papilliferum that apparently metastasized to a regional lymph node, but we have serious

Table 14–1. Anatomic Distribution of the Different Types of Ductal Papillomas
in the AFIP Registry

Anatomic Site	Number of Sialadenoma Papilliferums	Number of Intraductal Papillomas	Number of Inverted Ductal Papillomas
Major Glands			
Parotid gland	2	3	—
Submandibular gland	—	1	—
Sublingual gland	1	—	—
Minor Glands			
Palate (total)	7	5	—
Hard	(1)	(1)	—
Soft	(2)	(1)	—
Not specified	(4)	(3)	—
Lip (total)	—	10	5
Lower	—	(5)	(5)
Upper	—	(4)	—
Not specified	—	(1)	—
Oral cavity, NOS*	2	1	—
Buccal mucosa	1	4	1
Retromolar	1	—	—
Gingiva	1	—	—
Total†	15	24	6

*NOS = not otherwise specified
†Does not include numbers in parentheses

doubts about the diagnosis of this lesion and have not included it among acceptable reported cases. Nor have we included the cases that were noted among surveys of minor salivary tumors by Regezi and colleagues[15] and Waldron and colleagues.[14] We do not dispute the diagnoses of these latter cases, but we have not included them as reported cases simply because they were a part of general surveys with few specific details.

In the AFIP registry, we have an additional 15 cases of sialadenoma papilliferum (Table 14–1). These 15 tumors constitute only 0.1 percent of the 13,749 epithelial salivary gland tumors and 0.6 percent of the benign epithelial salivary gland tumors of the minor salivary glands in our registry. This is somewhat less than the 1.3 percent and 2.0 percent incidences of benign tumors of minor salivary glands reported by Regezi and colleagues[15] and by Waldron and colleagues,[14] respectively.

Clinical Features

The clinical presentation of sialadenoma papilliferum is quite unique among salivary gland neoplasms. Nearly all salivary gland neoplasms, both the benign and malignant neoplasms located in either the major or the minor salivary glands, manifest as subsurface nodular swellings or masses that are covered by smooth, intact mucosa or skin. Sialadenoma papilliferum, on the other hand, occurs as an exophytic, papillary surface lesion. The clinical impression in most cases is squamous papilloma of the mucosa.

Analysis of the combined data of the AFIP registry (Table 14–1) and of the literature reveals that only four tumors have involved the major salivary glands, including three parotid gland lesions and one sublingual gland lesion. Ironically, the initial tumor reported by Abrams and Finck[17] was a parotid gland tumor. All other tumors have involved minor salivary glands of the oral or pharyngeal mucosa, and nearly 65 percent of these have occurred on the posterior hard palate or soft palate. The junction of the hard and soft palates is a common site, typically located on one side of the midline. Less frequently involved sites include the buccal mucosa and the mandibular retromolar trigone. Rare lesions have occurred on the gingiva, faucial pillar, upper lip, and pharyngeal mucosa.

Like squamous papilloma, sialadenoma papilliferum is generally a small lesion. Although some oral tumors have reached 2.5 cm in diameter, most tumors are less than 1.0 cm in size. Again, contrary to nearly all subsequent reports of this tumor, the initial parotid tumor reported by Abrams and Finck[17] was 7.5 cm in diameter.

Many of these tumors have been discovered during routine oral examinations or as incidental findings without the patients' being aware of the presence of the lesions. These tumors are asymptomatic, and if the patients are aware of them, they have usually detected them as growths on the mucosa that they can feel with their tongues.

Although patients' ages have ranged from 2 to 87 years, only the 2-year-old patient reported by Masi and colleagues[32] was younger than 20 years. Sixty-eight percent of patients have been older than 50 years, and the average age is 56 years (Fig. 14–1). Male patients have outnumbered female patients by a ratio of about 1.5 to 1.0. There is no apparent racial predilection.

Histopathologic Features

Gross specimen examination usually reveals a round to oval, well-circumscribed lesion of the surface mucosa. The lesion may be broad based or pedunculated. The surface of the tumor appears rough, pebbly, verrucous, or, typically, overtly papillary. The lesion is often reddish. Sections reveal cauliflowerlike surfaces and circumscribed nodules of tumor tissue that extend below the level of the mucosa. Small cystic spaces may sometimes be seen upon close examination.

Microscopically, these tumors display both an exophytic and an endophytic proliferation of ductal epithelium (Fig. 14–2). The mucosal surface of the lesion, very similar to a typical papilloma, is formed by many papillary projections and folds of epithelium that are supported by fibrovascular cores that extend above the level of the adjacent mucosa. The surface of these epithelial fronds is covered by parakeratotic, acanthotic stratified squamous epithelium (Fig. 14–3). At the junction with the normal mucosa, the stratified squamous epithelium may have a pseudoepitheliomatous appearance with wide, rounded, rete ridges that push into the lamina propria. The normal mucosal surface epithelium may form part of the stalk of pedunculated tumors, or it may form a lip or rolled border with more broad-based tumors. The fibrovascular cores of the papillary projections have a mild to intense, mixed inflammatory cell infiltrate of lymphocytes, plasma cells, and neutrophils. Some exocytosis and intraepithelial microabscesses may be noted (Fig. 14–4).

Below the surface papillary formations, the stratified squamous epithelium merges into ductal epithelium. The ductal epithelium lines branching, often tortuous ductlike lumina that are contiguous with the interpapillary clefts of the surface stratified squamous epithelium (Fig. 14–5). The ductal structures are frequently dilated, and the lining epithelium may form additional papillary projections into the lumina. Typically, at the base of the lesion, a proliferation of small ducts develops, some of which may be cystically enlarged (Fig. 14–6). There is no capsule around the proliferative ductal structures. This feature might cause concern to someone unfamiliar with this tumor because it creates an appearance of ductal cells infiltrating the lamina propria and submucosa.

The ductal epithelium that lines the ducts, cysts, and papillary folds is usually composed of a double layer of cells. The luminal cells are tall columnar cells, and the basilar cells are smaller cuboidal cells. The cytoplasm of these cells is prominently eosinophilic, and they resemble striated and interlobular excretory duct cells. The cells of the glandular proliferations at the base of the tumor often have a deeply eosinophilic, oncocytic appearance. Scattered mucous cells may be seen among the ductal or stratified squamous epithelial cells in some tumors, and these cells can be highlighted with mucicarmine or periodic acid–Schiff stain.

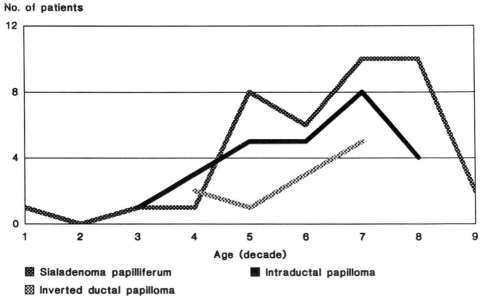

No. of patients

Age (decade)

▨ Sialadenoma papilliferum   ■ Intraductal papilloma

▨ Inverted ductal papilloma

Figure 14–1. The age distribution for patients with ductal papillomas in the AFIP registry and reported in the literature.

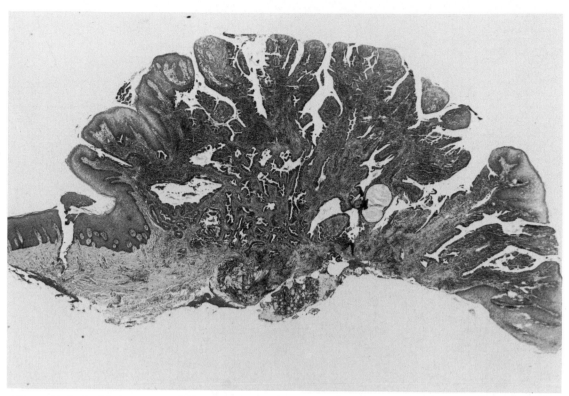

Figure 14–2. A sialadenoma papilliferum from the palate has papillary fronds that extend above the adjacent mucosal surface. Arborized, proliferative, salivary gland ducts are evident beneath the papillary fronds (× 15).

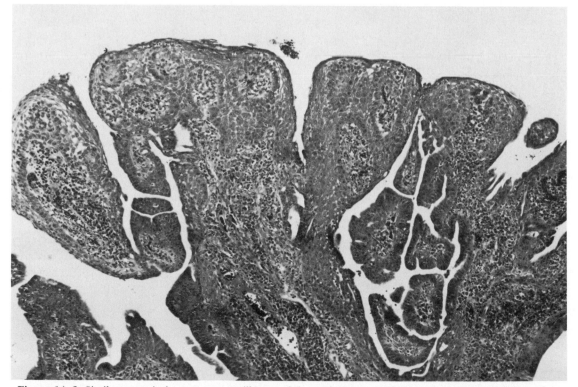

Figure 14–3. Similar to typical squamous papillomas of the oral mucosa, sialadenoma papilliferum has exophytic papillary projections with fibrovascular cores that are covered in the superficial portions by parakeratotic stratified squamous epithelium (× 75).

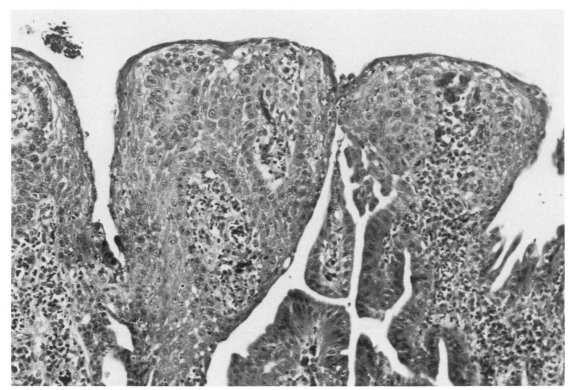

Figure 14–4. The fibrovascular cores of this sialadenoma papilliferum have a prominent inflammatory cell infiltrate with some exocytosis (× 150).

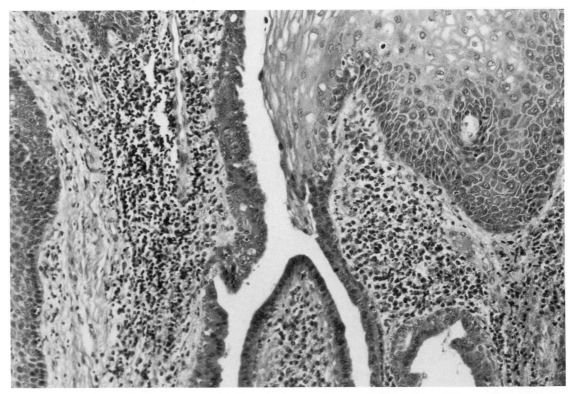

Figure 14–5. The stratified squamous epithelium that covers the superficial portions of the papillary projections of a sialadenoma papilliferum is contiguous with the columnar ductal epithelium that lines branching, proliferative ducts (× 150).

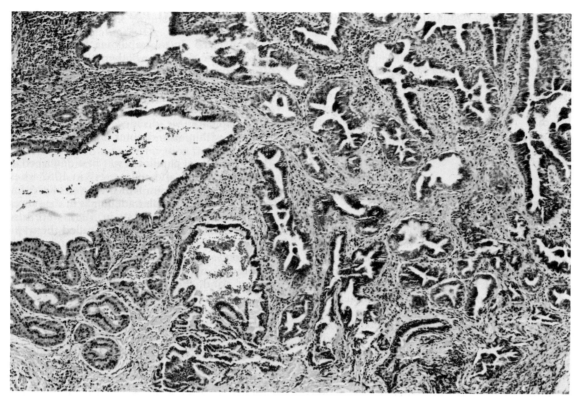

Figure 14–6. In the tissues beneath the surface papillations of a sialadenoma papilliferum is a proliferation of small and dilated ducts. Because no capsule surrounds this ductal proliferation, a false impression of invasion is possible (× 60).

Ultrastructural observations by Fantasia and colleagues[34] of cells at the tips of the papillary projections showed desmosomal attachments and bundles of tonofilaments in polygonal cells that are consistent with features of typical squamous epithelium. The ductal cells contained numerous mitochondria, nuclei in the apical half of the cell, junctional complexes near the luminal surface, and desmosomal attachments. Occasional infoldings of otherwise smooth plasma membranes were noted. The basal cells were separated from the connective tissues by a well-defined basal lamina.

Differential Diagnosis

Both the clinical and microscopic features of sialadenoma papilliferum have marked similarities to those of squamous papilloma. In addition, clinically, warty dyskeratoma and incipient verrucous carcinoma may be considered in a differential diagnosis. However, the ductal and glandular proliferations seen microscopically in sialadenoma papilliferum readily segregate it from these other exophytic and papillary lesions.

Mucous cells, squamous cells, ductal cells, cystic structures, and lack of encapsulation are features associated with both sialadenoma papilliferum and mucoepidermoid carcinoma. However, the unique exophytic, papillary configuration of sialadenoma papilliferum easily distinguishes it from mucoepidermoid carcinoma. In addition, the arrangement of the stratified squamous epithelium as caps on the papillary fronds of sialadenoma papilliferum is considerably different from the intermingling of epidermoid, mucous, and ductal cells that is seen in mucoepidermoid carcinoma.

If there is marked pseudoepitheliomatous hyperplasia of the mucosal surface epithelium, necrotizing sialometaplasia may have a superficial microscopic resemblance to sialadenoma papilliferum. Necrotizing sialometaplasia lacks the arborizing and papillary proliferation of ducts and the exophytic fronds covered by ductal and squamous epithelium. Sialadenoma papilliferum lacks the necrotizing lobules of salivary glands that are characteristic of necrotizing sialometaplasia.

Although the intraductal papilloma and inverted ductal papilloma (see later) share some features with sialadenoma papilliferum, neither exhibits the exophytic growth of sialadenoma papilliferum.

Prognosis and Treatment

The prognosis is exceptionally good, even for a benign tumor. Only one sialadenoma papilliferum

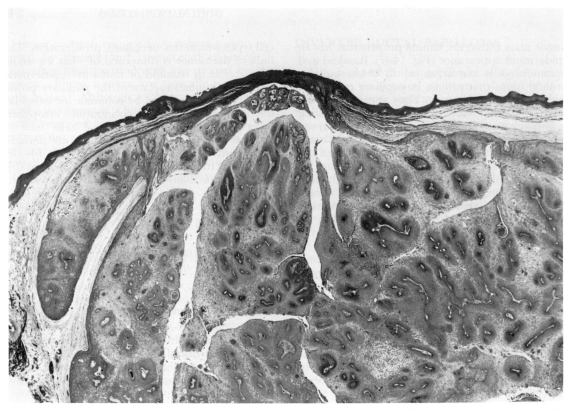

Figure 14–8. Inverted ductal papilloma of the buccal mucosa shows broad papillary projections that nearly fill a cystic cavity and push out into the adjacent lamina propria and submucosa just beneath the surface mucosa. The epithelium is predominantly stratified squamous (× 15).

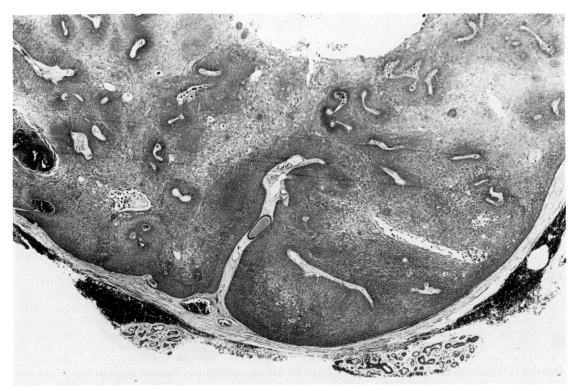

Figure 14–9. The normal tissue/tumor interface of this inverted ductal papilloma shows that the tumor is well-demarcated and extends by expansion rather than by invasion into the submucosa (× 30).

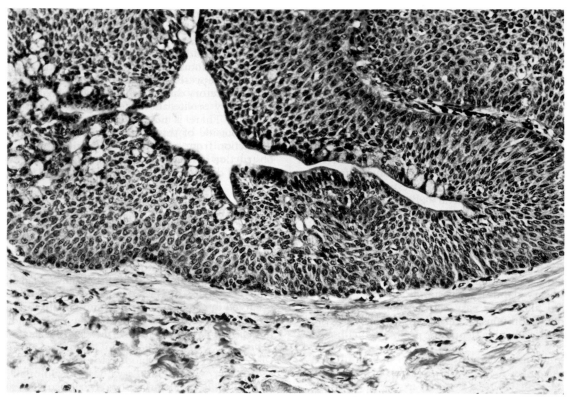

Figure 14–10. High magnification of an inverted ductal papilloma reveals several types of epithelial cells. Most of the epithelium is immature epidermoid or basaloid cells. A layer of columnar, duct-type cells is found on the luminal surface, and several ovoid, pale-staining mucous cells are interspersed (× 150).

ties.[45, 46] In fact, even the two terms invite some confusion. So-called *inverted papillomas of the oral cavity*, which are akin to the nasal and paranasal sinus papillomas, have been reported,[47, 48] but these appear to have arisen from surface epithelium rather than from the ductal system of minor salivary glands. Common histologic features between the two lesions include papillary, endophytic proliferation of stratified basal and epidermoid epithelium, intraepithelial microcysts, mucous cells, and columnar and cuboidal cells in areas along the luminal surface. Unlike sinonasal papillomas, inverted ductal papilloma is a small discrete mass that appears to grow by centripetal and centrifugal expansion. Sinonasal papillomas may be quite large and may involve extensive areas of the sinonasal mucosa, and recurrence is a problem that is not shared with inverted ductal papillomas. The most serious difference between the two is that sinonasal papillomas may undergo malignant transformation.[46]

As stated above, features that distinguish inverted ductal papilloma from sialadenoma papilliferum are the absence of exophytic papillary fronds, proliferation of ductal structures at the base of the lesion, and aborized ducts lined by a double layer of ductal epithelial cells. Although inverted ductal papilloma and mucoepidermoid

carcinoma both have mucous and epidermoid cells, inverted ductal papilloma lacks the multicystic and/or multinodular and infiltrative growth pattern of mucoepidermoid carcinoma.

INTRADUCTAL PAPILLOMA

Reports of intraductal papillomas in the English language scientific literature are rare. The rarity of these reports is only partly attributable to the fact that this is an uncommon salivary gland tumor. Within the literature, the terminology and the definition of this entity vary considerably. Abbey[49] reported a case in the upper lip and cited three other reports of intraductal papilloma. However, we disagree with the diagnosis in two of these other cases. As stated previously, we believe that the intraductal papilloma of the hard palate reported by Castigliano and Gold[19] had features consistent with those of sialadenoma papilliferum. Vellios and Davidson[50] provided no clinical data, a one sentence histologic description, and one photomicrograph that were inadequate to document a lesion that they called intraductal papilloma. Kerpel and colleagues[51] reported a papillary cystadenoma of the buccal mucosa that we believe was an example of an intraductal papilloma. Also,

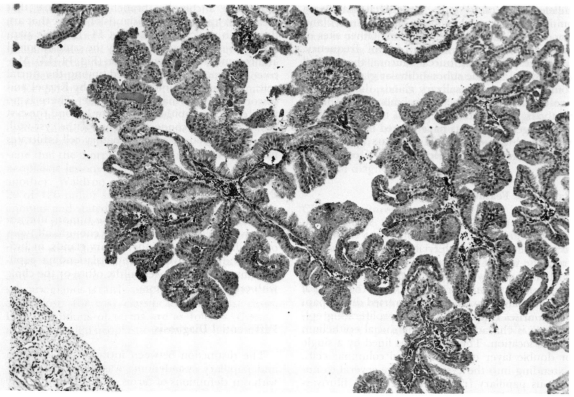

Figure 14–13. High magnification of an intraductal papilloma illustrates the branching, thin, fibrovascular cores that are covered with the columnar epithelium that is typical of salivary gland excretory ducts (× 75).

multiple, variable-sized, epithelium-lined cystic structures with linings that may form papillary folds, and unlike the intraductal papilloma, the multiple cysts of the cystadenoma appear to be proliferating in the supporting connective tissue stroma.

The character of the proliferating epithelium in inverted ductal papilloma is predominantly epidermoid, whereas in intraductal papilloma, it is columnar or cuboidal epithelium and/or mucous cells. The epidermoid epithelium in inverted papilloma appears to push into the surrounding stroma on a broad front. The intraductal papilloma is a well-demarcated cyst.

As noted by Eversole and Sabes,[11] salivary duct blockage may lead to ductal dilatation and hyperplasia of the ductal epithelium. Although this epithelial hyperplasia may produce some papillary folds and projections into the dilated duct, this epithelial proliferation is much less than that seen in intraductal papillomas. Also, in duct blockage reactions, the subjacent salivary gland lobules demonstrate inflammation, fibrosis, and atrophy.

REFERENCES

1. Eneroth C-M: Salivary gland tumors in the parotid gland, submandibular gland, and the palate region. Cancer 1971; 27:1415–1418.

2. Spiro RH, Koss LG, Hajdu SI, Strong EW: Tumors of minor salivary origin: A clinicopathologic study of 492 cases. Cancer 1973; 31:117–129.

3. Sharkey FE: Systematic evaluation of the World Health Organization classification of salivary gland tumors: A clinicopathologic study of 366 cases. Am J Clin Pathol 1977; 67:272–278.

4. Main JHP, Orr JA, McGurk FM, McComb RJ, Mock D: Salivary gland tumors: Review of 643 cases. J Oral Pathol 1976; 5:88–102.

5. Isacsson G, Shear M: Intraoral salivary gland tumors: A retrospective study of 201 cases. J Oral Pathol 1983; 12:57–62.

6. Theron EJ, Middlecote BD: Tumours of the salivary glands: The Bloemfontein experience. S Afr J Surg 1984; 22:237–242.

7. Eveson JW, Cawson RA: Salivary gland tumours: A review of 2410 cases with particular reference to histological types, site, age and sex distribution. J Pathol 1985; 146:51–58.

8. Eveson JW, Cawson RA: Tumours of the minor (oropharyngeal) salivary glands: A demographic study of 336 cases. J Oral Pathol 1985; 14:500–509.

9. Spiro RH: Salivary neoplasms: Overview of a 35-year experience with 2,807 patients. Head Neck Surg 1986; 8:177–184.

10. Ma DQ, Yu GY: Tumours of the minor salivary glands: A clinicopathologic study of 243 cases. Acta Otolaryngol (Stockh) 1987; 103:325–331.

11. Chaudhry AP, Labay GR, Yamane GM, Jacobs MS, Cutler LS, Watkins KV: Clinico-pathologic and histogenetic study of 189 intraoral minor salivary gland tumors. J Oral Med 1984; 39:58–78.

12. Seifert G, Miehlke A, Haubrich J, Chilla R: Diseases of the Salivary Glands: Pathology-Diagnosis-Treatment-Facial Nerve Surgery. Stuttgart, Georg Thieme Verlag, 1986; 206–211, 219.

13. Neville BW, Damm DD, Weir JC, Fantasia JE: Labial salivary gland tumors. Cancer 1988; 61:2113–2116.

14. Waldron CA, El-Mofty SK, Gnepp DR: Tumors of the intraoral minor salivary glands: A demographic and histologic study of 426 cases. Oral Surg Oral Med Oral Pathol 1988; 66:323–333.

15. Regezi JA, Lloyd RV, Zarbo RJ, McClatchey KD: Minor salivary gland tumors: A histologic and immunohistochemical study. Cancer 1985; 55:108–115.

16. Chau MNY, Radden BG: Intra-oral salivary gland neoplasms: A retrospective study of 98 cases. J Oral Pathol 1986; 15:339–342.

17. Abrams AM, Finck FM: Sialadenoma papilliferum: A previously unreported salivary gland tumor. Cancer 1969; 24:1057–1063.

18. Lever WF, Schaumburg-Lever G: Histopathology of the Skin, 6th Ed. Philadelphia, JB Lippincott Co, 1983; 544–546.

19. Castigliano SG, Gold L: Intraductal papilloma of the hard palate. Oral Surg Oral Med Oral Pathol 1954; 7:232–238.

20. Crocker DJ, Christ TF, Cavalaris CJ: Sialadenoma papilliferum: Report of case. J Oral Surg 1972; 30:520–521.

21. Jensen JL, Reingold IM: Sialadenoma papilliferum of the oral cavity. Oral Surg Oral Med Oral Pathol 1973; 35:521–525.

22. Whittaker JS, Turner EP: Papillary tumours of the minor salivary glands. J Clin Pathol 1976; 29:795–805.

23. Drummond JF, Giansanti JS, Sabes WR, Smith CR: Sialadenoma papilliferum of the oral cavity. Oral Surg Oral Med Oral Pathol 1978; 45:72–75.

24. Freedman PD, Lumerman H: Sialadenoma papilliferum. Oral Surg Oral Med Oral Pathol 1978; 45:88–94.

25. McCoy JM, Eckert EF: Sialadenoma papilliferum. J Oral Surg 1980; 38:691–693.

26. Nasu M, Tagagi M, Ishikawa G: Sialadenoma papilliferum. J Oral Surg 1981; 39:367–369.

27. Wertheimer FW, Bonk K, Ruskin WJ: Sialadenoma papilliferum. Int J Oral Surg 1983; 12:190–193.

28. Puts JJ, Voorsmit RA, van Haelst UJ: Sialocystadenoma papilliferum of the palate. J Maxillofac Surg 1984; 12:90–94.

29. Shirasuna K, Watatani K, Miyazaki T: Ultrastructure of a sialadenoma papilliferum. Cancer 1984; 53:468–474.

30. Rennie JS, MacDonald DG, Critchlow HA: Sialadenoma papilliferum: A case report and review of the literature. Int J Oral Surg 1984; 13:452–454.

31. Bass KD, Cosentino BJ: Sialadenoma papilliferum. J Oral Maxillofac Surg 1985; 43:302–304.

32. Masi JD, Hoang K-G, Sawyer R: Sialadenoma papilliferum of the adenoids in a 2-year-old child. Arch Pathol Lab Med 1986; 110:558–560.

33. Mitre BK: Sialadenoma papilliferum: Report of case and review of literature. J Oral Maxillofac Surg 1986; 44:469–474.

34. Fantasia JE, Nocco CE, Lally ET: Ultrastructure of sialadenoma papilliferum. Arch Pathol Lab Med 1986; 110:523–527.

35. Papanicolaou SJ, Triantafyllou AG: Sialadenoma papilliferum of the oral cavity: A case report and review of the literature. J Oral Med 1987; 42:57–60.

36. Grushka M, Podoshin L, Boss JH, Fradis M: Sialadenoma papilliferum of the parotid gland. Laryngoscope 1984; 94:231–233.

37. Chan KW, Ng WL, Lau WF: Sialadenoma papilliferum. Pathology 1985; 17:119–122.

38. Solomon MP, Rosen Y, Alfonso A: Intraoral papillary squamous cell tumor of the soft palate with features of sialadenoma papilliferum-? malignant sialadenoma papilliferum. Cancer 1978; 42:1859–1869.

39. Eversole LR: Histogenic classification of salivary tumors. Arch Pathol 1971; 92:433–442.

40. Batsakis JG: Salivary gland neoplasia: An outcome of modified morphogenesis and cytodifferentiation. Oral Surg Oral Med Oral Pathol 1980; 49:229–232.

41. Eversole LR, Sabes WR: Minor salivary gland duct changes due to obstruction. Arch Otolaryngol Head Neck Surg 1971; 94:19–24.

42. White DK, Miller AS, McDaniel RK, Rothman BN: Inverted ductal papilloma: A distinctive lesion of minor salivary gland. Cancer 1982; 49:519–524.

43. Batsakis JG, Brannon RB, Sciubba JJ: Monomorphic adenomas of major salivary glands: A histologic study of 96 tumours. Clin Otolaryngol 1981; 6:129–143.

44. Wilson DF, Robinson BW: Oral inverted ductal papilloma. Oral Surg Oral Med Oral Pathol 1984; 57:520–523.

45. Hyams VJ: Papillomas of the nasal cavity and paranasal sinuses: A clinicopathological study of 315 cases. Ann Otolaryngol 1971; 80:192–206.

46. Christensen WN, Smith RR: Schneiderian papillomas: A clinicopathologic study of 67 cases. Hum Pathol 1986; 17:3393–3400.

47. Moskow R, Moskow BS: Inverted papilloma: Report of a case. Oral Surg Oral Med Oral Pathol 1966; 15:918–922.

48. Greer RO: Inverted oral papilloma. Oral Surg Oral Med Oral Pathol 1973; 36:400–403.

49. Abbey LM: Solitary intraductal papilloma of the minor salivary glands. Oral Surg Oral Med Oral Pathol 1975; 40:135–140.

50. Vellios F, Davidson D: The natural history of tumors peculiar to the salivary glands. Am J Clin Pathol 1955; 25:147–157.

51. Kerpel SM, Freedman PD, Lumerman H: The papillary cystadenoma of minor salivary gland origin. Oral Surg Oral Med Oral Pathol 1978; 46:820–826.

52. Sher L: The papillary cystadenoma of salivary gland origin. Diastema 1982; 10:37–41.

53. Goldman RR: Melanogenic papillary cystadenoma of the soft palate. Am J Clin Pathol 1967; 48:49–52.

15

OTHER BENIGN EPITHELIAL NEOPLASMS

Paul L. Auclair, Gary L. Ellis, and Douglas R. Gnepp

CYSTADENOMA

Cystadenomas of the salivary glands are benign neoplasms in which the epithelium demonstrates adenomatous proliferation that is characterized by the formation of multiple cystic structures. The epithelial lining of these structures is frequently papillary. In our experience, cystadenomas are rare and have a frequency of occurrence similar to oncocytomas. Cystadenomas are well described in many other sites, including the ovary,[1] the biliary tree,[2] the appendix,[3] the epididymis,[4] and the pancreas;[5] cystadenomas at these sites share some morphologic similarities with those of the salivary glands.

It is noteworthy that no cystadenomas were included in several of the largest reviews of salivary gland tumors published during the last 50 years.[6-13] There may be several explanations for this, including the relative rarity of the lesion. However, we believe that many investigators have included these tumors under the general heading of *monomorphic adenoma* or consider them to be reactive rather than neoplastic. Chaudhry and coworkers[14] favor this latter assessment of the lesions and prefer the term *intraductal papillary hyperplasia*. Thackray and Lucas[10] suggested that cystadenomas were primarily cystic tumors in which the cyst formation is incidental; therefore, they concluded that these tumors were best classified according to the histologic structure of the solid nodules. Consequently, Thackray and Lucas did not regard cystadenomas as a separate entity.

Cystadenomas have been included in some reports on surveys of salivary gland tumors[15-22] and in many other reports that discuss them alone.[23-34] Nearly all tumors have occurred in the minor salivary glands, although at least two tumors arose in the parotid gland,[15, 34] and one developed in the submandibular gland.[34] Several reports[35-37]

of tumors that involved the larynx have also been published, including one report of a tumor that caused obstruction.[37]

The literature contains a number of conflicting interpretations and inconsistencies in terminology regarding these tumors. Based on published photomicrographs and descriptions, we interpret some cases reported as cystadenomas as more likely to be representative of canalicular adenoma,[20, 29] acinic cell adenocarcinoma,[25] mucoepidermoid carcinoma,[17] papillary cystadenocarcinoma,[26] intraductal papilloma,[30, 32, 34] and reactive ductal hyperplasia.[24, 28, 31] We agree wholeheartedly with those investigators[14, 32, 38] who have observed that some cystadenomas are difficult to distinguish from reactive ductal hyperplasia and metaplasia. In two reports,[39, 40] the terms *cystadenoma* and *papillary cystadenoma* have been used as synonymous with *papillary cystadenoma lymphomatosum* (*Warthin's tumor*). Other investigators[41, 42] have used the term *mucocyst adenoma* for tumors that we consider to be myoepitheliomas.

Several morphologic variants of cystadenomas have been described, including papillary oncocytic,[43] mucous cell,[32] and seromucous subtypes.[33] We include these subtypes under the general heading of cystadenoma and believe that they demonstrate the wide morphologic spectrum. Seifert and colleagues[44] prefer the term *cystic duct adenoma* to the term *cystadenoma* and include this type of tumor under their monomorphic adenoma heading. They also have noted that oncocytic differentiation and papillary structures may be present.

Clinical Features

The Armed Forces Institute of Pathology (AFIP) files contain 196 cystadenomas, and these

Percent

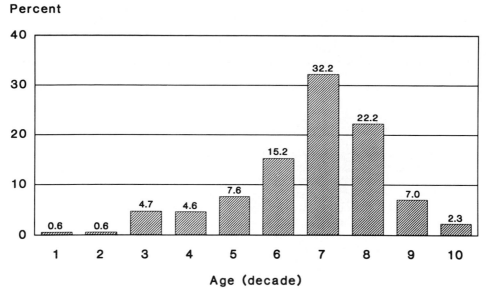

Figure 15–1. Distribution by age (in decades) of 193 patients with cystadenomas included in the AFIP salivary gland registry.

constitute 2.2 percent of all benign epithelial neoplasms. The patients' average and median ages are 53.5 and 55.0 years, respectively, and there is no difference in the average age of males and females. These tumors are most common in the eighth decade of life but are relatively frequent in the sixth through the eighth decades (Fig. 15–1).

If all patients are considered, nearly identical numbers of men and women are affected, but if the bias caused by predominantly male military/veterans is eliminated, there is nearly a 2 to 1 female predilection (96 women versus 53 men). The lesions are widely distributed among major (65 percent) and minor (35 percent) salivary glands (Table 15–1). We have noted a surprising discrepancy between the proportion of AFIP cases that involve the major glands and the few other previously published cases located in these sites.

Table 15–1. Anatomic Distribution of 196 Cases of Cystadenomas from the AFIP Registry

Anatomic Site	Number	Percentage
Major Glands		
Parotid gland	113	57.7
Submandibular gland	13	6.6
Sublingual gland	1	0.5
Minor Glands		
Lip (total)	21	10.7
Upper lip	(10)	(5.1)
Lower lip	(8)	(4.1)
Lip, NOS*	(3)	(1.5)
Cheek	16	8.2
Palate (total)	14	7.1
Palate, NOS*	(6)	(3.1)
Soft palate	(4)	(2.0)
Hard palate	(4)	(2.0)
Tonsil/oropharynx	11	5.6
Retromolar area	2	1.0
Floor of mouth	1	0.5
Other	1	0.5
Not Stated	3	1.5
Total†	196	100

*NOS = not otherwise specified
†Does not include numbers in parentheses

Because we believe that the number of cases in the AFIP files is sufficient to accurately represent the general population, the only plausible explanation involves differences in interpretation of these lesions. We therefore conclude that those lesions of the parotid gland that we consider cystadenomas are interpreted by others as cysts, ductal hyperplasias, or other benign or malignant salivary gland tumors. Our criteria for distinguishing among these are presented later with the discussion of differential diagnosis.

Most of the minor gland tumors are distributed among four sites that include the lips, the buccal mucosa, the palate, and the tonsillar area (Table 15–1). The 69 cases that involved the minor salivary glands constitute 4 percent of benign epithelial minor salivary gland tumors and 2 percent of benign and malignant cases combined. In comparison, Waldron and colleagues[21] reported 20 cystadenomas involving the minor glands that constituted 8.1 percent of the benign tumors and 4.7 percent of all cases in their files.

The minor salivary gland site distribution of this neoplasm is unusual when compared with that of other types of salivary gland tumors. Whereas palatal salivary gland tumors, in general, outnumber those of the lips (2:1) and the cheeks (4:1), cystadenomas involve the lips and cheeks more often than the palate (Table 15–1). Similarly, in the series of 20 cases reported by Waldron and coworkers,[21] 7 involved the buccal mucosa, 5 the lips, and 4 the palate. In the report by Kerpel and colleagues,[32] excluding one case that we considered an intraductal papilloma, there were two tumors in the buccal mucosa, two in the palate, and two in the floor of the mouth.

Cystadenomas of the major salivary glands usually present clinically as asymptomatic slowly enlarging swellings. Minor gland tumors produce smooth nodules that may be compressible. In the series reported by Waldron and coworkers,[21] only 2 of 20 lesions measured greater than 1 cm in diameter. Often, the clinical impression is that the swelling represents a mucocele.

Microscopic Features

The diagnostic histopathologic criteria for salivary gland cystadenomas have received little attention. We disagree with those who define this neoplasm as one in which the pattern of epithelial proliferation is identical to that of a papillary cystadenoma lymphomatosum (Warthin's tumor).[7, 20, 30, 45] Although we agree that the epithelium may occasionally resemble that seen in Warthin's tumor, the histopathology of cystadenomas has a much wider variation in cellular morphology and in the number of possible growth patterns.

The number and the size of the cystic structures vary dramatically among different tumors, but all of these tumors are multicystic. Cystadenomas are frequently well circumscribed and may have a thick, encapsulating band of fibrous connective tissue (Fig. 15–2 A). However, cystic structures are often haphazardly arranged over a background of fibrous connective tissue or salivary gland parenchyma, and evidence of encapsulation may be absent (Fig. 15–2B to D). In these cases, distinction between multifocal involvement and infiltration of surrounding fibrous connective tissue may be difficult and may require careful evaluation of the neoplastic epithelium.

The lining of the cystic structures varies from flattened to tall columnar epithelium (Fig. 15–3), and cuboidal, mucous, and oncocytic cells may all be seen. Rare cases may contain squamous cells (Fig. 15–4). Cystadenomas are usually predominantly or exclusively one type of cell but may infrequently show some variation from one area to the next. The cells show no morphologic atypia, but variation in the thickness and configuration of the epithelial lining may be conspicuous. The lining may be one to three epithelial cells thick and may then abruptly become focally thickened or form ramifying papillary projections with central cores of connective tissue (Fig. 15–4). Papillary proliferation was seen in 130 cases (66 percent) in the AFIP files. It is important to note that extraluminal, solid (noncystic) epithelial proliferation (Fig. 15–5) is usually limited in cystadenomas. Prominent solid growth should arouse suspicion of malignancy.

Some investigators[43] have designated the predominantly oncocytic papillary tumors as papillary oncocytic cystadenomas, a descriptively accurate term (Fig. 15–6). Thirty-two (16 percent) of the 196 cases in the AFIP files showed oncocytic change. It is the histopathology of these tumors that is most reminiscent of Warthin's tumor, especially if a double layer of cells is present; however, evidence of lymphoid tissue is lacking. If mucous cells dominate the cell population of lining epithelial cells, the tumor may be termed a *papillary mucous cystadenoma*.

Several cystadenomas in our files have had prominent lymphoid elements, including numerous germinal centers (Fig. 15–7). The epithelium in these tumors has been thin and predominantly cuboidal with focal squamous areas. Neither the bilayered oncocytic appearance nor the striking papillary growth characteristic of Warthin's tumor was observed.

In one recent case, the cytoplasm of many epithelial cells contained abundant melanin (Fig. 15–8). This phenomenon has been previously reported in a case[30] that we interpreted as intraductal papilloma.

Differential Diagnosis

In our consultative experience, cystadenomas are most often misinterpreted as ductal ectasias or

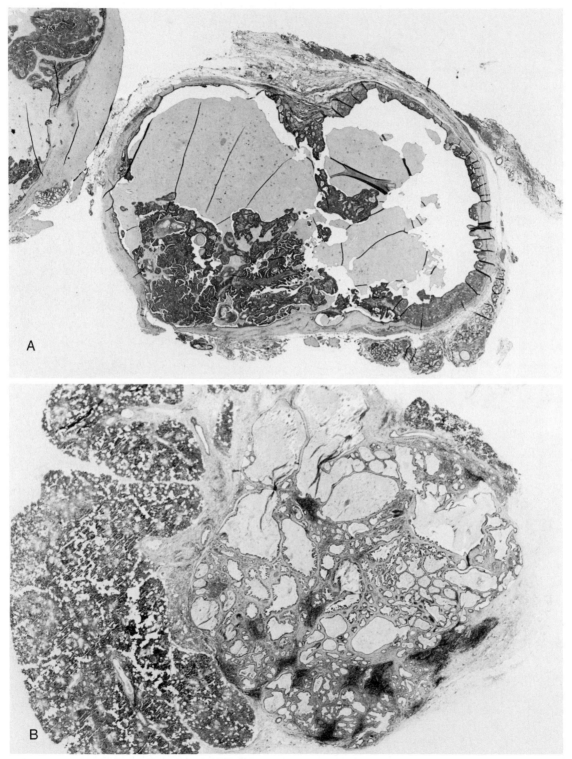

Figure 15–2. Low-power photomicrographs of four different cystadenomas showing multicystic epithelial proliferation. Capsular connective tissue is obvious in *(A)*, whereas in *(B)*, *Continued on following page*

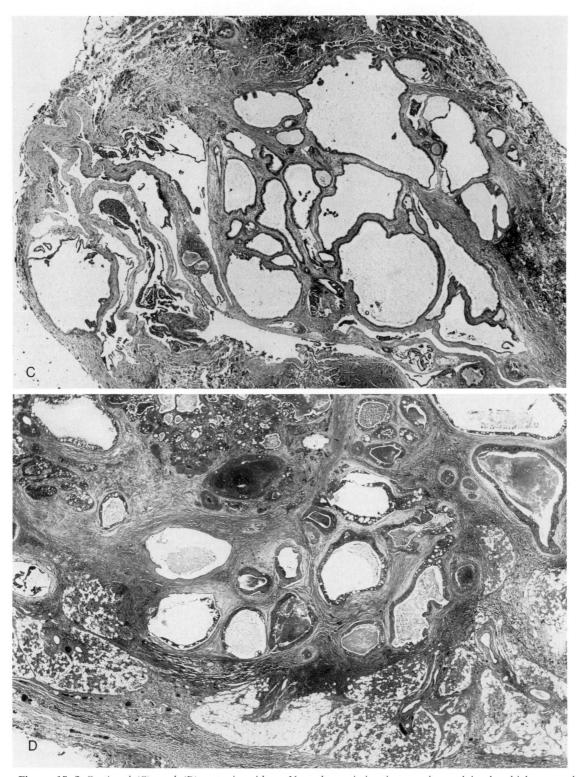

Figure 15–2 *Continued (C)*, and *(D)* none is evident. Note the variation in cyst size and in the thickness and configuration of the epithelium lining these structures (*A*, × 10; *B*, × 10; *C*, × 15; *D*, × 75).

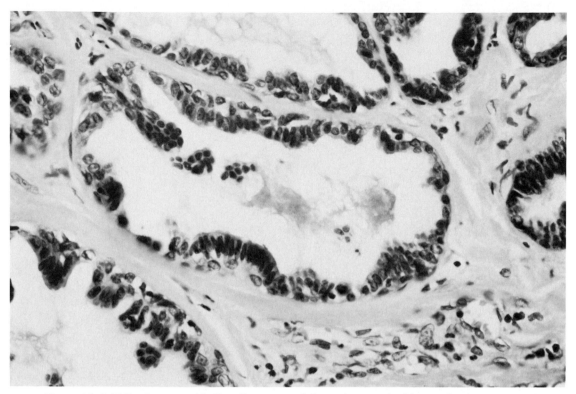

Figure 15–3. Tall columnar epithelium lines many of the cystic spaces in this cystadenoma (× 150).

cysts, Warthin's tumors, papillary cystic acinic cell adenocarcinomas, and mucoepidermoid carcinomas. Distinction from reactive changes secondary to obstruction is often most difficult, and we suspect that some lesions may be etiologically related to obstructive disease. However, the proliferative capacity of the epithelium in cystadenomas cannot be denied and is the most important feature supporting their designation as neoplasms.

Obstructive disease usually manifests fibrosis, acinar atrophy, and chronic inflammation, and the dilated ducts are normally widely spaced. In some cases, the course of the dilated duct is evident within the tissue section. Ectatic ducts and duct cysts rarely show prominent epithelial thickening, and well-formed papillary projections are ordinarily absent or very limited. Although squamous metaplasia may be seen in inflammatory conditions, it is rarely present in cystadenomas. However, in the minor glands in particular, mild chronic sialadenitis may occasionally be associated with cystadenomas, and adjacent tissue may contain ectatic ducts, which suggests a response to inflammation. Nonetheless, although the pathogenesis of these rare lesions remains in question, we do not doubt the neoplastic nature of the vast majority of tumors classified as cystadenomas. Their occasional large size and their ability to displace and to compress normal tissues support this interpretation. Additionally, morphologically

similar lesions in other sites are recognized as neoplastic, and in these sites, as well as in the salivary glands, a malignant counterpart (cystadenocarcinoma) occurs. Cystadenocarcinoma or papillary cystadenocarcinoma should be suspected any time cytomorphologic atypia is seen in the epithelial lining. The presence of extraluminal, solid, noncystic areas suggests the possibility of a cystadenocarcinoma or another malignant tumor and should lead to review of additional sections for infiltration.

As previously noted, cystadenomas show a greater variety of epithelial cell types than Warthin's tumors. Of the 32 cystadenomas that showed oncocytic epithelial cells, 9 were in the minor glands, and 23 were in the major glands, but none contained a lymphoid component. As noted by Fantasia and Miller,[46] if a heavy lymphocytic infiltrate is present, distinguishing among inflamed cystadenoma, obstructive sialadenitis with hyperplastic oncocytic ducts, and Warthin's tumor can be difficult. The epithelium within the few cystic lymphadenomas that we have reviewed does not resemble that seen within Warthin's tumor.

Low-grade mucoepidermoid carcinomas and cystadenomas may share many features and, in some cases, are very difficult to distinguish from one another. Mucoepidermoid carcinomas contain cell types, including epidermoid and basaloid intermediate cells, that are rarely seen in cystade-

Text continued on page 261

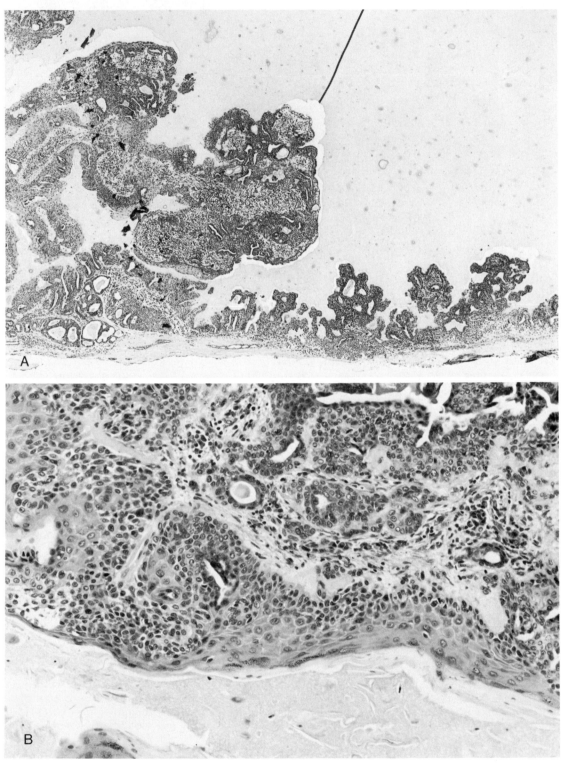

Figure 15–4. *A*, Cystadenoma is shown in which a mixture of cell types form papillae that project into a large central lumen (× 30). *B*, Higher magnification shows focal squamous epithelial lining and a population of smaller cells (× 150).

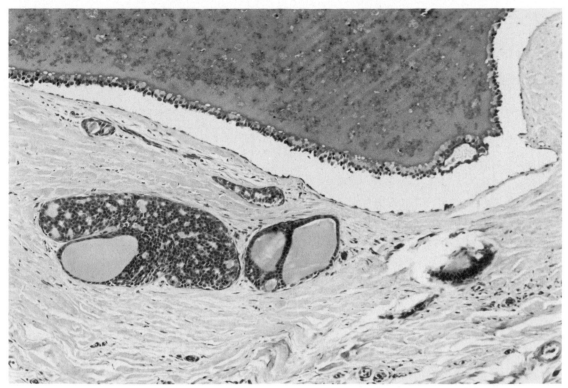

Figure 15–5. Small, solid epithelial proliferation in the wall of a cystadenoma is shown. Note the tendency for cyst formation (× 20).

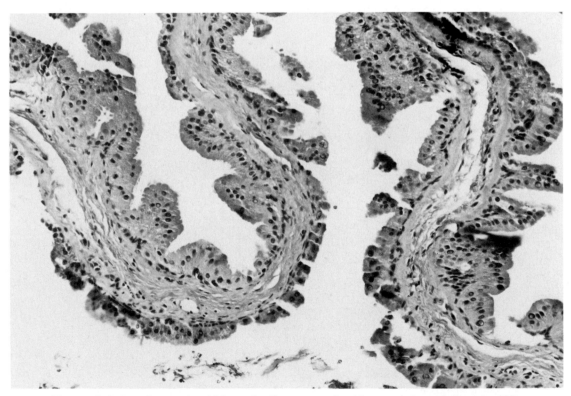

Figure 15–6. Cystadenoma in which nearly all areas were lined by oncocytic epithelium (× 150).

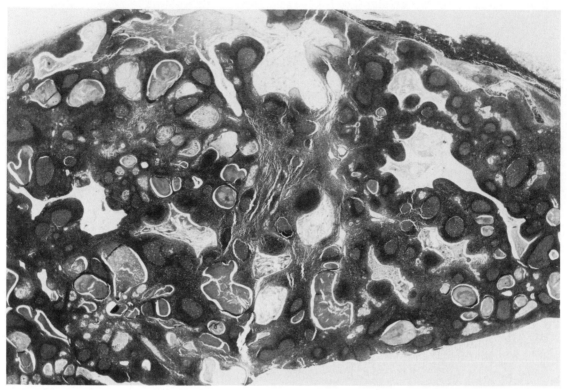

Figure 15–7. Intercystic lymphoid tissue with numerous germinal centers is prominent in this cystadenoma. We have referred to such tumors as cystic lymphadenomas. Uniformly thin cuboidal epithelium with focal squamous areas lines the cystic spaces (× 7.5).

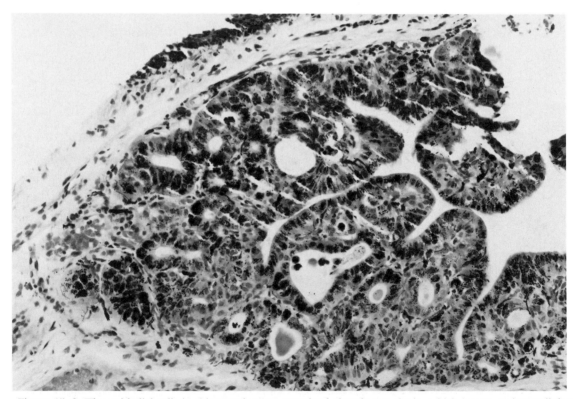

Figure 15–8. The epithelial cells in this cystadenoma contained abundant melanin, which is seen as intracellular and extracellular fine black granules (Fontana, × 150).

nomas. Marked, nonpapillary thickening of cyst lining cells is more characteristic of mucoepidermoid carcinoma, which often has areas of solid, proliferating, extraluminal cords and islands of tumor. If mucous cells are numerous in cystadenomas, they are of uniform size and shape and show no admixture with other cell types. The rare, low-grade mucoepidermoid carcinoma that is composed almost entirely of mucous cells usually contains larger, more irregular mucous cells than those seen in cystadenomas, and the cystic structures that these mucous cells line are found infiltrating beyond the confines of the salivary gland lobule.

Papillary cystic patterns are common in acinic cell adenocarcinomas. These tumors usually display multiple growth patterns, including the microcystic pattern that is characteristic of that tumor but that is not found in cystadenomas. Acinic cell adenocarcinomas also usually show less uniformity of the epithelium that lines the cystic structures, the presence of large serous, acinar cells, at least focally, and numerous solid islands and cords of tumor.

Polycystic disease of the parotid gland (see Chapter 2) is extremely rare but microscopically resembles cystadenoma. Polycystic disease is distinguished by more diffuse involvement of salivary gland lobules and focal apocrine-like lining epi-

thelial cells. Furthermore, congophilic and eosinophilic spheroliths with concentric laminations or radial structures are seen in polycystic disease.

Prognosis and Therapy

No large series of cystadenomas with follow-up information has been reported. At least one recurrence has been reported,[27] but it is not possible to substantiate the diagnosis of that case from the single photomicrograph. As previously noted, misinterpretation of other tumors as cystadenomas has occasionally led to the conclusion that cystadenomas were low-grade malignancies.[25] Data from case reports and from small series as well as the information from the cases in the AFIP files indicate that the likelihood of recurrence is low. Nonetheless, we recommend a conservative surgical procedure that ensures complete removal.

BENIGN SEBACEOUS NEOPLASMS

Sebaceous glands are commonly found in the parotid and submandibular glands and only rarely in the sublingual gland (Fig. 15–9). They were first described in four patients by Hamperl[47] in a

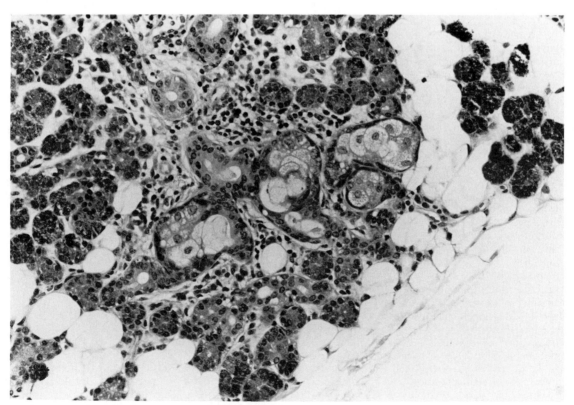

Figure 15–9. Sebaceous differentiation in a parotid gland is visible. Sebaceous foci are commonly associated with intercalated ducts (× 200).

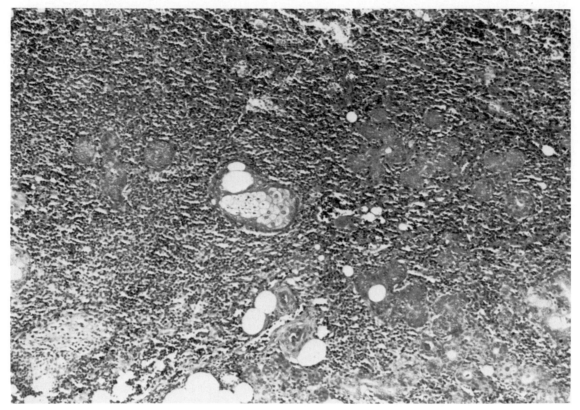

Figure 15–10. Intranodal sebaceous gland in a lymph node removed with a pleomorphic adenoma from the parotid. Note the adjacent islands of ectopic salivary gland tissue (× 100).

review of salivary glands from eighty-five subjects. Since Hamperl's initial description, other authors have described sebaceous glands in the normal submandibular[48–50] and parotid glands.[49–54] The youngest known patient with sebaceous foci in a parotid gland was a 14-month-old male, who was reported by Seifert and Geiler[54] in their series of 604 salivary gland lesions of children. From these studies, it can be concluded that sebaceous glands are normally found in the parotid and submandibular glands.

Sebaceous glands have also been observed in salivary gland tissue adjacent to benign and malignant tumors[50, 52, 55–62] and in inflammatory lesions.[50, 53, 61]

Intranodal inclusions of ectopic salivary gland tissue are commonly found in parotid and periparotid lymph nodes. However, intralymph node sebaceous glandular inclusions have only been described twice before.[50, 63] We have also recently observed a single sebaceous gland in an intraparotid lymph node (Fig. 15–10) in a patient with a pleomorphic adenoma.

Sebaceous glands are commonly found intraorally (in up to 80 percent of individuals) and are known as Fordyce's granules.[64, 65] These collections of sebaceous glands, which are thought to be developmental in origin, appear identical to those found in the skin.

Salivary gland sebaceous neoplasms are classified histologically into five categories: sebaceous adenoma, sebaceous lymphadenoma, sebaceous carcinoma, sebaceous lymphadenocarcinoma, and sebaceous differentiation in other tumors. Although sebaceous differentiation in the parotid and submandibular glands is relatively common, sebaceous neoplasms in these locations are extremely rare. Approximately 137 primary sebaceous tumors of salivary gland origin have been reported in the world literature.[63, 66–86] If we combine these 137 cases with the 11 AFIP cases not previously reported, there are 24 sebaceous adenomas, 39 sebaceous lymphadenomas, 29 sebaceous carcinomas, 3 sebaceous lymphadenocarcinomas, and 53 sebaceous lesions associated with other tumors. For a discussion of the malignant sebaceous tumors, the reader should refer to Chapter 27.

SEBACEOUS ADENOMA

The sebaceous adenoma is a rare, benign tumor that accounts for 0.1 percent of all salivary gland neoplasms and slightly less than 0.5 percent of all salivary adenomas.[86] The mean age at initial clinical presentation for the 23 literature and 1 AFIP

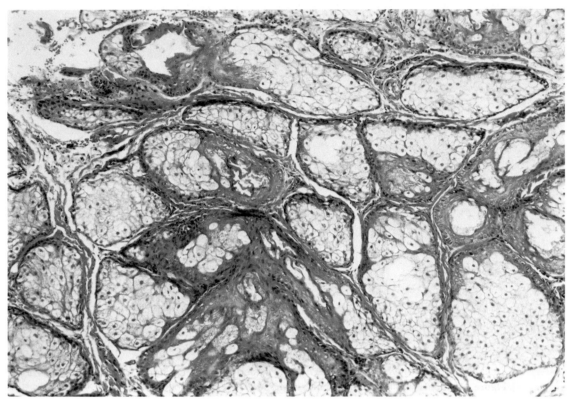

Figure 15–11. Sebaceous adenoma is composed of numerous well-defined nests of sebaceous cells that are surrounded by thin rims of connective tissue (× 100).

cases was 58 years (range 22 to 90 years). Gender information is available for 18 patients; 11 were men, and 7 were women. Twelve tumors were located in the parotid gland, four in the buccal mucosa, two in the submandibular gland, and three in the area of the lower molars or retromolar region. The site of origin is not available in three tumors. The tumors ranged in size from 0.4 to 3.0 cm in diameter.

On gross examination, the tumors are commonly encapsulated or sharply circumscribed, and they vary in color from grayish-white to pinkish-white to yellow or yellowish-gray. These tumors are composed of sebaceous cell nests with minimal atypia and pleomorphism and no tendency to invade local structures (Fig. 15–11). Many tumors are microcystic or may be composed predominantly of ectatic salivary ducts with focal sebaceous differentiation (Fig. 15–12). The sebaceous glands may vary markedly in size and in tortuosity and are usually embedded in a fibrous stroma. Occasionally, tumors demonstrate marked oncocytic metaplasia, and histiocytes and/or foreign body giant cells may be seen focally. Lymphoid follicles, cytologic atypia, cellular necrosis, and mitoses are not observed in sebaceous adenomas. Eight patients were stated to have had total excision of tumor, five a parotidectomy, and one a total sub-

mandibulectomy. The extent of the operative procedure was not recorded in ten cases. Follow-up information ranging from 3 months to 16 years (mean 4.5 years) was available in 13 patients. To date, none of the tumors has recurred.

SEBACEOUS LYMPHADENOMA

The sebaceous lymphadenoma is a rare, benign tumor composed of well-differentiated, variably shaped nests of sebaceous glands and ducts within a background of lymphocytes and lymphoid follicles. There is minimal cytologic atypia and no tendency to invade local structures. Twenty-six (74 percent) of the 35 reported cases and 3 of 4 previously unreported AFIP cases with stated patient age were first diagnosed in the sixth to eighth decades of life (range 25 to 89 years). Gender information was available in 34 patients; 19 were female, and fifteen were male. Thirty-six tumors occurred in the parotid gland or in the area of the parotid gland, and one tumor occurred in the anterior midline of the neck. The site was not stated in two patients.

Tumors have ranged in size from 1.3 to 6.0 cm in greatest dimension. Sebaceous lymphadenomas

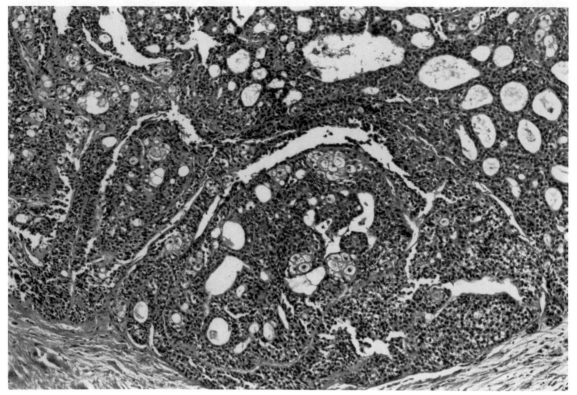

Figure 15–15. Adenoid cystic carcinoma with multiple small areas of sebaceous differentiation (× 100).

cent) and fifteen of the sebaceous lymphadenomas (43 percent) were associated with a foreign body inflammatory reaction to extravasated sebum. This foreign body reaction can be helpful in differentiating these tumors from mucoepidermoid carcinoma. This latter tumor may also be cystic and may contain nests of clear cells; however, foreign body inflammation is unusual in mucoepidermoid carcinomas. In addition, unlike mucoepidermoid carcinoma, which contains intracellular mucin in some clear cells, mucin positivity is never found in the clear sebaceous cells. However, it should be remembered that intracellular and extracellular mucin may be occasionally found within sebaceous tumors in ducts adjacent to sebaceous cells.

Several authors have recently emphasized the association of sebaceous neoplasms of the skin with an increased risk of developing visceral, predominantly colonic, carcinomas.[88, 89] Of the 81 primary salivary gland sebaceous neoplasms with clinical follow-up, only 4 were associated with a second primary carcinoma, and none of these were colonic carcinomas. Therefore, unlike sebaceous neoplasms in the skin, it would appear that there is no associated increased risk of developing a visceral carcinoma in patients with a salivary gland sebaceous tumor.

The origin of sebaceous lymphadenoma appears to be similar to that ascribed to Warthin's tumor by Bernier and Bhaskar.[15] They and others[90] have concluded that Warthin's tumors arise in lymph nodes from ectopic salivary tissue. This argument is strengthened by the description of two tumors with coexisting foci of Warthin's tumor and sebaceous lymphadenoma,[58, 75] the demonstration of normal sebaceous glands intermixed with ectopic salivary gland tissue in three parotid area lymph nodes, and the description of twelve Warthin's tumors with focal sebaceous differentiation. Therefore, it seems logical to conclude that sebaceous lymphadenoma arises from intranodal sebaceous rests.

REFERENCES

1. Scully RE: Tumors of the Ovary and Maldeveloped Gonads, Fascicle 16. Atlas of Tumor Pathology, 2nd Series. Washington DC, Armed Forces Institute of Pathology, 1978; 53–91.
2. March JL, Dahms B, Longmire WP Jr: Cystadenomas and cystadenocarcinomas of the biliary system. Arch Surg 1974; 109:41–43.
3. Wolff M, Ahmed N: Epithelial neoplasms of the vermiform appendix (exclusive of carcinoid): Cystadenomas, papillary adenomas, and adenoma-

tous polyps of the appendix. Cancer 1976; 37:2511–2522.

4. Price EB Jr: Papillary cystadenoma of the epididy-mis: A clinicopathologic analysis of 20 cases. Arch Pathol 1971; 91:456–470.

5. Cubilla AL, Fitzgerald PJ: Tumors of the Exocrine Pancreas, Fascicle 19. Atlas of Tumor Pathology, 2nd Series. Washington, DC, Armed Forces Institute of Pathology, 1978; 100–106.

6. Foote FW, Frazell EL: Tumors of the major salivary glands. Cancer 1953; 6:1065–1133.

7. Evans RW, Cruickshank AH: Epithelial Tumours of the Salivary Glands. Philadelphia, WB Saunders Co, 1970.

8. Woods JE, Chong GC, Beahrs OH: Experience with 1,360 primary parotid tumors. Am J Surg 1975; 130:460–462.

9. Richardson GS, Dickason WL, Gaisford JC, Hanna DC: Tumors of salivary glands: An analysis of 752 cases. Plast Reconstr Surg 1975; 55:131–138.

10. Thackray AC, Lucas RB: Tumors of the Major Salivary Glands, Fascicle 10. Atlas of Tumor Pathology, 2nd Series. Washington, DC, Armed Forces Institute of Pathology, 1974.

11. Eveson JW, Cawson RA: Salivary gland tumours: A review of 2410 cases with particular reference to histological types, site, age and sex distribution. J Pathol 1985; 146:51–58.

12. Spiro RH: Salivary neoplasms: Overview of a 35-year experience with 2,807 patients. Head Neck Surg 1986; 8:177–184.

13. Fitzpatrick PJ, Theriault C: Malignant salivary gland tumors. Int J Radiat Oncol Biol Phys 1986; 12:1743–1747.

14. Chaudhry AP, Labay GR, Yamane GM, Jacobs MS, Cutler LS, Watkins KV: Clinico-pathologic and histogenetic study of 189 intraoral minor salivary gland tumors. J Oral Med 1984; 39:58–78.

15. Bernier JL, Bhaskar SN: Lymphoepithelial lesions of salivary glands. Cancer 1958; 11:1156–1179.

16. Brown RL, Bishop EL, Girardeau HS: Tumors of the minor salivary glands. Cancer 1959; 12:40–46.

17. Bauer WH, Bauer JD: Classification of glandular tumors of salivary glands: Study of 143 cases. Arch Pathol 1958; 55:328–346.

18. Chaudhry AP, Vickers RA, Gorlin RJ: Intraoral minor salivary gland tumors: An analysis of 1,414 cases. Oral Surg Oral Med Oral Pathol 1961; 14:1194–1226.

19. Vellios F, Shafer WG: Tumors of the intraoral accessory salivary glands. Surg Gynecol Obstet 1959; 108:450–456.

20. Whittaker JS, Turner EP: Papillary tumors of the minor salivary glands. J Clin Pathol 1976; 29:795–805.

21. Waldron CA, El-Mofty SK, Gnepp DR: Tumors of the intraoral minor salivary glands: A demographic and histologic study of 426 cases. Oral Surg Oral Med Oral Pathol 1988; 66:323–333.

22. Chau MNY, Radden BG: Intra-oral salivary gland neoplasms: A retrospective study of 98 cases. J Oral Pathol 1986; 15:339–342.

23. Skorpil F: Über das Cystadenoma papillare der grosen und kleinen Speicheldrüsen. Frankfurt Z Path 1941; 5:39–59.

24. Akin RK, Kreller AJ, Walters PJ: Papillary cystadenoma of the lower lip; Report of a case. J Oral Maxillofac Surg 1973; 31:858–860.

25. Brooks HW, Hiebert AE, Pullman NK, Stofer BE. Papillary cystadenoma of the palate: Review of

the literature and report of two new cases. 1956; 9:1047–1050.

26. Chaudhry AP, Gorlin RJ, Mitchell DF: Papillary cystadenoma of minor salivary gland origin: Report of a case. Oral Surg Oral Med Oral Pathol 1960; 13:452–454.

27. Collins EM: Papillary cystadenoma of accessory salivary glands. Am J Surg 1958; 96:749–750.

28. Wilson DF, MacEntree MI: Papillary cystadenoma of minor salivary gland origin. Oral Surg Oral Med Oral Pathol 1974; 37:915–918.

29. Calhoun NR, Cerine FC, Mathews MJ: Papillary cystadenoma of the upper lip; report of a case. Oral Surg Oral Med Oral Pathol 1965; 20:810–813.

30. Goldman RR: Melanogenic papillary cystadenoma of the soft palate. Am J Clin Pathol 1967; 48:49–52.

31. Parnes EI: Papillary cystadenoma: Report of a case. Oral Surg Oral Med Oral Pathol 1966; 21:782–785.

32. Kerpel WM, Freedman PD, Lumerman H: The papillary cystadenoma of minor salivary gland origin. Oral Surg Oral Med Oral Pathol 1978; 46:820–826.

33. Greene GW, Lipani C, Woytash JJ, Meenaghan MA: Seromucous cystadenoma of the oral cavity. J Oral Maxillofac Surg 1984; 42:48–53.

34. Sher L: The papillary cystadenoma of salivary gland origin. Diastema 1982; 10:37–41.

35. Kroe DJ, Pitcock JA, Cocke EW: Oncocytic papillary cystadenoma of the larynx. Arch Pathol 1967; 84:429–432.

36. Donald PJ, Krause CJ: Papillary cystadenoma of the larynx. Laryngoscope 1973; 83:2024–2028.

37. Olesen LL, Spaun E: Obstruction of the larynx caused by an onocytic papillary cystadenoma. Ugeskr Laeger 1989; 151:100.

38. Eversole LR, Sabes WR: Minor salivary gland duct changes due to obstruction. Arch Otolaryngol 1971; 94:19–24.

39. Kuhn AJ: Cystadenoma of the parotid gland and larynx. Arch Otolaryngol 1961; 83:2024–2028.

40. Krogdahl AS, Bretlau P, Hastrup N: Multiple tumours of the parotid gland. J Laryngol Otol 1983; 97:1035–1037.

41. Bhaskar SN, Weinmann JP: Tumors of the minor salivary glands. Oral Surg Oral Med Oral Pathol 1955; 8:1278–1297.

42. Renstrup G, Pindborg JJ: Salivary gland tumors in the palate. Acta Pathol Microbiol Scand 1960; 49:417–425.

43. Cohen MA, Batsakis JG: Oncocytic tumors (oncocytomas) of minor salivary glands. Arch Otolaryngol 1958; 88:97–99.

44. Seifert G, Miehlke A, Haubrich J, Chilla R: Diseases of the Salivary Glands. Pathology-Diagnosis-Treatment-Facial Nerve Surgery. Stuttgart, Georg Thieme Verlag, 1986; 206–211.

45. Peel RL, Gnepp DR: Diseases of the salivary glands. *In* Barnes L (ed.): Surgical Pathology of the Head and Neck. New York, Marcel Dekker, Inc, 1985; 569–570.

46. Fantasia JE, Miller AS: Papillary cystadenoma lymphomatosum arising in minor salivary glands. Oral Surg Oral Med Oral Pathol 1981; 52:411–416.

47. Hamperl H: Beitrage zur normalen und pathologischen histologie menschlicher speicheldrusen. Zeit fur Mikroskopisch Anat Forschung 1931; 27:1–55.

surfaced mass that is often clinically mistaken for a mucocele (Fig. 16–2A). The magenta color of several cases in our files led to the clinical diagnosis of hemangioma or nevus. Mucus may be discharged through a small opening on the mucosal surface, and in these cases, the tumor may be misinterpreted as a draining dental abscess (Fig. 16–2B). Focal erythema or even ecchymosis may be seen. Some mucoepidermoid carcinomas have a granular or papillary surface and are thought to be papillomas or verrucous carcinomas, and we have also seen cases described as hard masses that were clinically interpreted as osteomas or tori. Large lesions at the base of the tongue or in the oropharynx may cause dysphagia, and one patient noted "throat" problems for 20 years before seeking medical attention. Ulceration is associated with lesions which, in most cases, have an aggressive clinical course. Numbness of teeth may occur when bone is involved. Cupping of bone, most often of the hard palate, is seen often enough to justify thorough radiographic evaluation of any mucoepidermoid carcinoma that involves mucosa that overlies bone. As noted previously by other investigators,[71-73] the differential diagnosis of any swelling of the hard or soft palates must include mucoepidermoid carcinoma as well as other salivary gland tumors, and clinicians must be keenly aware that these lesions often masquerade as benign or inflammatory conditions.

PATHOLOGIC FINDINGS

On macroscopic examination, most previously untreated mucoepidermoid carcinomas are relatively well circumscribed. They may appear at least partially encapsulated and, rarely, complete encapsulation is ostensibly noted. Nevertheless, it should be remembered that accurate delimitation of the borders may be difficult or impossible to determine by gross inspection and may, consequently, be seriously underestimated. The cut surface is usually firm and pinkish or yellowish tan. Extreme induration is occasionally present. Cyst formation may be readily evident, but the prominence of this element varies. The majority of the cut surface may be cystic or, more commonly, there may be such haphazard distribution of the cysts that only a fraction of the entire surface is cystic. The cystic spaces contain viscid, translucent mucoid material that may be blood-tinged. Focal hemorrhage is sometimes present and may be striking, particularly if a previous invasive procedure, such as an incisional biopsy or fine-needle aspiration, has been performed.

Cellular Composition

Mucoepidermoid carcinomas are characterized histologically by the presence of a variety of cell types and growth patterns, both of which form the basis for recognition and grading. It is not, however, merely the presence or absence of particular cell types or growth patterns that may help determine the grade of a given tumor but, rather, the proportion of each element relative to the other. As originally intended, the term "mucoepidermoid" emphasizes the presence of mucous and epidermoid cells, but the diagnosis can be established in the absence of epidermoid cells. The recognition of this tumor involves identification of mucous, epidermoid, intermediate, columnar, or clear cells, each proliferating alone or in many different combinations, in a cystic or solid pattern.

Mucous cells are those cells that contain epithelial mucin. Although special stains are required to verify identification of mucous cells in some mucoepidermoid carcinomas, they can often be recognized with only hematoxylin and eosin staining, just as easily as the cells that form mucous acini of normal salivary glands. These latter neoplastic mucous cells have abundant, pale, foamy cytoplasm, are usually relatively large, and may assume round, cuboidal, ovoid, columnar, or goblet shapes. Although easily recognized, they may be confused on low-power microscopic examination with sebaceous cells, seen in rare mucoepidermoid carcinomas. These foamy mucous cells often occur in small clusters or line cystic spaces into which mucin is deposited (Fig. 16–3). In many instances, mucous cells are scattered singly, vastly outnumbered by other cell types or, in high-grade lesions, they may be extremely rare. In some lesions, large edematous squamoid cells may be present that have pale, eosinophilic, granular cytoplasm, and care must be taken not to misinterpret these as mucous cells without histochemical verification. The epithelial mucin produced by mucous and other cell types stains positively for mucicarmine and periodic acid–Schiff and is resistant to diastase digestion. Mucous cells constitute a very limited proportion of most mucoepidermoid carcinomas, and we estimate that less than 5 percent of all cases contain a majority of mucous cells. Tumors with predominant mucous cells are found more commonly in the minor salivary glands.

A population of tumor cells that is often more important than mucous cells for the recognition of mucoepidermoid carcinomas is a group of highly prolific, basaloid cells, referred to as intermediate cells. The term "intermediate" was originally applied to cells that in size and appearance were classified between basal cells and those cells that possessed a more definite epidermoid appearance.[1] Currently, most pathologists use the term to also include the basal cells seen in this tumor, which are sporadically referred to as maternal cells.[21] Intermediate cells demonstrate gradual transitions in sizes from small basal cells, which are slightly larger than lymphocytes and have little to no discernible cytoplasm; to cells having a wide rim of cytoplasm, sometimes more pronounced toward one end of the cell; and finally, to cells

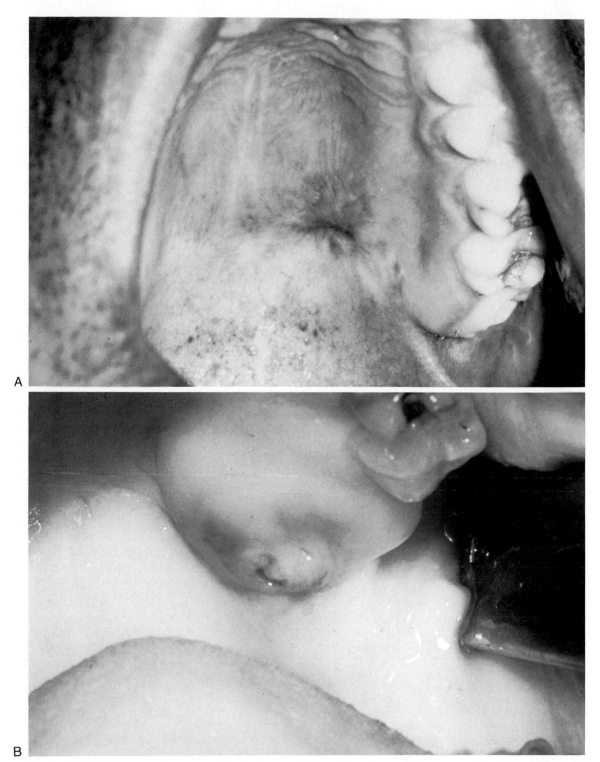

A

B

Figure 16–2. *A*, Common appearance of palatal mucoepidermoid carcinoma. This case was found in a 17-year-old male. The tumor was only slightly elevated and showed a characteristic bluish tinge. *B*, Mucoepidermoid carcinoma in a 52-year-old man. Initially, this chronically draining tumor was clinically interpreted as a sinus related to a dental infection.

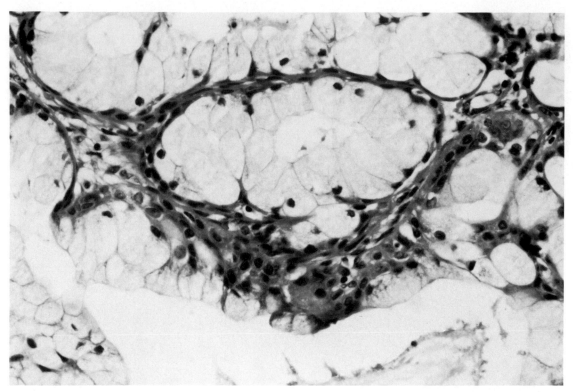

Figure 16–3. Large, foamy mucous cells that are lining either cystic structures or smaller ductal structures (×
300).

with ample, evenly distributed cytoplasm. The
larger forms of intermediate cells are perhaps two
to three times the size of their basaloid predeces-
sor, and further enlargement leads to their interpretation as epidermoid cells. This cellular maturation was originally referred to as "epidermoid
metaplasia."[1] The basaloid intermediate cells are
usually seen in clusters in which transformation
to the more mature forms is readily evident (Fig.
16–4). These smaller basal cells are usually vastly
outnumbered by the larger forms, which apparently have a capacity to further differentiate into
epidermoid, mucous, or clear cells, because the
latter cell types are also frequently present. There
is no clear distinction between the large intermediate cells and the epidermoid cells. As would be
expected, the two cell types are often amalgamated
into solid tumor islands, and they become very
difficult to distinguish from one another. The
cytoplasmic borders of intermediate cells are
sometimes sharply demarcated, notably so in areas
where cells are less cohesive; however, often the
cells have a more syncytial arrangement in which
individual borders can be appreciated only with
difficulty (Fig. 16–5). As basaloid cells mature,
their nuclei enlarge, although this enlargement is
proportionately smaller than their cytoplasmic increase, and the original condensed nuclear chromatin becomes more vesicular. Intermediate cells
may reveal cytoplasmic mucin and diastase labile
periodic acid–Schiff–positive particles that ultrastructural analysis has identified as glycogen.[74]
Dardick and coworkers[75] have suggested that the
majority of intermediate cells represent highly
modified myoepithelial cells that result from tumor induction.

Epidermoid cells, together with intermediate
and mucous cells, line cystic spaces or form solid
masses. Additional differentiation of the epidermoid cells may occur in the form of further
enlargement and the acquisition of distinctly polygonal cell outlines. The epidermoid or squamous
cell zones may be sharply demarcated from the
intermediate cells (Fig. 16–6), or they may blend
imperceptibly with other cells from which they
have apparently originated. Squamous cells only
occasionally form keratin pearls or become individually keratinized, but some degree of stratifi-
cation is normally evident.

Clear cells are large and polygonal and have
sharply defined cytoplasmic borders. In spite of
their clear cytoplasm, they often morphologically
resemble squamous cells, and transition from one
of these cell types to the other is sometimes obvious. Clear cells may dominate large areas of a
tumor, which complicates interpretation. Infrequently these cells contain abundant, demonstrable mucin (Fig. 16–7), but in most clear cells, only
traces are seen focally. Examination of multiple
sections of predominantly clear cell tumors often

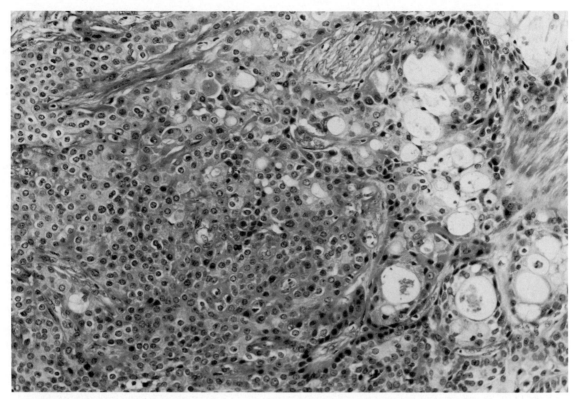

Figure 16–4. Small, basaloid intermediate cells are seen maturing into larger epidermoid cells (× 150).

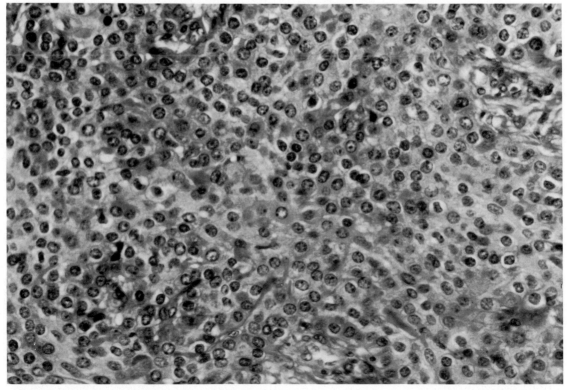

Figure 16–5. This frequently seen syncytial arrangement of intermediate and epidermoid cells illustrates the difficulty of identifying individual cell types (× 300).

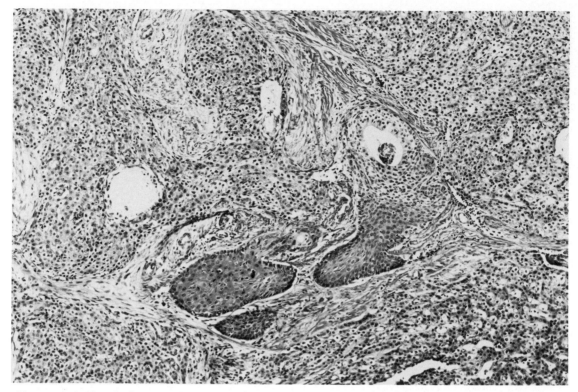

Figure 16–6. Sharply demarcated, large islands of squamous cells are surrounded by sheets of intermediate cells in this field (× 75).

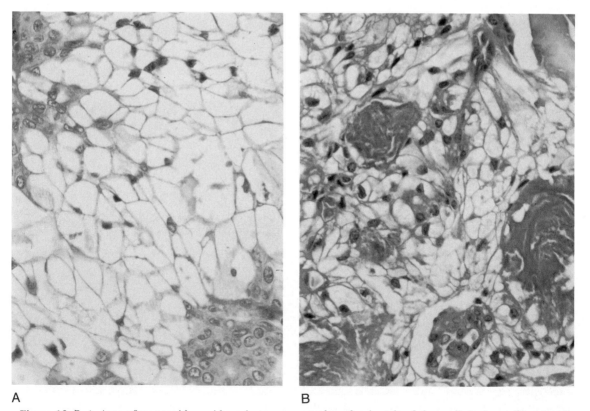

A   B

Figure 16–7. *A,* Area of mucoepidermoid carcinoma composed predominantly of clear cells is shown (hematoxylin & eosin, × 150). *B,* Mucicarmine stain of same tumor reveals presence of intracellular mucin within several clear cells and small pools of extracellular mucin (mucicarmine, × 150).

discloses the more characteristic blend of mucous, intermediate, and epidermoid cells and reveals the true nature of the tumor (Fig. 16–8).

Origin of mucoepidermoid carcinomas from cells of the salivary gland excretory and intercalated ducts has been discussed in Chapter 7. Microscopic sections that fortuitously reveal neoplastic proliferation from a terminal excretory duct support this histogenetic concept (Fig. 16–9). Although these neoplasms are of salivary duct origin, the epithelial element is often accompanied by a mild to moderate, sometimes desmoplastic, proliferation of dense, fibrous stroma. The prominent stroma and the lack of encapsulation may, indeed, make it impossible to determine whether epithelial tumor cells are invading normal peripheral fibrous tissues or if both epithelial and fibrous tissue are components of the neoplasm. This is especially true in tumors of the minor salivary glands, where fibrous tissue normally separates salivary gland lobules. Prominent lymphoid tissue, similar to that seen in acinic cell carcinomas, may also be evident (Fig. 16–10). This feature has led to the mistaken interpretation of primary tumors as metastatic disease and benign lymphoepithelial lesions. As previously noted, mucoepidermoid carcinoma may arise from ectopic salivary gland tissue located in cervical lymph nodes (Fig. 16–11).

Seven cases in our files were interpreted as arising from or as being closely associated with a benign salivary gland tumor, including mixed tumors, Warthin's tumors, and an oncocytoma. The information available is inadequate to establish any meaningful biologic significance in regard to this multiple tumor phenomenon. None of the mucoepidermoid carcinomas in our files were proved histologically to have occurred bilaterally or as separate foci within the same gland, although such phenomena have been reported.[76] Other combinations of unilateral synchronous and metachronous occurrences of mucoepidermoid carcinomas have also been reported.[77–81]

Grading Criteria

Our current understanding and application of grading concepts depend on both our experience and that of others. Although grading mucoepidermoid carcinomas is undeniably subjective, we believe a relatively strong consensus exists among pathologists who use similar criteria. Most differences of opinion involve low and intermediate grades. It is futile, however, to attempt grading unless an adequate amount of properly fixed and stained tumor tissue is available. Small, torn, or artifactually distorted fragments of tumor tissue are best left ungraded.

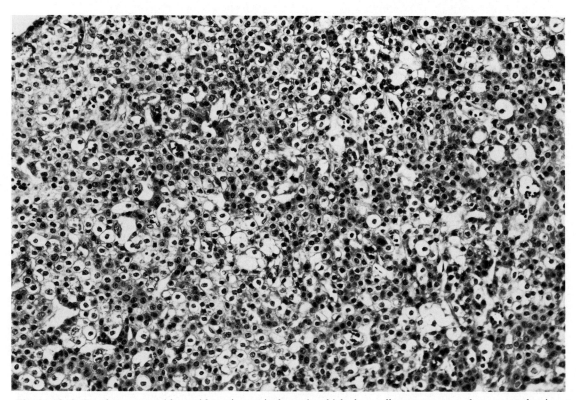

Figure 16–8. Another mucoepidermoid carcinoma is shown in which clear cells are numerous but not predominant and are more intimately associated with intermediate and epidermoid cells (× 150).

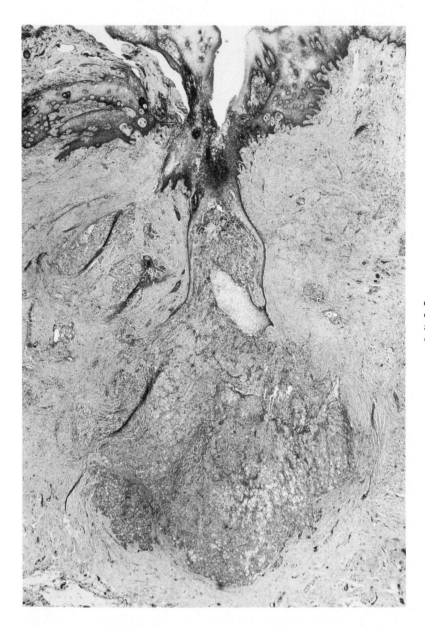

Figure 16–9. Mucoepidermoid carcinoma of oral cavity is shown originating from excretory duct as duct approaches the surface epithelium ($\times$ 15).

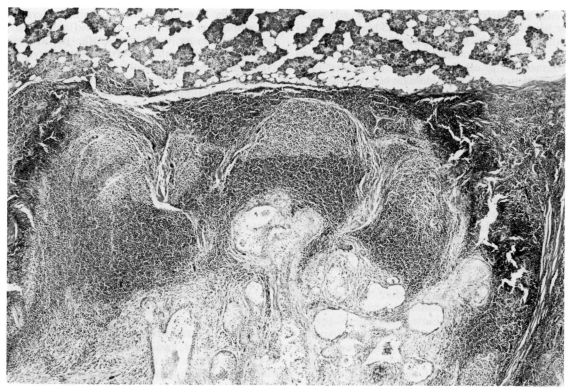

Figure 16—10. Mucoepidermoid carcinomas frequently incite a prominent lymphoid response. Occasionally, this response is misinterpreted as lymph node metastasis. Cases showing this feature have also mistakenly been thought to have arisen from ectopic intranodal salivary gland tissue (× 40).

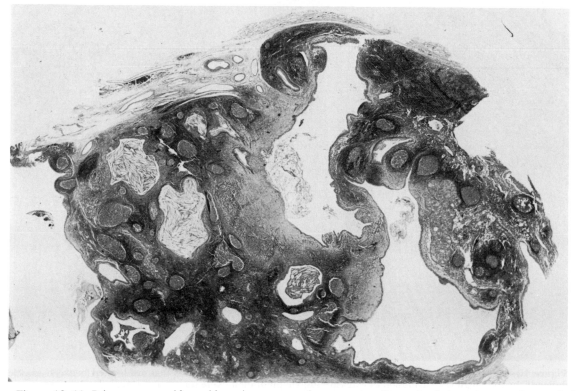

Figure 16—11. Primary mucoepidermoid carcinoma arose from ectopic salivary gland tissue in posterior cervical lymph node (× 7.5).

16–17). Squamous cells may rarely demonstrate keratin pearl formation. Mucous cells are usually readily evident, and mucin stains reveal numerous additional cells that stain positively for mucin. Nuclear atypia is not a necessary feature, but it may be focally evident (Fig. 16–18). Mitotic figures are quite rare, but nucleoli are noted more often in intermediate-grade lesions than in low-grade lesions. The distinction between the low and the intermediate grades is primarily based on the relative proportion of the cystic and solid cellular areas and the predominance of intermediate and epidermoid cells (Fig. 16–19). Intermediate-grade tumors are not a mixture of both low- and high-grade areas.

High Grade

High-grade mucoepidermoid carcinomas are characterized by nearly solid cellular proliferations of epidermoid and intermediate cells, which display a noticeable degree of cytologic atypia. The nuclear-cytoplasmic ratio of many cells is altered. Also, nucleoli are prominent, and mitoses may be numerous.

As discussed by other investigators,[16] high-grade mucoepidermoid carcinomas may show at least two different patterns. The first resembles a moderately differentiated squamous cell carcinoma because of a diffuse proliferation of epidermoid cells, which have a moderate degree of cellular pleomorphism (Fig. 16–20). The presence of glandular or small cystic structures can help separate high-grade mucoepidermoid carcinoma from squamous cell carcinoma but, when absent, histochemical demonstration of cells that test positively for mucin can also be diagnostic. The second pattern is characterized by a variety of cell types that are most often dominated by intermediate cells, but mucous, epidermoid, and squamous cells are often seen. Many cells demonstrate a moderate degree of anaplasia (Fig. 16–21). Assignment of the designation *high grade* depends on the solid, hypercellular proliferation of morphologically abnormal cells. In both patterns, sufficient cellular pleomorphism is present to allow distinction from low- and intermediate-grade tumors, and with either pattern, mitotic activity is usually prominent.

DIFFERENTIAL DIAGNOSIS

The diagnosis of mucoepidermoid carcinoma is based on the identification of a mixture of mucous, intermediate, epidermoid, and in some cases, clear cells; also, low- and intermediate-grade tumors have a characteristic cystic growth pattern. In some tumors, one cell type may dominate, and in

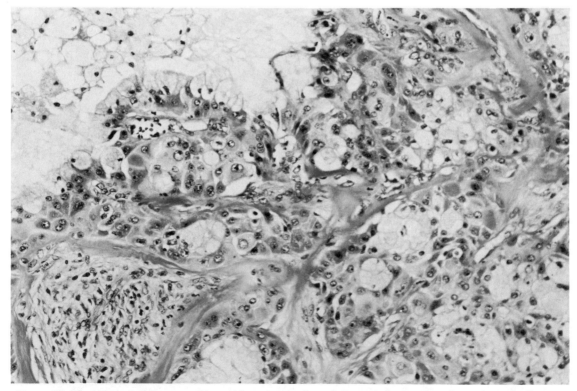

Figure 16–18. Although this mucoepidermoid carcinoma showed some cystic growth and a variety of cell types, a moderate degree of nuclear morphologic alteration makes it an intermediate-grade tumor (× 150).

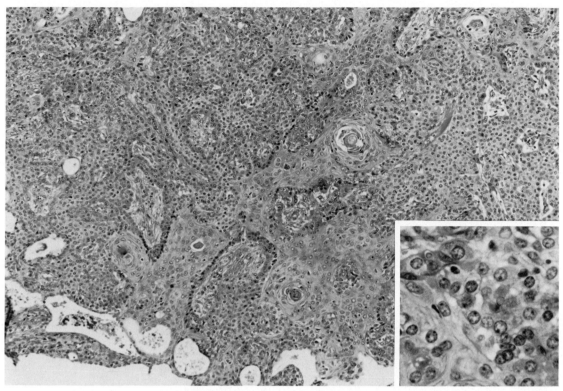

Figure 16–19. Sheetlike growth of intermediate and squamous cells is seen in this intermediate-grade mucoepidermoid carcinoma. Note bland nuclear morphologic character (× 75). *Inset,* × 300.

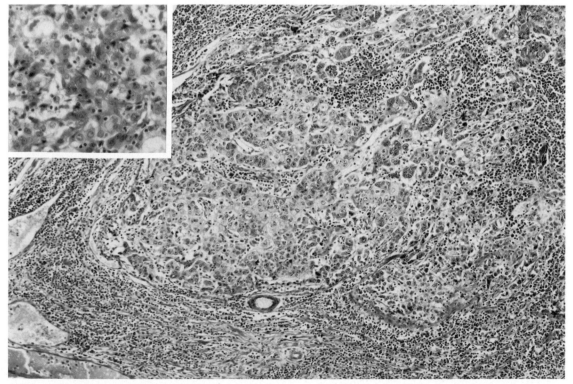

Figure 16–20. This high-grade mucoepidermoid carcinoma resembles a moderately differentiated squamous cell carcinoma. Cytoplasmic mucin was demonstrated in many cells (× 75). *Inset,* × 150.

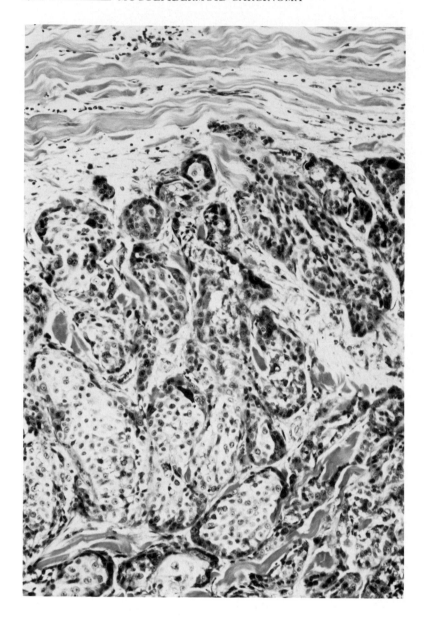

Figure 16–21. This high-grade mucoepidermoid carcinoma is composed predominantly of solid islands of intermediate and epidermoid cells that are focally pleomorphic (× 75).

these cases, review of other areas of the same section or additional sections usually reveals the more characteristic admixture of cells.

Distinguishing low-grade mucoepidermoid carcinomas from cystadenoma may cause considerable difficulty and may be impossible if a generous tissue sample has not been provided. Cystadenomas often have multiple large cystic structures that are lined, in most areas, by a thin layer of cuboidal cells. In contradistinction, the cystic structures in mucoepidermoid carcinomas have a wide range of sizes and are lined, at least focally, by proliferations of several cell types or, rarely, by mucous cells exclusively. Luminal papillary projections may be seen in both lesions, but the cell population characteristic of each is still retained. Mucoepidermoid carcinomas in a few instances

have occasionally appeared to develop from the epithelial lining of cystadenomas; thus, adequate sampling is critical.

Solid, sheetlike proliferations of intermediate cells are sometimes reminiscent of myoepithelial cell zones in mixed tumors. Mucoepidermoid carcinomas do not show the small, well-formed ducts with round central lumina that are characteristically seen in mixed tumors. Furthermore, mucoepidermoid carcinomas demonstrate neither chondroid nor myxoid areas. Occasionally, spillage of mucus may impart a "myxomatous" appearance, but the source of the mucus from a ruptured cyst is usually obvious.

Adenosquamous carcinoma of the minor glands reveals a squamous cell component that focally involves the overlying mucosal epithelium. The adenocarcinomatous component may closely resemble mucoepidermoid carcinoma; thus, the surface epithelium must be evaluated for the presence of dysplastic changes. In addition, intermediate cells are not a feature of adenosquamous carcinoma.

Polymorphous low-grade adenocarcinomas may have cellular proliferations that resemble intermediate cells, and they may produce pools of extracellular mucoid substances. However, the growth pattern of this tumor characteristically demonstrates concentrically arranged cords of tumor cells and prominent perineural invasion, which are both notably rare in mucoepidermoid carcinomas. In addition, polymorphous, low-grade adenocarcinoma does not show epidermoid differentiation, although it may contain focal clear cell areas.

Primary or metastatic squamous cell carcinomas of the major salivary glands can be difficult to differentiate from high-grade mucoepidermoid carcinomas without histochemical staining for mucin. Only in cases in which intracytoplasmic mucin can unquestionably be demonstrated within tumor cells should the diagnosis of mucoepidermoid carcinoma be made. Care must be taken to avoid misinterpreting mucin-positive cells in residual ducts or glands as evidence of mucin-positive tumor cells. In general, primary or metastatic squamous cell carcinomas demonstrate a greater degree of individual cell keratinization and keratin pearl formation than high-grade mucoepidermoid carcinomas.

Some cellular adenocarcinomas, not otherwise specified, and cystadenocarcinomas may resemble intermediate-grade mucoepidermoid carcinomas but lack the characteristic mixed-cell population of mucoepidermoid carcinoma. Similarly, mucoepidermoid carcinoma that is composed predominantly of clear cells focally shows small clusters of epidermoid, mucous, or intermediate cells, which allow this tumor to be separated from clear cell carcinomas.

CLINICAL BEHAVIOR AND PROGNOSIS

Recurrence

The overall recurrence rate of mucoepidermoid carcinoma is about 25 percent, but the value of this figure is relatively insignificant when differences by grade are considered. Thorvaldsson and colleagues,[83] for instance, have reported that the recurrence rate is 10 percent for low-grade lesions but 74 percent for high-grade tumors. Patients are much more likely to have recurrences if the margins of resection are positive, regardless of grade. Healey and colleagues[15] reported that none of 33 low- and intermediate-grade lesions re-

curred when the margins were free of tumor, but 6 of 12 of the same grades recurred when the margins were involved. Similarly, 13 of 16 high-grade lesions recurred when margins were positive for tumor.

Although most tumors that recur do so within 1 year of therapy, there are several cases of low- and intermediate-grade tumors in the AFIP files that recurred, or were reactivated, after much longer intervals; in one case this interval lasted as long as 22 years from the time of the original diagnosis. Delayed recurrences have been noted by others.[12, 15]

Metastasis

The rates of both regional and distant metastases are influenced by the histologic grade, the clinical stage, and the specific site of origin. Spiro and coworkers[12] have observed that metastases to regional lymph nodes appeared to be more frequent from submandibular tumors than from other major or minor gland sites. Although cervical metastases from the minor glands were usually not appreciated at the time of diagnosis, they also noted that over the course of the disease the parotid and minor glands had similar incidences of metastases. Distant metastases, however, occur less often with lesions of minor glands than with those of the parotid or submandibular glands. The distant sites most often involved are the lung, the skeleton, and the brain. No site is spared, however, and we have seen many high-grade tumors that disseminated widely throughout the body. Involvement of the intraparotid lymph nodes is much less significant than regional or distant metastasis.

Survival

Survival is closely related to the clinical stage and the histologic grade. We wholeheartedly concur with those investigators who give consideration to both when assessing prognosis. For staging of minor salivary gland tumors, Spiro and colleagues[12] have used criteria normally applied to squamous cell carcinoma of the oral cavity, the pharynx, the larynx, and the sinuses. Although staging and grading are inter-related, they appear to work independently of each other. Grade I lesions behave less aggressively than grade III lesions, regardless of stage, and conversely, a lower stage lesion has a better prognosis than stage III or IV lesions, regardless of grade.[17] The pathologist and the surgeon together must consider both the grade and the stage when determining treatment and prognosis.

Other factors reported to influence prognosis are the age and the sex of the patient and the site of involvement.[12, 17, 84] Better survival is seen among younger patients and among females. Conley and Tinsley[84] studied 15 patients under 17 years of age and discovered no deaths that were attributable to tumor. Although they concluded that the probability of death for children with this tumor is essentially zero, other investigators[63, 86] have reported aggressive or fatal cases in young patients. The need for thorough tumor removal, even in the younger population, obviously cannot be overemphasized.[62, 85–87] Furthermore, in a study of prognostic factors for all salivary gland tumor types, with the majority being mucoepidermoid carcinomas, univariate and multivariate analyses demonstrated that prognosis for patients over the age of 60 years, regardless of other factors, is significantly worse than that for younger patients.[88] This is probably related to a greater proportion of low-grade tumors in younger patients. Tumors in the submandibular gland and in the base of the tongue generally have a poorer outlook than those at other major and minor salivary gland sites. As might be expected, invasion into bone signifies a poorer prognosis.

The 5-year survival rate of patients with high-grade mucoepidermoid carcinomas is only a moderately meaningful indicator of long-term survival. Hickman and colleagues[89] reviewed the data on 749 patients from 27 reports and listed the 5-year and 10-year survival rates for all grades as 71 and 50 percent, respectively. Others have reported a continual decline in survival over a period of 10 to 15 years.[90] Because death from low-grade tumors is extremely rare, the implication is that intermediate-grade and, especially, high-grade tumors may follow a prolonged course. The experience of Memorial Sloan-Kettering Cancer Center[12] was 5-year, 10-year, and 15-year cure rates of 49, 42, and 33 percent, respectively, for intermediate- and high-grade tumors. Nevertheless, there is evidence from other studies[13, 17, 18, 23, 39, 40] that most deaths will occur before the tenth year after the initial diagnosis, and there is a dramatic reduction in the death rate between the eighth and the tenth years.

TREATMENT

Major Glands

Conservative excision with preservation of the facial nerve, if possible, is recommended for stage I and stage II mucoepidermoid carcinomas of the parotid gland.[12] It appears that, in these circumstances, patients who have partial parotidectomies with clear margins of resection do as well as those who have total parotidectomies.[91] The affected submandibular gland should be removed entirely. Radical neck dissection is performed in patients with clinical evidence of cervical node metastasis and is considered in any patient with a T3 lesion. Elective lymphadenectomy in patients with high-grade lesions but no apparent nodal involvement was deemed worthwhile in one series because occult metastases were found in two-thirds of the patients.[12]

In the past, patients with facial nerve paralysis were considered incurable,[92, 93] but recent studies have shown that this presentation does not necessarily signify incurable disease.[91, 94] Patients were treated by reducing the nerve back to the histologically tumor-negative nerve trunk, and in some cases, this was followed by postoperative radiation. The 5-year disease-free rate in patients receiving this aggressive treatment was about 60 percent.

Minor Glands

Treatment of minor salivary gland mucoepidermoid carcinomas is also primarily surgical. In general, wide surgical excision is recommended, with the goal of ensuring tumor-free margins.[14] The wound is often left open to heal secondarily. If the tumor erodes or invades underlying bone, a portion of the mandible or maxilla should be excised to obtain a margin free of tumor. Mucoepidermoid carcinoma of the retromolar mucosa often involves bone; therefore, this site, in particular, should be evaluated radiographically prior to surgery.

Optimal treatment of lesions of the hard palate remains controversial. Olsen and coworkers[14] state that regardless of tumor grade or size, partial maxillectomy should be accomplished, and Tran and colleagues[73] advocate radical palatectomy and postoperative radiation therapy for high-grade tumors or if margins are questionable. Melrose and coinvestigators[19] believe that treatment involving local excision with a modest margin of clinically normal tissue or, if there is evidence of bone destruction, block removal of underlying bone is adequate for well-differentiated tumors. We and others[33, 95, 96] agree with this latter approach for small, low-grade tumors and suggest, in the absence of bone involvement, wide excision down to periosteum with 1- or 2-cm tumor-free lateral margins as adequate therapy. We know of no previously untreated, low-grade lesion from this site less than 2 cm in maximum dimension that has caused serious difficulty. Several patients who underwent partial maxillectomies for these small, low-grade lesions have written to us to bemoan the misery and the poor quality of their lives over the past 20 to 40 years because of their operation. On the other hand, high-grade and advanced-stage tumors must be treated aggressively at this and other sites. Enucleation of these high-grade lesions is to be condemned.[97]

Indications for neck dissection are similar to those for the major salivary glands, but primary tumors of the tongue are of particular concern, especially lesions larger than 2 cm. In these cases, neck dissection, followed by resection of the primary tumor through the mandible, has been recommended.[14] Lymph node dissection may also be indicated if lymphadenopathy is present in cases of high-grade tumors from any site and in cases with lesions larger than 4 cm.

Radiotherapy

In 1970, Jakobsson and Eneroth[98] considered mucoepidermoid carcinoma as one of the types of salivary gland cancer that was not radiosensitive, but the radiation doses delivered at that time are low if compared to those used today. More recent reports suggest that higher dose therapeutic radiation is beneficial for high-grade and advanced stage tumors and for those tumors that involve the facial nerve.[99–103] The exact role of radiotherapy remains somewhat controversial, in large part because of limited data from large, multi-institutional studies. Additionally, many studies have failed to report results specifically for histologic type, grade, and stage.

Some investigators have recommended postoperative irradiation only for high-grade malignancies, including high-grade mucoepidermoid carcinomas of the parotid glands;[104] however, others[105] have proposed it be routinely used postoperatively for all malignant parotid salivary gland tumors. We do not support this latter view.

In a recent study of tumors in the major glands, including 49 mucoepidermoid carcinomas, Tran and colleagues[91] concluded that adjuvant radiation therapy offered no increase in local control or survival among patients who had surgical excision with margins free of tumor. They noted that radiation may improve local control and survival if residual disease is found at the surgical margins in a patient no longer amenable to surgery, but that radiation therapy was not an adequate substitute for leaving clear surgical margins. The data from studies by Fu and colleagues,[60] King and Fletcher,[106] Chung and coworkers,[107] and McNaney and coinvestigators[108] indicated that 5,000 to 7,000 rad (50 to 70 Gy) of postoperative irradiation given over 5 to 6 weeks may improve the local control rate for cases with gross or microscopic disease at the margins of resection.

There is some evidence that fast neutron radiotherapy may have more success than conventional photon therapy, especially for tumors in advanced stages.[109, 110] One study reported a 74 percent local control rate for patients with unresectable tumors with facial nerve involvement,[110] and some patients maintained function of the facial nerve.

Data defining the proper role of radiotherapy for mucoepidermoid carcinomas of the minor glands are limited. In a study[14] of six patients with minor salivary gland lesions who received radiation therapy at the Mayo Clinic, no tumors regressed, and all the patients died from their disease. Ellis and colleagues[111] studied seven mucoepidermoid carcinomas in advanced stages and reported local control of one with radiation alone and of three others with combined surgery and radiation therapy. Because of the relatively poor prognosis of the base of the tongue lesions, it has been recommended that lesions at that site receive combined surgery and postoperative radiation.[112–115]

The possible late sequelae of radiation therapy, especially when used in younger patients, should discourage its indiscriminate use in the treatment of mucoepidermoid carcinomas. In addition to radiation-induced sarcomas, anaplastic transformation of irradiated mucoepidermoid carcinoma has been reported.[13] Primary therapy should be directed at complete resection of tumor. The information that is currently available supports the view that combined therapy should be reserved for patients with unresectable and high-grade tumors, especially in sites where complete surgical removal is difficult.

Few studies have assessed the role of chemotherapy.[116–120] Kaplan and colleagues[116] and Suen and Johns[117] have suggested that high-grade mucoepidermoid carcinoma may show sensitivity similar to that of squamous cell carcinoma.

CENTRAL MUCOEPIDERMOID CARCINOMAS

Of the 1,701 cases of mucoepidermoid carcinoma in the AFIP files, 61 and 13 cases originated centrally within the mandible and maxilla, respectively. Together they represented 4.3 percent of mucoepidermoid carcinomas from all sites. There are no epidemiologic findings in these 74 patients that are markedly different from the 1,627 cases involving other, more typical sites. The uniqueness of these cases pertains to their origin from sites that do not normally contain salivary gland tissue and to their clinical presentation as radiolucent lesions.

The exact site was specified in 22 patients with mandibular tumors, and, of those, 19 were in the third molar region. The other three mandibular lesions were in the anterior mandible. Of the maxillary lesions, the molar area was most often specified.

Many patients with central mucoepidermoid carcinomas are asymptomatic, and a unilocular or multilocular radiolucent lesion is found during routine dental examination. Several patients whose records are in our files noted a painless swelling and, occasionally, facial asymmetry. Some lesions destroyed a large portion of the jaw, and in several cases the mandibular ramus appeared almost entirely occupied by tumor. Pain was present in about one half of the cases studied by

Gingell and coworkers,[121] and paresthesia and dysphagia occurred rarely.

The radiographic differential diagnosis usually includes dentigerous or other odontogenic cysts, ameloblastoma, and odontogenic keratocyst. Many tumors in our files were associated with impacted third molars (Fig. 16–22A), and a few were seen periapically (Fig. 16–22B). The lesions were most often relatively well circumscribed, belying the true nature of the neoplasm.

A subject that has attracted attention is the pathogenesis of these neoplasms.[122] Sources for the epithelium that gives origin to these central jaw tumors have been theorized as (1) ectopic salivary gland tissue resulting from (a) developmentally entrapped minor salivary glands in the mandibular retromolar area, (b) inclusions of embryonic rests of the submandibular or sublingual glands, or (c) salivary glands displaced from the maxillary sinus lining; and (2) neoplastic transformation of the epithelial lining of odontogenic cysts.

We suspect that origin from entrapped minor salivary glands in either jaw is extremely rare. Ectopic salivary gland tissue is rarely discovered in biopsies of the mandible or maxilla, and in our experience, it is a rarer occurrence than the discovery of mucoepidermoid carcinomas in these sites. Additionally, although a few reports of other types of intraosseous salivary gland tumors do exist, they are exceedingly unusual, and some originated from odontogenic cysts rather than ectopic salivary tissue.[123–128]

Although origin from ectopic salivary gland tissue has not been confirmed, there is direct and irrefutable histologic evidence that some cases arise from the lining of odontogenic cysts. In some cases, transition from cyst lining to proliferating carcinoma has been evident histologically (Fig. 16–23). The pluripotential capacity of odontogenic cyst epithelium is further supported by the frequent occurrence of mucous cell prosoplasia, particularly in dentigerous cysts. Most central mucoepidermoid carcinomas occur in the third molar region of the mandible, which is also the most common location for dentigerous cysts. The lining of these cysts has the capacity to give rise to other neoplasms, including ameloblastomas and squamous cell carcinomas. The inclusion of mucoepidermoid carcinoma as another type of primary intra-alveolar (odontogenic) carcinoma has been suggested.[129] Eversole and coworkers[130] have re-

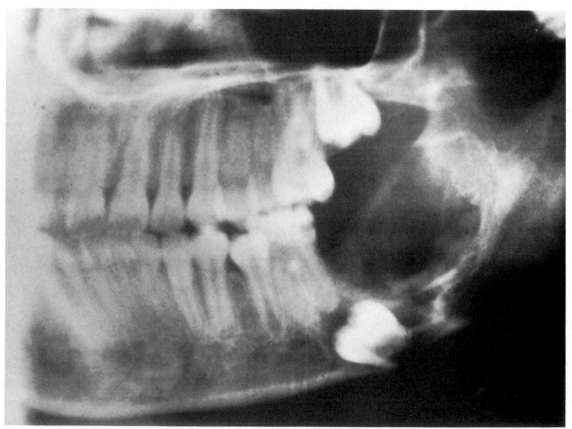

Figure 16–22. These radiographs show mandibular mucoepidermoid carcinomas associated with (A) cyst displacing impacted third molar.

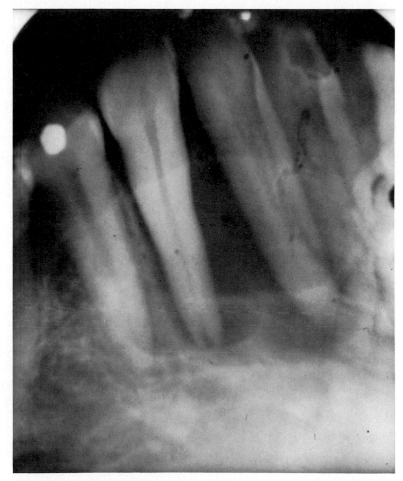

Figure 16–22 *Continued* (*B*) Roots of lateral incisor and canine teeth, mimicking an inflammatory process.

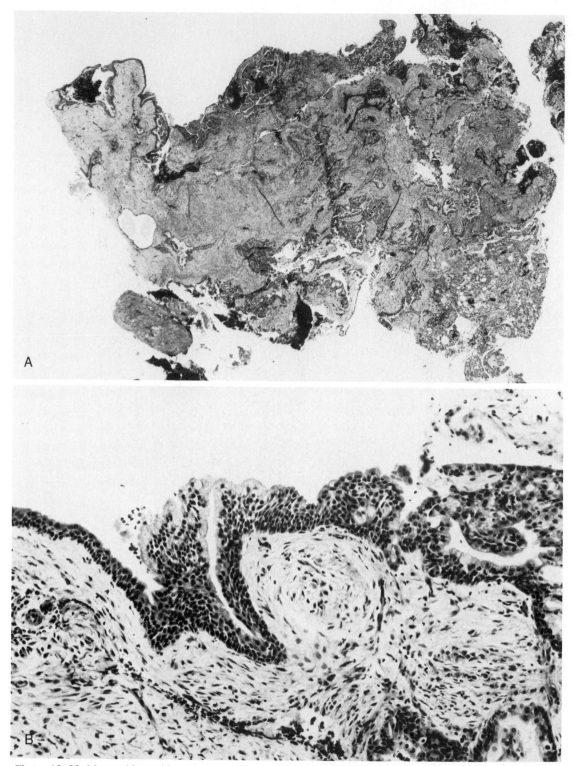

Figure 16–23. Mucoepidermoid carcinoma arising from odontogenic cyst that is associated with an impacted third molar is shown. *A*, Odontogenic cyst lining epithelium is seen along the top left edge of the tissue. Increased epithelial proliferation is present in adjacent epithelium, and infiltrating tumor is seen just to the left of center. Neoplastic islands are seen throughout the connective tissue at right and bottom (× 7.5). *B*, Higher power showing neoplastic transformation of cyst lining. Mucous prosoplasia and focal proliferation of cells that resemble intermediate cells (seen in the center) were in the transition zone between the cyst lining (far left) and the edge of the tumor (far right) (× 150).

ported that nearly 50 percent of central mucoepidermoid carcinomas are associated with a cyst or unerupted tooth.

In one case in our files, the patient had synchronous mucoepidermoid carcinomas of both the mandible and maxilla and was also found to have adenomatous hyperplasia of the palatal salivary glands. Another patient's mandibular mucoepidermoid carcinoma was associated with an ameloblastoma, which illustrates the proliferative and pluripotent capacities of odontogenic cystic epithelium.

Most central mucoepidermoid carcinomas histologically are low-grade lesions, but too few cases with long-term follow-up have been reported to confidently characterize their clinical behavior. En bloc resection with preservation of the inferior border of the mandible has been suggested as proper treatment.[130] More radical surgery for higher grade lesions, possibly including neck dissection, may be indicated. In Eversole and coworkers' study,[130] the recurrence rate was 30 percent and the survival rate at both 2 and 5 years was 100 percent. However, one patient died at 14 years, and at least one other patient was alive with disease at 10 years.

REFERENCES

1. Stewart FW, Foote FW, Becker WF: Mucoepidermoid tumors of salivary glands. Ann Surg 1945; 122:820–844.
2. Lecene P: Adenomes et kystes de la parotide. Rev de Chir, Paris 1908; 27:1–17.
3. Masson P, Berger L: Epitheliomas a double metaplasie, del la partoide. Bull Assoc Franc p L'etude du Cancer. 1924; 13:366–373.
4. Volkmann R: Üeber endotheliale Geschwülste zugleich ein Beitrag zu den Speicheldrüsen- und Gaumentumoren. Deutsche Zeitschrift fur Chirurgie 1895; 41:1–180.
5. De MN, Tribedi BP: A mixed epidermoid and mucus-secreting carcinoma of the parotid gland. J Pathol Bact 1939; 49:432–433.
6. Krompecher E: Üeber den Ausgang und Einteilung der Epitheliome der Speichel- und Schleimdrüsen. Beitrage zur pathologischen Anatomie und zur Allgemeinen Pathologie 1922; 70:489–509.
7. Ewing J: Neoplastic Diseases, 2nd Ed. Philadelphia, WB Saunders Co, 1922; 727.
8. Schilling F: Beitrag zur Kenntnis der Parotidgeschwülstele. Beitr Pathol Anat 1921; 68:139–160.
9. Lang J: Pathologische Anatomie der grossen Kopfspeicheldrüsen. Henke-Lubarsch, Handb. d. spez. Pathol. Anat. u. Histol. Vol 2. Berlin, Julius Springer, 1929; 1.
10. Foote FW Jr, Frazell EL: Tumors of the major salivary glands. Cancer 1953; 6:1065–1133.
11. Rawson AJ, Howard JM, Royster HP, Horn RC Jr: Tumors of the salivary glands: A clinicopathologic study of 160 cases. Cancer 1950; 3:445–458.
12. Spiro RH, Huvos AG, Berk R, Strong EW: Mucoepidermoid carcinoma of salivary gland origin: A clinicopathologic study of 367 cases. Am J Surg 1978; 136:461–468.
13. Evans HL: Mucoepidermoid carcinoma of salivary glands: A study of 69 cases with special attention to histologic grading. Am J Clin Pathol 1984; 81:696–701.
14. Olsen KD, Devine KD, Weiland LH: Mucoepidermoid carcinoma of the oral cavity. Otolaryngol Head Neck Surg 1981; 89:783–791.
15. Healey WV, Perzin KH, Smith L: Mucoepidermoid carcinoma of salivary gland origin: Classification, clinical-pathologic correlation, and results of treatment. Cancer 1970; 26:368–388.
16. Woolner LB, Pettet JR, Kirklin JW: Mucoepidermoid tumors of major salivary glands. Am J Clin Pathol 1954; 24:1350–1362.
17. Nascimento AG, Amaral AL, Prado LA, Kligerman J, Silveira RP: Mucoepidermoid carcinoma of salivary glands: A clinicopathologic study of 46 cases. Head Neck Surg 1986; 8:409–417.
18. Acetta PA, Gray GF Jr, Hunter RM, Rosenfeld L: Mucoepidermoid carcinoma of salivary glands. Arch Pathol Lab Med 1984; 108:321–325.
19. Melrose RJ, Abrams AM, Howell FV: Mucoepidermoid tumors of the intraoral minor salivary glands: A clinicopathologic study of 54 cases. J Oral Pathol 1973; 2:314–325.
20. Bhaskar SN, Bernier JL: Mucoepidermoid tumors of major and minor salivary glands; clinical features, histology, variations, natural history and results of treatment for 144 cases. Cancer 1962; 15:801–817.
21. Sikorowa L: Mucoepidermoid carcinomas of salivary glands. Pol Med J 1964; 3:1345–1367.
22. Eversole LR: Mucoepidermoid carcinoma: A review of 815 cases. J Maxillofac Surg 1970; 28:490–494.
23. Eneroth CM, Hjertman L, Moberger G: Mucoepidermoid carcinoma of the palate. Acta Otolaryngol 1970; 70:408–418.
24. Eneroth CM, Hjertman L, Moberger G, Soderberg G: Mucoepidermoid carcinomas of the salivary glands, with special reference to the possible existence of a benign variety. Acta Otolaryngol 1972; 73:68–74.
25. Glassman LM: The mucoepidermoid tumour of the minor salivary glands. Diastema 1983; 11:11–16.
26. Shrikande SS, Sirsat MV: Histologic differences between benign and malignant mucoepidermoid tumors of salivary glands. Indian J Cancer 1970; 7:200–206.
27. Chomette G, Auriol M, Tereau Y, Vaillant JM: Mucoepidermoid tumors of minor salivary glands. Clinical and pathologic correlations. Histoenzymologic and ultrastructural studies. Ann Pathol 1982; 2:29–40.
28. Jakobsson PA, Blanck C, Eneroth CM: Mucoepidermoid carcinoma of the parotid gland. Cancer 1968; 22:111–124.
29. Gray JM, Hendrix RD, French AJ: Mucoepidermoid tumors of salivary glands. Cancer 1963; 16:183–194.
30. Acetta PA, Evans HL: Mucoepidermoid carcinoma—the real enemy among them. Letter to the editor. Am J Clin Pathol 1984; 82:512–513.
31. Thackray AC, Sobin LH: Histological Typing of Salivary Gland Tumors. Geneva, World Health Organization, 1972.

32. Sharkey FE: Systematic evaluation of the World Health Organization classification of salivary gland tumors. Am J Clin Pathol 1977; 67:272–278.

33. Eversole LR, Rovin S, Sabes WR: Mucoepidermoid carcinoma of minor salivary glands: Report of 17 cases with follow-up. J Oral Surg 1972; 30:107–112.

34. Eversole LR: Glycoprotein heterogeneity in mucoepidermoid carcinoma. A histochemical evaluation. Arch Otolaryngol 1972; 96:426–432.

35. Kumasa S, Yuba R, Sagara T, Okutomi T, Okada Y, Mori M: Mucoepidermoid carcinomas: immunohistochemical studies on keratin, S-100 protein, lactoferrin, lysozyme and amylase. Bas Appl Histochem 1988; 32:429–441.

36. Laudadio P, Caliceti PT, Rinaldi CA: Mucoepidermoid tumour of the parotid gland: A very difficult prognostic evaluation. Clin Otolaryngol 1987; 12:177–182.

37. Eneroth CM, Zetterberg A: A cytochemical method of grading the malignancy of salivary gland tumours preoperatively. Acta Otolaryngol 1976; 81:489–495.

38. Hamper K, Schimmelpenning H, Caselitz J, Arps H, Berger J, Askensten U, Auer G, Seifert G: Mucoepidermoid tumors of the salivary glands. Correlation of cytophotometrical data and prognosis. Cancer 1989; 63:708–717.

39. Jensen OJ, Poulsen T, Schiodt T: Mucoepidermoid tumors of salivary glands: A long term follow-up study. APMIS 1988; 96:421–427.

40. Spitz MR, Batsakis JG: Major salivary gland carcinoma. Descriptive epidemiology and survival of 498 patients. Arch Otolaryngol 1984; 110:45–48.

41. Katz AD: Thyroid and associated polyglandular neoplasms in patients who received head and neck irradiation during childhood. Head Neck Surg 1979; 1:417–422.

42. Katz AD, Preston-Martin S: Salivary gland tumors and previous radiotherapy to the head or neck. Report of a clinical series. Am J Surg 1984; 147:345–348.

43. Spitz MR, Tilley BC, Batsakis JG, Gibeau JM, Newell GR: Risk factors for major salivary gland carcinoma. A case-comparison study. Cancer 1984; 54:1854–1859.

44. Benninger MS, Lavertu P, Linden MD, Sebek B: Multiple parotid gland primary neoplasms after radiation therapy. Otolaryngol Head Neck Surg 1988; 98:250–253.

45. Rice DH, Batsakis JG, McClatchey KD: Postirradiation malignant salivary gland tumor. Arch Otolaryngol 1976; 102:699–701.

46. Ju DM: Salivary gland tumors occurring after radiation of the head and neck area. Am J Surg 1968; 116:518–523.

47. Batsakis JG, Regezi JA: The pathology of head and neck tumors: Salivary glands, Part 1. Head Neck Surg 1978; 1:59–68.

48. Schneider AB, Favus MJ, Stachura ME, Arnold MJ, Frohman LA: Salivary gland neoplasms as a late consequence of head and neck irradiation. Ann Intern Med 1977; 87:160–164.

49. Eveson JW, Cawson RA: Salivary gland tumours. A review of 2410 cases with particular reference to histological types, site, age and sex distribution. J Pathol 1985; 146:51–58.

50. Eveson JW, Cawson RA: Tumours of the minor (oropharyngeal) salivary glands: A demographic study of 336 cases. J Oral Pathol 1985; 14:500–509.

51. Thackray T, Lucas RB: Tumors of the Major Salivary Glands, Fascicle 10. Atlas of Tumor Pathology, 2nd series. Washington DC, Armed Forces Institute of Pathology, 1974.

52. Morgan MN, Mackenzie DH: Tumors of salivary glands. A review of 204 cases with 5-year follow-up. Br J Surg 1968; 55:284–288.

53. Ma DQ; Yu GY: Tumours of the minor salivary glands. A clinicopathologic study of 243 cases. Acta Otolaryngol (Stockh) 1987; 103:325–331.

54. Yu GY, Ma DQ: Carcinoma of the salivary gland: A clinicopathologic study of 405 cases. Semin Surg Oncol 1987; 3:240–244.

55. Bhargava S, Sant MS, Arora MM: Histomorphologic spectrum of tumours of minor salivary glands. Indian J Cancer 1982; 19:134–140.

56. Isacsson G, Shear M: Intraoral salivary gland tumors: A retrospective study of 201 cases. J Oral Pathol 1983; 12:57–62.

57. Fitzpatrick PJ, Theriault C: Malignant salivary gland tumors. Int J Radiat Oncol Biol Phys 1986; 12:1743–1747.

58. Seifert G, Rieb H, Donath K: Classification of the tumours of the minor salivary glands. Pathohistologic analysis of 160 cases. Laryngol Rhinol Otol 1980; 59:379–400.

59. Friedman M, Levin B, Grybauskas V, Strorigl T, Manaligod J, Hill JH, Skolnik E: Malignant tumors of the major salivary glands. Otolaryngol Clin North Am 1986; 19:625–636.

60. Fu KK, Leibel SA, Levine ML, Friedlander LM, Boles R, Phillips TL: Carcinoma of the major and minor salivary glands. Analysis of treatment results and sites and causes of failure. Cancer 1977; 40:2882–2890.

61. Spiro RH: Salivary neoplasms: Overview of a 35-year experience with 2,807 patients. Head Neck Surg 1986; 8:177–184.

62. Castro EB, Huvos AG, Strong EW, Foote FW, Jr: Tumors of the major salivary glands in children. Cancer 1972; 29:312–317.

63. Krolls SO, Trodahl JN, Boyers RC: Salivary gland lesions in children. A survey of 430 cases. Cancer 1972; 30:459–469.

64. Myer C, Cotton RT: Salivary gland disease in children: A review. Part 1: Acquired non-neoplastic disease. Clin Pediatr 1986; 25:314–322.

65. Seifert G, Okabe H, Caselitz J: Epithelial salivary gland tumors in children and adolescents. Analysis of 80 cases (Salivary Gland Registry 1965–1984). ORL J 1986; 48:137–149.

66. Gnepp DR, Heffner DK: Mucosal origin of sinonasal tract adenomatous neoplasms. Mod Pathol 1989; 2:365–371.

67. Neville BW, Damm DD, Weir JC, Fantasia JE: Labial salivary gland tumors. Cancer 1988; 61:2113–2116.

68. Owens OT, Calcaterra TC: Salivary gland tumors of the lip. Arch Otolaryngol 1982; 108:45–47.

69. Goldblatt LI, Ellis GL: Salivary gland tumors of the tongue. Analysis of 55 new cases and review of the literature. Cancer 1987; 60:74–81.

70. Spiro RH, Huvos AG, Strong EW: Cancer of the parotid gland. A clinicopathologic study of 288 primary cases. Am J Surg 1975; 130:452–459.

71. Coates HL, Devine KD, DeSanto LW, Weiland LH: Glandular tumors of the palate. Surg Gynecol Obstet 1975; 140:589–593.

72. Chung CK, Rahman SM, Constable WC: Malignant salivary gland tumors of the palate. Arch Otolaryngol 1978; 104:501–504.

73. Tran L, Sadeghi A, Hanson D, Ellerbroek N, Calcaterra TC, Parker RG: Salivary gland tumors of the palate: The UCLA experience. Laryngoscope 1987; 97:1343–1345.

74. Chen SY: Ultrastructure of mucoepidermoid carcinoma in minor salivary glands. Oral Surg Oral Med Oral Pathol 1979; 47:247–255.

75. Dardick I, Daya D, Hardie J, van Nostrand AWP: Mucoepidermoid carcinoma: Ultrastructural and histogenetic aspects. J Oral Pathol 1984; 13:342–358.

76. Catania VC, Bandieramonte G, Salvadori B: Tumori bilaterali della parotide. Tumori 1975; 61:39–44.

77. Janecka IP, Perzin KH, Sternschein MJ: Rare synchronous parotid tumors of different histologic types. Plast Reconst Surg 1983; 72:798–802.

78. Pontilena N, Rankow RM: Coexisting benign mixed tumor and mucoepidermoid carcinoma of the parotid gland. Ann Otolaryngol 1979; 88:327–330.

79. Tanaka N, Chen W: Muco-epidermoid papillary cystadenoma lymphomatosum: A case of bilateral papillary cystadenoma lymphomatosum (Warthin's tumor) of the parotid complicated with muco-epidermoid tumor. Gann 1953; 44:229–231.

80. Gnepp DR, Schroeder W, Heffner D: Synchronous tumors arising in a single major salivary gland. Cancer 1989; 63:1219–1224.

81. Schilling JA, Block BL, Speigel JC: Synchronous unilateral parotid neoplasms of different histologic types. Head Neck 1989; 11:179–183.

82. Spiro RH, Koss LG, Hajdu SI, Strong EW: Tumors of minor salivary origin. A clinicopathologic study of 492 cases. Cancer 1973; 31:117–129.

83. Thorvaldsson SE, Beahrs OH, Woolner LB, Simons JH: Mucoepidermoid tumors of the major salivary glands. Am J Surg 1970; 120:432–438.

84. Conley J, Tinsley PP: Treatment and prognosis of mucoepidermoid carcinoma in the pediatric age group. Arch Otolaryngol 1985; 111:322–324.

85. Lack EE, Upton MP: Histopathologic review of salivary gland tumors in childhood. Arch Otolaryngol Head Neck Surg 1988; 114:898–906.

86. Dahlqvist A, Ostberg Y: Malignant salivary gland tumours in children. Acta Otolaryngol 1981; 94:175–179.

87. Baker SR, Malone B: Salivary gland malignancies in children. Cancer 1985; 55:1730–1736.

88. O'Brien CJ, Soong SJ, Herrera GA, Urist MM, Maddox WA: Malignant salivary tumors—analysis of prognostic factors and survival. Head Neck Surg 1986; 9:82–92.

89. Hickman RE, Cawson RA, Duffy SW: The prognosis of specific types of salivary gland tumors. Cancer 1984; 54:1620–1624.

90. Rosenfeld L, Sessions DG, McSwain B, Graves H Jr: Malignant tumors of salivary gland origin: 37-year review of 184 cases. Ann Surg 1966; 163:726–735.

91. Tran L, Sadeghi A, Hanson D, Juillard G, Mackintosh R, Calcaterra TC, Parker RG: Major salivary gland tumors: Treatment results and prognostic factors. Laryngoscope 1986; 96:1139–1144.

92. Eneroth CM: Facial nerve paralysis: A criterion of malignancy in parotid tumors. Arch Otolaryngol 1972; 95:300–304.

93. Eneroth CM, Hamberger CA: Principles of treatment of different types of parotid tumors. Laryngoscope 1974; 84:1732–1740.

94. Byun YS, Faos JV, Kin YH: Management of malignant salivary gland tumors. Laryngoscope 1980; 90:1052–1060.

95. Frable WJ, Elzay RP: Tumors of minor salivary glands: A report of 73 cases. Cancer 1970; 25:932–941.

96. Spiro RH: The management of salivary neoplasms: An overview. Auris Nasus Larynx (Tokyo)12 (Suppl II) 1985; 2:S122–S127.

97. Stuteville OH, Corley RD: Surgical management of tumors of intraoral minor salivary glands. Report of eighty cases. Cancer 1967; 20:1578–1586.

98. Jakobsson PA, Eneroth CM: Variations in radiosensitivity of various types of malignant salivary gland tumors. Acta Otolaryngol Suppl (Stockh) 1969; 263:186–188.

99. Connell HC, Evans JC: Mucoepidermoid carcinoma of the salivary glands. Am J Surg 1972; 124:519–521.

100. Guillamondegui OM, Byers RM, Luna MA, Chiminazzo H Jr, Jesse RH, Fletcher GH: Aggressive surgery in treatment for parotid cancer: The role of adjunctive postoperative radiotherapy. Am J Roentgenol 1975; 123:49–54.

101. Reddy SP, Marks JE: Treatment of locally advanced, high-grade, malignant tumors of major salivary glands. Laryngoscope 1988; 98:450–454.

102. Shidnia H, Hornback NB, Hamaker R, Lingeman R: Carcinoma of major salivary glands. Cancer 1980; 45:693–697.

103. Tu G, Hu Y, Jiang P, Qin D: The superiority of combined therapy (surgery and postoperative irradiation) in parotid cancer. Arch Otolaryngol 1982; 108:710–713.

104. Rossman KJ: The role of radiation therapy in the treatment of parotid carcinomas. Am J Roentgenol Radium Ther Nucl Med 1975; 123:492–499.

105. Kagan AR, Nussbaum H, Handler S, Shapiro R, Gilbert HA, Jacobs M, Miles JW, Chan PY, Calcaterra T: Recurrences from malignant parotid salivary gland tumors. Cancer 1976; 37:2600–2604.

106. King JJ, Fletcher GH: Malignant tumors of the major salivary gland. Radiology 1971; 199:381–384.

107. Chung CT, Sagerman RH, Ryoo MC, King GA, Yu WS, Dalal PS: The changing role of external-beam irradiation in the management of malignant tumors of the major salivary glands. Radiology 1982; 145:175–177.

108. McNaney D, McNeese MD, Guillamondegui OM, Fletcher GH, Oswald MJ: Postoperative radiation in malignant epithelial tumors of the parotid. Int J Radiat Oncol Biol Phys 1983; 9:1289–1295.

109. Henry LW, Blasko JC, Griffin TW, Parker RG: Evaluation of fast neutron teletherapy for ad-

vanced carcinomas of the major salivary glands. Cancer 1979; 44:814–818.

110. Catterall M, Errington RD: The implications of improved treatment of malignant salivary gland tumors by fast neutron radiotherapy. Int J Radiat Oncol Biol Phys 1987; 13:1313–1318.

111. Ellis ER, Million RR, Mendenhall WM, Parsons JT, Cassisi NJ: The use of radiation therapy in the management of minor salivary gland tumors. Int J Radiat Oncol Biol Phys 1988; 15:613–617.

112. Kessler DJ, Mickel RA, Calcaterra TC: Malignant salivary gland tumors of the base of the tongue. Arch Otolaryngol 1985; 111:664–666.

113. Devries EJ, Johnson JT, Myers EN, Barnes EL, Mandell-Brown M: Base of tongue salivary gland tumors. Head Neck Surg 1987; 9:329–331.

114. Roper PR, Wolf PF, Luna MA, Goepfert H: Malignant salivary gland tumors of the base of the tongue. South Med J 1987; 80:605–608.

115. Goepfert H, Giraldo AA, Byers RM, Luna MA: Salivary gland tumors of the base of tongue. Arch Otolaryngol 1976; 102:391–395.

116. Kaplan MJ, Johns ME, Cantrell RW: Chemotherapy for salivary gland cancer. Otolaryngol Head Neck Surg 1986; 95:165–170.

117. Suen JY, Johns ME: Chemotherapy for salivary gland cancer. Laryngoscope 1982; 92:235–239.

118. Posner MR, Ervin TJ, Weichselbaum RR, Fabian RL, Miller D: Chemotherapy of advanced salivary gland neoplasms. Cancer 1982; 50:2261–2264.

119. Venook AP, Tseng A Jr, Meyers FJ, Silverberg I, Boles R, Fu KK, Jacobs CD: Cisplatin, doxorubicin, and 5-fluorouracil chemotherapy for salivary gland malignancies: A pilot study of the Northern California Oncology Group. J Clin Oncol 1987; 5:951–955.

120. Belani CP, Eisenberger MA, Gray WC: Preliminary experience with chemotherapy in advanced sal-

ivary gland neoplasms. Med Pediatr Oncol 1988; 16:197–202.

121. Gingell JC, Beckerman T, Levy BA, Snider LS: Central mucoepidermoid carcinoma. Review of the literature and report of a case associated with an apical periodontal cyst. Oral Surg Oral Med Oral Pathol 1984; 57:436–440.

122. Browand BC, Waldron CA: Central mucoepidermoid tumors of the jaws. Report of nine cases and review of the literature. Oral Surg Oral Med Oral Pathol 1975; 40:631–643.

123. Slavin F, Mitchell RM: Adenoid cystic carcinoma of the mandible. Br J Surg 1971; 58:546–548.

124. Breitenecker G, Wepner F: A pleomorphic adenoma (so-called mixed tumor) in the wall of a dentigerous cyst. Oral Surg Oral Med Oral Pathol 1973; 36:63–71.

125. Dhawan IK, Bhargava S, Nayak NC, Gupta RK: Central salivary gland tumors of the jaws. Cancer 1970; 26:211–217.

126. Freedman SI, Van de Velde RL, Kagan AR, Perzik SL: Primary malignant mixed tumor of the mandible. Cancer 1972; 30:167–173.

127. Ito H, Soda T, Asakura A, Nakajima T, Kobayashi Y, Miyazawa M: Central acinic cell tumor of the mandible. Bull Tokyo Med Dent Univ 1970; 17:239–247.

128. Morgan JG, Thoma KH: Mandibular mixed tumor of the salivary type. Am J Orthod 1940; 26:602–605.

129. Waldron CA, Mustoe TA: Primary intraosseous carcinoma of the mandible with probable origin in an odontogenic cyst. Oral Surg Oral Med Oral Pathol 1989; 67:716–724.

130. Eversole LR, Sabes WR, Rovin S: Aggressive growth and neoplastic potential of odontogenic cysts. With special reference to central epidermoid and mucoepidermoid carcinomas. Cancer 1975; 35:270–282.

17

ACINIC CELL ADENOCARCINOMA

Gary L. Ellis and Paul L. Auclair

The existence of acinic cell adenocarcinoma apparently has been recognized for about a century; Nasse,[1] in 1892, described four parotid adenomas composed of cells that closely resembled the normal acinar cells.[2-4] For the first half of the twentieth century, these acinar cell-like tumors were believed to be benign, and such terms as *glandular epitheliomas, adenoma, salivary adenoma, parotid adenoma,* and *serous cell adenoma* were applied.[5-10] In 1953, Buxton and colleagues[10] were the first to ascribe a malignant potential to many of these tumors, which they designated as *serous cell adenocarcinomas;* shortly after this first report, Foote and Frazell[11, 12] and Godwin and coworkers[2] reported series of parotid gland tumors that they classified as *acinic cell adenocarcinomas.* For many years, controversy over the biologic potential of these tumors persisted because some investigators believed that many of the acinic cell neoplasms were biologically benign with only an occasional unpredictable malignancy.[4, 13-16] The term *acinic cell tumor* was often used to indicate the ambiguity in biologic behavior. The argument presented in favor of this terminology stated that classification of tumors as malignant because they only occasionally metastasized was no more correct than classification of tumors known to be highly malignant as benign because they occasionally did not metastasize. The fallacy of this argument is evident from the accumulated reports and studies that document many cases of metastases and death from acinic cell adenocarcinomas. Although the frequency of metastasis is low, it is not rare. At this time, most investigators recognize these tumors as adenocarcinomas with low-grade malignant potential.

In most surveys in the literature since the classification of this tumor in the early 1950s, the acinic cell adenocarcinoma has been the least common of the four most frequently encountered types of traditionally recognized salivary gland carcinomas, which include mucoepidermoid carcinoma, adenoid cystic carcinoma, malignant mixed tumor, and acinic cell adenocarcinoma.[11, 17-28] This comparatively lower rate of occurrence has frequently been observed even in analyses limited to the major salivary glands where acinic cell adenocarcinomas occur most frequently.[17-22, 25, 27] One of the earliest surveys of salivary gland tumors was conducted at New York's Memorial Center for Cancer and Allied Diseases by Foote and Frazell,[11] who studied cases accessioned up to 1949; they found that 2.3 percent of 877 major salivary gland tumors and 7.8 percent of 268 malignant major salivary gland tumors were acinic cell adenocarcinoma. This was compared with an incidence of 36.5 and 12.7 percent of malignant tumors for mucoepidermoid carcinoma and adenoid cystic carcinoma, respectively. However, in this early classification, miscellaneous and unclassified malignancies made up 26.5 percent of the malignant group of tumors. In a subsequent analysis of the Memorial Cancer Center experience that was published 33 years later and is one of the largest series reported, Spiro[27] found that acinic cell adenocarcinomas constituted 3.0 percent of 2,807 salivary gland tumors from all sites and 3.8 percent of 1,965 parotid gland tumors. This was less than the incidences of mucoepidermoid carcinoma (15.7 percent); adenoid cystic carcinoma (10.0 percent); adenocarcinoma, not otherwise specified (NOS, 8.0 percent); and malignant mixed tumor (5.7 percent). However, if only parotid gland tumors were considered, acinic cell adenocarcinoma was more prevalent than adenoid cystic carcinoma and adenocarcinoma, NOS. Other published large series of salivary gland tumors have shown the incidence of acinic cell adenocarcinoma to range from 2.0 to 3.2 percent of all benign and malignant salivary gland tumors,

2.7 to 15.8 percent of all malignant salivary gland tumors, 0.4 to 4.4 percent of all parotid gland tumors, and 1.4 to 20.0 percent of all malignant parotid gland tumors.[11, 15, 17–33] These include studies from the United States,[11, 15, 17–22, 27, 29–31] Canada,[25] Britain,[24] Germany,[26] South Africa,[23] China,[28] and Sweden.[33] Among these series, the number of salivary gland tumors that were reviewed ranged from a minimum of 100 to as many as 2,913 and averaged about 950. The rather broad ranges for the incidence of acinic cell adenocarcinoma may reflect actual variances in incidence among different populations of patients who were seen in different hospitals, institutions, or countries; however, it is more likely that they reflect differences among some pathologists regarding criteria for and/or experiences with the spectrum of histopathologic features of acinic cell adenocarcinoma. The extensive cellular and tissue polymorphism that may be encountered in the histopathologic spectrum of this neoplasm is often not appreciated by pathologists with limited experience in reviewing salivary gland tumors in general and acinic cell adenocarcinomas specifically. On the basis of the cases submitted for consultation to the Armed Forces Institute of Pathology (AFIP), it has been our impression that in regard to diagnosis, our referring pathologists experience more difficulty with acinic cell adenocarcinoma than with any of the other common malignant salivary gland neoplasms.

At the time of preparation of this text, the files of the AFIP contained 886 acinic cell adenocarcinomas among 13,749 primary epithelial salivary gland neoplasms. This is a frequency of occurrence of 6.5 percent. These cases constitute 17.5 percent of the 5,054 malignant epithelial salivary gland tumors in the registry. This compares to a frequency of occurrence among all salivary epithelial malignancies of 34 percent for mucoepidermoid carcinoma, 12 percent for adenoid cystic carcinoma, and 6.5 percent for malignant mixed tumor. A heterogeneous group of adenocarcinomas that were not classified into one of the more specific categories of carcinoma constitutes approximately 17 percent of the malignant neoplasms. Acinic cell adenocarcinoma is the second most common malignant neoplasm of salivary glands in our experience. Why should our rate of occurrence exceed that of other investigators? A couple of explanations would seem to be most likely. First, the AFIP receives consultation material from all types and sizes of hospitals, institutions, and laboratories throughout the United States and around the world within both the military and civilian communities. This collection of cases may be a more representative experience than that of the large therapeutic centers where many of the previous studies originated. On the other hand, since the AFIP is a consultative center, our higher incidence may be indicative of the difficulty encountered in the diagnosis of this

tumor. Actually, both explanations, in part, are probably responsible for the frequency with which we encounter this tumor.

Because of the similarity of many tumor cells to normal serous acinar cells, some investigators have believed that acinic cell adenocarcinomas originate from the serous acini.[4, 34] However, many other investigators have not accepted that these tumors develop by neoplastic transformation and proliferation of functionally differentiated acinar cells.[35–40] The histogenetic theory discussed by Eversole[39] and, later, by Regezi and Batsakis[40] and by Batsakis[41] hypothesizes that the acinic cell adenocarcinoma develops from stem or reserve epithelial cells located at the tubuloacinar terminal of the salivary gland duct unit, that is, the intercalated duct region. Accordingly, the variety of cellular and tissue morphologic features observed in these tumors is a reflection of the neoplastic proliferation of these reserve cells at different stages of differentiation toward the acinar cell. Recent electron microscopic, immunohistochemical, and experimental studies lend some support to this hypothesis.[42–48] In an ultrastructural analysis of two acinic cell adenocarcinomas from the glossopalatine glands, Inoue and coworkers[42] observed serous-type and ductlike cells. Since the glossopalatine glands are pure mucous glands, it is difficult to conceive that this tumor's serous-type cells arose from neoplastic proliferation of differentiated mucous cells. Sato and colleagues[48] and Hayashi and coworkers[47] have shown that intercalated duct cell lines can be induced to transform into acinar type cells that produce acinic cell adenocarcinomas. Nonetheless, Dardick and others[49] have recently found evidence that differentiated acinar and ductal cells are capable of cell division and proliferation and, therefore, could participate in tumorigenesis. Whatever the cell or cells of origin, the important point of these studies is that these tumors manifest multidirectional differentiation with both ductal and acinar type cells.

CLINICAL FEATURES

Consistent with results from previous studies,* the parotid gland was found to be the predominant site of occurrence (83 percent) of the 869 cases of acinic cell adenocarcinoma in the AFIP salivary gland registry in which the site was known (Table 17–1). Only 3.8 percent occurred in the submandibular gland, and 13 percent developed in the minor salivary glands. The buccal mucosa, upper lip, and palate, in that order, are the most frequent minor salivary gland sites of occurrence. Twelve tumors stated to be in the neck and three tumors in the auricular region are presumed to have originated in the parotid gland or, less likely,

---

*See references 15, 18, 19, 21, 23–28, 35, 43, 50–53.

Table 17–1. Anatomic Distribution of 886 Cases of Acinic Cell Adenocarcinoma in the AFIP Registry

Anatomic Site	Number of Cases	Percentage
Major Glands		
Parotid gland	718	81.0
Submandibular gland	33	3.7
Sublingual gland	2	0.2
Minor Glands		
Buccal mucosa	43	4.9
Lip (total)	38	4.3
Upper	(24)	(2.7)
Lower	(8)	(0.9)
Not specified	(6)	(0.7)
Palate (total)	22	2.5
Hard	(7)	(0.8)
Soft	(4)	(0.5)
Not specified	(11)	(1.2)
Tongue	5	0.6
Oral cavity, NOS*	3	0.3
Retromolar	2	0.2
Floor of mouth	1	0.1
Tonsillar area	1	0.1
Mandible	1	0.1
Site not stated	17	1.9
Total†	886	100.0

*NOS = not otherwise specified.
†Does not include numbers in parentheses.

the submandibular gland; however, no normal salivary gland tissue was present in the surgical specimens. The sublingual gland is a rare site of occurrence; only two tumors were located in this gland. The proportion of acinic cell adenocarcinomas in minor salivary glands in our registry is considerably greater than that reported at the Memorial Center for Cancer and Allied Diseases in New York by Spiro and colleagues,[51] but it is the same as that reported by Perzin and LiVolsi.[52] Others have found the proportion of these tumors that occur in minor salivary glands to vary from 0 to 33 percent.* In our experience, acinic cell adenocarcinomas account for about 30 percent of all primary malignancies in the parotid gland, but only 7 percent of submandibular gland, 6 percent of sublingual gland, and 8 percent of minor gland malignant neoplasms. The frequency of minor salivary gland tumors in our series is the same as that reported by Waldron and colleagues[54] but is greater than that described in other investigations of minor salivary gland tumors.[55–58] Only a few studies of minor salivary gland acinic cell adenocarcinomas have been performed.[16, 59–61] In the parotid gland, acinic cell adenocarcinoma is just behind mucoepidermoid carcinoma (33 percent) as the most frequently encountered salivary gland malignant tumor. Gustafsson and Carlsoo[62] have described synchronous acinic cell adenocarcino-

*See references 15, 18, 19, 21, 23–28, 35, 43, 50.

mas of the left parotid and right submandibular glands, and they found 14 examples of bilateral parotid gland acinic cell adenocarcinomas in the literature. However, we believe that at least one of these reports[63] clearly illustrates clear cell oncocytoma[64] and oncocytosis rather than acinic cell adenocarcinomas. We have only one case of bilateral acinic cell adenocarcinomas in our files at the AFIP.

When the male bias of cases involving military personnel and veterans (about 17 percent of cases) is eliminated, women constitute 59 percent of the patients with acinic cell adenocarcinomas in the registry. This is consistent with a female predominance that has been observed by many[2, 3, 21, 22, 24, 35, 51, 65, 66] but not all.[50, 52] Of the patients whose race was recorded, 90 percent were white, and 8 percent were black. At the time of diagnosis, the ages of patients ranged from 3 to 91 years (Fig. 17–1). The mean age was 44 years. Patients under 20 years made up 12.5 percent of the total patients, and the incidence among adult patients was evenly spread throughout the decades of life.

These tumors, which have ranged in size up to 13 cm, are generally less than 3 cm in diameter when excised. Tumor growth is usually slow, although occasional tumors may have a more rapid enlargement. Patients have typically been aware of their tumor masses for less than a year, but some patients have reported being aware of the presence of the lesion for up to 30 years. Swelling, the principal symptom, is noted in nearly all cases; however, pain or tenderness is also experienced rather frequently. Facial nerve paralysis is infrequent but is an ominous prognostic sign.[53]

PATHOLOGIC FEATURES

Gross examination of parotidectomy specimens typically demonstrates that primary (first occurrence) acinic cell adenocarcinomas are mononodular, well circumscribed, and 2 to 4 cm in diameter. However, multinodularity is not infrequent. Some tumors may appear to be encapsulated. In tissue sections, they are grayish white to reddish gray and lack the slimy texture of myxoid-type mixed tumors. They vary in consistency from firm to soft, may be somewhat friable, and may be solid or cystic. The cystic tumors usually have numerous small to microscopic cystic spaces, but larger cysts are occasionally present and may dominate the lesion.

Although the descriptive terminology varies, most descriptions from various investigators are similar and include a wide spectrum of histopathologic features. In 1965, Abrams and colleagues[36] provided one of the classic histologic descriptions of acinic cell adenocarcinomas, which we believe is still applicable; we used Abrams and colleagues' descriptive categorizations for a quantitative histologic analysis and clinicopathologic correlation

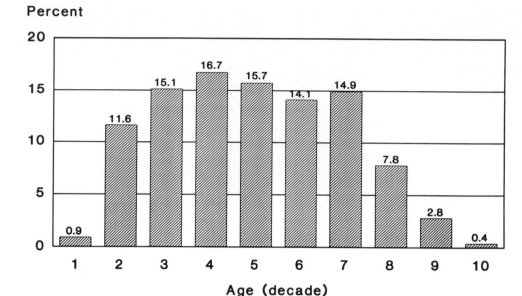

Figure 17–1. The distribution by age of 886 patients with acinic cell adenocarcinoma in the AFIP registry of salivary gland pathology.

of 294 cases.[53] The morphologic growth patterns can be described as solid, microcystic, papillary-cystic, and follicular. The individual cell characteristics can be categorized as acinar, intercalated ductlike, vacuolated, clear, and nonspecific glandular. Any and all of these morphologic patterns and cell types may be seen in any specific tumor. In fact, 45 percent of these neoplasms manifest more than one growth pattern, and it is unusual for a tumor to be composed of only one cell type. Actually, it has been the occurrence of well-differentiated acinar cells in association with these other cell types and morphologic patterns that has enabled us to define the broad spectrum of acinic cell adenocarcinoma.

Obviously, the well-differentiated acinar cell is the basis for the nosologic designation of these tumors as *acinic cell adenocarcinomas*. These cells are usually readily identified by their relatively large size, round to polygonal shape, basophilic to amphophilic cytoplasm, and dark-staining cytoplasmic granules that are similar to those of normal parenchymal acinar cells (Figs. 17–2 and 17–3). The amount of cytoplasmic granules varies from a few to many. The nuclei are round, eccentrically located, darkly stained, and very uniform from cell to cell. Periodic acid–Schiff stain highlights the cytoplasmic granules. The acinar cell is the predominant cell type observed in about 43 percent of the tumors, but some of these cells can be found in nearly all acinic cell adenocarcinomas.

The intercalated ductlike cells are smaller than acinar cells and cuboidal (Figs. 17–3 and 17–4). Their cytoplasm is amphophilic to acidophilic. The nuclei are centrally placed and about the same size as the acinar cells; thus, the ratio of nuclei to cytoplasm is increased. The nuclei also appear hyperchromatic like the acinar cell nuclei. Often, these cells surround small lumina. Intercalated duct cells are the predominant cell type in approximately 32 percent of these neoplasms but can be seen in a very high percentage of cases.

The vacuolated cells are peculiar cells and seem rather unique to acinic cell adenocarcinomas among salivary gland neoplasms. We are not aware of any other type of salivary gland tumor in which vacuolated cells may be so conspicuous. These cells are typically about the size of the well-differentiated acinar cells, although some appear to be distended by the cytoplasmic vacuoles (Figs. 17–4 and 17–5). They have eccentric nuclei that are less chromatic and more pleomorphic than those of acinar or intercalated ductlike cells. If evident, the cytoplasm is amphophilic to eosinophilic. However, the cytoplasmic compartment is punctuated by clear vacuoles that occupy most of the cytoplasm. Several vacuoles or a single large vacuole may be present. Stains for lipids and glycogen demonstrate no material in the vacuoles, but there may be some mucopolysaccharides. The vacuolated cells are most evident in the microcystic and papillary cystic growth patterns, where it appears that many of the cystic spaces may form by rupture of the cell membranes and coalescence of the vacuoles. Although the vacuolated cells are the predominant cell type in fewer than 10 percent of tumors, they are seen in about one third of the neoplasms.

It is our opinion that clear cells in acinic cell adenocarcinomas have been overemphasized.[3, 4, 37, 50] Some of our referring pathologists associate clear cells in salivary gland tumors with acinic cell

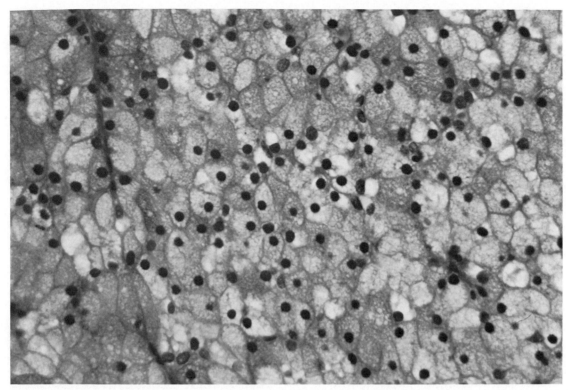

Figure 17–2. This group of moderately well-differentiated acinar type cells in an acinic cell adenocarcinoma of the parotid gland have uniform, dark, round, eccentric nuclei and a basophilic cytoplasm. Occasional cells have cytoplasmic vacuoles (× 400).

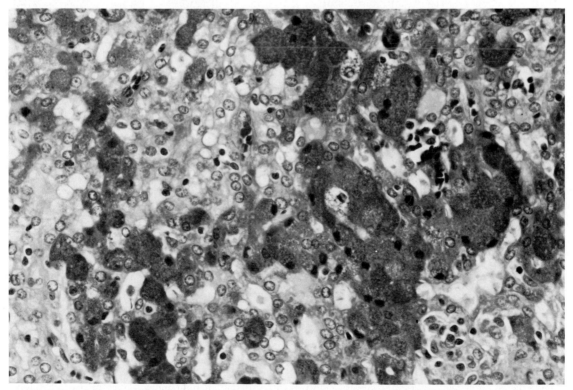

Figure 17–3. The large, dark, granular acinar type cells stand out from the smaller, paler staining, intercalated ductlike and nonspecific glandular cells in this acinic cell adenocarcinoma (× 300).

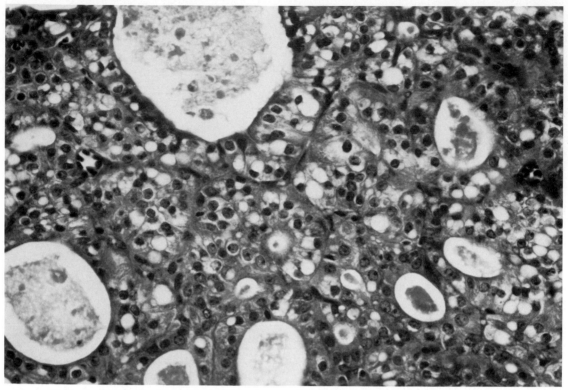

Figure 17–4. In this field, most of the cells appear to be intercalated ductlike cells. They are cuboidal and amphophilic staining. Several lumina are evident, and some cells have cytoplasmic vacuoles (× 150).

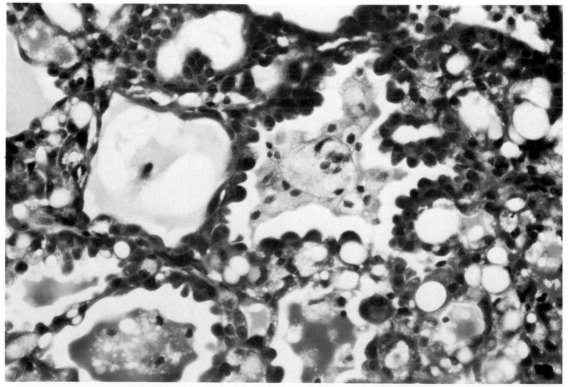

Figure 17–5. High magnification of a microcystic area in acinic cell adenocarcinoma. Many of the lumen-lining cells bulge into the lumina and create a hobnail-like configuration. Variably sized vacuoles distend the cytoplasmic compartment of many cells (× 300).

adenocarcinoma, and when they encounter a salivary gland tumor dominated by clear cells, they incorrectly conclude that it is an acinic cell adenocarcinoma. In our experience, clear cells occur more frequently in mucoepidermoid carcinoma than in acinic cell adenocarcinoma, and epithelial-myoepithelial carcinoma, which is predominantly composed of clear cells, is more common than "clear cell" acinic cell adenocarcinoma. In our studies, clear cells have been found in only 6 percent of acinic cell adenocarcinomas and make up more than one half of the cell population in only 1 percent of tumors. They typically occur in sheets, but they may be seen as isolated cells (Fig. 17–6). They do not appear to be vacuolated cells that have become completely distended with vacuoles, but they have morphologic features more like those of acinar or intercalated ductlike cells that have lost their cytoplasmic staining. Faintly staining wisps of basophilic or amphophilic cytoplasm may be seen in some cells. The nuclei are round and darkly staining.

The nonspecific glandular cells are perhaps the most difficult to describe of the various cell types and are defined by the absence of features that are characteristic of the other four cell types. They usually form a syncytium of cells with indistinct cell boundaries and amphophilic cytoplasm (Fig. 17–7, see also Fig. 17–3). The nuclei are typically larger and more vesicular and pleomorphic than those of the other cell types. Although mitotic figures are infrequent in acinic cell adenocarcinomas, they are most evident in the nonspecific glandular cells. These cells can be found in over one half of all acinic cell adenocarinomas and make up the most prevalent cell type in about 15 percent of these cases.

A solid growth pattern is the most easily recognized morphologic variant of acinic cell adenocarcinoma because it usually contains large numbers of well-differentiated acinar cells and most closely resembles the normal parotid gland parenchyma. In fact, on occasion, a consulting pathologist has misinterpreted this tumor pattern as a glandular hyperplasia or as a normal parotid gland. The absence of striated ducts should distinguish the solid growth pattern of acinic cell adenocarcinoma from normal parenchyma. The solid pattern is composed of sheets of tumor cells that frequently have an organoid configuration (Fig. 17–8). Groups of the tumor's acinar cells are separated and surrounded by very thin fibrous septa that contain small, nearly invisible capillaries. Clear cells often grow in solid sheets also, but they are rarely the dominant cell type. Sometimes these solid tumor masses are surrounded by an ostensible capsule, and this feature surely helped to delude early investigators into interpreting these

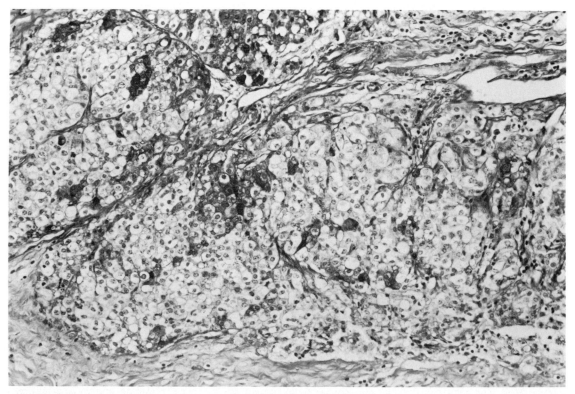

Figure 17–6. A focus of clear cells in an acinic cell adenocarcinoma. In this section stained with periodic acid–Schiff stain the well-differentiated acinar type cells, with their dark cytoplasmic granules, stand out from the clear cells, whose cytoplasm also failed to stain with hematoxylin and eosin (× 75).

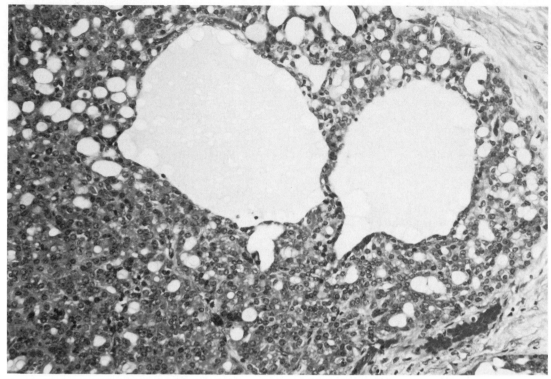

Figure 17–7. An area of nonspecific glandular cells is associated with a microcystic pattern in this acinic cell adenocarcinoma. Unlike acinic, intercalated ductlike, vacuolated, and clear cells, the individual cell boundaries are difficult to discern (× 150).

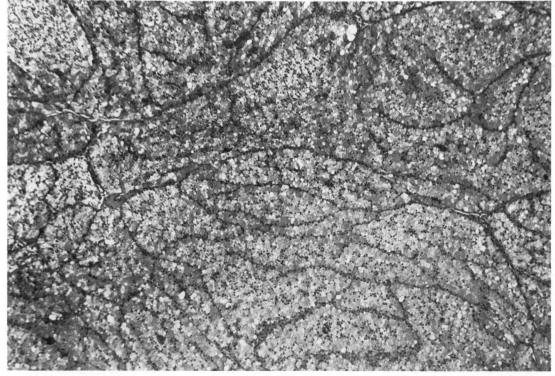

Figure 17–8. This solid growth pattern of acinic cell adenocarcinoma has sheets of well-differentiated acinar cells arranged in irregular organoid formations that are separated by thin fibrovascular septa (× 60).

lesions as being benign. A solid growth pattern is the dominant pattern in around 38 percent of the tumors.

Although the solid pattern may be considered the "classic" pattern of acinic cell adenocarcinoma, the microcystic pattern is actually seen more commonly than the solid pattern. The microcystic pattern is extensive in one third of acinic cell adenocarcinomas and can be found to a lesser extent in nearly another one third of these neoplasms. The microcystic pattern has numerous small cystic spaces, most of which are about three to ten times the size of acinar cells (Fig. 17–9). Well-differentiated acinar cells are still quite frequent and may even be the dominant cell type in this pattern; however, vacuolated and intercalated ductlike cells can also be prominent. Actually, it appears that the microcystic spaces may result from the coalescence of intracellular vacuoles of ruptured cells. Proteinaceous or mucinous material may pool in the microcystic spaces, but papillary projections of tumor cells into the cysts are absent.

The papillary-cystic growth pattern is characterized by one or more cystic structures that contain proliferations of epithelium. The cysts may be small with a few folds of lining epithelium pro-jecting into the lumina. Other cystic structures can be quite large with long stalks, fronds, or masses of glandular epithelium within the lumina (Fig. 17–10). Some of the epithelial projections have thin fibrovascular cores, whereas others appear to be masses of epithelium without apparent supporting stroma. These epithelial proliferations can vary in thickness from just a few cells to many cells and may assume a cystic or microcystic appearance of their own. Intercalated ductlike and nonspecific glandular cells usually predominate; however, vacuolated cells are often numerous, and acinar cells can be seen. The apical portions of many of the lumen-lining cells bulge into the lumen and produce a tombstone or hobnail-like conformation (see Fig. 17–5). Occasionally, these tumors present as single cysts that are lined by cuboidal epithelium with scattered papillary projections. In these cases, the tumors give the impression that they may have arisen from the epithelial lining of parotid cysts. The papillary-cystic pattern occurs less frequently than the microcystic or solid growth pattern, and since well-differentiated acinar cells are frequently not conspicuous, we have found this configuration often to be difficult for pathologists to recognize as acinic cell adenocarcinoma.

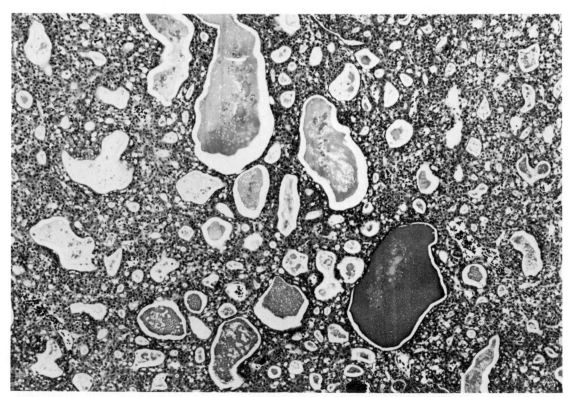

Figure 17–9. Microcystic pattern is characterized by numerous very small but variably sized spaces within the epithelial cell proliferation. A few of the larger cysts contain an amorphous, eosinophilic material that is reminiscent of thyroid follicles. In this particular case, most of the tumor cells appear to be intercalated ductlike and nonspecific glandular cells. In other tumors, acinar-type cells can be dominant in the microcystic pattern (× 75).

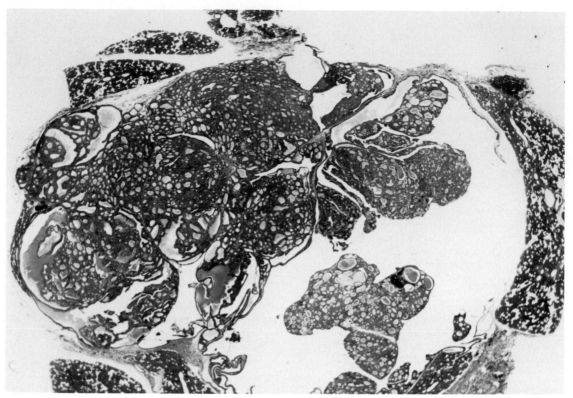

Figure 17–10. Several contiguous, large cystic structures contain papillary masses of tumor cells in this example of the papillary-cystic growth pattern. Some of the individual tumor masses appear to have a follicular configuration (× 7.5).

The follicular pattern of acinic cell adenocarcinoma is the least frequently encountered. It is observed in only 10 percent of acinic cell adenocarcinomas, and it is the dominant pattern in only about one half of those. This pattern has a definite thyroidlike appearance (Figs. 17–9 to 17–11). Variable-sized, ovoid to round cystic spaces are lined by cuboidal to low columnar epithelial cells. Many of the cystic spaces contain an eosinophilic proteinaceous material that simulates the appearance of colloid. The intercystic areas are usually occupied by epithelial cells that are mostly nonspecific glandular cells with some vacuolated and acinic type cells.

One of the curious features of acinic cell adenocarcinomas is their frequent association with a lymphoid infiltrate in the supporting stroma. Although this feature has frequently been described in the literature,[2, 3, 4, 35, 36, 65] we have found that some pathologists can be perplexed by this lymphoid tissue. This infiltrate is not just a scattering of inflammatory cells but a dense collection of lymphocytes in which even germinal centers may be evident (Fig. 17–12). If the tumor is well circumscribed, the lymphoid pattern suggests that the acinic cell adenocarcinoma has arisen within an intraparotid lymph node. Although, in some cases, this may actually be the truth, in most cases,

the lymphoid stroma accompanies the infiltrating carcinoma into the adjacent parotid parenchyma and tissues, much like a lymphoepithelial lesion. The extent of the infiltrate can vary from focal to diffuse. In fact, in one tumor that was composed predominantly of well-differentiated acinar cells, the lymphoid infiltrate was so extensive that the referring pathologist was led to misinterpret the lesion as a lymphoma infiltrating normal parotid parenchyma.

As we have already stated, on gross examination many of these tumors are well circumscribed, but microscopic examination demonstrates that most are infiltrative. However, even microscopically it is not rare for these tumors to be well circumscribed, and some even appear encapsulated, which tends to impugn their malignant potential. About one half of the tumors have a fine vascularized fibrous connective stroma, whereas the rest have areas of collagenization that may produce extensive hyalinization in a few tumors. Prominent vascularity and hemorrhage may be associated with some of the collagenous regions. Psammoma-type calcifications, similar to those seen in thyroid papillary carcinoma, are occasionally found.

Stanley and colleagues[67] have reported six cases that had histopathologic features of acinic cell adenocarcinoma associated with poorly differen-

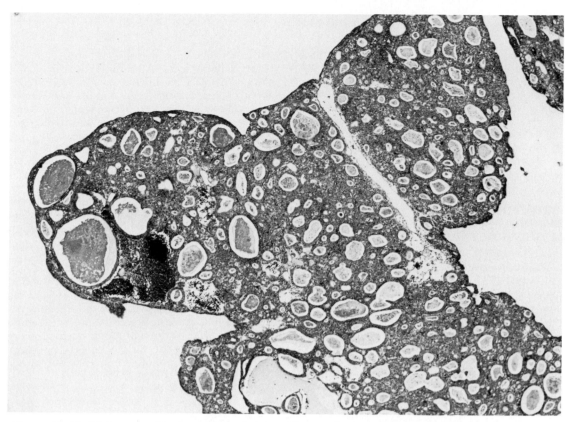

Figure 17–11. Higher magnification of one of the papillary projections seen in Figure 17–10 reveals that the tumor cells surround many small cystic spaces that contain an eosinophilic precipitate. This so-called follicular pattern resembles thyroid follicular tissue (× 30).

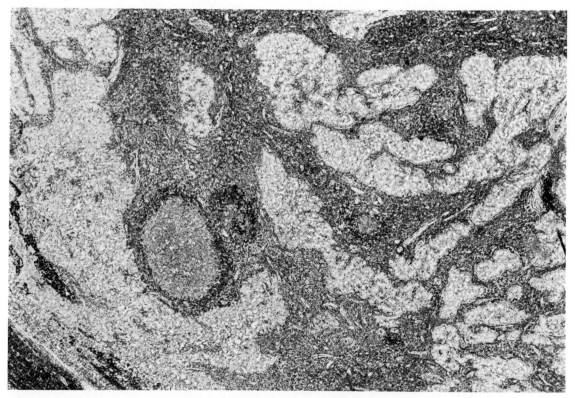

Figure 17–12. Irregularly shaped islands and masses of acinic cell adenocarcinoma are surrounded by an intense lymphoid infiltrate, which even has a focal germinal center (lower left). Although this lymphoid stroma may suggest that this tumor arose in or metastasized to a lymph node, in many cases the lymphoid tissue accompanies the adenocarcinoma as it infiltrates adjacent tissue and parotid parenchyma (× 30).

tiated carcinoma in the same tumor. We also have had experience with two similar cases (Fig. 17–13). Whether these cases are examples of collision tumors or represent dedifferentiation of a clone of cells within the acinic cell adenocarcinoma is speculative; however, we would recommend that therapeutic considerations in these cases be made on the basis of the high-grade poorly differentiated carcinoma.

HISTOCHEMISTRY, IMMUNOHISTOCHEMISTRY, AND ULTRASTRUCTURE

As already mentioned, staining with periodic acid–Schiff (PAS) stain for cytoplasmic granules may be helpful in the identification of well-differentiated acinar cells in tumors in which they are not conspicuous; however, once an appreciation for the morphologic spectrum of acinic cell adenocarcinomas is developed, it is usually not necessary. Periodic acid–Schiff stain also demonstrates the neutral mucopolysaccharides that may be present in many of the cystic and microcystic

structures. Diastase digestion of tissue sections before staining with PAS shows that little or none of the PAS reactivity is due to glycogen. This is also true for the clear cell regions and demonstrates that the clear cytoplasm seen with hematoxylin and eosin staining is not due to glycogen. Stains for salivary mucus, like mucicarmine and alcian blue, are usually negative in the solid areas of the tumors but may show some reactivity in the cystic, microcystic, and vacuolated areas. Usually, this staining is not very intense in contrast to the deeply stained mucous cells in mucoepidermoid carcinomas, and most of the mucinous material is seen extracellularly. The presence of some mucinous material does not preclude a diagnosis of acinic cell adenocarcinoma.

Some of the immunohistochemical studies of acinic cell adenocarcinomas reported in the literature have been somewhat contradictory, and caution should be exercised when interpreting the results of immunohistochemistry.[45, 46, 68–79] We have found that the use of immunohistochemistry to distinguish among the various types of parenchymal salivary gland tumors is not really worthwhile. As an example, it is a good idea to keep in mind that cells with both ductal and myoepithelial dif-

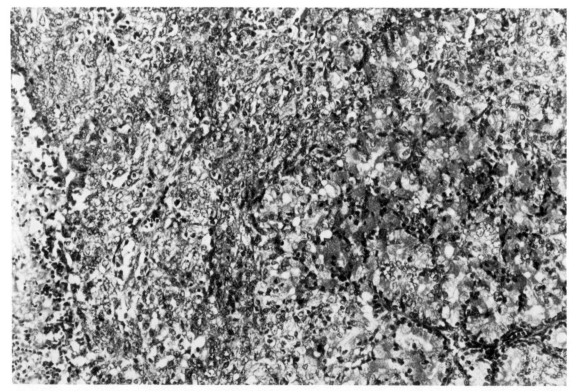

Figure 17–13. In the right middle part of this photomicrograph well-differentiated acinar cells with dark, granular cytoplasm and small, dark nuclei can be seen. Adjacent to these acinar cells are poorly differentiated epithelial cells with indistinct cell borders and large, vesicular nuclei. Examination of large portions of this tumor indicated that the acinar cells were not residual normal parotid gland parenchyma but were proliferative tumor cells. It is uncertain whether this rare tumor pattern represents collision of undifferentiated carcinoma and acinic cell adenocarcinoma or dedifferentiation of acinic cell adenocarcinoma (× 150).

ferentiation can be found in mixed tumors, adenoid cystic carcinomas, and polymorphous low-grade adenocarcinomas, as well as in others. Yet, each of the three examples has distinct and different histomorphologic features and biologic behavior. In the normal parotid gland, the acinar cells do not demonstrate immunoreactivity for keratin, epithelial membrane antigen, S-100 protein, actin, or glial fibrillary acidic protein, but they do show reactivity for amylase, lysozyme, lactoferrin, secretory piece, and proline-rich protein. The intercalated duct cells are immunoreactive for keratin, epithelial membrane antigen, secretory piece, and, occasionally, S-100 protein. The normal myoepithelial cells are immunoreactive for keratin and actin, and in mixed tumors, these cells may demonstrate S-100 protein and glial fibrillary acidic protein reactivity. Well-differentiated acinar cells in acinic cell adenocarcinomas have been shown to be immunoreactive for amylase and lactoferrin and, to a lesser extent, secretory piece and lysozyme.[45, 72, 78] However, contrary to other reports, Morley and coworkers[70] could not demonstrate amylase immunoreactivity in three acinic cell adenocarcinomas that they studied. Most acinic cell adenocarcinomas manifest reactivity with anti-keratin antibodies, but the reactive cells are thought to be ductal differentiated cells. Some studies have found no immunoreactivity for S-100 protein, whereas others have detected S-100 protein in intercalated ductlike cells in acinic cell adenocarcinomas.[69, 71, 73–75] Hayashi and colleagues[47] located immunoreactive vasoactive intestinal polypeptide, typically associated with neuroendocrine or neuroepithelial differentiation, in 11 acinic cell adenocarcinomas. Even vimentin has been immunohistochemically demonstrated in acinic cell adenocarcinoma.[77] Except for perhaps antiamylase to help identify acinar cell differentiation, use of these immunohistochemical reactions is probably of little practical help in the diagnostic differentiation of acinic cell adenocarcinomas from other epithelial salivary gland tumors.

In general, observations with electron microscopy have paralleled those of light microscopy, and both acinar and ductal types of cells have been noted.[34, 38, 42–44, 59, 75, 80, 81] The most notable ultrastructural feature of cells with acinar differentiation is the presence of cytoplasmic, electron-dense, round to oval, membrane-bound granules analogous to the zymogen granules of normal serous cells (Fig. 17–14). In general, the secretory type granules in the cells of acinic cell adenocarcinomas are smaller and more variable in size than those of normal serous cells. The granules may range in size from about 80 to 800 nm. In addition, rough endoplasmic reticulum and mitochondria can be prominent in the acinarlike cells. In contrast, the intercalated ductlike cells and nonspecific glandular cells are smaller and have relatively fewer organelles with few or no secretory granules (Fig. 17–15). The intercalated ductlike cells tend to line lumina and may have lipid inclusions. Tight, intermediate, and desmosomal junctional complexes connect cells to one another. On the basis of his ultrastructural analysis, Echevarria[80] concluded that the clear cells were the result of artifact. Chaudhry and coinvestigators,[44] on the other hand, found that the cytoplasmic vacuoles represented dilatations of rough endoplasmic reticulum, enzymatic degradation of secretory granules, lipid inclusions, and intracytoplasmic pseudolumina as well as artifact. Although it has traditionally been thought that myoepithelial differentiated cells were not a part of acinic cell adenocarcinomas, some recent electron microscopic studies have identified occasional myoepithelial type cells in these neoplasms.[44, 75] These cells, of course, are characterized by cytoplasmic extensions, numerous cytoplasmic filaments with dense bodies, desmosomal attachments, and basal laminae.

PROGNOSIS AND THERAPY

In an analysis of the follow-up status of 244 patients with acinic cell adenocarcinomas in the files of the AFIP, Ellis and Corio[53] found that 12 percent of the patients had one or more tumor recurrences, 8 percent of patients experienced metastasis of their tumors, and 6 percent died because of their tumors. These figures are lower than those reported by others, in whose series on average there was a recurrence rate of about 35 percent, a metastatic rate of 16 percent, and a death rate as a result of disease of 16 percent.[2, 35, 36, 51, 52, 65, 66] Unlike the observations of some previous investigators, Ellis and Corio[53] discovered that most recurrences and metastases occurred within 5 years of the initial therapy. They also found that tumors with the poorest clinical course had the shortest mean duration. Although acinic cell adenocarcinomas occur in the minor salivary glands infrequently, the prognosis for the minor gland tumors has been better than for those in the parotid gland.[16, 59–61]

Acinic cell adenocarcinomas are regarded as low-grade malignancies. In an analysis of 2,298 salivary gland malignancies reported in the literature, Hickman and colleagues[82] found the 5-year and 10-year survival rates for acinic cell adenocarcinoma to be 82 and 68 percent, respectively. This was the best of the tumor types studied, which included mucoepidermoid carcinoma, adenoid cystic carcinoma, and malignant mixed tumor. The results of other investigators have been similar.[20, 22, 25, 27, 31, 51, 52] We have not found any of the four histomorphologic growth patterns or predominance of any one of the five cell types to be reliably predictive of a more favorable or worse clinical course. All microscopic variations have been expressed among tumors with both favorable

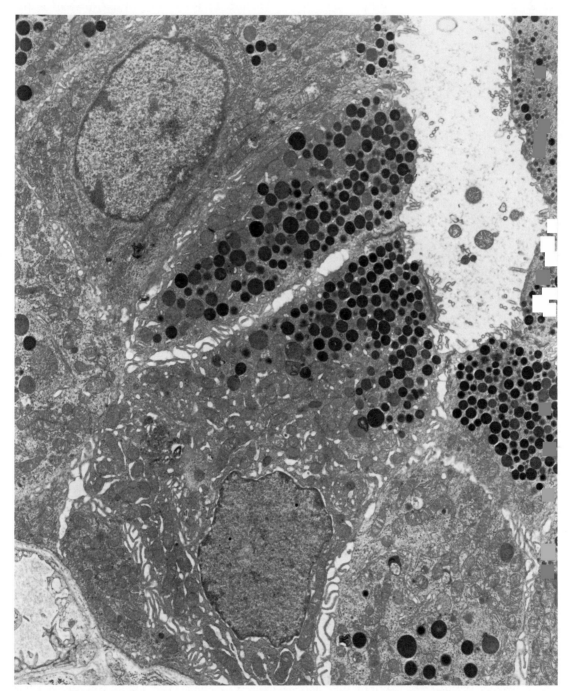

Figure 17–14. Electron micrograph of an acinic cell adenocarcinoma shows several well-differentiated acinar type cells that contain many electron-dense membrane-bound granules. Some of the cells border a small lumen (upper right), have a few microvilli on their luminal surface, and are connected by tight junctions along their apical portions (× 7,300).

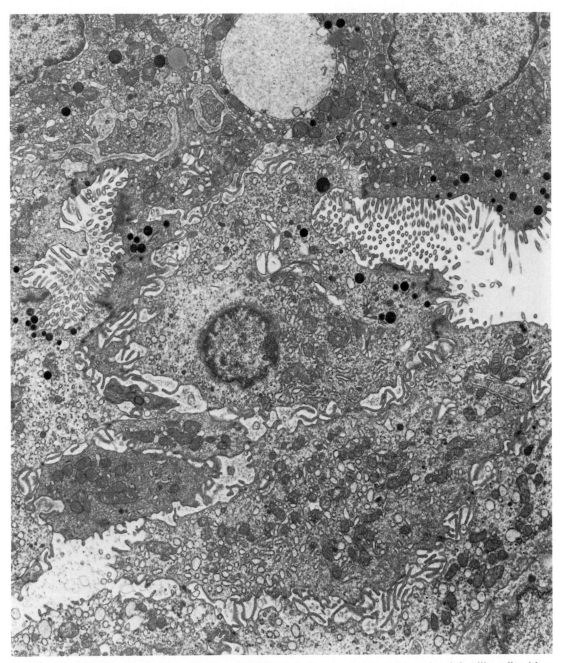

Figure 17–15. Electron micrograph of acinic cell adenocarcinoma demonstrates intercalated ductlike cells with rare electron-dense membrane-bound granules, a few mitochondria, some rough endoplasmic reticulum, and microvilli that project into small lumina (× 8,600).

and poor clinical outcomes, although an intercalated ductlike cell type has been more frequent in tumors that metastasized. About one half of the tumors that have recurred or metastasized have been well circumscribed without substantial infiltrative growth. On the other hand, multinodularity and stromal hyalinization have evinced in 70 and 60 percent, respectively, of acinic cell adenocarcinomas that recurred or metastasized. The clinical stage of the disease seems to be a more important prognostic factor than histopathologic features.[20, 51]

Some investigators have suggested segregating acinic cell adenocarcinomas into low-grade and high-grade neoplasms. In 1979, Batsakis and coworkers[35] defined high-grade acinic cell adenocarcinomas as having infiltrative growth, a medullary pattern, ductulotubular architecture, and prominence of undifferentiated cells that we believe are equivalent to our nonspecific glandular cells. Their low-grade carcinomas manifested acinolobular, microcystic, and papillary growth patterns and were composed of cells that had no ductuloglandular or tubular elements. However, it appeared that the extent of invasion and the scope of surgery best correlated with the outcome for the patients. In fact, the authors commented that the fallibility of such a grading system is evident by the occasional patient with a low-grade carcinoma who follows the same postoperative course as a patient with a high-grade carcinoma.

If the tumor is confined to the superficial lobe of the parotid gland, at least superficial lobe parotidectomy is suggested. When the deep lobe is involved, total parotidectomy is probably necessary. Local enucleation is to be avoided. If the facial nerve is uninvolved by tumor, preservation of the facial nerve is desirable. When the submandibular gland is the site of occurrence, complete resection of the gland is necessary. In the minor salivary glands, ensured complete local excision is needed. Radical neck dissection need not be performed routinely but is used when there is clinical evidence of cervical lymph node involvement. Radiation as the only therapy is not recommended. Tu and colleagues[83] have stated that postoperative radiation therapy does not increase the survival for patients with low-grade malignant parotid tumors, but in cases where there is doubt about the completeness of removal, and further surgery is not feasible because of extensive local disease, postoperative radiotherapy may be advantageous.

DIFFERENTIAL DIAGNOSIS

Acinic cell adenocarcinomas that are made up of numerous well-differentiated acinar cells pose few problems in differential diagnosis unless an occasional small tumor is confused with normal serous parenchyma. As we stated, striated ducts are found in normal salivary glands but not in acinic cell adenocarcinoma, and the normal parotid gland has considerable interlobular adipose tissue that is absent in acinic cell adenocarcinomas.

When well-differentiated acinar cells are inconspicuous, papillary cystic and follicular patterns can be quite similar in appearance to papillary and follicular thyroid carcinomas. Also, we have seen thyroid carcinomas that have metastasized to parotid lymph nodes, although the primary thyroid carcinoma was still undiagnosed. Immunostaining for thyroglobulin should readily identify thyroid carcinoma.

The rare cystadenocarcinoma of the salivary gland may be difficult to distinguish from papillary cystic acinic cell adenocarcinomas. When papillary cystic carcinomas occur in the parotid gland, our first consideration is acinic cell adenocarcinoma; however, in the minor salivary glands where acinic cell adenocarcinomas are uncommon, we usually first think about cystadenocarcinoma or polymorphous low-grade adenocarcinoma. If we can convincingly identify well-differentiated acinar cells, the diagnosis of acinic cell adenocarcinoma is confirmed. Periodic acid–Schiff and anti-amylase staining may help. The presence of numerous vacuolated areas and/or areas of microcyst formation, certainly, favors acinic cell adenocarcinoma. The demonstration of intensely stained mucous cells with mucicarmine or alcian blue argues strongly against acinic cell adenocarcinoma. It should be remembered, however, that the distinction between cystadenocarcinoma and acinic cell adenocarcinoma is more academic than therapeutic because treatment is essentially the same.

The rare acinic cell adenocarcinoma with numerous clear cells may be difficult to segregate from other clear cell tumors, such as mucoepidermoid carcinoma, epithelial-myoepithelial carcinoma, clear cell variant of oncocytoma, and metastatic renal cell carcinoma. We believe that Nelson and colleagues'[63] report of "bilateral acinous cell tumors of the parotid gland" is an example that illustrates this confusion. Their photomicrographs and microscopic description convince us that their tumors were actually clear cell oncocytomas and oncocytosis, which only recently has been adequately described.[64] Unlike in many clear cell oncocytomas, the clear cells in acinic cell adenocarcinoma do not contain significant glycogen and are unreactive with phosphotungstic acid–hematoxylin stain. Nor does the tumor contain foci of intensely eosinophilic oncocytes. Mucoepidermoid carcinomas have intensely mucicarminophilic cells that are not seen in acinic cell adenocarcinoma. Epithelial-myoepithelial carcinomas contain glycogen, are more immunoreactive for S-100 protein, and have a distinctive biphasic pattern of eosinophilic, cuboidal, duct-lining cells surrounded by clear cells, in this case myoepithelial cells. Metastatic renal cell carcinoma typically has demonstrable glycogen by PAS staining before and after diastase digestion, and the vascular pattern of the tumor is usually dramatically more noticeable than that of acinic cell adenocarcinoma. If we cannot locate any of the morphologic or cytologic patterns of typical acinic cell adenocarcinoma, we do not classify a tumor as acinic cell adenocarcinoma.

There are many similarities between polymorphous low-grade adenocarcinoma of minor salivary gland and acinic cell adenocarcinoma that predominantly occurs in the parotid gland. Both are low-grade adenocarcinomas, have fairly bland cytologic features, and manifest various morphologic configurations, both within a single tumor and from tumor to tumor. However, although there may be some overlap of morphologic features, the variety of cell types as well as the distinctive acinar cell serves to discriminate the acinic cell adenocarcinoma.

REFERENCES

1. Nasse D: Die Geschwulste der Speicheldrusen und verwandte Tumoren des Kopfes. Arch Klin Chir 1892; 44:233–302.
2. Godwin JT, Foote FW Jr, Frazell EL: Acinic cell adenocarcinoma of the parotid gland: Report of twenty-seven cases. Am J Pathol 1954; 30:465–477.
3. Fox NM Jr, ReMine WH, Woolner LB: Acinic cell carcinoma of the major salivary glands. Am J Surg 1963; 106:860–867.
4. Evans RW, Cruickshank AH: Epithelial Tumours of the Salivary Glands. Philadelphia, WB Saunders Co, 1970; 98–119.
5. Masson P: Tumeurs des glandes anneses des muquiuses de la face et du cou. VII. Serie A. Plate I, Figs. A,B,C,D. Atlas du Cancer. Assoc Franc pour L'Etude du Cancer, Fascicles 3 and 4, 1924.
6. Schutz CB: Adenoma of the salivary gland. Am J Pathol 1926; 2:153–157.
7. Lloyd OC: Salivary adenoma and adenolymphoma. J Pathol Bacteriol 1946; 58:699–710.
8. Godwin JT, Colvin SH Jr: Adenoma of the parotid gland. Arch Pathol 1948; 46:187–189.
9. Bauer WH, Bauer JD: Classification of glandular tumors of salivary glands: Study of 143 cases. Arch Pathol 1953; 55:328–346.
10. Buxton RW, Maxwell JH, French AJ: Surgical treatment of epithelial tumors of the parotid gland. Surg Gynecol Obstet 1953; 97:401–416.
11. Foote FW Jr, Frazell EL: Tumors of the major salivary glands. Cancer 1953; 6:1065–1133.
12. Foote FW Jr, Frazell EL: Tumors of the Major Salivary Glands, Section IV, Fascicle 11. Atlas of Tumor Pathology. Washington, DC, Armed Forces Institute of Pathology, 1954.
13. Thackray AC, Sobin LH: Histological Typing of Salivary Gland Tumours. Geneva, World Health Organization, 1972; 23–24.
14. Thackray AC, Lucas RB: Tumors of the Major Salivary Glands, Fascicle 10. Atlas of Tumor Pathology, 2nd Series. Washington, DC, Armed Forces Institute of Pathology, 1974; 18–90.
15. Sharkey FE: Systematic evaluation of the World Health Organization classification of salivary gland tumors: A clinicopathologic study of 366 cases. Am J Clin Pathol 1977; 67:272–278.
16. Abrams AM, Melrose RJ: Acinic cell tumors of minor salivary gland origin. Oral Surg Oral Med Oral Pathol 1978; 46:220–233.
17. Friedman M, Levin B, Grybauskas V, Strorigl T, Manaligod J, Hill JH, Skolnik E: Malignant tumors of the major salivary glands. Otolaryngol Clin North Am 1966; 19:625–636.
18. Rosenfeld L, Sessions DG, McSwain B, Graves H Jr: Malignant tumors of salivary gland origin: 37-year review of 184 cases. Ann Surg 1966; 165:726–734.
19. Fu KK, Leibel SA, Levine ML, Friedlander LM, Boles R, Phillips TL: Carcinoma of the major and minor salivary glands: An analysis of treatment results and sites and causes of failures. Cancer 1977; 40:2882–2890.
20. Levitt SH, McHugh RB, Gomez-Marin O, Hyams VJ, Soules EH, Strong EW, Sellers AH, Woods JE, Guillamondegui OM: Clinical staging system for cancer of the salivary gland: a retrospective study. Cancer 1981; 47:2712–2724.
21. Hunter RM, Davis BW, Gray GF Jr, Rosenfeld L: Primary malignant tumors of salivary gland origin: A 52-year review. Am Surgeon 1983; 49:82–89.
22. Spitz MR, Batsakis JG: Major salivary gland carcinoma: Descriptive epidemiology and survival of 498 patients. Arch Otolaryngol 1984; 110:45–49.
23. Theron EJ, Middlecote BD: Tumours of the salivary glands: The Bloemfontein experience. S Afr J Surg 1984; 22:237–242.
24. Eveson JW, Cawson RA: Salivary gland tumours: A review of 2410 cases with particular reference to histological types, site, age and sex distribution. J Pathol 1985; 146:51–58.
25. Fitzpatrick PJ, Theriault C: Malignant salivary gland tumors. Int J Radiat Oncol Biol Phys 1986; 12:1743–1747.
26. Seifert G, Miehlke A, Haubrich J, Chilla R: Diseases of the Salivary Glands: Pathology-Diagnosis-Treatment-Facial Nerve Surgery. Stuttgart, Georg Thieme Verlag, 1986; 171, 224–230.
27. Spiro RH: Salivary neoplasms: Overview of a 35-year experience with 2,807 patients. Head Neck Surg 1986; 8:177–184.
28. Yu GY, Ma DQ: Carcinoma of the salivary gland: A clinicopathologic study of 405 cases. Semin Surg Oncol 1987; 3:240–244.
29. Spiro RH, Huvos AG, Strong EW: Cancer of the parotid gland: A clinicopathologic study of 288 primary cases. Am J Surg 1975; 130:452–459.
30. Woods JE, Chong GC, Beahrs OH: Experience with 1,360 primary parotid tumors. Am J Surg 1975; 130:460–462.
31. O'Brien CJ, Herrera GA, Maddox WA: Malignant salivary tumors—Analysis of prognostic factors and survival. Head Neck Surg 1986; 9:82–92.
32. Beahrs OH, Woolner LB, Carveth SW, Devine KD: Surgical management of parotid lesions: Review of seven hundred sixty cases. Arch Surg 1960; 80:890–904.
33. Eneroth C-M: Salivary gland tumors in the parotid gland, submandibular gland, and the palate region. Cancer 1971; 27:1415–1418.
34. Kay S, Schatzki PF: Ultrastructure of acinic cell

carcinoma of the parotid salivary gland. Cancer 1972; 29:235–244.

35. Batsakis JG, Chinn EK, Weimert TA, Work WP, Krause CJ: Acinic cell carcinoma: A clinicopathologic study of thirty-five cases. J Laryngol Otol 1979; 93:325–340.

36. Abrams AM, Cornyn J, Scofield HH, Hansen LS: Acinic cell adenocarcinoma of the major salivary glands: A clinicopathologic study of 77 cases. Cancer 1965; 18:1145–1162.

37. Bhaskar SN: Acinic cell carcinoma of salivary glands: Report of twenty-one cases. Oral Surg Oral Med Oral Pathol 1964; 17:62–74.

38. Erlandson RA, Tandler B: Ultrastructure of acinic cell carcinoma of the parotid gland. Arch Pathol 1972; 93:130–140.

39. Eversole LB: Histogenic classification of salivary tumors. Arch Pathol 1971; 92:433–443.

40. Regezi JA, Batsakis JG: Histogenesis of salivary gland neoplasms. Otolaryngol Clin North Am 1977; 10:297–307.

41. Batsakis JG: Salivary gland neoplasia: An outcome of modified morphogenesis and cytodifferentiation. Oral Surg Oral Med Oral Pathol 1980; 49:229–232.

42. Inoue T, Shimono M, Yamamura T, Saito I, Watanabe O, Kawahara H: Acinic cell carcinoma arising in the glossopalatine glands: A report of two cases with electron microscopic observations. Oral Surg Oral Med Oral Pathol 1984; 57:398–407.

43. Chomette G, Auriol M, Vaillant JM: Acinic cell tumors of salivary glands. Frequency and morphological study. J Biol Buccale 1984; 12:157–169.

44. Chaudhry AP, Cutler LS, Leifer C, Satchidanand S, Labay G, Yamane G: Histogenesis of acinic cell carcinoma of the major and minor salivary glands: An ultrastructural study. J Pathol 1986; 148:307–320.

45. Warner TF, Seo IS, Azen EA, Hafez GR, Zarling TA: Immunocytochemistry of acinic cell carcinomas and mixed tumors of salivary glands. Cancer 1985; 56:2221–2227.

46. Daley TD, Tolson ND, Wysocki GP: Lectin probes of glycoconjugates in human salivary gland neoplasms: 2. J Oral Pathol 1985; 14:531–538.

47. Hayashi Y, Yoshida H, Nagamine S, Yanagawa T, Yura Y, Azuma M, Sato M: Induction of cells with acinar cell phenotype including presence of intracellular amylase: Treatment with 12-O-tetradecanoyl-phorbol-13-acetate in a neoplastic human salivary intercalated duct cell line grown in athymic nude mice. Cancer 1987; 60:1000-1008.

48. Sato M, Azuma M, Hayashi Y, Yoshida H, Yanagawa T, Yura Y: 5-Azacytidine induction of stable myoepithelial and acinar cells from a human salivary intercalated duct cell clone. Cancer Res 1987; 47:4453–4459.

49. Dardick I, Byard RW, Carnegie JA: A review of the proliferative capacity of major salivary glands and the relationship to current concepts of neoplasia in salivary glands. Oral Surg Oral Med Oral Pathol 1990; 69:53–67.

50. Gorlin RJ, Chaudhry A: Acinic cell tumor of the major and minor salivary glands. J Oral Surg 1957; 15:304–306.

51. Spiro RH, Huvos AG, Strong EW: Acinic cell carcinoma of salivary origin: A clinicopathologic study of 67 cases. Cancer 1978; 41:924–935.

52. Perzin KH, LiVolsi VA: Acinic cell carcinomas arising in salivary glands: A clinicopathologic study. Cancer 1979; 44:1434–1457.

53. Ellis GL, Corio RL: Acinic cell adenocarcinoma: A clinicopathologic analysis of 294 cases. Cancer 1983; 52:542–549.

54. Waldron CA, El-Mofty SK, Gnepp DR: Tumors of the intraoral minor salivary glands: A demographic and histologic study of 426 cases. Oral Surg Oral Med Oral Pathol 1988; 66:323–333.

55. Spiro RH, Koss LG, Hajdu SI, Strong EW: Tumors of minor salivary origin: A clinicopathologic study of 492 cases. Cancer 1973; 31:117–129.

56. Isacsson G, Shear M: Intraoral salivary gland tumors: A retrospective study of 201 cases. J Oral Pathol 1983; 12:57–62.

57. Eveson JW, Cawson RA: Tumours of the minor (oropharyngeal) salivary glands: A demographic study of 336 cases. J Oral Pathol 1985; 14:500–509.

58. Ma DQ, Yu GY: Tumours of the minor salivary glands: A clinicopathologic study of 243 cases. Acta Otolaryngol (Stockh) 1987; 103:325–331.

59. Chen S-Y, Brannon RB, Miller AS, White DK, Hooker SP: Acinic cell adenocarcinoma of minor salivary glands. Cancer 1978; 42:678–685.

60. Ferlito A: Acinic cell carcinoma of minor salivary glands. Histopathology 1980; 4:331–343.

61. Castellanos JL, Lally ET: Acinic cell tumor of the minor salivary glands. J Oral Maxillofac Surg 1982; 40:428–431.

62. Gustafsson H, Carlsoo B: Multiple acinic cell carcinoma: Some histological and ultrastructural features of a case. J Laryngol Otol 1985; 99:1183–1193.

63. Nelson DW, Nichols RD, Fine G: Bilateral acinous cell tumors of the parotid gland. Laryngoscope 1978; 88:1935–1941.

64. Ellis GL: "Clear cell" oncocytoma of salivary gland. Hum Pathol 1988; 19:862–867.

65. Eneroth C-M, Jakobsson PA, Blanck C: Acinic cell carcinoma of the parotid gland. Cancer 1966; 19:1761–1772.

66. Chong GC, Beahrs OH, Woolner LB: Surgical management of acinic cell carcinoma of the parotid gland. Surg Gynecol Obstet 1974; 138:65–68.

67. Stanley RJ, Weiland LH, Olsen KD, Pearson BW: Dedifferentiated acinic cell (acinous) carcinoma of the parotid gland. Otolaryngol Head Neck Surg 1988; 98:155–161.

68. Gusterson BA, Lucas RB, Ormerod MG: Distribution of epithelial membrane antigen in benign and malignant lesions of the salivary glands. Virchows Arch [A] 1982; 397:227–233.

69. Hara K, Ito M, Takeuchi J, Iijima S, Endo T, Hidaka H: Distribution of S-100 protein in normal salivary glands and salivary gland tumors. Virchows Arch [A] 1983; 401:237–249.

70. Morley DJ, Hodes JE, Calland J, Hodes ME: Immunohistochemical demonstration of ribonuclease and amylase in normal and neoplastic parotid glands. Hum Pathol 1983; 14:969–973.

71. Kahn HJ, Baumal R, Marks A, Dardick I, van Nostrand AW: Myoepithelial cells in salivary gland tumors: An immunohistochemical study. Arch Pathol Lab Med 1985; 109:190–195.

72. Caselitz J, Seifert G, Grenner G, Schmidtberger R: Amylase as an additional marker of salivary gland neoplasms: An immunoperoxidase study. Pathol Res Pract 1983; 176:276–283.

73. Nakazato Y, Ishida Y, Takahashi K, Suzuke K: Immunohistochemical distribution of S-100 protein and glial fibrillary acidic protein in normal and neoplastic salivary glands. Virchows Arch [A] 1985; 405:299–310.

74. Zarbo RJ, Regezi JA, Batsakis JG: S-100 protein in salivary gland tumors: An immunohistochemical study of 129 cases. Head Neck Surg 1986; 8:268–275.

75. Dardick I, George D, Jeans D, Wittkuhn JF, Skimming L, Rippstein P, van Nostrand AW: Ultrastructural morphology and cellular differentiation in acinic cell carcinoma. Oral Surg Oral Med Oral Pathol 1987; 63:325–334.

76. Hayashi Y, Nishida T, Yoshida H, Yanagawa T, Yura Y, Sato M: Immunoreactive vasoactive intestinal polypeptide in acinic cell carcinoma of the parotid gland. Cancer 1987; 60:962–968.

77. Gustafsson H, Virtanen I, Thornell LE: Expression of cytokeratins and vimentin in salivary gland carcinomas as revealed with monoclonal antibodies. Virchows Arch [A] 1988; 412:515–524.

78. Seifert G, Caselitz J: Epithelial salivary gland tumors: Tumor markers. *In* Fenoglio-Preiser CM, Wolff M, Rilke F: Progress in Surgical Pathology. Vol 10. New York, Field & Wood Medical Publishers, 1989; 157–187.

79. Egan M, Crocker J, Nar P: Localization of salivary amylase and epithelial membrane antigen in salivary gland tumours by means of immunoperoxidase and immunogold-silver techniques. J Laryngol Otol 1988; 102:242–247.

80. Echevarria RA: Ultrastructure of the acinic cell carcinoma and clear cell carcinoma of the parotid gland. Cancer 1967; 20:563–571.

81. Ghadially FN: Diagnostic Electron Microscopy of Tumours. Boston, Butterworth Inc, 1980; 215–219.

82. Hickman RE, Cawson RA, Duffy SW: The prognosis of specific types of salivary gland tumors. Cancer 1984; 54:1620–1624.

83. Tu G, Hu Y, Jiang P, Qin D: The superiority of combined therapy (surgery and postoperative irradiation) in parotid cancer. Arch Otolaryngol 1982; 108:710–713.

18

ADENOCARCINOMA, NOT OTHERWISE SPECIFIED

Paul L. Auclair and Gary L. Ellis

There are 19 specific types of malignant epithelial salivary gland tumors in our classification system (see Chapter 8) that have unique and generally well-described histopathologic features. Nonetheless, a substantial number of tumors occur that lack the histomorphologic features necessary to permit their meaningful classification into one of these defined groups. In the past, some investigators[1-3] have used the unqualified term *adenocarcinoma* to designate a group of miscellaneous, unclassifiable salivary gland adenocarcinomas. However, because most epithelial malignancies of the salivary glands are also adenocarcinomas of one type or another, we believe that an additional modifying term should be used to denote this particular group. We prefer to add the defining and explanatory qualifier *not otherwise specified* (*NOS*).

HISTORICAL REVIEW

Review of the literature reveals marked differences among various investigators regarding miscellaneous adenocarcinomas. The inconsistency may be mainly attributed to differences in classification schemes and, to a lesser degree, to variations in the methods for reporting newly recognized types of adenocarcinoma. These differences among investigators make it impossible to adequately evaluate the purported frequency of occurrence and the expected biologic behavior of these neoplasms. The morphologic heterogeneity seen in this group of tumors, although substantial, is somewhat exaggerated by this reporting variability.

In one of the earliest reviews of a large number of salivary gland tumors of major glands, Foote and Frazell[1] classified 39 of 877 (4.4 percent) as miscellaneous adenocarcinomas. In a review of tumors of the major glands by Thackray and Lucas,[2] only 1 percent of parotid and 1.7 percent of submandibular gland tumors were coded as unclassified adenocarcinomas. Spiro and coworkers[26] reviewed 2,807 cases of salivary gland tumors in 1986 and reported a frequency of occurrence of 8 percent for these adenocarcinomas. Many other published reports[4-32] of salivary gland tumors have included a group of unclassified adenocarcinomas that constituted a significant proportion of the tumors. The unclassified group of adenocarcinomas ranged in frequency between 1.9 and 11.8 percent of both benign and malignant tumors and between 8.8 and 44.7 percent of the malignant tumors.

Some investigators have subclassified these tumors according to several different observed morphologic growth patterns. Foote and Frazell[1] distinguished anaplastic, trabecular or solid, mucous cell, and pseudoadamantine patterns. Bauer and Bauer[8] included papillary and acanthomatous patterns. Main and coworkers,[11] in a series published in 1976, described solid anaplastic, trabecular, cystic, mucinous, and oncocytic subtypes. Seifert and coworkers[33] distinguished between solid, papillary, and tubular subtypes. Spiro and associates[26] reported 204 cases of adenocarcinoma of both major and minor salivary gland origin, subclassified them by their characteristic growth patterns, and graded them. These cases represented about 9 percent of all salivary gland neoplasms on file at the Memorial Sloan-Kettering Cancer Center. Sixty-eight percent of the cases involved the minor glands; nearly one half of these cases involved the glands of the sinonasal and laryngeal areas, whereas 28 and 4 percent occurred in the parotid and submandibular glands, respectively. They simply referred to this entire group of neoplasms as adenocarcinomas but recognized seven growth patterns that they described as (1) typical, (2) mucinous, (3) papillary, (4) trabecular, (5) papillary and mucinous, (6) sebaceous, and (7) others. About 95 percent of the cases demonstrated one of the first three morphologic patterns. They noted that most of their so-called typical adenocarcinomas occurred in the parotid gland. Many of the mucinous or other unusual variants of adenocarcinomas occurred in the area of the nasal sinuses, and papillary adenocarcinomas usually involved oral sites or the parotid gland. Most of the tumors were divided into one of three histologic grades based on cytomorphologic criteria. The majority of the papillary tumors were classified as low grade, whereas most of the typical adenocarcinomas were classified as high grade.

A few investigators, applying different classifications, categorized some tumors as specific subtypes that in other reports had been included under the heading of miscellaneous adenocarcinomas. For instance, Chaudhry and colleagues[6] distinguished the tumor categories papillary cystadenocarcinoma and mucus-producing adenocarcinoma as separate from unclassifiable adenocarcinoma. Several other investigators[6–8, 28, 34–41] have published cases of papillary adenocarcinoma that they considered different from any of the more commonly recognized types of salivary gland adenocarcinoma that may have a papillary component, such as acinic cell and mucoepidermoid carcinomas. Most of these reports concerned cases that affected the minor salivary glands, especially those located in the palate.

Some reports included tumors that currently could be classified as other specific types. Stene and Koppang's[7] study in 1981 included a micrograph that we interpret as polymorphous low-grade adenocarcinoma, a tumor first described in 1983.[42] Apparently, this micrograph was representative of 8 of their 13 cases, which were characterized by the authors as containing focal resemblance to adenoid cystic carcinoma and the presence of small groups of mucus-producing cells. Other cases in their series included examples of clear cell carcinoma, sebaceous carcinoma, and epithelial-myoepithelial carcinoma, which are tumors that at this time would be included under their own respective categories. In 1982, Spiro and colleagues[26] reported a case of trabecular adenocarcinoma that we would now classify as basal cell adenocarcinoma, a tumor first described as such in 1990.[43]

We use the term *not otherwise specified* literally, meaning that we cannot categorize a tumor as one of the specific types listed in our classification. Actually, this approach probably renders a greater degree of homogeneity to our cases than to those reported in most other series, but we estimate that a fair degree of similarity exists between our material and the 144 cases (59 percent) reported by Spiro and coworkers[26] as "typical" adenocarci-

nomas. However, we classify their papillary and adenopapillary adenocarcinomas as cystadenocarcinomas but recognize that sometimes cystadenocarcinomas may not have a papillary component. We also classify sebaceous and clear cell adenocarcinomas and malignant myoepitheliomas under their respective headings.

Although we recognize a unique type of adenocarcinoma that we designate as *mucinous adenocarcinoma* because of its morphologic similarity to the skin tumor with a similar name, it is, in our opinion, not equivalent to most of the tumors termed *mucin-producing adenocarcinoma* by other investigators.[6, 7, 26, 44] Many different types of salivary gland adenocarcinomas produce cytoplasmic or extracellular mucins in various amounts, and this feature alone does not by itself constitute a single group of tumors.

CLINICAL FINDINGS

Incidence

At the time of the preparation of this manuscript, 881 cases in the salivary gland registry of the Armed Forces Institute of Pathology (AFIP) have been categorized as adenocarcinoma, NOS. These 881 cases constitute 6.4 percent of all benign and malignant epithelial tumors and 17.4 percent of all malignant epithelial salivary gland tumors. Adenocarcinoma, NOS, is the third most common malignant tumor of the salivary glands; only mucoepidermoid and acinic cell carcinomas are more common. We have not retrospectively reviewed every case of adenocarcinoma, NOS, in our files, and we expect that some of the older cases may represent tumors that should be reclassified as one of the more recently defined types of tumors, such as polymorphous low-grade adenocarcinoma and basal cell adenocarcinoma. However, because of the relative rarity of these latter types, we suspect that only a small number of the 881 cases would qualify for reclassification.

Without disregarding the reporting inconsistencies previously discussed, many other investigators have noted that adenocarcinoma, NOS, ranks as one of the three most common types of malignant salivary gland tumors.[6, 10, 12, 15, 23, 24, 27] Rosenfeld and coinvestigators[4] have reported adenocarcinoma, NOS, as the most common type of malignant epithelial tumor among all salivary gland sites.

The frequency rates of the AFIP material are similar to those reported at Memorial Sloan-Kettering Cancer Center,[3, 26] which houses the laboratory with the largest previously published series, when it is recognized that their figures included several tumors that can be classified as other specific types. Additionally, 61 of their 204 cases (30 percent) were from the area of the nasal sinuses or the laryngeal areas. Tumors from these sites are not included among our 881 cases, and we discuss them separately in Chapter 31.

Age, Sex, and Race

Adenocarcinoma, NOS, affects patients primarily in the fourth through the eighth decades of life (Fig. 18–1). Over 75 percent of the patients were between the ages of 40 and 79 years, and only 2.6 percent of patients were under 20 years of age. The mean and median ages of the 881 patients were 55.6 and 58.0 years, respectively. The age range of patients at the time of the initial diagnosis was 9 months to 94 years. Occurrence in children is very unusual in our experience and in that of other investigators.[33, 45, 46]

The mean age of patients with lesions of the submandibular and sublingual glands was 5 years greater than the average for all patients, and the mean age of patients with tongue lesions was nearly 10 years older than the overall mean age. Conversely, patients with lesions of the buccal mucosa and lower lip, on average, were younger (44.7 and 48.0 years, respectively) than the whole group. However, for tumors of nearly every site, the greatest number of patients was in the sixth or seventh decades of life.

The mean age of women and men was 54.6 and 55.8 years, respectively. Women with submandibular tumors averaged 63.7 years, almost 7.0 years greater than their male counterparts with tumors in the same site. The data for cases occurring at all other sites that involved substantial numbers of cases showed men and women to be of similar ages.

Of the 767 cases in the AFIP files for which the sex of the patient was stated, 475 (61.9 percent) were males and only 292 (38.1 percent) were females. However, when only the 513 civilian patients were considered, 55 percent were females and 45 percent were males. Because the combined military and veteran population is overwhelmingly male, only the data regarding relative sex predilection for civilian patients are useful. Among civilian patients, there was a particularly high predominance of female patients with tumors of the buccal mucosa (82 percent) and the lower lip (73 per cent).

The race was stated for 459 of the 881 patients (52.1 percent). Just over 83 percent were white, about 14 percent were black, and nearly 3 percent were Asian. In one series,[9] 42.9 percent of all patients were Hispanic, a much higher proportion than for other types of malignant salivary gland tumors reported in that study.

Localization

The site distribution of adenocarcinoma, NOS, is shown in Table 18–1. Of the 819 cases for which the site was stated, the major salivary glands accounted for 66.2 percent, and the minor salivary glands accounted for 33.8 percent. This contrasts with the findings of Spiro and coworkers,[26] who reported that 68 percent involved the minor glands and 32 percent affected the parotid or submandibular glands. This difference is largely explained by the fact that 30 percent of the cases in their series were from the minor glands of the antrum, ethmoid, nasopharynx, nasal cavity, or

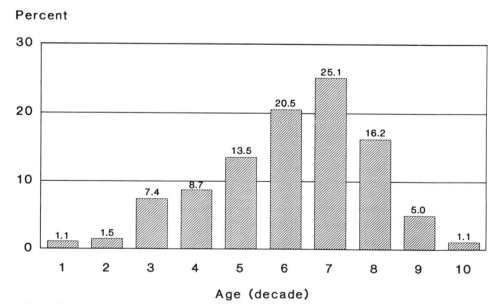

Figure 18–1. Distribution by age (in decades) of 757 patients with adenocarcinoma, NOS, in the AFIP files.

Table 18–1. Distribution by Anatomic Site of 881 Cases of Adenocarcinoma, NOS,* from the AFIP Registry

Anatomic Site	Number of Cases	Percentage
Major Glands		
Parotid gland	433	49.1
Submandibular gland	101	11.5
Sublingual gland	5	0.6
Neck, not specified	3	0.3
Minor Glands		
Palate (total)	126	14.3
Palate, not specified	(85)	(9.6)
Hard palate	(23)	(2.6)
Soft palate	(18)	(2.0)
Lip (total)	42	4.8
Upper lip	(18)	(2.0)
Lower lip	(14)	(1.6)
Lip, not specified	(10)	(1.1)
Tongue	29	3.3
Cheek	24	2.7
Floor of mouth	8	0.9
Tonsil/oropharynx	8	0.9
Retromolar area	4	0.4
Other	36	4.1
Not Stated	62	7.0
Total†	881	100

*NOS = not otherwise specified
†Does not include numbers in parentheses

larynx, which are all sites that we excluded from our series and that we discussed separately (see Chapter 31).

The parotid gland is clearly the most commonly involved site and is involved in about 50 percent of all cases. Adenocarcinoma, NOS, accounts for about 12 percent of all sublingual malignancies, which is a figure comparable to that reported in a 50-year review of the literature of tumors involving that site.[47] The minor glands of the palate give rise to about 15 percent of all cases, and a slightly smaller proportion arises from the submandibular gland. The upper and lower lips, the tongue, and the buccal mucosa are sites of most of the other tumors.

Patients with adenocarcinoma, NOS, of the major glands most often present with a solitary, asymptomatic mass, but about 25 percent of patients complain of pain or the effects of nerve involvement. A few patients present with skin involvement.[26] The size of the tumors at initial presentation ranges from about 2 to 10 cm. Although most patients are aware of a swelling for less than 2 years, some patients confess to tolerating their tumors for more than a decade. Our impression is that the duration of adenocarcinoma, NOS, prior to initial diagnosis, in general, is shorter than that reported for mucoepidermoid, acinic cell, and adenoid cystic carcinomas. Patients with tumors of the intraoral minor salivary glands most often present with an asymptomatic submu-

cosal mass. In the series reported by Spiro and coworkers,[26] 36 percent of the intraoral tumors were ulcerated, and 25 percent involved underlying bone.

PATHOLOGIC FEATURES

The macroscopic appearance of adenocarcinoma, NOS, is no different than other types of solid adenocarcinomas of the salivary glands. A firm to hard mass replaces glandular parenchyma and compresses surrounding adjacent tissues. Large tumors of the parotid and submandibular glands insinuate themselves into extraglandular tissues. Tumors at any site may demonstrate some degree of focal circumscription, but normally the borders are irregular and often indiscernible from surrounding tissues. Tumor extension into muscle and bone may be recognized. The cut surface of the mass is white or yellow-white and may reveal focal areas of hemorrhage and necrosis. Cystic spaces are not recognized grossly.

The histologic diagnosis of adenocarcinoma, NOS, depends more on the exclusion of other characteristic types of salivary carcinomas than on the recognition of histomorphologic features that are specific to adenocarcinoma, NOS. During review and study of the microscopic morphologic details of one of these cases, mental comparison to the characteristic microscopic images of other salivary gland adenocarcinomas must be made.

Like other investigators who have studied this group of tumors, we have observed that they show a wide range in the degree of cellular differentiation so that different grades are relatively easily discerned on a cytomorphologic basis. Spiro and colleagues[26] have presented convincing evidence that grading these tumors is feasible and worthwhile for determining prognosis. Adenocarcinoma, NOS, as a group, includes low- and intermediate-grade tumors as well as high-grade, lethal tumors. Low-grade tumors are less common than either intermediate- or high-grade tumors.

A seemingly endless number of growth patterns make characterization of this group of tumors impossible; even within a single tumor, strikingly different patterns may be seen (Fig. 18–2). The cells in some tumors have abundant cytoplasm with distinct borders; thus, these cells focally resemble myoepithelial cells. However, in other tumors, the cells are so closely packed together that the cytoplasmic borders are not discernible. Scattered clear cells are frequently present. Tumor cells may proliferate as individual clusters or islands; as ramifying and anastomosing cords; and in diffuse, sheetlike arrangements. Variable amounts of intervening connective tissue add to the morphologic heterogeneity. Typically, there is a complete lack of epidermoid differentiation. Common to all cases of adenocarcinoma, NOS, is the formation of glandular or ductlike structures,

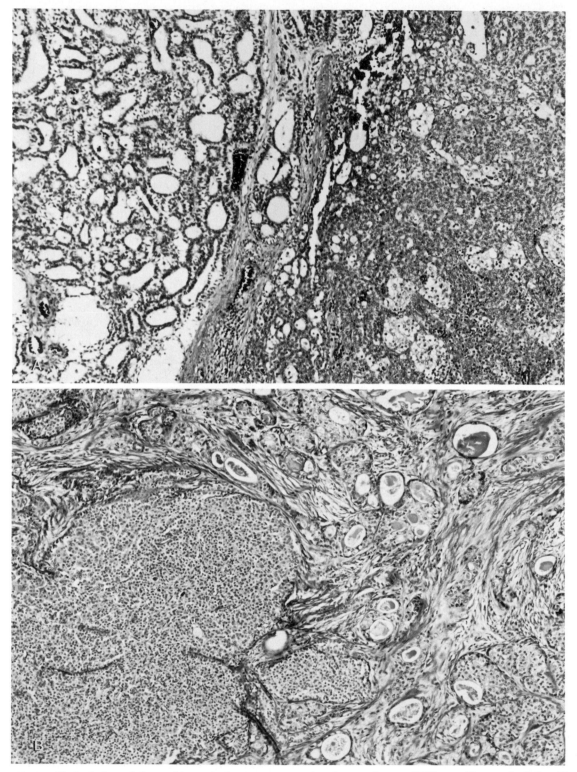

Figure 18–2. A few of the various growth patterns seen in adenocarcinoma, NOS, are illustrated. *A,* In this example, relatively solid and tubular growth patterns are distinctly separate (× 75). *B,* A different tumor shows solid islands intermixed with numerous ductlike structures (× 75).

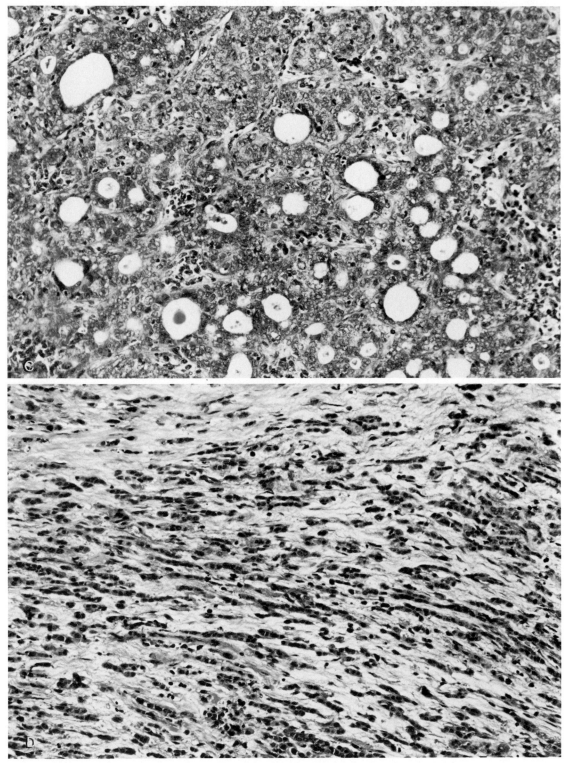

Figure 18–2 *Continued C,* This example shows a more even distribution of ductal differentiation among solid nests of tumor (× 150). *D,* Streaming of tumor cells is seen in this tumor which involves the submandibular gland (× 150).

although in some high-grade tumors even this feature is not immediately obvious. In poorly differentiated carcinomas that lack glandular differentiation, we prefer the diagnosis of undifferentiated carcinoma (see Chapter 25).

Low-grade (grade I) tumors are often relatively well circumscribed, but at least focally, they reveal infiltration (Fig. 18–3). These tumors contain numerous well-formed ductlike structures with central lumina, and they have cells with such bland cytomorphologic features that they often suggest an incorrect benign interpretation. The tumor cells reveal few mitoses and nuclei that show minimal variation in size, shape, and staining characteristics. Central lumina may be lined by cuboidal cells with slightly enlarged nuclei that are evenly spaced and palisaded (Figs. 18–4 and 18–5). The tumor cells usually contain a moderate amount of eosinophilic cytoplasm and round-to-ovoid vesicular nuclei, but occasionally larger oncocytoid cells are present focally. The impressively bland cytologic appearance of the tumor cells and the circumscription seen via low-power examination obviously conflict with the presence of parenchymal infiltration (Fig. 18–6) and the broad, pushing borders of the tumor that extend into fibrous connective tissue and muscle.

Grade II tumors also demonstrate obvious glandular differentiation and are readily recognized as adenocarcinomas. However, they show greater morphologic variability and more frequent mitoses than are seen in grade I tumors (Fig. 18–7). Grade III tumors reveal more solid growth and contain obviously enlarged, pleomorphic nuclei and numerous mitoses (Fig. 18–8). Small cohesive clusters of cells may show primitive attempts at glandular or ductal formation, but a thorough search may be required before identification of glandular differentiation is made. Intracytoplasmic mucin may be demonstrable with the mucicarmine stain, and small accumulations of extracellular mucus are often evident. Necrosis and hemorrhage may be prominent. The cells may be so closely packed that nuclear molding is evident; also, tumor giant cells may be seen.

Although in all grades small intercellular spaces may be evident between tumor cells, neither large cystic spaces nor papillary elements are observed. In some cases, however, we have noted small, focal zones of tumor that exhibited features of specific types of salivary gland adenocarcinomas. These zones most often simulate adenoid cystic carcinoma, but features of acinic cell adenocarcinoma have also been observed. However, the very limited proportion of the entire tumor that shows these features precludes definitive subclassification and warrants the *NOS* designation.

DIFFERENTIAL DIAGNOSIS

Because the diagnosis of adenocarcinoma, NOS, is largely one of exclusion, all adenocarcinomas and some adenomas must be considered in the differential diagnosis. The bland cytologic features of low-grade adenocarcinomas, NOS, often lead to their misinterpretation as mixed tumors or other types of adenomas. The frequency of this error highlights the importance of ensuring thorough evaluation of the tumor interface with non-neoplastic tissues. The only evidence of malignancy is often focal infiltration by tumor cells in the form of glandular or ductlike structures. Although some adenomas of the upper lip often show a characteristic canalicular growth pattern that is not found in adenocarcinoma, NOS, many adenomas of the parotid gland are usually not equally distinctive; thus, determination of biologic potential largely depends on assessment of the peripheral interface.

Because adenocarcinoma, NOS, may contain clear cells, the diagnoses of epithelial-myoepithelial carcinoma and clear cell adenocarcinoma may be considered. The characteristic biphasic pattern of epithelial-myoepithelial carcinoma is not present in adenocarcinoma, NOS, nor is the overwhelming prominence of clear cells that is required for diagnosis of clear cell adenocarcinoma. The presence of cystic and papillary structures could lead to consideration of cystadenocarcinoma, acinic cell adenocarcinoma, and mucoepidermoid carcinoma; however, adenocarcinoma, NOS, does not contain large cystic spaces or reveal the presence of features characteristic of each of these other tumors.

Low-grade adenocarcinoma, NOS, and polymorphous low-grade adenocarcinoma have similar bland cytomorphologic features and well-formed glandular and ductal structures. However, polymorphous, low-grade adenocarcinoma contains characteristic concentric whorling of tumor cells, greater variability of cell types and growth patterns within the same tumor, and often has focal myxoid areas. Furthermore, nearly all cases reported have occurred in the minor salivary glands.

Metastatic adenocarcinomas occasionally simulate primary parotid neoplasms and may present difficulties in separation from adenocarcinoma, NOS, because of their relatively nonspecific histologic appearance. A high index of suspicion and a thorough medical history are required to establish an accurate interpretation. Morphologic features may suggest the primary site, and sometimes this suspicion can be confirmed or ruled out with immunohistochemical studies.

CLINICAL BEHAVIOR AND PROGNOSIS

Our knowledge of the biologic behavior of adenocarcinomas, NOS, is relatively limited because few studies have involved long-term follow-up of large numbers of these tumors. The greatest amount of information is found in the report by Spiro and coworkers.[26] According to these inves-

Text continued on page 330

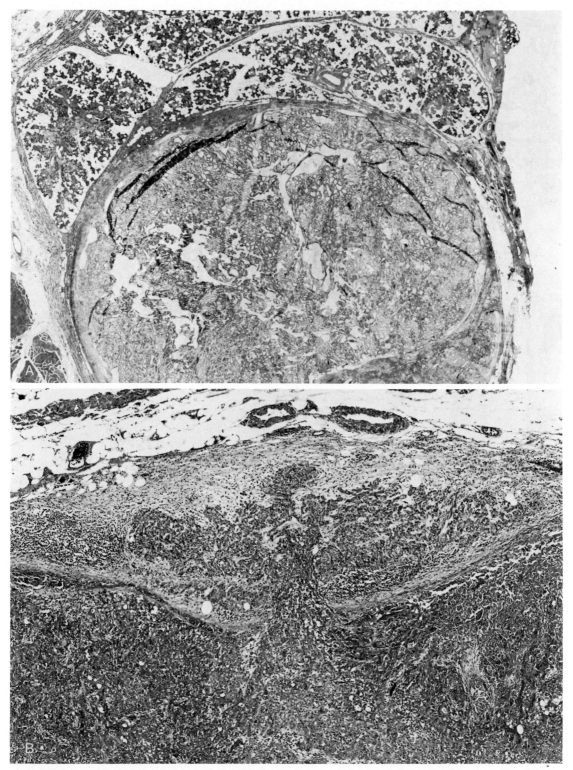

Figure 18–3. *A,* Well-circumscribed low-grade tumor is seen in the parotid gland (× 7.5). *B,* Another tumor is shown that was generally well circumscribed but that focally, as shown here, revealed infiltrative growth (× 40).

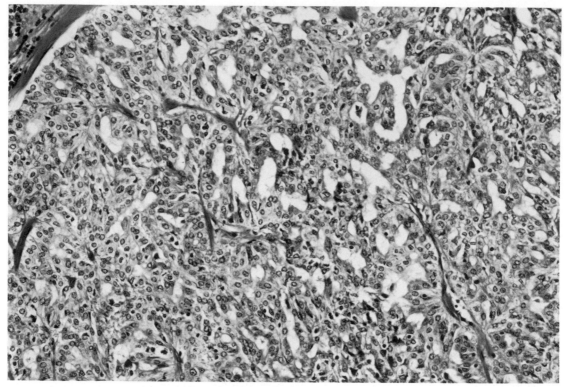

Figure 18–4. Low-grade adenocarcinoma, NOS, composed of a morphologically monotonous population of cells shows formation of many ductal structures (× 150).

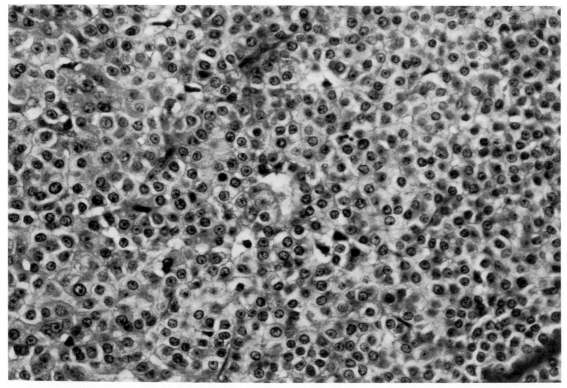

Figure 18–5. High-power magnification of low-grade adenocarcinoma, NOS. Although nucleoli are evident, minimal morphologic alterations are evident. Mitotic figures are extremely rare, which is typical for this group of tumors (× 150).

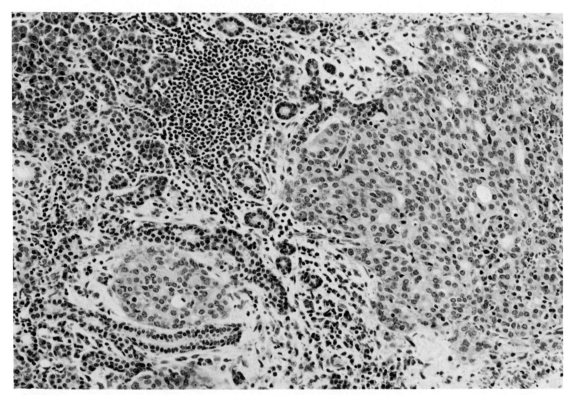

Figure 18–6. Infiltration and acinar replacement are evident focally in this low-grade adenocarcinoma, NOS. These findings allow distinction from adenomas that may have similar nuclear features. Note inflammatory response at leading edge of tumor (× 150).

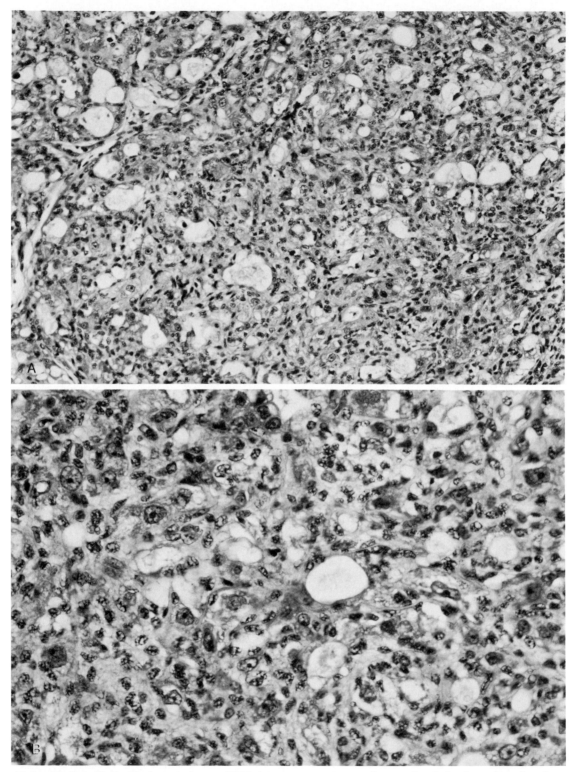

Figure 18–7. *A,* Grade II adenocarcinoma, NOS, demonstrates a greater degree of variation in nuclear size, shape, and staining characteristics than is seen in low-grade tumors (× 150). *B,* Higher magnification of the same case. Note scattered large vesicular nuclei, with enlarged nucleoli and irregular nuclear contours (× 300).

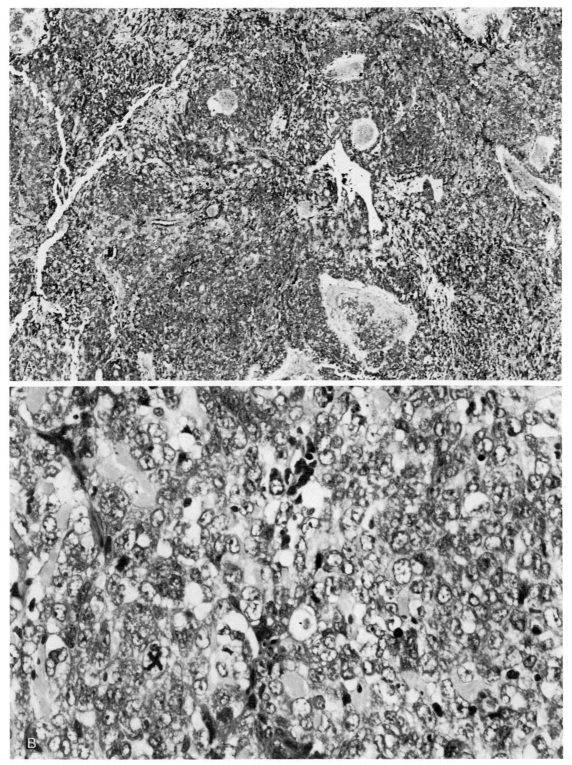

Figure 18–8. *A,* High-grade adenocarcinoma, NOS, shows hypercellularity and relatively solid growth that is interrupted by a few primitive attempts at duct formation (× 40). *B,* Higher magnification reveals pleomorphic, closely packed nuclei, limited glandular differentiation, and an abnormal mitotic figure (× 300).

tigators, the biologic behavior is influenced by the clinical stage, the histologic grade, and the site of involvement.

They reported that the overall cure rates at 5, 10, and 15 years were 41, 34, and 28 percent, respectively. Direct correlation with this data to our cases is not possible because of the previously mentioned differences in site distribution (30 percent of their cases were from the areas of the nasal sinuses and the larynx) and because of their inclusion of tumors that we subclassify as other specific subtypes. However, most of their cases (144 of 204) were apparently morphologically similar to ours, and this group of tumors is easily the largest reported series with follow-up information. The 5-, 10-, and 15-year cure rates of tumors from the area of the nasal sinuses were 21, 15, and 10 percent, respectively, which is considerably worse than the overall average. Laryngeal tumors had a similarly poor outlook. If these two sites were excluded from consideration, somewhat better rates, overall, would be seen. Tu and colleagues[48] have reported 5-, 10-, and 15-year survival rates of 85, 71, and 60 percent, respectively.

Local recurrences were found in 51 percent of the patients followed by Spiro and colleagues,[26] and in some patients, multiple episodes of recurrence were experienced. Cervical metastases were seen in 27 percent of the patients, and slightly more than half of those were found at the time of initial diagnosis. Distant metastases occurred in 26 percent of all the patients in their study. The lungs were the most commonly affected distant sites, but metastases to the skeleton, abdomen, and skin also occurred. Wide dissemination of tumor was not unusual in their series nor in the AFIP material. Metastatic tumor usually retains the morphologic features of the primary tumor.

The histologic grade of the tumor correlated with the rate of recurrence, the amount of cervical and distant metastases, and, ultimately, the rate of survival.[26] Only 5 percent of patients with grade I tumors were found to have cervical metastases, compared with 49 percent of those with grade III tumors. About one third of patients with high-grade lesions experienced distant metastases. The cure rates for grades I, II, and III tumors at 5 years were 69, 46, and 8 percent, respectively, and at 15 years, the rates were 54, 31, and 3 percent, respectively. These findings emphasize the inadequacy of 5-year follow-up. The treatment results for grade I tumors were similar to the results for acinic cell adenocarcinomas and intermediate-grade mucoepidermoid carcinomas. High-grade tumors had the worst 5-, 10-, and 15-year prognoses of all salivary gland adenocarcinomas.

The site involved appeared to have an important role in determining prognosis. In the series by Spiro and coworkers,[26] the survival rates were found to vary, in descending order, for tumors of the oral cavity, the parotid glands, and the sub-

mandibular glands. Less than 14 percent of tumors of the parotid gland were high-grade, which is in contrast to the 50 percent of high-grade submandibular gland tumors. Submandibular gland lesions were more likely to metastasize to cervical lymph nodes than lesions of the parotid glands or the intraoral minor salivary glands.

The most accurate predictor of the ultimate outcome of the disease appeared to be the clinical stage. The 15-year cure rates for disease stages I, II, and III were 67, 35, and 8 percent, respectively. Patients with a higher clinical stage were much more likely to have higher grade lesions. Only 8 percent of patients with stage I disease had high-grade tumors, which contrasts with the 33 percent of those with stage III disease.

TREATMENT

Surgery remains the primary therapeutic modality for adenocarcinoma, NOS, and both the stage and grade of the tumor should play a role in determining therapeutic decisions for tumors of either the major or the minor glands. Radical parotid gland resection is indicated in patients with stage III disease. At one cancer center,[26] 90 percent of the patients with lymphadenopathy were found to have lymph node metastases, and metastases were also confirmed in three of seven patients who received an elective lymphadenectomy. Patients with less extensive disease had subtotal parotidectomies with or without preservation of the facial nerve, depending on the extent of the tumor. Submandibular gland tumors were treated by gland resection with neck dissection in about one half of the cases.

Tumors of the minor salivary glands were either locally excised (presumably in patients with low-stage and low-grade tumors), or palatectomies or mandibulectomies were performed.

Although there is only limited information available regarding the efficacy of using radiotherapy for the treatment of this group of salivary gland tumors, there is at least some evidence that certain patients benefit from its use. It appears that the particularly poor long-term survival of patients with high-grade or stage III or IV tumors may warrant postoperative irradiation.

Some investigators[49] have reported that adenocarcinoma, NOS, appeared to be of relatively low radiosensitivity. However, Tran and colleagues[12] noted that only three of nine patients with adenocarcinoma, NOS, had their tumors locally controlled by surgery alone, but six of eight patients had control with combined therapy that included 4,000 to 6,000 rad of postoperative radiation.

Other reports are less specific regarding the efficacy of radiotherapy for specific histologic grades of tumor. Shidnia and colleagues[50] and Tu and coworkers[48] reported improved results with postoperative radiation in high-grade tumors but not in low-grade tumors. Reddy and co-investigators[51] achieved improved results in patients with stages III and IV tumors of high histologic grade. Authors of other studies also have advocated the use of postoperative radiotherapy.[13, 14, 15, 20, 23, 52–54] Many of these studies emphasize the importance of attempting total gross tumor removal with surgery rather than reliance on radiation therapy to control residual neoplasm. Treatment failure often appears to be related to the presence of residual tumor at the tumor margin. Limited information is available regarding the role of chemotherapy.[55, 56]

REFERENCES

1. Foote FW Jr, Frazell EL: Tumors of the major salivary glands. Cancer 1953; 6:1065–1133.
2. Thackray AC, Lucas RB: Tumors of the Major Salivary Glands. Fascicle 10. Atlas of Tumor Pathology, 2nd series. Washington DC, Armed Forces Institute of Pathology, 1974.
3. Spiro RH: Salivary neoplasms: Overview of a 35-year experience with 2,807 patients. Head Neck Surg 1986; 8:177–184.
4. Rosenfeld L, Sessions DG, McSwain B, Graves H Jr: Malignant tumors of salivary gland origin: 37-year review of 184 cases. Ann Surg 1966; 163:726–735.
5. Sharkey FE: Systematic evaluation of the World Health Organization classification of salivary gland tumors. Am J Clin Pathol 1977; 67:272–278.
6. Chaudhry AP, Vickers RA, Gorlin RJ: Intraoral minor salivary gland tumors-analysis of 1,414 cases. Oral Surg Oral Med Oral Pathol 1961; 14:1194–1226.
7. Stene T, Koppang HS: Intraoral adenocarcinomas. J Oral Pathol 1981; 10:216–225.
8. Bauer WH, Bauer JD: Classification of glandular tumors of salivary glands. Study of one hundred forty-three cases. Arch Pathol 1953; 55:328–346.
9. Spitz MR, Batsakis JG: Major salivary gland carcinoma. Arch Otolaryngol 1984; 110:45–49.
10. Eveson JW, Cawson RA: Salivary gland tumours: A review of 2410 cases with particular reference to histological types, site, age and sex distribution. J Pathol 1985; 146:51–58.
11. Main JH, Orr JA, McGuirk FM, McComb RJ, Mock D: Salivary gland tumors: Review of 643 cases. J Oral Pathol 1976; 5:88–102.
12. Tran L, Sadeghi A, Hanson D, Juillard G, MacKintosh R, Calcaterra TC, Parker RG: Major salivary gland tumors: Treatment results and prognostic factors. Laryngoscope 1986; 96:1139–1144.
13. Guillamondegui OM, Byers RM, Luna MA, Chiminazzo H Jr, Jesse RH, Fletcher GH: Aggressive surgery in treatment for parotid cancer: The role of adjunctive postoperative radiotherapy. Am J Roentgenol 1975; 123:49–54.
14. Byun YS, Faos JV, Kin YH: Management of malignant salivary gland tumors. Laryngoscope 1980; 90:1052–1060.
15. Fu KK, Leibel SA, Levine ML, Friedlander LM, Boles R, Phillips TL: Carcinoma of the major and minor salivary glands: Analysis of treatment results and sites and causes of failure. Cancer 1977; 40:2882–2890.
16. Bissett RJ, Fitzpatrick PJ: Malignant submandibular gland tumors: A review of 91 patients. Am J Clin Oncol 1988; 11:46–51.
17. Owens OT, Calcaterra TC: Salivary gland tumors of the lip. Arch Otolaryngol 1982; 108:45–47.
18. Richardson GS, Dickason WL, Gaisford JC, Hanna DC: Tumors of salivary glands: An analysis of 752 cases. Plast Reconst Surg 1975; 55:131–138.
19. Isacsson G, Shear M: Intraoral salivary gland tumors: A retrospective study of 201 cases. J Oral Pathol 1983; 12:57–62.
20. Ellis ER, Million RR, Mendenhall WM, Parsons JT, Cassisi NJ: The use of radiation therapy in the management of minor salivary gland tumors. Int J Radiat Oncol Biol Phys 1988; 15:613–617.
21. Woods JE, Chong GC, Beahrs OH: Experience with 1,360 primary parotid tumors. Am J Surg 1975; 130:460–462.
22. Ma DQ, Yu GY: Tumours of the minor salivary glands: A clinicopathologic study of 243 cases. Acta Otolaryngol (Stockh) 1987; 103:325–331.
23. Fitzpatrick PJ, Theriault C: Malignant salivary gland tumors. Int J Radiat Oncol Biol Phys 1986; 12:1743–1747.
24. Friedman M, Levin B, Grybauskas V, Strorigl T, Manaligod J, Hill JH, Skolnik E: Malignant tumors of the major salivary glands. Otolaryngol Clin North Am 1986; 19:625–636.
25. Theron EJ, Middlecote BD: Tumours of the salivary glands: The Bloemfontein experience. S Afr J Surg 1984; 22:237–242.
26. Spiro RH, Huvos AG, Strong EW: Adenocarcinoma of salivary origin: Clinicopathologic study of 204 patients. Am J Surg 1982; 144:423–431.
27. Yu GY, Ma DQ: Carcinoma of the salivary gland: A clinicopathologic study of 405 cases. Semin Surg Oncol 1987; 3:240–244.
28. Wyatt AP, Henry L, Curwen MP: Salivary tumours: A clinicopathological study and follow-up of 156 cases. Br J Surg 1967; 54:636–645.
29. Morgan MN, MacKenzie DH: Tumours of salivary glands: A review of 204 cases with 5-year follow-up. Br J Surg 1968; 55:284–288.
30. Seifert G, Miehlke A, Haubrich J, Chilla R: Diseases of the Salivary Glands: Pathology-Diagnosis-Treatment-Facial Nerve Surgery. Stuttgart, Georg Thieme Verlag, 1986; 171–274.
31. Bardwil JM, Reynolds CT, Ibanez ML, Luna AM: Report of one hundred tumors of the minor salivary glands. Am J Surg 1966; 112:493–497.
32. Chau MNY, Radden BG: Intra-oral salivary gland neoplasms: A retrospective study of 98 cases. J Oral Pathol 1986; 15:339–342.
33. Seifert G, Okabe H, Caselitz J: Epithelial salivary gland tumors in children and adolescents: Analysis of 80 cases (Salivary Gland Registry 1965–1984). ORL J 1986; 48:137–149.
34. Burbank PM, Dockerty MB, Devine KD: Clinicopathologic study of 43 cases of glandular tumor of the tongue. Surg Gynecol Obstet 1959; 109:573–582.
35. Cady B, Hutter RVP: Nonepidermoid cancer of the gum. Cancer 1969; 23:1318–1324.
36. Whittaker JS, Turner EP: Papillary tumours of the

minor salivary glands. J Clin Pathol 1976; 29:795–805.

37. Brooks HW, Hiebert AE, Pullman AE, Stofer BE: Papillary cystadenoma of the palate: A review of the literature and report of two new cases. Oral Surg Oral Med Oral Pathol 1956; 9:1047–1050.

38. Calhoun NR, Cerine FC, Mathews MJ: Papillary cystadenoma of the upper lip: Report of a case. Oral Surg Oral Med Oral Pathol 1965; 20:810–813.

39. Edwards EG: Tumors of the minor salivary glands. Am J Clin Pathol 1960; 34:455–463.

40. Allen MS Jr, Fitz-Hugh GS, March WL: Low-grade papillary adenocarcinoma of the palate. Cancer 1974; 33:153–158.

41. Mills SE, Garland TA, Allen MS Jr: Low-grade papillary adenocarcinoma of palatal salivary gland origin. Am J Surg Pathol 1984; 8:367–374.

42. Freedman PD, Lumerman H: Lobular carcinoma of intraoral minor salivary gland origin: Report of twelve cases. Oral Surg Oral Med Oral Pathol 1983; 56:157–165.

43. Ellis GL, Wiscovitch JG: Basal cell adenocarcinomas of the major salivary glands. Oral Surg Oral Med Oral Pathol 1990; 69:461–469.

44. Blanck C, Eneroth C-M, Jakobsson PA: Mucus-producing adenopapillary (non-epidermoid) carcinoma of the parotid gland. Cancer 1971; 28:676–685.

45. Castro EB, Huvos AG, Strong EW, Foote FW Jr: Tumors of the major salivary glands in children. Cancer 1972; 29:312–317.

46. Baker SR, Malone B: Salivary gland malignancies in children. Cancer 1985; 55:1730–1736.

47. Nishijima W, Tokita N, Takooda S, Tsuchiya S, Watanabe I: Adenocarcinoma of the sublingual gland: Case report and 50 year review of the literature. Laryngoscope 1984; 94:96–101.

48. Tu G, Hu Y, Jiang P, Qin D: The superiority of combined therapy (surgery and postoperative irradiation) in parotid cancer. Arch Otolaryngol 1982; 108:710–713.

49. Jakobsson PA, Eneroth CM: Variations in radiosensitivity of various types of malignant salivary gland tumours. Acta Otolaryngol 1970; 263:186–188.

50. Shidnia H, Hornback NB, Hamaker R, Lingeman R: Carcinoma of major salivary glands. Cancer 1980; 45:693–697.

51. Reddy SP, Marks JE: Treatment of locally advanced, high-grade, malignant tumors of major salivary glands. Laryngoscope 1988; 98:450–454.

52. Chung CT, Sagerman RH, Ryoo MC, King GA, Yu WS, Dalal PS: The changing role of external-beam irradiation in the management of malignant tumors of the major salivary glands. Radiology 1982; 145:175–177.

53. King JJ, Fletcher GH: Malignant tumors of the major salivary glands. Radiology 1971; 100:381–384.

54. Matsuba HM, Mauney M, Simpson JR, Thawley SE, Pikul FJ: Adenocarcinomas of major and minor salivary gland origin: A histopathologic review of treatment failure patterns. Laryngoscope 1988; 98:784–788.

55. Dreyfuss AI, Clark JR, Fallon BG, Posner MR, Norris CM Jr, Miller D: Cyclophosphamide, doxorubicin, and cisplatin combination chemotherapy for advanced carcinomas of salivary gland origin. Cancer 1987; 60:2869–2872.

56. Belani CP, Eisenberger MA, Gray WC: Preliminary experience with chemotherapy in advanced salivary gland neoplasm. Med Pediatr Oncol 1988; 16:197–202.

19

ADENOID CYSTIC CARCINOMA

Charles E. Tomich

Adenoid cystic carcinoma is a clinically and pathologically well-defined entity that has been described extensively in the literature. It occurs primarily in the major salivary glands and relatively frequently in the oral accessory salivary glands, particularly the palate. It occurs less commonly in other glandular areas of the head and neck. In the head and neck areas, the tumor has been found in the ceruminal glands of the ears and in the lacrimal glands of the eyes.

Theodor Billroth[1] is generally credited with the initial description of this tumor and with the suggestion that it be called *cylindroma*. In 1945, Bauer and Fox's[2] suggested use of the term *adeno-myoepithelioma* was based on their theory that the lesion was histogenetically derived from intercalated duct and myoepithelial cells. Dockerty and Mayo[3] used the designation *adenocarcinoma, cylindroma type*. Foote and Frazell proposed the currently accepted appellation *adenoid cystic carcinoma* in their classic paper in 1953[4] and in their fascicle on major salivary gland tumors in 1954.[5] Thus, the term adenoid cystic carcinoma has persisted for nearly 4 decades, and virtually no recent attempts have been made to alter it.

At the Armed Forces Institute of Pathology (AFIP) during a 48-year period (1940–1988), 600 examples of the tumor have been observed. It is the fourth most common malignant salivary gland tumor in these files, following mucoepidermoid carcinoma, acinic cell carcinoma, and adenocarcinoma, not otherwise specified (NOS). Adenoid cystic carcinoma accounts for 11.8 percent of the 5,054 malignant salivary gland tumors studied during that period.

The incidence of adenoid cystic carcinoma varies widely in reported series. In 1961, Chaudhry and colleagues[6] reported that adenoid cystic carcinoma was the most common histologic type among 520 malignant salivary gland tumors studied and that it accounted for 41.3 percent. On the other hand, Eneroth[7] encountered 119 cases among 528 malignant salivary gland tumors (22.5 percent). Regezi and Sciubba[8] compiled data from nine reported series, including the report by Chaudhry that was just cited. The series totaled 3,150 malignant salivary gland tumors; 723 (22.9 percent) were histologically classified as adenoid cystic carcinomas. Waldron and coworkers[9] encountered 40 adenoid cystic carcinomas among 476 oral minor salivary gland tumors (9.4 percent). Considering only malignant tumors (181), adenoid cystic carcinoma accounted for 22.1 percent.

The histologic features that have been considered to be within the spectrum of adenoid cystic carcinoma have varied, depending on the investigators. Indeed, based on more current criteria, tumors originally classified as adenoid cystic carcinoma proved to be polymorphous low-grade adenocarcinomas, epithelial-myoepithelial carcinomas and even canalicular and basal cell adenomas. However, several histologic types are recognized, including (1) the classic *cribriform* type, which is composed of small, deeply basophilic, uniform cells resembling basal cells that are arranged in anastomosing cords or ductlike patterns; (2) the *tubular* type, which is composed of single or multiple layers of small basaloid cells that are arranged in small ducts with a single lumen; and (3) the *solid* type, which is composed of sheets of basaloid cells with scanty cytoplasm and, at times, central areas of necrosis.[10, 11]

CLINICAL FINDINGS

Age and Sex Incidence

Adenoid cystic carcinoma occurs most often in adults in the fifth, sixth, and seventh decades of life. In the AFIP series, 60 percent of all cases

Percent

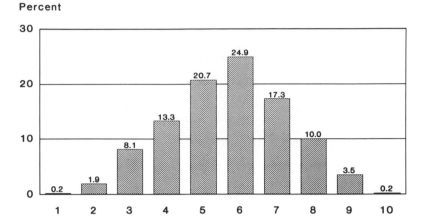

Age (decade)

Figure 19–1. Distribution by age of 600 patients with adenoid cystic carcinoma reported by the AFIP during a 48-year period. Although the tumor may occur at any age, it is not common in the first two decades of life.

occurred within these 3 decades (Fig. 19–1). Although the tumor is uncommon in young persons, occasional cases are encountered in the first 2 decades of life.[12-14]

Most series show an equal distribution of cases between the sexes. Overall, 53.3 percent of the patients with adenoid cystic carcinoma in the AFIP series were male. Interestingly, when civilian cases alone were analyzed, a total of 417 cases, 62 percent (259 cases) were found to occur in women. The vast majority of patients were white (84.4 percent); only 11 percent of the patients affected were black.

Clinical Complaints

Typically, adenoid cystic carcinoma is apparent in the major salivary glands as a swelling or as a mass (Fig. 19–2). Characteristically, the tumor grows slowly; patients may be aware of the lesion for months and even years in some instances. Pain and tenderness generally occur during the course of tumor growth. Fixation to skin and to surrounding deeper structures develops in the later stages of tumor growth. An ominous feature of adenoid cystic carcinoma of the parotid gland as

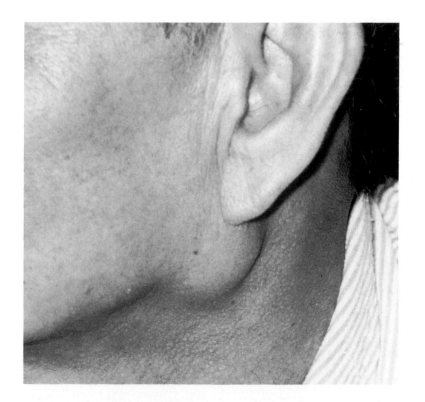

Figure 19–2. Adenoid cystic carcinoma of the parotid gland in an adult woman. (Courtesy of Dr. Edward C. Weisberger, Indiana University Medical Center.)

well as of other malignant salivary gland neoplasms in this location is paralysis of the facial nerve.

Adenoid cystic carcinoma of the intraoral accessory salivary glands presents typically as a swelling or mass. Pain is a variable finding, particularly in the early stages of development. As tumor growth progresses, pain and ulceration develop (Fig. 19–3).

Symptoms of facial pain and swelling characterize adenoid cystic carcinoma of the maxillary antrum, but these symptoms are not specific for this particular tumor. Radiographic examination is valuable in assessing the extent of osseous destruction (Fig. 19–4). Symptoms may have been present for months or years and are generally of longer duration than those associated with squamous carcinoma, which is the most frequent malignancy of this location. Adenoid cystic carcinomas of the nasal cavity and ear canal produce symptoms of obstruction and deafness, respectively.

Anatomic Location

Adenoid cystic carcinomas occur predominantly in the parotid and submandibular glands. They are only rarely observed in the sublingual gland owing to the uncommon occurrence of tumors in this gland. In the AFIP series of 600 cases, 312 tumors (52 percent) occurred in the major glands, including the sublingual gland (Table 19–1). Similar findings have been reported in other series. In the cases compiled by Regezi and Sciubba,[8] 335 of 723 tumors (46.3 percent) occurred in the major glands.

From another point of view, however, adenoid cystic carcinomas may be viewed as uncommon. Spiro and colleagues[15] reported that only 1.6 percent of *all* parotid tumors are adenoid cystic carcinomas; Eneroth[7] reported a comparable rate of occurrence of 2.2 percent. Eneroth and Hjertman[16] found that 12 percent of *all* submandibular salivary gland tumors are of this histologic type. Relative to the sublingual glands, adenoid cystic carcinomas account for 40 percent of the tumors in this particular gland;[17] however, numerically they are encountered rarely. Nonetheless, this carcinoma does account for 20 percent of the malignant parenchymal tumors of the sublingual gland in the AFIP series.

Virtually all reported series reflect the relatively frequent occurrence of adenoid cystic carcinoma in the minor salivary glands, particularly the palate. Although 42.5 percent of adenoid cystic carcinomas occurred in the minor glands, 20.5 percent were in the palate (see Table 19–1). Adenoid

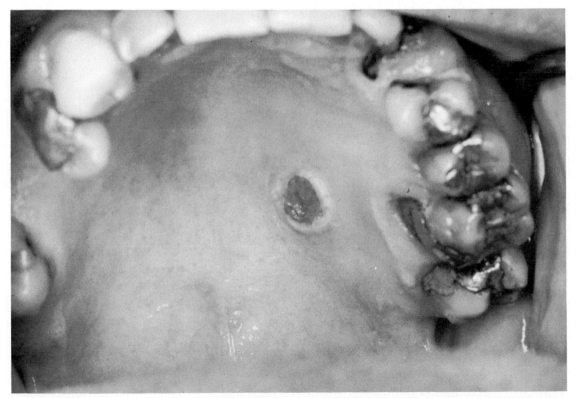

Figure 19–3. Adenoid cystic carcinoma of the palate in an adult male. Ulceration developed fairly early in the course of the disease.

Table 19–1. Distribution by Anatomic Site of 600 Patients with Adenoid Cystic Carcinoma from the AFIP Salivary Gland Registry

Anatomic Site	Number of Cases	Percentage
Major Glands		
Parotid gland	161	26.8
Submandibular gland	144	24.0
Sublingual gland	7	1.2
Minor Glands		
Palate (total)	123	20.5
Palate, not specified	(79)	(13.2)
Hard palate	(24)	(4.0)
Soft palate	(20)	(3.3)
Lip (total)	22	3.7
Upper lip	(18)	(3.0)
Lower lip	(4)	(0.6)
Tongue	30	5.0
Cheek	23	3.8
Floor of mouth	14	2.3
Tonsil/oropharynx	8	1.3
Retromolar area	5	0.8
Other	30	5.0
Not Stated	33	5.5
*Total**	600	100.0

*Does not include numbers in parentheses

cystic carcinoma accounts for 8.3 percent of *all* palatal salivary gland tumors and 17.7 percent of the *malignant* palatal salivary gland tumors (AFIP series). Batsakis[17] reported that 44.7 percent of 510 adenoid cystic carcinomas occurred in the

intraoral minor glands, a figure comparable to the 42.5 percent based on the AFIP series (see Table 19–1).

Besides occurring in the palatal salivary glands, adenoid cystic carcinoma is noted in other intraoral sites. Of particular interest are those cases occurring in the tongue. In a study by deVries and his colleagues,[18] 22 salivary gland tumors, all malignant, were found in the base of the tongue. Six (27 percent) were classified as adenoid cystic carcinoma. Goldblatt and Ellis[19] studied 50 malignant salivary gland tumors of the tongue, 5 (10 percent) of which were adenoid cystic carcinomas. In an extensive study, Spiro and coworkers[20] reviewed 27 such neoplasms of the tongue. Thus, adenoid cystic carcinoma appears to be the third most common malignancy of the tongue; it is exceeded in frequency of occurrence only by epidermoid and mucoepidermoid carcinomas.

Adenoid cystic carcinoma of the salivary glands of the buccal mucosa is encountered with some frequency. In the AFIP series (see Table 19–1), 23 were found in this anatomic location. Waldron and colleagues[9] observed seven cases in this site.

In their study of labial salivary gland tumors, Neville and colleagues[21] observed four adenoid cystic carcinomas of the upper lip; none were encountered in the lower lip. Waldron's group[9] encountered two such tumors in the upper lip. Surprisingly, in the AFIP series, 18 were found in the upper lip, and 4 were encountered in the lower lip (see Table 19–1).

As may be noted in Table 19–1, adenoid cystic carcinoma is encountered in any intraoral location in which salivary glands normally occur. Besides

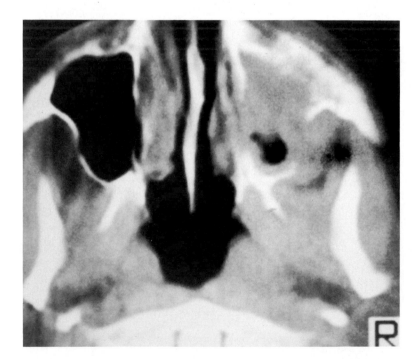

Figure 19–4. Computed tomographic scan of antral adenoid cystic carcinoma. The tumor has destroyed the lateral nasal/medial antral wall. (Courtesy of Dr. Homayoon Shidnia, Indiana University Medical Center.)

occurring in salivary glands, adenoid cystic carcinomas arise in the mucous glands of the upper airway (including the paranasal sinuses) and in the bronchial glands (see Chapter 31).[17, 20] Finally, adenoid cystic carcinomas are known to occur in other anatomic sites that contain exocrine or eccrine glands, particularly sweat glands or variants thereof. Noteworthy are those arising in the ceruminal glands of the ear,[22] the breast,[23] and the vulva.[24]

GROSS FINDINGS

Adenoid cystic carcinoma usually presents as a fairly well-defined mass within the substance of the involved gland. On cut section, the tumor lacks encapsulation, although it may appear to be demarcated from the surrounding salivary gland tissue. Close inspection typically shows infiltration into the surrounding parenchymal tissue. The tumor is firm, white, or grayish-white and is not usually "cystic." Grossly observable "cystic" zones are uncommon, as are areas of hemorrhage.

MICROSCOPIC FINDINGS

Like many salivary gland tumors, adenoid cystic carcinoma has been described as having varied microscopic patterns. However, the actual cells that form these "patterns" are remarkably uniform in size, shape, and staining qualities. Thus, the tumor is composed of isomorphic cells that are arranged in various morphologic patterns. Depending on the relative prominence of these morphologic patterns, adenoid cystic carcinoma is seen to exist in (1) the *cribriform pattern*, (2) the *tubular pattern*, and (3) the *solid pattern*.

Cribriform Type. The cribriform pattern is the most important and most recognized microscopic type. This classic pattern of adenoid cystic carcinoma is generally recognized by the arrangement of the tumor cells in the so-called "Swiss cheese" configuration (Fig. 19–5). The tumor cells are characterized by dark, deeply basophilic nuclei and scanty cytoplasm. Nucleoli are seldom observed, and division figures are rarely encountered. The cells are arranged in nests of variable size and shape that contain many circular or ovoid spaces; these spaces impart the Swiss cheese pattern. The spaces may contain either a faintly basophilic mucinous substance or hyalinized eosinophilic zones (Fig. 19–6). Other microscopic fields may show cords of the same isomorphic tumor cells within the hyalinized material (Fig. 19–7). Both such fields may occur concomitantly in the same tumor field. The stroma of the tumor is typically fibrous; however, at times, it may be somewhat hyalinized. Prominent stromal features of chondroid, myxomatous, and hyalinized areas

are not typically encountered; thus, their presence should suggest another diagnosis, such as mixed tumor. Most important to the differential diagnosis, however, is the fact that the supporting stroma does not contain the individual tumor cells that are observed in the mixed tumor.[25]

Tubular Type. The second major microscopic pattern of adenoid cystic carcinoma is the tubular type. The tumor cells are identical to those observed in the cribriform pattern; however, the arrangement of these cells is different. Single ductal structures are formed by layers of the isomorphic cells (Fig. 19–8). In longitudinal section (Fig. 19–9), these ductal structures are viewed as ducts or tubules, a feature that is responsible for the designation of this histologic pattern. It is obvious that the ducts or tubules in cross-section and in longitudinal section may be viewed in the same tumor. The lumina may contain a mucinous substance that is faintly eosinophilic (Fig. 19–10). This material typically stains positively with periodic acid–Schiff (PAS) stain before and after diastase digestion. Cribriform areas may coexist with the tubular pattern, and transitions may be observed (Fig. 19–11).

Solid Type. The third major microscopic pattern of adenoid cystic carcinoma is the solid type. The isomorphic tumor cells characteristic of the cribriform and tubular types are arranged in nests or sheets of varying size and shape (Fig. 19–12). There is no, or only a minimal, tendency to form the circular or ovoid spaces that characterize the cribriform type, and no ducts or tubular structures like those observed in the tubular type are formed. Occasionally, areas of necrosis may be found centrally within some of the solid nests.[11, 26] In addition to foci of necrosis, cellular pleomorphism and mitoses may be observed in this pattern, which are features that are not usually found in the other patterns of adenoid cystic carcinoma.[26]

Multiple Patterns

It is recognized that most adenoid cystic carcinomas do not occur in "pure" cribriform, tubular, or solid types. Rather, all three patterns can be observed in the majority of tumors.[10] Generally, tumors are classified according to the histologic pattern that predominates. The main reason for histologically typing adenoid cystic carcinoma, or any other malignancy, is to assess any clinical or prognostic differences between the histologic types. In this regard, numerous observers have reported prognostic differences between the three morphologic patterns (see later).

Perzin and colleagues[10] studied 62 cases of adenoid cystic carcinoma that occurred in both major and minor salivary glands. The classic cribriform pattern predominated in 27 tumors (43.5 percent), the tubular pattern in 22 tumors (35.5 percent),

Text continued on page 342

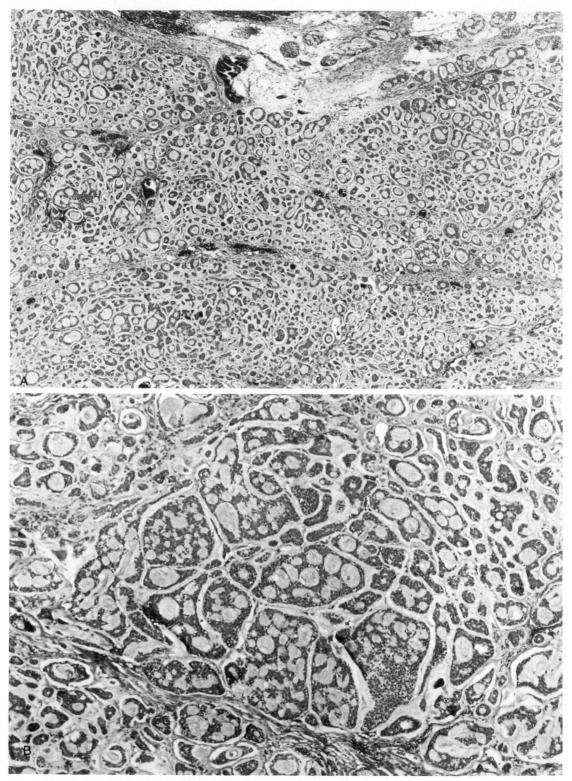

Figure 19–5. *A* Example of the cribriform pattern of adenoid cystic carcinoma. *B*, Higher magnification shows variable-sized cribriform spaces formed by small, deeply basophilic cells. (A, × 30; B, × 75.)

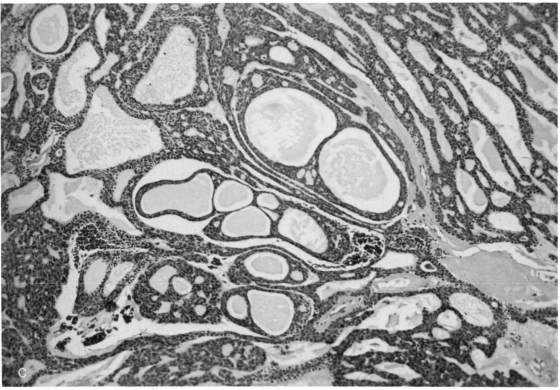

Figure 19–5 *Continued C,* This adenoid cystic carcinoma demonstrates variation in size and shape of the cystic spaces (× 100).

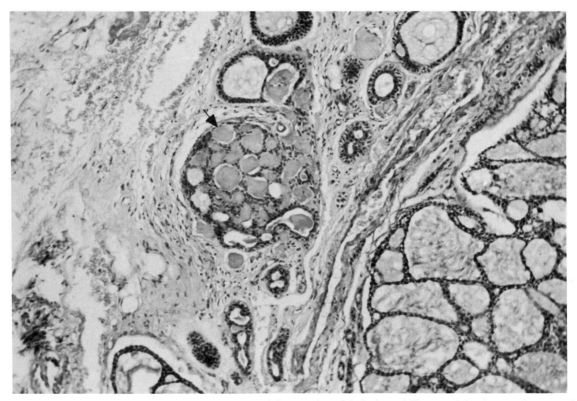

Figure 19–6. The large cribriform spaces at the right contain a faintly basophilic material, whereas the nest of tumor cells in the center (arrow) contains eosinophilic hyalinized material (× 100).

Blanck and coworkers[42] reported a 70 percent 5-year survival rate for patients with parotid gland tumors; however, the 20-year survival rate was only 13 percent. Conley and Dingman[39] emphasized the need for long-term evaluation that lasts up to 20 years. In their group of 34 patients with 5 years' follow-up after initial treatment, 30 (88.2 percent) were alive. In their 10-year follow-up group of 40 patients, 19 survived (47.5 percent), but 8 had persistent disease. The 15-year group of 35 patients had 15 survivors (42.8 percent), 8 of whom had persistent tumor. In the group with over 20-years' follow-up that involved 25 patients, only 5 (20 percent) were alive with no evidence of disease. Their data showed a more favorable prognosis in patients with major salivary gland tumors than in those with minor salivary gland tumors. Overall, 64 percent of 56 patients with parotid and submandibular gland tumors were alive with no evidence of disease, whereas only 28 percent of 78 patients with minor gland tumors were alive and free of disease. Significantly, none of the 13 patients with minor salivary gland tumors in the 20-year study group were alive and free of disease.

In addition to recurrence rate, a relationship also has been made between the histologic pattern of the tumor and survival. Perzin and coworkers[10] reported a favorable outcome for 50 percent of those patients with tumors that have a tubular pattern and for 26 percent of those patients with tumors that have a cribriform pattern; none of those with a solid pattern had a favorable outcome. All patients with the solid pattern had died of, or were living with, their tumor. Conversely, Nascimento and coworkers[26] reported a more favorable prognosis for patients with the cribriform pattern. Five-year survival rates for the cribriform, tubular, and solid patterns were 52.3, 33.3, and 13.3 percent, respectively. In the 10-year study, no one with tubular or solid patterns survived, and only 14.3 percent of those with a cribriform pattern survived.

The study by Matsuba and colleagues[40] supported the findings of Nascimento's group. Those patients with a cribriform pattern had the longest survival time, followed by those with tubular and solid patterns. In the study of 20-plus years, the longest surviving patient with a solid pattern was 8 years, whereas 4 patients with the cribriform pattern survived over 20 years.

Hickman and colleagues[43] reviewed 30 reported series of adenoid cystic carcinoma, which consisted of 1,065 patients. Based on this review, the expected 5-year survival rate is 62.4 percent, and the expected 10-year survival rate is 38.9 percent.

Salivary gland adenoid cystic carcinoma has a dismal ultimate prognosis for cure, although long-term survivors, even with persistent disease, are not uncommon. Factors that indicate a poor prognosis include failure of local disease control at the initial surgical procedure, a solid pattern histologically, recurrent disease, and distant metastasis.

There is general agreement that surgery is the preferred treatment for adenoid cystic carcinoma.[41] Complete excision at the first surgical procedure has been shown to offer the patient the best chance for long-term survival and cure.[10, 39, 40] Elective regional lymph node dissection is not indicated,[39] because distant metastasis is more common than cervical (regional) node involvement.[41] With submandibular gland tumors, however, some type of node dissection is performed, since this conforms to established principles of surgery. Although complete surgical removal is a necessity relative to any chance for cure, Matsuba and colleagues[40] have cautioned against extremely radical or mutilating surgery, particularly in the presence of distant metastasis.

Adenoid cystic carcinoma is a radiosensitive tumor, and radiation therapy does play a role in the management of this disease, particularly in the control of microscopic disease after initial surgery or in treating local recurrent disease. Radiation therapy also has been recommended for palliation of unresectable disease.[39]

REFERENCES

1. Billroth T: Beobachtungen uber Geschwulste der Speicheldrusen. Virchows Arch [A] 1859; 17:357–375.
2. Bauer WH, Fox RA: Adenomyoepithelioma (cylindroma) of palatal mucous glands. Arch Pathol 1945; 39:96–102.
3. Dockerty MB, Mayo CW: Primary tumors of submaxillary gland with special reference to mixed tumors. Surg Gynecol Obstet 1942; 74:1033–1045.
4. Foote FW Jr, Frazell EL: Tumors of the major salivary glands. Cancer 1953; 6:1065–1133.
5. Foote FW Jr, Frazell EL: Tumors of the Major Salivary Glands, Section IV, Fascicle 11. Atlas of Tumor Pathology. Washington, D.C., Armed Forces Institute of Pathology, 1954.
6. Chaudhry AP, Vickers RA, Gorlin RJ: Intraoral minor salivary gland tumors. Oral Surg Oral Med Oral Pathol 1961; 14:1194–1226.
7. Eneroth C-M: Salivary gland tumors in the parotid gland, submandibular gland and the palate region. Cancer 1971; 27:1415–1418.
8. Regezi JA, Sciubba JJ: Oral Pathology. Clinical-Pathologic Correlations. Philadelphia, WB Saunders Co, 1989.
9. Waldron CA, El-Mofty SK, Gnepp DR: Tumors of the intraoral minor salivary glands: A demographic and histologic study of 426 cases. Oral Surg Oral Med Oral Pathol 1988; 66:323–333.
10. Perzin KH, Gullane P, Clairmont AC: Adenoid cystic carcinoma arising in salivary glands: A correlation of histologic features and clinical course. Cancer 1978; 42:265–282.
11. Tarpley TM, Giansanti JS: Adenoid cystic carcinoma. Oral Surg Oral Med Oral Pathol 1976; 41:484–497.
12. Krolls SO, Trodahl JN, Boyers RC: Salivary gland lesions in children: A survey of 430 cases. Cancer 1972; 30:459–469.

13. Castro EB, Huvos AG, Strong EW, Foote FW Jr: Tumors of the major salivary glands in children. Cancer 1972; 29:312–317.

14. Baker SR, Malone B: Salivary gland malignancies in children. Cancer 1985; 55:1730–1736.

15. Spiro RH, Huvos AG, Strong EW: Cancer of the parotid gland: A clinicopathologic study of 288 primary cases. Am J Surg 1975; 130:452–459.

16. Eneroth C-M, Hjertman L: Adenoid cystic carcinoma of the submandibular gland. Laryngoscope 1966; 76:1639–1661.

17. Batsakis JG: Tumors of the Head and Neck. Clinical and Pathologic Considerations, 2nd edition. Baltimore, Williams & Wilkins Co, 1979.

18. deVries EJ, Johnson JT, Myers EN, Barnes EL, Mandell-Brown M: Base of tongue salivary gland tumors. Head Neck Surg 1987; 9:329–331.

19. Goldblatt LI, Ellis GL: Salivary gland tumors of the tongue. Analysis of 55 new cases and review of the literature. Cancer 1987; 60:74–81.

20. Spiro RH, Koss LG, Hajdu SI, Strong EW: Tumors of minor salivary origin. A clinicopathologic study of 492 cases. Cancer 1973; 31:117–129.

21. Neville BW, Damm DD, Weir JC, Fantasia JE: Labial salivary gland tumors. Cancer 1988; 61:2113–2116.

22. Hyams VJ, Batsakis JG, Michaels L: Tumors of the Upper Respiratory Tract and Ear, Fascicle 25. Atlas of Tumor Pathology, 2nd Series. Washington, D.C., Armed Forces Institute of Pathology, 1988.

23. Ro JY, Silva EG, Gallagher HS: Adenoid cystic carcinoma of the breast. Hum Pathol 1987; 18:1216–1281.

24. Abrao FS, Marques AF, Marziona F, Abrao MS, Junqueira LC, Torloni H: Adenoid cystic carcinoma of Bartholin's gland: Review of the literature and report of two cases. J Surg Oncol 1985; 30:132–137.

25. Evans RW, Cruickshank AH: Epithelial Tumours of the Salivary Glands. Philadelphia, WB Saunders Co, 1970.

26. Nascimento AG, Amaral ALP, Prado LAF, Kligerman J, Silveira TRP: Adenoid cystic carcinoma of salivary glands: A study of 61 cases with clinicopathologic correlation. Cancer 1986; 57:312–319.

27. Batsakis JG, Pinkston GR, Luna MA, Byers RM, Sciubba JJ, Tillery GW: Adenocarcinoma of the oral cavity: A clinicopathologic study of terminal duct carcinoma. J Laryngol Otol 1983; 97:825–835.

28. Fayemi AO, Toker C: Salivary duct carcinoma. Arch Otolaryngol 1974; 366–368.

29. Qizilbash AH, Sianos J, Young JEM, Archibald SD: Fine-needle aspiration biopsy of major salivary glands. Acta Cytol 1985; 29:503–512.

30. Eneroth C-M, Zajicek J: Aspiration biopsy of salivary gland tumors. IV. Morphologic studies on smears and histologic sections from 45 cases of adenoid cystic carcinoma. Acta Cytol 1969; 13:59–63.

31. Chen J-C, Gnepp DR, Bedrossian CWM: Adenoid cystic carcinoma of the salivary glands: An immunohistochemical study. Oral Surg Oral Med Oral Pathol 1988; 65:316–326.

32. Schmitt FC, Filho CZ, Bacchi MM, Castilho ED, Bacchi CE: Adenoid cystic carcinoma of trachea metastatic to placenta. Hum Pathol 1989; 20:193–195.

33. Morinaga S, Nakajima T, Shimosato Y: Normal and neoplastic myoepithelial cells in salivary gland: An immunohistochemical study. Hum Pathol 1987; 18:1218–1226.

34. Hoshino M, Yamamoto I: Ultrastructure of adenoid cystic carcinoma. Cancer 1970; 25:186–198.

35. Chaudhry AP, Leifer C, Cutler LS, Satchidanand S, Laday GR, Yamane GM: Histogenesis of adenoid cystic carcinoma of the salivary glands: Light and electron-microscopic study. Cancer 1986; 58:72–82.

36. Corio RL, Sciubba JJ, Brannon RB, Batsakis JG: Epithelial-myoepithelial carcinoma of intercalated duct origin: A clinicopathologic and ultrastructural assessment of sixteen cases. Oral Surg Oral Med Oral Pathol 1982; 53:280–287.

37. Evans HL, Batsakis JG: Polymorphous low-grade adenocarcinoma of the minor salivary glands: A study of 14 cases of a distinctive neoplasm. Cancer 1984; 53:935–942.

38. Eby LS, Johnson DS, Baker HW: Adenoid cystic carcinoma of the head and neck. Cancer 1972; 29:1160–1168.

39. Conley J, Dingman DL: Adenoid cystic carcinoma in the head and neck (cylindroma). Arch Otolaryngol 1974; 100:81–90.

40. Matsuba HM, Spector GJ, Thawley SE, Simpson JR, Mauney M, Pikul FJ: Adenoid cystic salivary gland carcinoma: A histopathologic review of treatment failure patterns. Cancer 1986; 57:519–524.

41. Spiro RH, Armstrong J, Harrison L, Geller NL, Lin S-Y, Strong EW: Carcinoma of major salivary glands: Major trends. Arch Otolaryngol Head Neck Surg 1989; 115:316–321.

42. Blanck C, Eneroth C-M, Jacobsson F, Jakobsson PA: Adenoid cystic carcinoma of the parotid gland. Acta Radiol 1967; 177–196.

43. Hickman RE, Cawson RA, Duffy SW: The prognosis for specific types of salivary gland tumors. Cancer 1984; 54:1620–1624.

20

MALIGNANT MIXED TUMORS

Douglas R. Gnepp and Bruce M. Wenig

Malignant mixed tumors of salivary gland origin are relatively uncommon neoplasms. However, the broad heading *malignant mixed tumor* includes three different clinical and pathologic entities: carcinoma ex mixed tumor (carcinoma arising in a mixed tumor), carcinosarcoma (true malignant mixed tumor), and metastasizing mixed tumor. The first accounts for the vast majority of malignant mixed tumors, whereas the last two are extremely uncommon and account for only a small percentage of tumors in this group.

This chapter reviews the literature and AFIP experiences with malignant mixed tumors involving the upper aerodigestive tract. Malignant mixed tumors arising in the lacrimal glands,[1, 2] skin,[3–5] lower respiratory tract,[6, 7] and other more unusual anatomic locations[8, 9] are not considered in this chapter.

CARCINOMA EX MIXED TUMOR

Carcinoma ex mixed tumor, also known as carcinoma ex pleomorphic adenoma or carcinoma arising in a mixed tumor, is a mixed tumor in which a second neoplasm develops from the epithelial component that fulfills the criteria for malignancy. These criteria include invasiveness, destruction of normal tissues, cellular anaplasia, cellular pleomorphism, atypical mitoses, and abnormal architectural patterns, such as back-to-back glands and sheets of cells. Necrosis and increased numbers of normal-appearing mitotic figures always are worrisome but, by themselves, should not be considered as indicative or diagnostic of malignancy. Also, it is important to be aware that benign mixed tumors may, on occasion, have focal areas of marked epithelial atypia. Therefore, cellular atypia alone is insufficient for making a definitive diagnosis of malignancy and must be combined with other criteria before malignancy can be firmly established. When carcinoma ex mixed tumor metastasizes, only the carcinoma component metastasizes; the benign mixed tumor component is not found in the metastases.

Incidence

In the Armed Forces Institute of Pathology (AFIP) registry, there are 326 carcinoma ex mixed tumors, which account for 2.2 percent of all types of tumors, 4.5 percent of all mixed tumors (benign and malignant combined), and 6.5 percent of all malignant tumors. Slightly higher than those reported in the AFIP series, the average incidence rates for carcinoma ex mixed tumor in 58 recent series in the literature[10–70] are 3.6 percent of all salivary gland tumors (range 0.9 to 14.0 percent), 6.2 percent of all mixed tumors (range 1.9 to 23.3 percent), and 11.7 percent of all malignant salivary gland tumors (range 2.8 to 42.4 percent).

The National Institutes of Health issued a report on the Surveillance, Epidemiology, and End Results program in 1981.[36] This report tabulated 301,972 malignant tumors from all body sites for a 5-year period from 1973 to 1977 in an estimated population of 100,672,758. Seventy-two malignant mixed tumors (most likely carcinoma ex mixed tumors since carcinosarcomas were tabulated separately) were found in the major salivary glands, 9 in the oral cavity, 3 in the lips, and 1 in the nasal cavity, which resulted in a prevalence rate of 5.6 cases per 100,000 malignant tumors per year and an annual incidence rate of 0.17 tumor per 1,000,000 people.

Clinical Findings

Analysis of the 304 patients in the AFIP files whose ages were stated indicates an incidence peak that spans a single broad age range with 64 percent of cases occurring in the sixth to eighth decades (Fig. 20–1). The mean patient age at the time of occurrence was 56.4 years; the mean ages for men and women were equivalent. Similar mean ages have been recorded by other authors;[10, 28, 42] however, Gerughty and colleagues[71] recorded a younger average age of 40 years. Occurrence of this tumor is exceptional in patients under 20 years. Only four cases were recorded in the AFIP material. The youngest patient was 8 years old, and the oldest was 95 years old. This lower incidence in children has been previously recorded by others. Krolls and colleagues[72] reviewed 430 salivary gland lesions in children, including 54 malignant tumors, and Lack and Upton[73] reviewed 80 salivary gland tumors, including 15 carcinomas. Carcinoma ex mixed tumor was conspicuously absent from both of these series.

Data on gender were available for 308 patients. Men outnumbered women by a ratio of 58:42; however, if the military bias is eliminated, there is a slight predominance of female patients, with 55 percent of tumors occurring in women. Similar data on gender distribution have been demonstrated in other series.[10] Information on race does not indicate any significant predominance.

Localization

Data from the 326 AFIP cases are summarized in Table 20–1. Eighty percent of the tumors in these cases arose in the major salivary glands and 17.5 percent in the minor glands. Of the 260 major gland tumors, 81 percent involved the parotid gland, 16.5 percent the submandibular gland, and 0.4 percent (1 tumor) the sublingual

Table 20–1. Distribution by Anatomic Site of 326 Patients with Carcinoma Ex Mixed Tumor from the AFIP Registry

Anatomic Site	Number of Cases	Percentage
Major Glands		
Parotid gland	210	64.4
Submandibular gland	43	13.2
Sublingual gland	1	0.3
Neck, not otherwise specified	6	1.8
Total major glands	(260)	(79.8)
Minor Glands		
Palate	36	11.0
Upper lip	6	1.8
Tongue	4	1.2
Cheek	4	1.2
Tonsil/oropharynx	4	1.2
Minor glands, not otherwise specified	3	0.9
Total, minor glands	(57)	(17.5)
Not Stated	9	2.7
*Total, All Glands**	326	100.0

*Does not include numbers in parentheses

gland. The specific major gland was unknown in six patients. In the minor glands, 63 percent of tumors involved the palate; 10.5 percent the upper lip; 7 percent each the tongue, cheek, and oropharyngeal regions; and 5 percent other minor gland sites.

Presenting Symptoms

The presenting symptoms are variable. The most frequent symptom is a painless mass;[10, 42] 15 percent of patients note recent rapid growth, occasionally with ulceration.[42] Pain has been described in 4 to 55 percent of patients[10, 42, 48] and

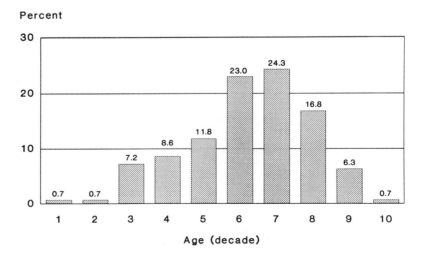

Figure 20–1. Distribution by age (in decades) of 304 patients with carcinoma ex mixed tumors from the AFIP salivary gland registry.

appears to be more common in submandibular gland tumors.[69] Development of facial nerve palsy and skin fixation is variable. Palsy develops in up to 38 percent of patients, and fixation of tumors to adjacent tissues occurs in up to 65 percent of patients.[10, 48] The tumors are characteristically present for long periods of time. Beahrs and coworkers[48] stated that tumors had been found to be present for up to 52.0 years, with an average duration of 23.3 years. However, LiVolsi and colleagues[42] indicated that 45 percent of carcinoma ex mixed tumors may be present for less than 3 years; and Spiro and coworkers[10] mentioned that swelling had been present for 2 years or less in one half of the patients in their series. Eneroth and Zetterberg[74] reviewed 623 patients with benign and malignant mixed tumors in the parotid gland and found that the incidence of malignancy progressively increased with the preoperative duration of the tumor from 1.6 percent for tumors present for less than 5 years to 9.4 percent for tumors present for periods longer than 15 years.

Pathology

In general, the average size of carcinoma ex mixed tumor is more than twice that of its benign counterpart,[69] ranging from 1.5 to 25.0 cm in greatest dimension.[59, 69] Nagao and coworkers[65] found that more than 83 percent of 282 benign mixed tumors were less than 5 cm in maximum diameter, whereas 50 percent of 48 carcinoma ex mixed tumors were greater than 5 cm in maximum dimension. In addition, LiVolsi and Perzin[42] noticed that tumors arising in minor salivary gland sites are smaller, on the average, than their major gland counterparts. Grossly, carcinoma ex mixed tumor is usually poorly circumscribed, and many are extensively infiltrative. Occasional tumors, especially in the major glands, may be well circumscribed or completely encapsulated.[42, 65] The tumors have been described as hard and white or tan-gray.[42, 65] The proportion of benign to malignant regions in each tumor varies considerably. In some tumors, only small foci of residual benign mixed tumor may be found, whereas in others, the majority of the tumor is composed of typical benign mixed tumor with only a small area of carcinomatous tissue. Most tumors fall between these two extremes.

The malignant areas in carcinoma ex mixed tumor consist of epithelial cells with an increased nuclear cytoplasmic ratio, prominent nucleoli, and prominent numbers of mitoses. The most common histologic pattern in these areas is poorly differentiated adenocarcinoma (Fig. 20–2) or undifferentiated carcinoma, but tumors with epidermoid carcinoma, mucoepidermoid carcinoma (Fig. 20–3), myoepithelial carcinoma, adenoid cystic carcinoma, clear cell carcinoma, papillary carci-

noma, and terminal duct carcinoma (polymorphous low-grade adenocarcinoma) have also been described.[10, 42, 59, 75–77]

Destructive infiltrative growth is the most reliable histologic criterion for the diagnosis of a carcinoma ex mixed tumor. Gerughty and colleagues[71] suggested that histologic evidence of an invasive growth pattern, neural or vascular invasion, necrosis, and focal calcification implied a poor prognosis. The number of patients with neural involvement has varied among different series from a small percentage of tumors up to 55 percent of tumors.[42] Vascular invasion is observed somewhat less frequently, with up to 19 percent of tumors demonstrating vascular invasion.[65] Mitotic figures are usually common, and in some studies, all tumors contain mitotic figures.[65] Mitoses are much more commonly found in carcinoma ex mixed tumors than in benign mixed tumors. In addition, there seems to be a positive correlation between the increasing frequency of occurrence of mitotic figures and more invasive growth patterns.[65]

Carcinoma ex mixed tumor seems to arise in two different situations: in primary or in recurrent mixed tumor. Beahrs and coinvestigators[48] described a benign mixed tumor that recurred as a carcinoma ex mixed tumor after 24 years. Other authors have documented numerous carcinoma ex mixed tumors that have arisen from recurrent, histologically benign mixed tumors.[10,42] Supporting the de novo origin for many of these tumors, Gerughty and coworkers[71] found that 64 percent (16 of 25) of their tumors had a short clinical history, and Spiro and coworkers[10] found 30 percent of patients in their series had symptoms of swelling for less than 1 year before diagnosis. This second group included six of eight palatal tumors in which swelling had been apparent for only a few months. In addition, Eneroth and Zetterberg[74] examined the nuclear DNA content of mixed tumors of varying ages (preoperative duration of less than 1 year and more than 5 years) and in two carcinoma ex mixed tumors with preoperative durations of 15 and 16 years. They found only a diploid population of cells in the mixed tumors with a preoperative duration of less than 1 year; however, tetraploid populations of cells were found in mixed tumors with a preoperative duration of greater than 5 years as well as in the carcinomatous component of both the carcinoma ex mixed tumors. This suggests that as mixed tumors age, a population of cells may undergo transformation that could give origin to the carcinomatous component of carcinoma ex mixed tumor.

Many carcinoma ex mixed tumors may have only small areas of residual mixed tumor. Therefore, a thorough examination of a carcinoma may be necessary to find these small foci for proper histologic classification. Although we consider it somewhat extreme, Foote and Frazell[69] stated that looking for the benign mixed tumor component

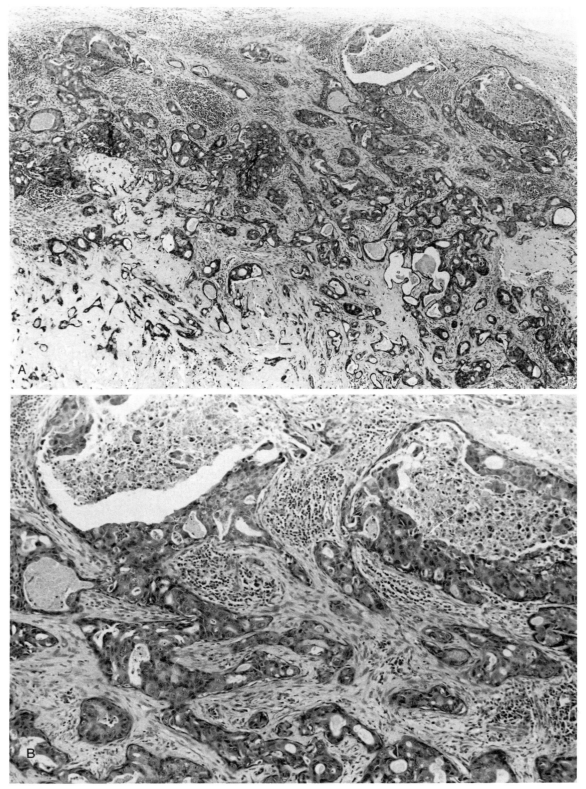

Figure 20–2. Carcinoma ex mixed tumor. *A,* Note the benign mixed tumor (lower left) with adenocarcinoma (upper half) (× 40). *B,* Higher magnification of *A* demonstrates irregular foci of adenocarcinoma composed of back-to-back glands, with focal necrosis set in a desmoplastic background (× 100).

Percent

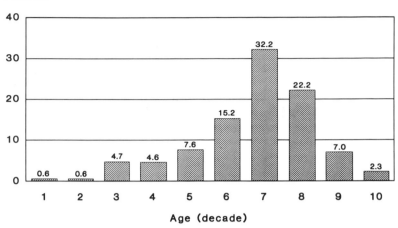

Figure 21–1. Distribution by ages (in decades) of 171 patients with primary squamous cell carcinoma of salivary glands reported in the salivary gland registry of the AFIP.

years. Females average 62.0 years of age and males 60.3 years. Figure 21–1 shows the age distribution by decade. Nearly 80 percent of the patients were in their fifth decade of life or older, and only 2 patients were under 20 years of age. The average age of patients with parotid tumors was 61.6 years—about 5 years older than the average of those with submandibular tumors. A similar age difference between patients with tumors at these sites has been previously noted.[24] Figure 21–2 compares the age distribution of patients with primary squamous cell carcinoma, squamous cell carcinoma metastatic to the major glands, and mucoepidermoid carcinoma. A nearly identical distribution is seen for primary and metastatic squamous cell carcinoma.

The sex is known for 175 patients, and these data show a marked male predilection (86.3 percent male to 13.7 percent female). However, of the 103 military patients, none are female. Therefore, a more significant reflection of the general population is shown by data for the 71 civilian patients whose sex is known. Of these patients, there were 47 males and 24 females, which is almost a 2 to 1 male predilection. A nearly identical male to female ratio has been observed by others.[24]

The race is known for 126 patients. Just over 87 percent were white, 5.6 percent were black, and about 2.5 percent were either Asian, Native American, or Malaysian.

LOCALIZATION

The 224 cases seen in our consultation service account for 6.3 percent of primary parotid, 8.3 percent of submandibular, and 3 percent of sublingual epithelial malignancies. The anatomic distribution of these cases includes 169 cases (75.5 percent) in the parotid gland, 42 cases (18.8 percent) in the submandibular gland, and 1 case (0.4 percent) in the sublingual gland. Twelve cases (5.3

Percent

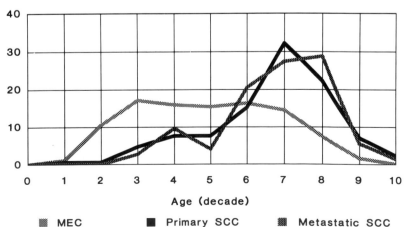

Figure 21–2. Age comparison of patients with primary salivary gland squamous cell carcinoma (SCC), metastatic squamous cell carcinoma, and mucoepidermoid carcinoma (MEC).

 MEC   ■ Primary SCC   Metastatic SCC

percent) were simply referred to as primary squamous cell carcinoma of major glands. This distribution is very similar to the experience of the Memorial Sloan-Kettering Cancer Center, which reported that 42 of 50 cases (84 percent) occurred in the parotid gland, and 8 (16 percent) occurred in the submandibular gland.[24] We agree with Batsakis,[2] who has stressed that because of the number of lymph nodes normally located in the submandibular area, great care must be taken to ensure that the submandibular gland is the primary site and is not secondarily involved by extension of metastatic disease from adjacent lymph nodes.

In the review by Shemen and colleagues,[24] the most common presenting symptom of patients with parotid tumors was an asymptomatic mass. Nonetheless, 19 percent of their patients with squamous cell carcinoma suffered pain, and 11 percent had facial nerve palsy. The size of the masses was greater than 3 cm in all but 8 of the 42 patients with measurable tumors. Submandibular squamous cell carcinoma often replaced the entire gland. In two thirds of the patients, a painful mass was present, whereas one third of the patients were asymptomatic. In either gland, symptoms were present for less than 1 year in about 75 percent of the patients and rarely were present for more than 2 years. These investigators also found fixation to skin and/or deep structures in 69 percent of the patients and ulceration in 5 percent.

PATHOLOGIC FINDINGS

On gross examination, these tumors appear unencapsulated, and the tumor interface is often difficult to distinguish from the salivary gland parenchyma. As with other squamous cell carcinomas, these tumors are firm or hard, and the cut surface is light gray or white.

Histologically, these tumors are similar to squamous cell carcinomas from other sites. Cytoplasmic mucin is not found in this tumor. Special stains for mucus should be routinely performed to ensure that the tumor is not a high-grade mucoepidermoid carcinoma. Most tumors are well- or moderately differentiated keratinizing squamous cell carcinomas (Fig. 21–3). Trabeculae of desmoplastic fibrous connective tissue often separate the tumor into multiple nodules (Fig. 21–4). Origin in dysplastic salivary ducts is fortuitously evident in some cases (Fig. 21–5). Squamous cell carcinomas often overrun the glandular parenchyma, which leaves small remnants of metaplastic ducts or degenerating acini surrounded by desmoplastic fibrous tissue. Desmoplasia may be so pronounced that entire salivary gland lobules

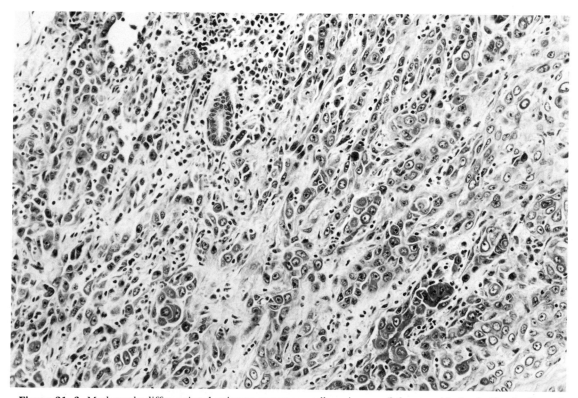

Figure 21–3. Moderately differentiated primary squamous cell carcinoma of the parotid gland. Nearly the entire salivary gland lobule has been replaced by tumor. Two small ducts remain (× 150).

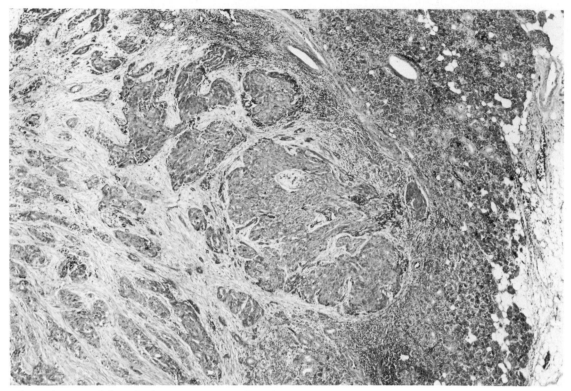

Figure 21–4. Nodules of primary squamous cell carcinoma are seen separated by dense fibrous connective tissue. Tumor has infiltrated an adjacent salivary gland lobule (right side) (× 30).

are replaced by fibrous connective tissue that contains scattered tumor islands (Fig. 21–6). Intracellular keratin and keratin pearl formation are normally prominent, and intercellular bridges are evident. Only 15 of the 224 cases (6.7 percent) in the AFIP files were interpreted as high-grade squamous cell carcinomas (Fig. 21–7), and several of these had foci of nonkeratinizing squamous cell carcinoma. One carcinoma was associated with a separate focus of Warthin's tumor in the same gland; this association was previously reported by others.[25, 26] Three carcinomas have occurred in the same gland with separate foci of parotid cysts and benign mixed tumors.

It has been our experience that islands of squamous cell carcinoma occasionally have marked infiltrates of lymphoid tissue in close apposition (Fig. 21–8); this is similar to the phenomenon seen in acinic cell adenocarcinoma and mucoepidermoid carcinomas. However, this phenomenon poses problems in differential diagnosis when it occurs with this tumor because it suggests metastatic disease to a lymph node, and metastatic carcinoma is foremost among differential diagnostic considerations. Furthermore, primary squamous cell carcinomas of the parotid gland may metastasize to intraglandular lymph nodes. Although distinction from lymph node metastasis

may occasionally be impossible, the haphazard arrangement of the lymphoid tissue and lack of typical lymph node architecture assist in the proper interpretation.

Occasionally, extensive parenchymal invasion is accompanied by extension of tumor into the dermis overlying the gland, which suggests possible epidermal origin. If the surgical specimen in these cases includes epidermis, it should be evaluated for dysplasia, and a thorough review of the clinical presentation should be undertaken.

DIFFERENTIAL DIAGNOSIS

Ductal squamous metaplasia is relatively common and can be misinterpreted as squamous cell carcinoma. Islands of metaplastic ductal epithelium may have nearly indiscernible lumina but show neither the infiltrative growth pattern nor the degree of cytomorphologic atypia normally present in islands and cords of squamous cell carcinoma. However, rarely, during early ductal regeneration, a significant degree of atypia may be found. Additionally, small, uniformly round metaplastic ducts, acinar atrophy, and an inflammatory cell infiltrate suggest a degenerative rather than a neoplastic process.

Text continued on page 377

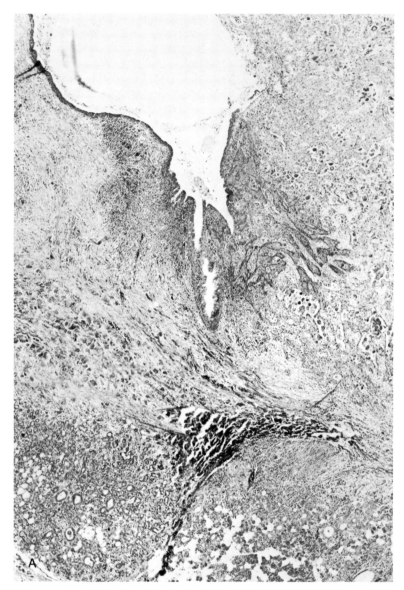

Figure 21–5. *A,* Primary squamous cell carcinoma is shown arising from large excretory duct. Note the normal epithelial lining (upper left) and the abrupt malignant transformation. Tumor occupies the entire upper right side of the photograph (× 30).

clinically evident or suspected. Because locoregional failure was overall the most significant problem, it was suggested that a composite resection might be appropriate for most sizeable tumors that involve the capsule of the submandibular gland.

Although, in general, evidence from studies assessing the effectiveness of postoperative radiotherapy for salivary gland tumors has been inconclusive, there is mounting evidence that combined therapy may improve local control and, at least for some tumors, including squamous cell carcinomas, also improve survival.[29-33] Limited evidence that some salivary gland cancers may be sensitive to chemotherapeutic drugs exists,[34-36] but further studies are needed to assess their adjuvant and palliative roles.

REFERENCES

1. Foote FW Jr, Frazell EL: Tumors of the major salivary glands. Cancer 1953; 6:1065–1133.
2. Batsakis JG: Primary squamous cell carcinomas of major salivary glands. Ann Otol Rhinol Laryngol 1983; 92:97–98.
3. Batsakis JG, McClatchey KD, Johns M, Regezi J: Primary squamous cell carcinoma of the parotid gland. Arch Otolaryngol 1976; 102:355–357.
4. Batsakis JG, Regezi JA: Selected controversial lesions of salivary tissues. Otolaryngol Clin North Am 1977; 10:309–328.
5. Fu KK, Leibel SA, Levine ML, Friedlander LM, Boles R, Phillips TL: Carcinoma of the major and minor salivary glands: Analysis of treatment results and sites and causes of failure. Cancer 1977; 40:2882–2890.
6. Seifert G, Okabe H, Caselitz J: Epithelial salivary gland tumors in children and adolescents: Analysis of 80 cases (Salivary Gland Registry 1965–1984). ORL J 1986; 48:137–149.
7. Fitzpatrick PJ, Theriault C: Malignant salivary gland tumors. Int J Radiat Oncol Biol Phys 1986; 12:1743–1747.
8. Wyatt AP, Henry L, Curwen MP: Salivary tumours: A clinicopathological study and follow-up of 156 cases. Br J Surg 1967; 54:636–645.
9. Bissett RJ, Fitzpatrick PJ: Malignant submandibular gland tumors: A review of 91 patients. Am J Clin Oncol 1988; 11:46–51.
10. Spitz MR, Batsakis JG: Major salivary gland carcinoma: Descriptive epidemiology and survival of 498 patients. Arch Otolaryngol 1984; 110:45–48.
11. Rosenfeld L, Sessions OG, McSwain B, Graves H Jr: Malignant tumors of salivary gland origin: 37-year review of 184 cases. Ann Surg 1966; 163:726–735.
12. Eneroth CM: Salivary gland tumors in the parotid gland, submandibular gland, and the palate region. Cancer 1971; 27:1415–1418.
13. Friedman M, Levin B, Grybauskas V, Strorigl T, Manaligod J, Hill JH, Skolnik E: Malignant tumors of the major salivary glands. Otolaryngol Clin North Am 1986; 194:625–636.
14. Eveson JW, Cawson RA: Salivary gland tumours: A review of 2,410 cases with particular reference to histological types, site, age and sex distribution. J Pathol 1985; 146:51–58.
15. Woods JE, Chong GC, Beahrs OH: Experience with 1,360 primary parotid tumors. Am J Surg 1975; 130:460–462.
16. Yu GY, Ma DQ: Carcinoma of the salivary gland: A clinicopathologic study of 405 cases. Semin Surg Oncol 1987; 3:240–244.
17. Conley J, Meyers E, Cole R: Analysis of 115 patients with tumors of the submandibular gland. Ann Otol Rhinol Laryngol 1972; 81:323–330.
18. Richardson GS, Dickason WL, Gaisford JC, Hanna DC: Tumors of salivary glands: An analysis of 752 cases. Plast Reconst Surg 1975; 55:131–138.
19. Trail ML, Lubritz J: Tumors of the submandibular gland. Laryngoscope 1974; 84:1225–1232.
20. Spiro RH, Huvos AG, Strong EW: Cancer of the parotid gland: A clinicopathologic study of 288 primary cases. Am J Surg 1975; 130:452–459.
21. Spiro RH, Hajdu ST, Strong EW: Tumors of the submaxillary gland. Am J Surg 1976; 132:463–468.
22. Spiro RH: Salivary neoplasms: Overview of a 35-year experience with 2,807 patients. Head Neck Surg 1986; 8:177–184.
23. Skolnik EM, Friedman M, Becker S, Sisson GA, Keyes GR: Tumors of the major salivary glands. Laryngoscope 1977; 87:843–861.
24. Shemen LJ, Huvos AG, Spiro RH: Squamous cell carcinoma of salivary gland origin. Head Neck Surg 1987; 9:235–240.
25. Volmer VJ: Multiple unilaterale tumoren der glandula parotis. Zbl Allg Pathol u Pathol Anat 1982; 126:327–334.
26. Schilling JA, Block BL, Speigel JC: Synchronous unilateral parotid neoplasms of different histologic types. Head Neck 1989; 11:179–183.
27. Ridenhour CE, Spratt JS Jr: Epidermoid carcinoma of the skin involving the parotid gland. Am J Surg 1966; 112:504–507.
28. Marks MW, Ryan RF, Litwin MS, Sonntag BV: Squamous cell carcinoma of the parotid gland. Plast Reconst Surg 1987; 79:550–554.
29. Tu GY, Hu YH, Jiang PJ: The superiority of combined therapy (surgery and postoperative irradiation) in parotid cancer. Arch Otolaryngol 1982; 108:710–713.
30. Shidnia H, Hornback NB, Hamaker R, Lingeman R: Carcinoma of major salivary glands. Cancer 1980; 45:693–697.
31. Tran L, Sadeghi A, Hanson D, Juillard G, Mackintosh R, Calcaterra TC, Parker RG: Major salivary gland tumors: Treatment results and prognostic factors. Laryngoscope 1986; 96:1139–1144.
32. Guillamondegui OM, Byers RM, Luna MA, Chiminazzo H Jr, Jesse RH, Fletcher GH: Aggressive surgery in treatment for parotid cancer: The role of adjunctive postoperative radiotherapy. Am J Roentgenol 1975; 123:49–54.
33. Reddy SP, Marks JE: Treatment of locally advanced, high-grade, malignant tumors of major salivary glands. Laryngoscope 1988; 98:450–454.
34. Suen JY, Johns ME: Chemotherapy for salivary gland cancer. Laryngoscope 1982; 92:235–239.
35. Kaplan MJ, Johns ME, Cantrell RW: Chemotherapy for salivary gland cancer. Otolaryngol Head Neck Surg 1986; 95:165–170.
36. Eisenberger MA: Supporting evidence for an active treatment program for advanced salivary gland carcinomas. Cancer Treat Rev 1985; 69:319–321.

22

CLEAR CELL CARCINOMA

Gary L. Ellis and Paul L. Auclair

The failure of cytoplasm to appear stained with hematoxylin and eosin when examined via light microscopy may result from one or more mechanisms. These mechanisms include the intracellular accumulation of nonstaining compounds, such as glycogen, lipids, and mucins; a true sparsity of cell organelles; and artifact induced during tissue fixation and/or processing. For example, artifact is the principal factor in the clear cells seen in acinic cell adenocarcinomas.[1] The clear cells in epithelial-myoepithelial carcinoma are the result of glycogen accumulation, whereas the clear cells in renal cell carcinoma are produced by the accumulation of cytoplasmic glycogen and lipid.[2, 3]

Clear cell neoplasms of salivary glands have created diagnostic dilemmas and challenges as well as controversy over their classification for decades.[1, 2, 4–8] These uncommon neoplasms have been classified as both adenomas and carcinomas. The terminology employed for these neoplasms has reflected this diagnostic diversity and includes such terms as *adenomyoepithelioma,*[4] *clear cell adenoma,*[9–12] *glycogen-rich adenoma,*[5, 6] *glycogen-rich carcinoma* or *adenocarcinoma,*[13–16] *clear cell carcinoma,*[8] *glycogen-rich tumor,*[17] *clear cell tumor,*[18] *monomorphic clear cell tumor,*[19] and *epithelial-myoepithelial carcinoma.*[2, 20] Even metastatic clear cell tumors, such as renal cell carcinoma, can be difficult to differentiate from primary clear cell neoplasms of the salivary glands. Despite the many reports of clear cell adenomas of salivary gland origin in the literature, Batsakis and Regezi,[7] in 1977, stated that they believed that the majority of, if not all, nonmucinous epithelial clear cell neoplasms of the salivary gland should be considered to be at least low-grade malignant tumors. Although their statement seemed controversial at the time, on the basis of both our experience and that subsequently reported in the literature, we believe they were essentially correct, but with at least one exception. The one exception we have identified is the clear cell variant of oncocytoma (see Chapter 13), which

has recently been more clearly described.[21] Dardick and colleagues[22] have identified a single case of a clear cell variant of myoepithelioma in their analysis of myoepitheliomas.

Many different types of benign and malignant salivary gland neoplasms, such as mixed tumors, oncocytoma, mucoepidermoid carcinoma, acinic cell adenocarcinoma, and polymorphous low-grade adenocarcinoma, may contain foci of clear cells as a part of their cytopathologic spectrum. When these clear cell foci are a minor component, appropriate identification of the tumor can nearly always be accomplished on the basis of the predominant histopathologic features. In rare instances, clear cells may be a major component of such tumors as mucoepidermoid carcinoma, acinic cell adenocarcinoma, and oncocytoma. Although more difficult, proper classification of such tumors can usually be made by the experienced observer on the basis of their morphologic growth patterns and foci with histopathologic features "typical" of these tumors. Unfortunately, because a few mucoepidermoid carcinomas or acinic cell adenocarcinomas contain a prominent number of clear cells, many clear cell tumors in the salivary glands have been inappropriately classified as mucoepidermoid carcinoma or acinic cell adenocarcinoma. The fallacy of this practice is highlighted by the recent definitive delineation of the epithelial-myoepithelial carcinoma, a clear cell dominant tumor with distinctive biphasic cytologic features (see Chapter 24).[2, 20, 23–25] In fact, it is evident from the photomicrographs and/or histologic descriptions provided that many reports in the literature of so-called clear cell adenoma, glycogen-rich adenoma, clear cell tumor, glycogen-rich adenocarcinoma, clear cell carcinoma, or other similar terminology were what we now prefer to categorize as the bimorphic epithelial-myoepithelial carcinoma.[4, 6, 8–10, 13, 18, 19, 26]

Notwithstanding the statements just made about the refinement of our concepts of clear cell tumors and the categorization of a large group of these tumors as epithelial-myoepithelial carcinomas, there remains a small group of clear cell tumors that do not have the distinctive morphology of epithelial-myoepithelial carcinoma. Batsakis and others[27, 28] have suggested that these monomorphous clear cell tumors are variants of epithelial-myoepithelial carcinoma in which the ductal differentiated cells are inconspicuous. We speculate that in many cases, their assumption may be correct; however, some monomorphous clear cell carcinomas seem to have a morphologic growth pattern that is distinct from epithelial-myoepithelial carcinoma. Chen[8] actually segregated clear cell carcinomas into two groups: bimorphic tumors that equate to epithelial-myoepithelial carcinoma and monomorphic tumors. Lattanzi and colleagues[14] went further and defined three groups of clear cell tumors: monomorphic, bimorphic, and a combination of both. Assessment of this last category indicates that these tumors may be a single pathologic entity with varying morphologic patterns. Nevertheless, since it remains to be definitively determined whether these monomorphous clear cell tumors belong within the spectrum of epithelial-myoepithelial carcinomas, we continue to identify a group of clear cell carcinomas distinct from epithelial-myoepithelial carcinoma. Echoing the thoughts of Batsakis and Regezi,[7] we believe that either most or all of these epithelial clear cell tumors are malignant.

The registry of salivary gland disease at the Armed Forces Institute of Pathology (AFIP) contains 92 cases that have been diagnosed simply as clear cell carcinoma or adenocarcinoma. However, pathologists at the AFIP did not begin routinely using the diagnosis *epithelial-myoepithelial carcinoma* until 1979; thus, we suspect that at least a small number of these tumors could be reclassified if evaluated today. Therefore, in our analysis, we have not included data from the 32 cases diagnosed before 1979.

Of those tumors entered into the registry since 1979, the remaining 60 cases make up 1.5 percent of all the salivary gland tumors and 3.2 percent of all the malignant tumors. It is nearly impossible to evaluate meaningful data on the frequency and incidence of clear cell tumors from the literature, because hardly any major surveys of salivary gland tumors have included clear cell tumors as a separate group and because the classification of this group of tumors has been significantly modified over the last decade.

CLINICAL FEATURES

Fifty-seven percent of these 60 cases occurred in the intraoral minor salivary glands, whereas 28 and 12 percent occurred in the parotid and submandibular glands, respectively (Table 22–1). The palate was the most frequently involved intraoral

Table 22–1. Anatomic Distribution of 60 Cases of Clear Cell Carcinoma of Salivary Gland in the AFIP Registry from 1979 to 1989

Anatomic Site	Number	Percentage
Major Glands		
Parotid gland	17	28.3
Submandibular gland	7	11.7
Neck	2	3.3
Minor Glands		
Palate (total)	16	26.7
Hard	(4)	(6.7)
Soft	(6)	(10.0)
Not specified	(6)	(10.0)
Lip (total)	8	13.3
Lower	(6)	(10.0)
Not specified	(2)	(3.3)
Tonsillar area	3	5.0
Floor of mouth	2	3.3
Tongue	2	3.3
Buccal mucosa	2	3.3
Pharynx	1	1.7
*Total**	60	100.0

*Does not include numbers in parentheses

site. Although the number of female patients slightly outnumbered the number of male patients, no significant sex predilection was evident, even when only nonmilitary cases (88 percent) were analyzed. Nor was any race preference indicated by the data. Patients' ages have ranged from 18 to 86 years, and the mean age was 56 years. The peak incidence occurred during the sixth to eighth decades of life (Fig. 22–1).

Similar to most salivary gland neoplasms, swelling is the principal clinical manifestation.

PATHOLOGIC FEATURES

At gross specimen examination, these tumors may appear to be circumscribed, but they are usually not encapsulated. The cut surfaces are grayish-white to grayish-tan.

The dominant microscopic feature, of course, is tumor cells with cytoplasm that does not stain with hematoxylin and eosin (Fig. 22–2). Although clear cells are the most conspicuous feature, a number of cells can be found with pale eosinophilic or amphophilic cytoplasm. The tumor cells are round to polygonal and vary in size. The nuclei are generally fairly uniform with little pleomorphism and few or no mitotic figures. The chromatin is evenly dispersed, and nucleoli are not prominent. The demonstration of cytoplasmic glycogen with periodic acid–Schiff staining before and after digestion of the tissue sections with diastase can vary considerably from tumor to tumor, although at least some glycogen can be seen in most clear cell carcinomas (Fig. 22–3). The amount of glycogen visualized may also be influ-

No. of patients

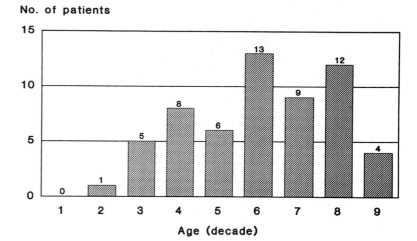

Figure 22–1. The distribution by age of 58 patients with clear cell carcinoma reported in the AFIP registry from 1979 to 1989.

enced by tissue fixation, since formalin is not the best fixative for preservation of glycogen.

Clear cell carcinomas manifest several growth patterns, but any one neoplasm is usually reasonably uniform in appearance. The tumors may grow as solid sheets, small nests, or cords of epithelial cells (Figs. 22–4 through 22–6). The tumors that occur as large sheets most closely resemble epithelial-myoepithelial carcinoma ex-

cept, of course, for the absence of eosinophilic ductal cells that line small lumina. Some of these tumors may have an organoid arrangement with groups of clear cells surrounded by thin vascular channels, whereas in other tumors, anastomosing bands of fibrous connective tissue crisscross the tumor (Figs. 22–5, 22–7). The tumors that grow as small nests or cords are usually associated with a collagenous stroma that varies from loose to

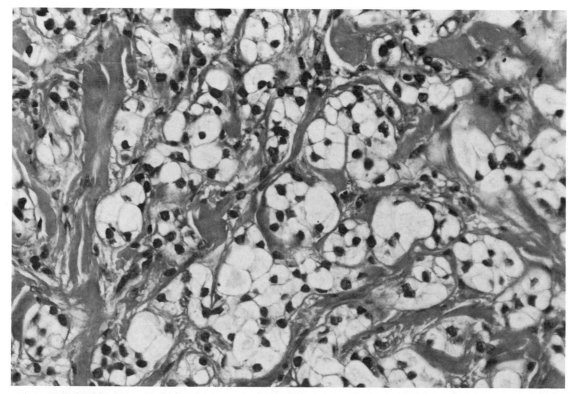

Figure 22–2. This clear cell carcinoma from the lower lip consists of irregularly shaped aggregates of round and polygonal cells with dark, round nuclei and water-clear cytoplasm. Little pleomorphism is visible, and no mitotic figures are seen (× 300).

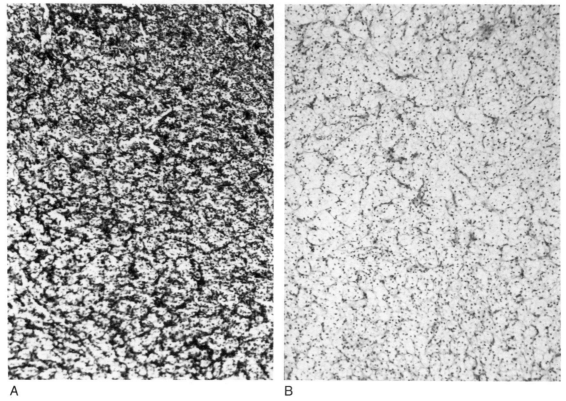

A   B

Figure 22–3. Glycogen is prominent in this clear cell carcinoma. This is demonstrated by *(A)* significant staining via periodic acid–Schiff stain before digestion of the tissue section with diastase and by *(B)* little staining via periodic acid–Schiff stain after digestion. The amount of demonstrable glycogen varies among tumors *(A, B, × 60)*.

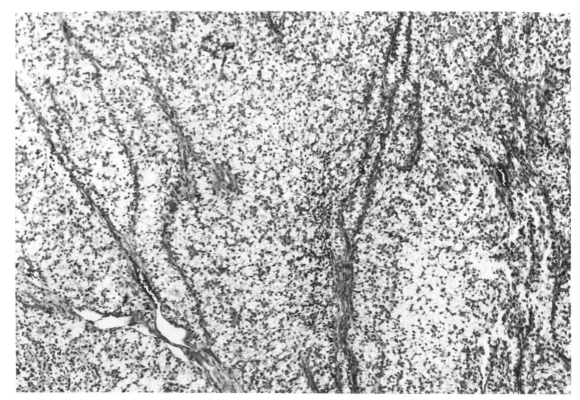

Figure 22–4. Clear cell carcinoma of the tongue is composed of sheets of clear cells. This tumor resembles epithelial-myoepithelial carcinoma, except for the conspicuous absence of ductal cells (× 75).

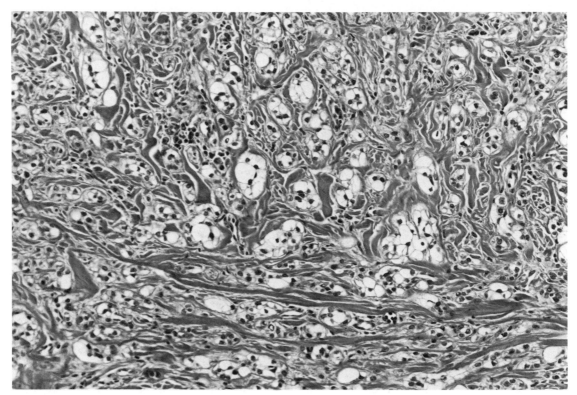

Figure 22–5. Small nests of clear cells are supported by a dense collagenous stroma in a clear cell carcinoma of the lip (× 150).

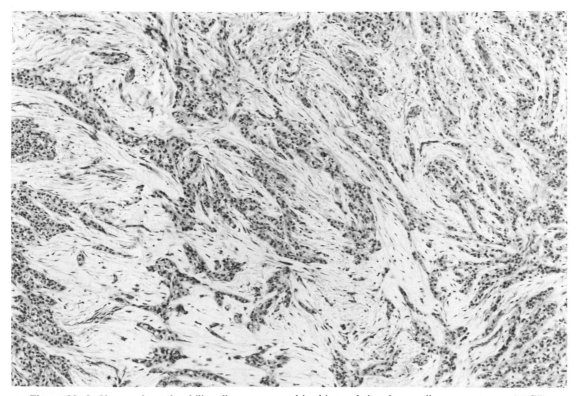

Figure 22–6. Clear and amphophilic cells are arranged in thin cords in a loose collagenous stroma (× 75).

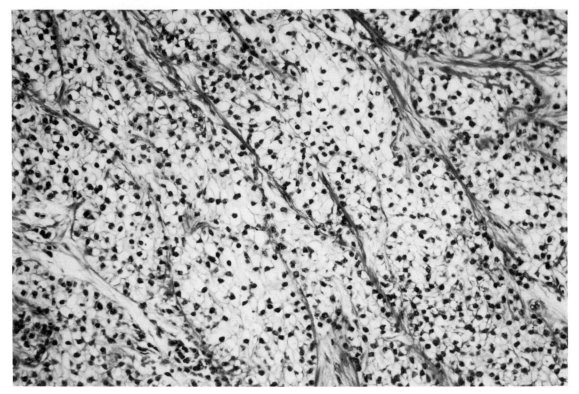

Figure 22–7. Groups of clear cells are separated by thin fibrovascular septa (× 160).

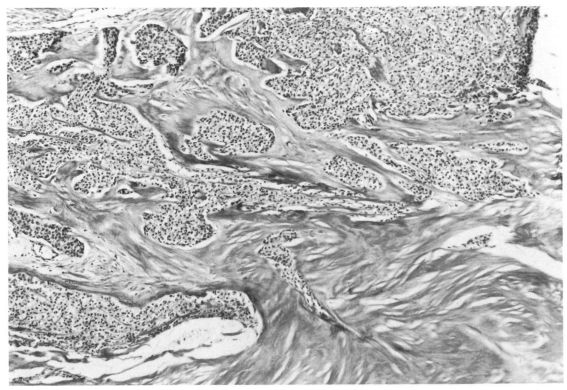

Figure 22–8. Marked hyalinization of the thick collagenous stroma gives this clear cell carcinoma of the minor salivary gland a scirrhous appearance (× 75).

hyalinized and that sometimes produces a scirrhous appearance (Fig. 22–8). Infiltration is characteristic (Fig. 22–9). When these tumors develop as small nests or cords in an extensive fibrous stroma, they are usually easily recognized as carcinomas because of their obvious infiltrative appearance. When these tumors are composed of large sheets of cells and occur in the major salivary glands, a condensation of fibrous tissue frequently occurs at the tumor periphery and imparts an encapsulated appearance (Fig. 22–10). These are the tumors that are probably most often mistaken for clear cell "adenomas." Extensive tissue sectioning may be needed to demonstrate the infiltrative growth in some cases.

Stains for cytoplasmic mucin, such as mucicarmine, are ordinarily negative in clear cell carcinomas, but the presence of a rare mucous cell does not preclude the diagnosis of clear cell carcinoma. However, more than an occasional mucous cell should suggest the possibility of a "clear cell" mucoepidermoid carcinoma. As already stated, most, but not all, clear cell carcinomas demonstrate cytoplasmic glycogen with staining by periodic acid–Schiff stain with and without diastase digestion.

Many investigators believe that the lumen-lining cells in epithelial-myoepithelial carcinoma are intercalated ductlike cells and that the surrounding clear cells are of myoepithelial differentiation.[2, 20] Some pathologists also suggest that the clear cells in monomorphous clear cell carcinomas are neoplastic modified myoepithelial cells.[29] Immunohistochemical studies of epithelial-myoepithelial carcinoma have shown antikeratin immunoreactivity of the luminal cells and anti S 100 protein immunoreactivity but little or no antikeratin immunoreactivity of the clear cells.[10, 25] Our immunohistochemical results with monomorphous clear cell carcinomas and those results of others[12, 15, 16, 18, 30] have been inconsistent. Both antikeratin and anti–S-100 protein immunoreactivity have varied from strong to either weak or nonexistent. The electron microscopic findings in two cases of apparent monomorphous clear cell carcinoma supported an epithelial origin and demonstrated the presence of cytoplasmic glycogen but failed to substantiate myoepithelial differentiation.[16, 17]

PROGNOSIS AND TREATMENT

As a result of the relatively uncommon occurrence of these tumors and the confusion in terminology and definition of clear cell neoplasms of salivary glands that has plagued the literature, it is difficult to draw definitive conclusions about their biologic behavior. However, their infiltrative growth and the incidence of recurrence and of regional lymph node metastases indicate that it is appropriate to consider them low-grade adenocarcinomas. Consistent with their low-grade malignant status, partial or complete parotidectomy or sublingual glandectomy, complete submandibular glandectomy, and wide local excision of minor gland tumors are recommended forms of treatment.

DIFFERENTIAL DIAGNOSIS

As mentioned, mucoepidermoid carcinoma and acinic cell adenocarcinoma are two common malignant salivary gland tumors that may occasionally contain a significant number of clear cells. Mucous cells, which can be identified with the mucicarmine stain, and epidermoid cells can nearly always be found in mucoepidermoid carcinoma (see Chapter 16) and are not seen in clear cell carcinoma. The clear cells in both mucoepidermoid carcinoma and clear cell carcinoma may contain glycogen, but the clear cells in acinic cell adenocarcinoma do not. In addition, acinar, intercalated ductal, and vacuolated cells that can be recognized in acinic cell adenocarcinoma (see Chapter 17) are not a component of clear cell carcinoma.

As already stated, clear cell carcinoma may be one extreme end of the histopathologic spectrum of epithelial-myoepithelial carcinoma (see Chapter 24). However, we continue to distinguish the biphasic epithelial-myoepithelial carcinoma from the monophasic clear cell carcinoma, especially those that infiltrate as small cords or nests of clear cells. Therefore, the clear cell carcinoma lacks the small, cuboidal, eosinophilic, lumen-lining cells that are surrounded by clear cells in epithelial-myoepithelial carcinoma.

Although metastatic carcinoma in the salivary glands from primary tumors located below the clavicle is uncommon, metastatic renal cell carcinoma must always be considered in the differential diagnosis of clear cell tumors. The kidney is one of the more common infraclavicular primary sites for tumors that metastasize to the head and neck,[31] and several metastatic renal cell carcinomas have been reported in the salivary glands.[32–36] Discovery of metastatic tumor may be the first indication of a primary renal carcinoma. Both primary clear cell carcinoma and metastatic renal cell carcinoma may be glycogen-positive; may have a solid, organoid growth pattern; exhibit infiltration; frequently have little cytologic atypia; have few mitoses; and may be composed of nearly all clear cells, although other cell types are also seen in renal cell carcinoma. A positive reaction to mucicarmine would preclude the possibility of renal cell carcinoma, but primary clear cell carcinoma of the salivary gland is usually negative for intracytoplasmic mucin as well. Demonstration of intracytoplasmic lipid would favor renal cell carcinoma, but frozen tissue sections are needed because lipids are usually eluted during tissue

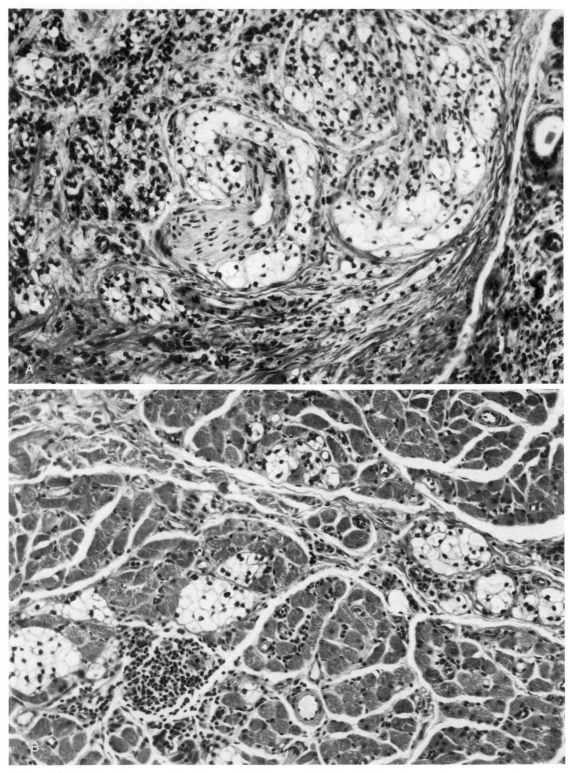

Figure 22–9. Infiltration, one of the characteristic features of salivary gland carcinomas, is evident in this clear cell carcinoma with perineural invasion *(A)* and intramuscular growth *(B)*. *(A* and *B*, × 160.)

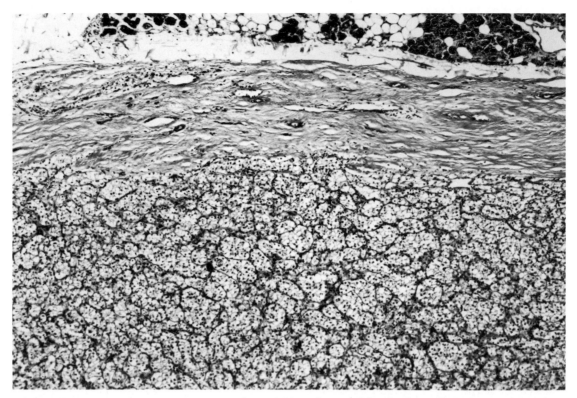

Figure 22–10. A pseudocapsule is present at the periphery of one nodule of a clear cell carcinoma of the parotid gland. Examination of multiple sections demonstrated infiltrative growth, and infiltration through the pseudocapsule can be seen in the upper left portion of this photomicrograph (× 60.)

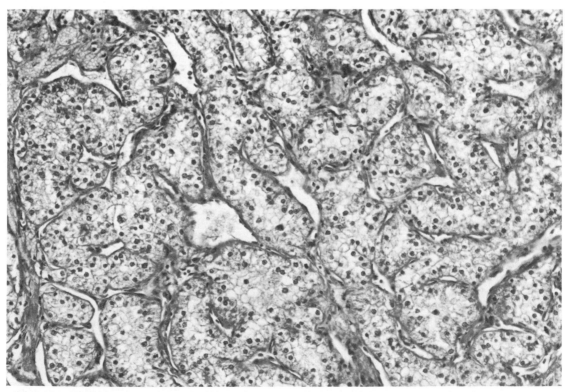

Figure 22–11. Metastatic renal cell carcinoma in the parotid gland has prominent vascular channels between islands and cords of tumor cells, which have mostly clear cytoplasm.

processing. In our experience, renal cell carcinomas usually present a more heterogeneous architecture and are more vascular than primary clear cell carcinomas. Small capillaries may be evident in clear cell carcinoma; however, in renal cell carcinoma, the vascular channels are often conspicuous, dilated, and even sinusoidal (Fig. 22–11). Hemorrhage and hemosiderin are generally more prominent in metastatic renal cell carcinoma. As the pleomorphism and cytologic atypia become more evident, the likelihood that the tumor is a primary clear cell carcinoma decreases. In some cases, it may not be possible to confidently differentiate between primary and metastatic carcinoma; therefore, further clinical evaluation for a renal primary tumor must be performed.

The clear cell variant of oncocytoma (see Chapter 13) that occurs in the parotid and submandibular glands may be the most difficult tumor to differentiate from clear cell carcinoma by light-microscopic examination. Both tumors contain glycogen, and clear cell carcinoma may have an organoid pattern that is similar to that of oncocytoma, although the organoid pattern is usually more poorly organized in clear cell carcinoma. Clear cell oncocytoma is not infiltrative, but it is frequently multifocal (oncocytosis). A distinction between the two must be made. In fact, the pattern of scattered, discrete foci, as seen in oncocytosis, can be very helpful in distinguishing between oncocytoma and clear cell carcinoma. Often, if a diligent search is made, foci of typical, intensely eosinophilic oncocytes can be found in clear cell oncocytoma. Cytoplasmic staining of mitochondria with phosphotungstic acid-hematoxylin can be useful for the demonstration of oncocytes, and electron microscopy can be diagnostic in this regard.

REFERENCES

1. Echevarria RA: Ultrastructure of the acinic cell carcinoma and clear cell carcinoma of the parotid gland. Cancer 1967; 20:563–571.
2. Corio RL, Sciubba JJ, Brannon RB, Batsakis JG: Epithelial-myoepithelial carcinoma of intercalated duct origin: A clinicopathologic and ultrastructural assessment of sixteen cases. Oral Surg Oral Med Oral Pathol 1982; 53:280–287.
3. Bennington JL, Beckwith JB: Tumors of the Kidney, Renal Pelvis, and Ureter, Fascicle 12. Atlas of Tumor Pathology, 2nd Series. Washington, DC, Armed Forces Institute of Pathology, 1975; 148.
4. Bauer WH, Fox RA: Adenomyoepithelioma (cylindroma) of palatal mucous glands. Arch Pathol 1945; 39:96–102.
5. Corridan M: Glycogen-rich clear-cell adenoma of the parotid gland. J Pathol Bacteriol 1956; 72:623–626.
6. Goldman RL, Klein H: Glycogen-rich adenoma of the parotid gland: An uncommon benign clear-cell tumor resembling certain clear-cell carcinomas of salivary origin. Cancer 1972; 30:749–754.
7. Batsakis JG, Regezi JA: Selected controversial lesions of salivary tissue. Otolaryngol Clin N Am 1977; 10:309–328.
8. Chen KTK: Clear cell carcinoma of the salivary gland. Hum Pathol 1983; 14:91–93.
9. Saksela E, Tarkkanen J, Wartiovaara J: Parotid clear-cell adenoma of possible myoepithelial origin. Cancer 1972; 30:742–748.
10. Hara K, Ito M, Takeuchi J, Iijima S, Endo T, Hidaka H: Distribution of S-100b protein in normal salivary glands and salivary gland tumors. Virchows Arch [A] 1983; 401:237–249.
11. Matsumura K, Sasaki K, Tsuji T, Shinozaki F: The nucleolar organizer regions associated protein (Ag-NORs) in salivary gland tumors. Int J Oral Maxillofac Surg 1989; 18:76–78.
12. Mori M, Ninomiya T, Okada Y, Tsukitani K: Myoepitheliomas and myoepithelial adenomas of salivary gland origin. Immunohistochemical evaluation of filament proteins, S-100 α and β, glial fibrillary acidic proteins, neuron-specific enolase, and lactoferrin. Pathol Res Pract 1989; 184:168–178.
13. Mohamed AH, Cherrick HM: Glycogen-rich adenocarcinoma of minor salivary glands. Cancer 1975; 36:1057–1066.
14. Lattanzi DA, Polverini P, Chin DC: Glycogen-rich adenocarcinoma of a minor salivary gland. J Oral Maxillofac Surg 1985; 43:122–124.
15. Uri AK, Wetmore RF, Iozzo RV: Glycogen-rich clear cell carcinoma in the tongue: A cytochemical and ultrastructural study. Cancer 1986; 57:1803–1809.
16. Hayashi K, Ohtsuki Y, Sonobe H, Takahashi K, Iwata J, Nishioka E, Kawakami T: Glycogen-rich clear cell carcinoma arising from minor salivary glands of the uvula: A case report. Acta Pathol Jpn 1988; 38:1227–1234.
17. Chaudhry AP, Cutler LS, Satchidanand S, Labay G, Sunder M, Lin C: Glycogen-rich tumor of the oral minor salivary glands: A histochemical and ultrastructural study. Cancer 1983; 52:105–111.
18. Matsushima R, Nakayama I, Shimizu M: Immunohistochemical localization of keratin, vimentin and myosin in salivary gland tumors. Acta Pathol Jpn 1988; 38:445–454.
19. Adlam DM: The monomorphic clear cell tumour: A report of two cases. Br J Oral Maxillofac Surg 1986; 24:130–136.
20. Donath K, Seifert G, Schmitz R: Zur diagnose und Ultrastruktur des tubularen Speichelgangcarcinoms: Epithelial-myoepitheliales Schaltsuckcarcinom. Virchows Arch [A] 1972; 356:16–31.
21. Ellis GL: "Clear cell" oncocytoma of salivary gland. Hum Pathol 1988; 19:862–867.
22. Dardick I, Thomas MJ, van Nostrand AWP: Myoepithelioma—new concepts of histology and classification: A light and electron microscopic study. Ultrastruct Pathol 1989; 13:187–224.
23. Daley TD, Wysocki GP, Smout MS, Slinger RP: Epithelial-myoepithelial carcinoma of salivary glands. Oral Surg Oral Med Oral Pathol 1984; 57:512–519.
24. Lampe H, Ruby RR, Greenway RE, DeRose G, Wysocki GP: Epithelial-myoepithelial carcinoma of the salivary gland. J Otolaryngol 1984; 13:247–251.
25. Luna MA, Ordonez NG, Mackay B, Batsakis JG, Guillamondegui O: Salivary epithelial-myoepithe-

lial carcinomas of intercalated ducts: A clinical, electron microscopic, and immunohistochemical study. Oral Surg Oral Med Oral Pathol 1985; 59:482–490.

26. Thackray AC, Lucas RB: Tumors of the Major Salivary Glands, Fascicle 10. Atlas of Tumor Pathology, 2nd Series. Washington, DC, Armed Forces Institute of Pathology, 1974; 62–63.

27. Batsakis JG: Clear cell tumors of salivary glands. Ann Otol 1980; 89:196–197.

28. Batsakis JG, Regezi JA, Bloch D: The pathology of head and neck tumors: Salivary glands, Part 3. Head Neck Surg 1979; 1:260–273.

29. Batsakis JG, Kraemer B, Sciubba JJ: The pathology of head and neck tumors: The myoepithelial cell and its participation in salivary gland neoplasia, Part 17. Head Neck Surg 1983; 5:222–233.

30. Zarbo RJ, Regezi JA, Batsakis JG: S-100 protein in salivary gland tumors: An immunohistochemical study of 129 cases. Head Neck 1986; 8:268–275.

31. Batsakis JG: Tumors of the Head and Neck: Clinical and Pathological Considerations, 2nd Ed. Baltimore, Williams & Wilkins, 1979; 240–251.

32. Bedrosian SA, Goldman RL, Dekelboum AM: Renal carcinoma presenting as a primary submandibular gland tumor. Oral Surg Oral Med Oral Pathol 1984; 58:699–701.

33. Seifert G, Hennings K, Caselitz J: Metastatic tumors to the parotid and submandibular glands—analysis and differential diagnosis of 108 cases. Pathol Res Pract 1986; 181:684–692.

34. Harrison DJ, McLaren K, Tennant W: A clear cell tumour of the parotid. J Laryngol Otol 1987; 101:633–635.

35. Madison JF, Frierson HF Jr: Pathologic quiz case 2. Clear cell carcinoma, consistent with metastatic renal cell carcinoma. Arch Otolaryngol Head Neck Surg 1988; 114:570–571.

36. Melnick SJ, Amazon K, Dembrow V: Metastatic renal cell carcinoma presenting as a parotid tumor: A case report with immunohistochemical findings and review of the literature. Hum Pathol 1989; 20:195–197.

23

POLYMORPHOUS LOW-GRADE ADENOCARCINOMA OF MINOR SALIVARY GLANDS

Bruce M. Wenig and Douglas R. Gnepp

The classification of neoplastic diseases is continuously being amended. Techniques, such as immunohistochemistry, flow cytometry, in-situ DNA hybridization, and polymerase chain reaction, have contributed to a more profound understanding of the phenotypic and genotypic characteristics of various cell lines and of their neoplastic mutations. The classification of salivary gland tumors has been part of this nosologic expansion, and over the past decade, additional neoplasms have been recognized as distinct entities that are separate from general categories, such as adenocarcinoma, not otherwise specified. One of these more recently recognized neoplasms is the polymorphous low-grade adenocarcinoma (PLGA).

In 1983, two separate groups of investigators reported on low-grade adenocarcinomas of minor salivary gland origin termed *terminal duct carcinoma* and *lobular carcinoma*.[1, 2] *Terminal duct carcinoma* was used to emphasize the proposed histogenesis of the tumor, which was thought to be the progenitor cell of the distal or terminal duct portions of the salivary gland unit, that is, the intercalated duct reserve cell. *Lobular carcinoma* was used because these salivary gland adenocarcinomas demonstrated areas of an infiltrative single-file growth pattern that is similar to that of the lobular carcinoma of the breast. In reality, these reports, although using different names, were describing the same neoplasm. Prior to these reports, a number of large series on upper aerodigestive tract minor salivary gland tumors included descriptions of neoplasms that today could be classified as PLGA.[3–5] In 1984, Evans and Batsakis described a

group of oral minor salivary gland neoplasms and used the term *polymorphous low-grade adenocarcinoma*, which emphasized the salient features of these tumors, namely, the varied histomorphology and the malignant, albeit indolent, behavior.[6] The authors stated that this group of neoplasms included those tumors previously termed terminal duct carcinoma,[1] lobular carcinoma,[2] papillary carcinoma[7, 8] and trabecular carcinoma.[4] At present, *polymorphous low-grade adenocarcinoma* is the accepted term for this neoplasm. Controversy exists in regard to the classification of the low-grade papillary adenocarcinoma of minor salivary gland origin.[9] Some authors include it in the general category PLGA, and identify papillary and nonpapillary variants separately on the basis of morphology as well as by apparent differences in biologic behavior.[10, 11] We believe that the low-grade papillary adenocarcinoma of minor salivary glands should be classified as a papillary cystadenocarcinoma and not as a subclassification of PLGA because of its more aggressive biologic potential. As such, our discussion of PLGA excludes those tumors with an exclusive or predominant papillary component.

CLINICAL FEATURES

Since 1984 an increasing number of tumor series and case reports describing PLGA have been included in the scientific literature. To date, there are 135 cases of PLGA cited in the literature,[1, 2, 6, 10–23] and 75 cases identified in the registry of salivary gland pathology at the Armed Forces Institute of Pathology (AFIP). The age distribution of patients from cases in the AFIP files is seen in Figure 23–1. For all 210 cases of PLGA, the patients' ages range from 21 to 94 years (median, 60 years), and these tumors occur most frequently in patients in the seventh decade of life. There is a decided sex predilection, with 67 percent of the tumors affecting women. The most common complaint from patients involves the presence of a painless mass or swelling that is occasionally associated with bleeding, increase in size, or discomfort. Other less frequently identified symptoms include otalgia, odynophagia, tinnitus, and airway obstruction. The AFIP experience (Table 23–1) parallels that of the literature in that the tumor is almost exclusively identified in the oral cavity where the palate represents the most frequent site of occurrence (58.5 percent of all cases). In descending order of frequency, the other intraoral sites include the following: buccal mucosa (14 percent), lip (13 percent), retromolar pad (3.5 percent), cheek (3 percent), tongue (2.5 percent), maxillary area (2 percent), mandibular mucosal area (1.5 percent), and posterior trigone region (0.5 percent). Involvement of nonoral sites is rare and has included only the nasal cavity (1 percent)[13, 17] and the nasopharynx (0.5 percent).[21] Two cases from the AFIP registry that were initially thought to involve the neck and the oropharynx actually primarily involved the floor of the mouth and the soft palate, respectively, with secondary extension to the neck and the oropharynx. Similarly, PLGA is a tumor of minor salivary glands and has not been identified in major salivary glands except as the malignant epithelial component in nine cases of carcinoma ex pleomorphic adenoma.[24] The duration of symptoms was quite variable, ranging from 2 weeks to a 20- to 30-year history of a mass lesion. No predisposing factors associated with this neoplasm are known to exist.

Table 23–1. Anatomic Distribution of 75 Cases of Polymorphous Low-Grade Adenocarcinoma in the AFIP Salivary Gland Registry

Anatomic Site	Number of Cases	Percentage
Palate (total)	44	58.6
Palate, not specified	(26)	(34.6)
Hard palate	(7)	(9.3)
Soft palate	(11)	(14.6)
Lip (total)	14	18.7
Upper lip	(12)	(16)
Lower lip	(1)	(1.3)
Lip, not specified	(1)	(1.3)
Cheek	12	16
Tongue	1	1.3
Floor of mouth	1	1.3
Pharynx	1	1.3
Minor, other	2	2.7
*Total**	75	100

*Does not include numbers in parentheses

PATHOLOGIC FEATURES

The tumors are variously described as polypoid or raised, round to oval, mucosal covered masses, ranging in size from 1.0 to 6.0 cm in greatest dimension. In general, the mucosa remains intact; however, scattered descriptions of ulcerated lesions exist.

Microscopically, polymorphous low-grade adenocarcinoma is characterized by infiltrative growth, morphologic diversity, and cytologic uniformity. The tumors are often well circumscribed, but unencapsulated, and they infiltrate surrounding tissues, including the surface epithelium, residual minor salivary glands, and connective tissue components (Fig. 23–2). The polymorphic nature of these lesions refers to the variety of growth patterns that may be identified within the same lesion and among different lesions, including

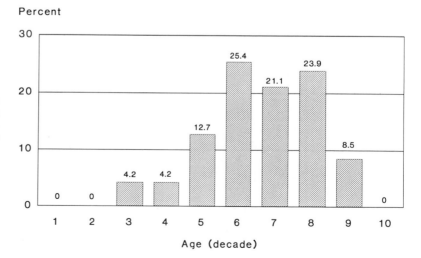

Figure 23–1. Age distribution by decade of 71 patients with polymorphous low-grade adenocarcinoma in the AFIP salivary gland registry.

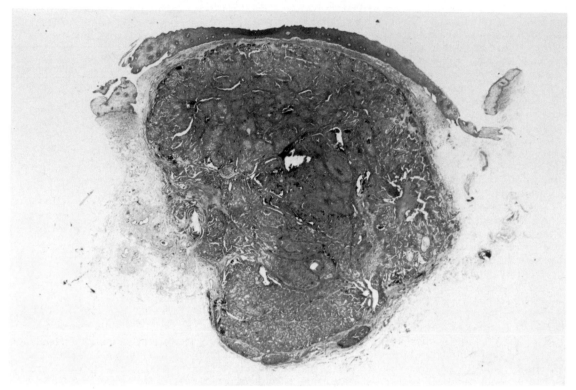

Figure 23–2. Low-power microscopy of a polymorphous low-grade adenocarcinoma shows a well-circumscribed but infiltrating tumor with a variety of growth patterns (× 7.5).

solid, glandular, cribriform, ductular, tubular, trabecular, or cystic lesions (Figs. 23–3 and 23–4). A single-file pattern is commonly seen and often located at the periphery of the tumor. Occasionally, a focal papillary pattern can be identified (see Fig. 23–4F). Neurotropism (peri- and intraneural) is found in the majority of tumors, and perivascular invasion may be identified, with tumor nests often arranged in concentric fashion around these structures (Fig. 23–5). In addition, invasion of bone, cartilage, muscle, and adipose tissue can be seen.

The tumor is composed of cuboidal to columnar isomorphic cells that have uniform ovoid to spindle-shaped nuclei. The chromatin varies from vesicular to stippled, but basophilic nuclei can also be identified (Fig. 23–6). Nucleoli are small and inconspicuous. Scant to moderate amounts of eosinophilic to amphophilic cytoplasm can be seen, and occasionally, clear cytoplasmic changes are focally predominant (see Fig. 23–6). Cell borders are typically indistinct. Mitotic figures are rare, and necrosis is not seen. The tumor stroma varies from mucoid to hyaline to mucohyaline, and in some cases, tumor nests are separated by a fibrovascular stroma (Fig. 23–7). In addition to the above findings, other changes that may sometimes be identified include intratubular calcifications (psammomalike bodies), pseudoepitheliomatous

hyperplasia of the surface epithelium, and squamous metaplasia within the tumor. The last change can be found in tumors of patients who have undergone fine-needle aspiration biopsy. Intraluminal mucin can be identified by periodic acid–Schiff stain after diastase digestion; however, only focal intracytoplasmic mucin is seen.

IMMUNOCYTOCHEMISTRY

The immunohistochemical reactivity in PLGA includes consistent demonstration of cytokeratin (high and low molecular weight), epithelial membrane antigen (EMA), and S-100 protein (Fig. 23–8).[21, 23, 25–27] Both the luminal and nonluminal cells are reactive for these antigens. Carcinoembryonic antigen (CEA) and muscle-specific actin are variably immunoreactive.[21, 23, 25] Glial fibrillary acidic protein (GFAP) immunoreactivity has not been consistently evaluated in PLGA. One report did not identify any immunoreactivity for GFAP in seven cases of PLGA,[23] whereas other studies identified focal positive immunoreactivity in limited cases.[21, 28]

The antigenic profile of PLGA is consistent with its proposed derivation from the intercalated duct region of the salivary duct system (see Chapter

Text continued on page 408

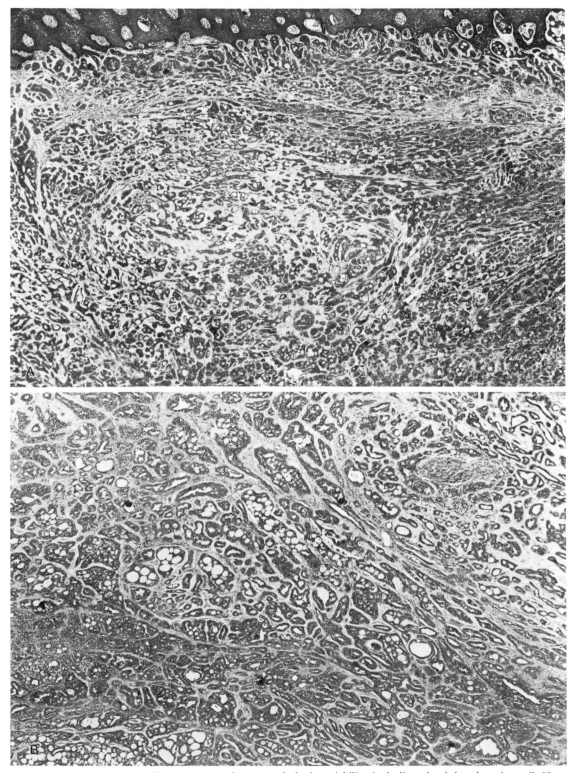

Figure 23–3. *A–D,* These infiltrating tumors have morphologic variability, including glandular, ductular, cribriform, cystic, trabecular, solid, and tubular patterns (*A, B:* × 30).

Illustration continued on following page

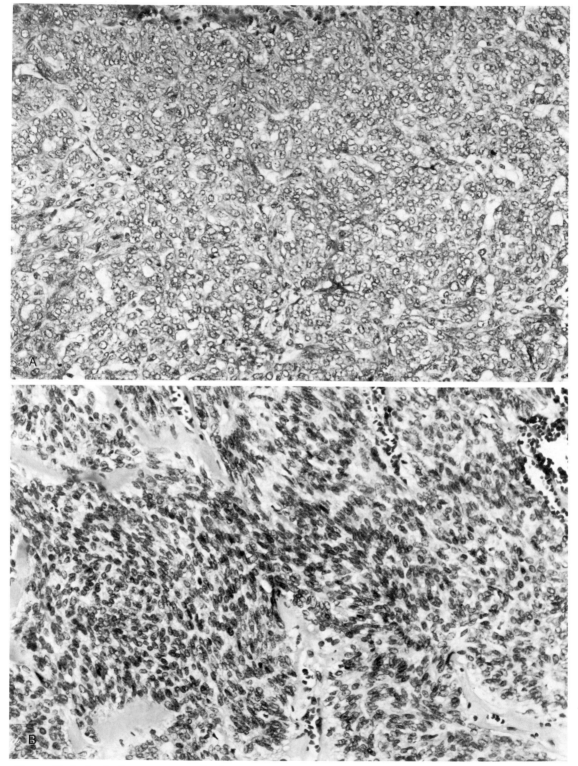

Figure 23–6. Cytologic appearance of polymorphic low-grade adenocarcinoma shows generally isomorphic cells with *(A)* round to oval and *(B)* spindle-shaped nuclei. *(A, B:* × 150.)

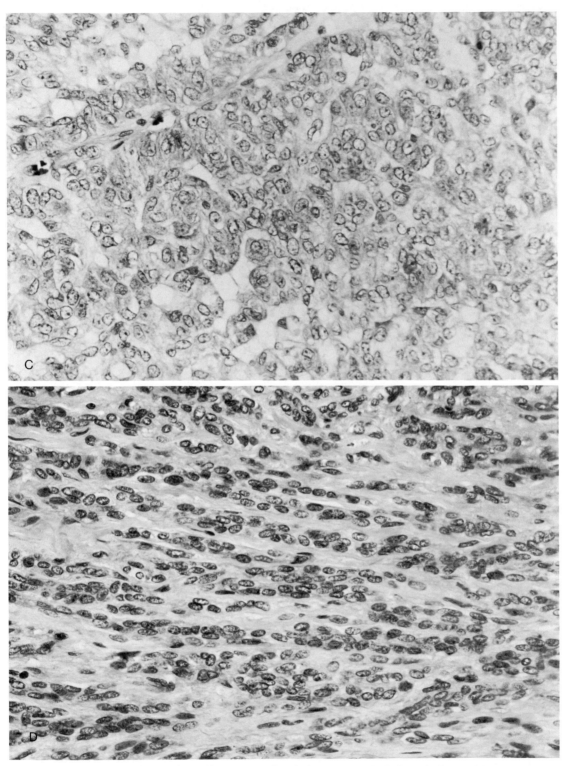

Figure 23–6 *Continued* At higher magnification cytoplasmic features may include vesicular nuclei *(C)* and stippled nuclei *(D)*. *(C, D, × 300.)*

Illustration continued on following page

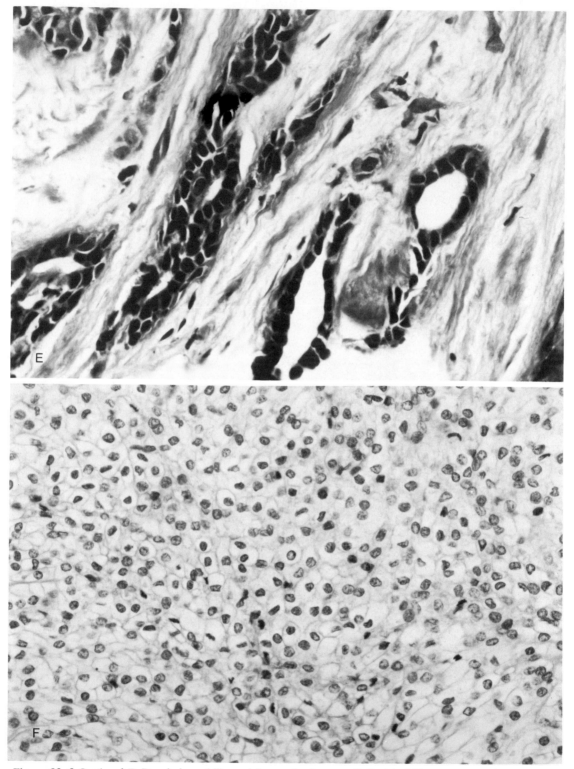

Figure 23–6 *Continued E,* Deeply basophilic nuclei may also be seen. *F,* Eosinophilic or amphophilic cytoplasm is usually indistinct, but on occasion clear cytoplasm with more distinct cell borders may be focally predominant. (*E, F:* × 300.)

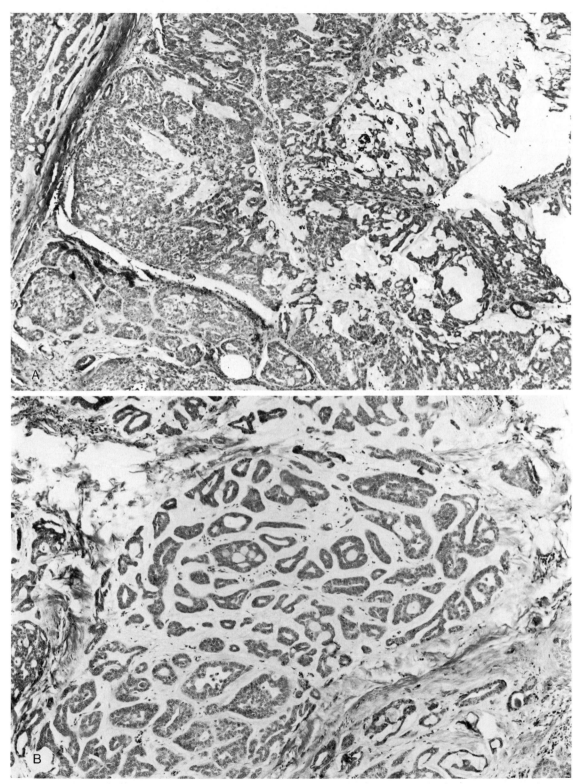

Figure 23–7. Tumor stroma may vary and includes the following types: *(A)* mucoid, *(B)* hyaline, and
Illustration continued on following page

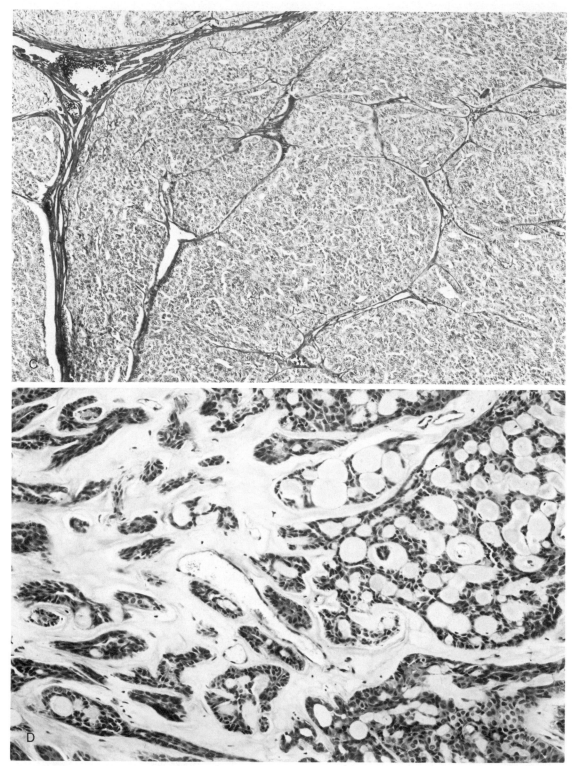

Figure 23–7 *Continued C,* fibrovascular, which forms thin septa in this tumor. The eosinophilic hyalinized stroma in (*D*) adds to the adenoid cystic-like appearance of this cribriform PLGA. (*A–C:* × 75; *D:* × 150.)

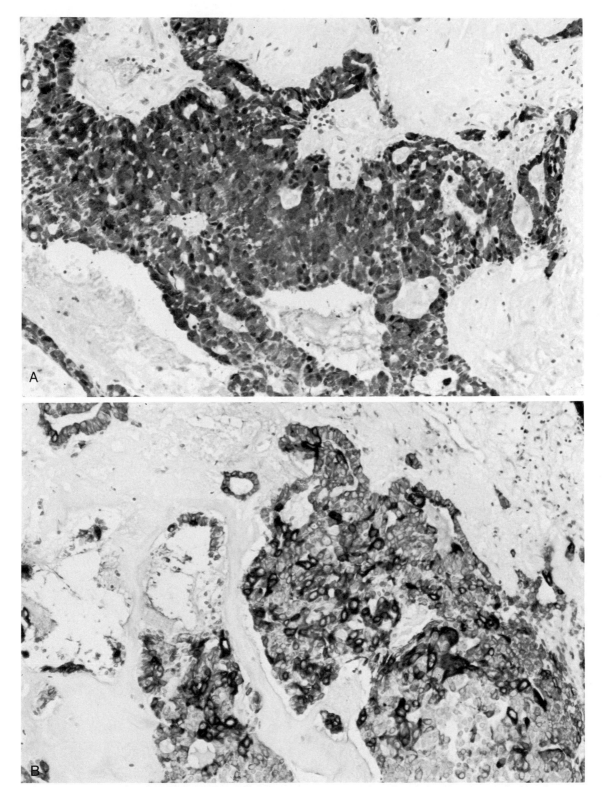

Figure 23–8. The immunocytochemical antigenic profile of polymorphous low-grade adenocarcinoma includes consistent diffuse reactivity for *(A)* cytokeratin, *(B)* epithelial membrane antigen,

Illustration continued on following page

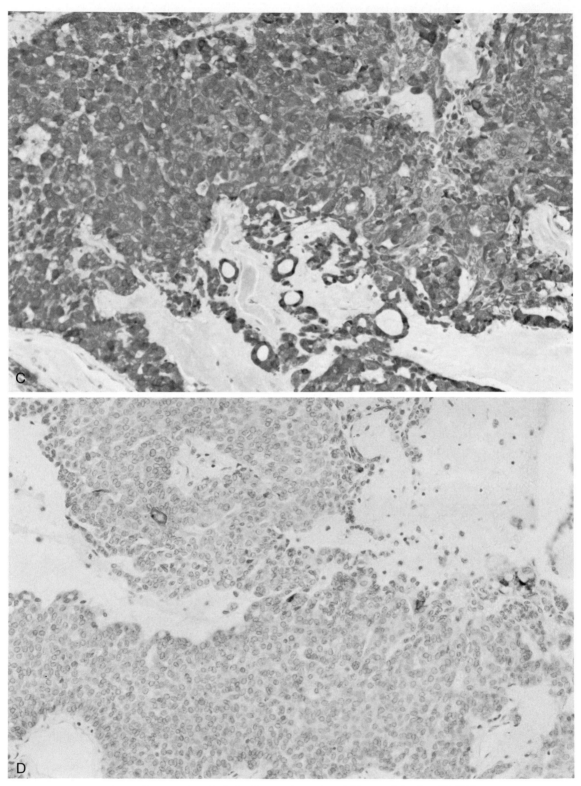

Figure 23–8 *Continued (C)* S-100 protein, and variable reactivity for *(D)* CEA,

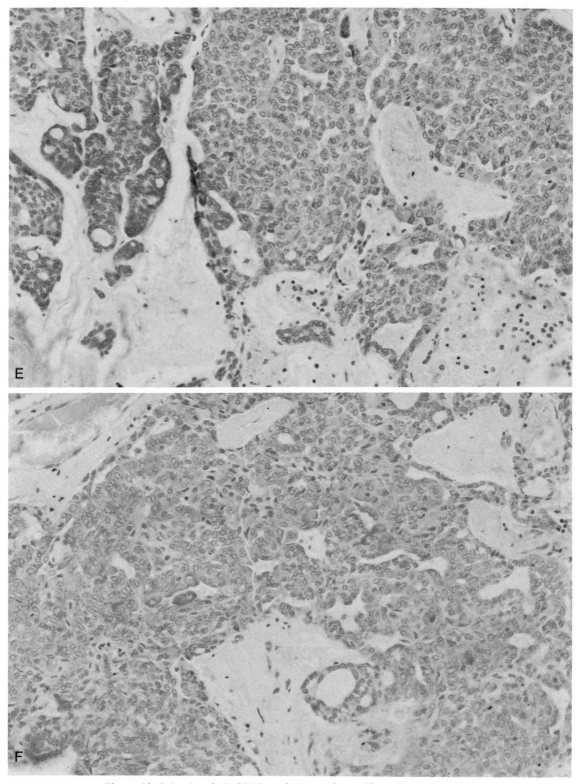

Figure 23–8 *Continued (E)* GFAP, and *(F)* muscle-specific actin. *(A–F:* × 150.)

7).[1, 25, 26] Numerous reports detail the immunohistochemical staining of the normal salivary gland duct system and its associated neoplasms.[25–33] To date, only a limited number of cases of PLGA have had detailed immunohistochemical evaluation.[21, 23, 25–27] In conjunction with the immunohistochemical profile of other tumors thought to arise from the intercalated duct region, the accumulated immunohistochemical data support the presence of at least two populations of tumor cells in PLGA, including those forming ductal structures and those with myoepithelial features.

ELECTRON MICROSCOPY

The ultrastructural features of PLGA have been documented in four reports.[10, 17, 18, 26] The findings were cuboidal or polygonal cells with high nuclear to cytoplasmic ratios, dispersed chromatin, and small nucleoli that were often in direct contact with the nuclear membrane. The cytoplasm contained abundant intermediate filaments. Mitochondria were scant, Golgi complexes were inconspicuous, and a variable amount of rough endoplasmic reticulum was seen. Well-formed junctional complexes joined cells that were surrounded by basal lamina. Areas of glandular differentiation displayed cells that were joined by desmosomes and apical tight junctions and that projected prominent microvilli into the luminal spaces. Pseudoglands consisted of cells with similar ultrastructural features, but well-formed junctional complexes were not seen. The cells at the outer aspect of cords were invested by glycosaminoglycans and by excessive basal lamina, which essentially formed a continuous layer around these cells. Associated with the basal lamina were micropinocytotic vesicles and microfilaments. These findings add support to the concept that PLGA has both ductal and myoepithelial differentiation.

DIFFERENTIAL DIAGNOSIS

The neoplasms that present the most difficulties in differentiation from PLGA are benign mixed tumor and adenoid cystic carcinoma.

Benign mixed tumors (BMT) of minor salivary glands can be seen in virtually all sites in the upper aerodigestive tract. Among the more than 3,000 intraoral salivary gland tumors in the AFIP registry, the BMT is the most common neoplasm; it accounts for 38 percent of all (benign and malignant) tumors and 74 percent of all benign tumors. They occur slightly more frequently in women, and the palate is the most frequently involved site. The benign mixed tumor of minor salivary glands is well circumscribed, often unencapsulated, and may have a pushing margin. Architectural patterns vary, and myxochondroid stromal features

are seen. The cytologic appearance is uniform without atypia. Squamous metaplasia is sometimes present. The benign mixed tumors that arise in the oral cavity tend to be more cellular than their major salivary gland counterparts.[16, 23] As such, differentiation from PLGA may prove difficult. However, in contrast to PLGA, BMTs are not infiltrative. Furthermore, BMTs do not display neurotropism nor do they demonstrate perivascular, osseous, or cartilaginous infiltration. Some authors have pointed to subtle differences in the cytologic features of BMT and PLGA;[23] however, relying on cytologic features alone in differentiating these tumors may lead to diagnostic errors. Immunocytochemistry may have some value in separating BMT from PLGA. Both tumors are thought to arise from the distal portions of the salivary duct system,[33, 34] and they share many of the same immunohistochemical features,[33] including immunoreactivity for cytokeratin, S-100 protein, muscle-specific actin, EMA, and CEA. GFAP immunoreactivity has been reported in PLGA, but this immunoreactivity has only been documented in limited cases and is usually focal in nature.[21, 28] In contrast, Anderson and colleagues[23] found no GFAP immunoreactivity in seven cases of PLGA, whereas GFAP immunoreactivity was demonstrated in all eleven cases of BMT. Only limited numbers of PLGA have been analyzed for the presence of GFAP staining; thus, although the data derived are potentially useful, a definitive conclusion cannot be drawn from these findings until the results are substantiated with a larger series.

Like their pleomorphic counterparts, the various monomorphic adenomas can be seen throughout the upper aerodigestive tract. Although usually encapsulated or well circumscribed, these lesions may be unencapsulated or multifocal or may demonstrate extension of tumor beyond the capsule. Furthermore, the array of morphologic varieties may be confused with PLGA. However, like BMT and unlike PLGA, invasion of nerves, vascular spaces, or other connective tissue components is not a feature of monomorphic adenomas.

Perhaps the most difficult tumor to differentiate histologically from PLGA is adenoid cystic carcinoma (ACC). Adenoid cystic carcinomas are frequently found in the oral cavity, occurring most often on the palate. Other sites include the buccal mucosa, floor of the mouth, lip, and retromolar trigone. ACCs are unencapsulated, infiltrating tumors that have a well-documented propensity for neural invasion. Other qualities ACCs have in common with PLGAs include an array of morphologic patterns identified as cribriform, solid, and tubular. The cells are small and basophilic with only minimal pleomorphism and mitotic activity. In general, the distinction between ACC and PLGA can be based on histologic examination. The nuclei of ACC are usually more hyperchromatic and more angular than those of PLGA. Cribriform areas with accumulation of basophilic pools of glycosaminoglycans, which are frequent in ACC, are not typical of PLGA. Cytoplasmic staining of PLGA is eosinophilic to amphophilic, whereas that of ACC is very pale to clear staining. Immunohistochemistry may assist in their differentiation. Although PLGA shares some common immunohistochemical features with ACC, studies have shown that EMA and CEA may assist in differentiating these tumors.[25, 35] Epithelial membrane antigen and carcinoembryonic antigen stained the true luminal cells of ACC in equal proportion and intensity. However, in PLGA, the staining qualities of EMA and CEA were dissimilar. Reactivity to EMA was seen in more than 90 percent of the tumor cells, and reactivity to CEA was seen in from fewer than 15 percent of cells in three cases to as many as 75 percent of cells in one case.[25, 35, 36]

The distinction between ACC and PLGA is important because ACC has a much more aggressive clinical course. In general, ACCs are slow-growing tumors with prolonged survivals, even in the face of metastatic disease.[8] However, ACCs are frequently relentless tumors with multiple recurrences, and these tumors decrease patients' long-term survival rates, despite all attempts at therapeutic intervention.[8]

TREATMENT AND PROGNOSIS

The treatment of PLGA should be conservative wide surgical excision. In the literature, the extent of surgical intervention has varied from excisional biopsy to wide local excision to more radical procedures, including maxillectomy, hemimandibulectomy, and orbital exenteration. The more radical procedures were used in cases that were erroneously diagnosed as carcinoma ex pleomorphic adenoma or in the period prior to appropriate identification of this tumor as a low-grade malignancy or in cases in which the tumor was extensively invading adjacent structures. Postoperative radiotherapy and chemotherapy have been used, but no evidence exists to substantiate any benefit from these modalities in conjunction with surgery. Similarly, although radical neck dissections have been performed, they appear unwarranted unless clinical evidence of cervical lymph node metastases is present.

Polymorphous low-grade adenocarcinoma is an indolent neoplasm. Although the tumor can recur, sometimes multiple times over many years, distant metastases have not been reported. In the cases with adequate follow-up in the literature, 80 percent of the patients are alive and well, without evidence of tumor in periods ranging from a few months to as long as 25 years after excision.[1, 2, 6, 10–12, 17–19, 21–23] Twenty-four percent of the patients

have tumor recurrence, which necessitates additional surgical intervention. In 5 of 84 cases (6 percent), metastasis to cervical lymph nodes occurred, and only one patient (1 percent) died as a result of direct extension of tumor to vital structures of the head.[12] This case represents the only death reported as a direct result of PLGA. The other patients with metastatic disease are free of tumor after excision of these metastatic foci.

DISCUSSION

Polymorphous low-grade adenocarcinoma has been established as a distinct type of minor salivary gland adenocarcinoma with characteristic clinicopathologic findings. The origin for this tumor is proposed as arising from the intercalated duct system, with light microscopic, immunohistochemical, and ultrastructural findings showing derivation from both ductal and myoepithelial cell lines. These findings support the multicellular theory of salivary gland tumor histogenesis.[37, 38] Polymorphous low-grade adenocarcinoma is a slow-growing, indolent, malignant tumor that can recur over long periods of time and may even metastasize to regional cervical lymph nodes; however, distant metastases do not occur, and death attributable to PLGA is extremely rare. In 1984, Mills and coworkers[9] described a group of lesions that they termed *low-grade papillary adenocarcinoma of minor salivary gland origin* (LPASO). In total, there are 21 cases in the literature acceptably labeled as LPASO.[9, 11, 39–44] Similarities between PLGA and LPASO include the predilection for the palate, the occurrence in middle age, and the apparent low-grade behavior. Based on these similarities, some investigators advocate grouping the papillary adenocarcinomas under the rubric of PLGA to include papillary and nonpapillary variants.[10, 11] However, we do not agree with this subclassification and, instead, consider these tumors to be papillary cystadenocarcinomas. Aside from the cumbersome terminology of PLGA of papillary and nonpapillary types, differences exist between these tumor types that warrant separate classification. LPASO affects men more frequently. Morphologically, the LPASOs are predominantly or exclusively composed of a papillary growth (see Chapter 27). In contrast, only a small percentage of cases of PLGA demonstrate any papillary component and, when present, it is limited in extent. Finally and perhaps most importantly, the behavior of LPASO differs from that of PLGA. In LPASO, local recurrence and cervical lymph node metastases occurred in 38 and 24 percent of the cases, respectively. Furthermore, a distant metastasis as well as three deaths directly related to tumor was reported to be associated with LPASO. Similar findings are not attributed to PLGA. Therefore, although in a large percentage of the cases LPASO behaved in a rather indolent manner, it has a greater tendency toward aggressive and even lethal behavior in contrast to PLGA.

Some investigators believe that PLGA may represent the low-grade variant of ACC.[1, 12, 18] There may be validity in this argument. Like PLGA, ACC arises from the intercalated duct region.[1, 25, 45] Morphologic similarities between these tumors further support this argument. However, cytologic, immunocytochemical, and biologic differences do not support this contention, and we believe that these tumors should be classified separately.

REFERENCES

1. Batsakis JG, Pinkston GR, Luna MA, Byers RM, Sciubba JJ, Tillery GW: Adenocarcinomas of the oral cavity: A clinicopathologic study of terminal duct carcinomas. J Laryngol Otol 1983; 97:825–835.
2. Freedman PD, Lumerman H: Lobular carcinoma of intraoral minor salivary glands. Oral Surg Oral Med Oral Pathol 1983; 56:157–165.
3. Chaudhry AP, Vickers RA, Gorlin RJ: Intraoral minor salivary gland tumors: An analysis of 1,414 cases. Oral Surg Oral Med Oral Pathol 1961; 14:1194–1226.
4. Stene T, Koppang HS: Carcinomas of intraoral salivary glands. Histopathology 1978; 2:19–29.
5. Stene T, Koppang HS: Intraoral adenocarcinomas. J Oral Pathol 1981; 10:216–225.
6. Evans HL, Batsakis JG: Polymorphous low-grade adenocarcinoma of minor salivary glands: A study of 14 cases of a distinctive neoplasm. Cancer 1984; 53:935–942.
7. Allen MS, Fitz-Hugh GS, Marsh WL: Low-grade papillary adenocarcinoma of the palate. Cancer 1974; 33:153–158.
8. Spiro RH, Koss LG, Hajdu SI, Strong EW: Tumors of minor salivary origin: A clinicopathologic study of 492 cases. Cancer 1973; 31:117–129.
9. Mills SE, Garland TA, Allen MS: Low-grade papillary adenocarcinoma of palatal salivary gland origin. Am J Surg Pathol 1985; 8:367–374.
10. Frierson HF, Mills SE, Garland TA: Terminal duct carcinoma of minor salivary glands: A nonpapillary subtype of polymorphous low-grade adenocarcinoma. Am J Clin Pathol 1985; 84:8–14.
11. Slootweg PJ, Muller H: Low-grade adenocarcinoma of the oral cavity: A comparison between the terminal duct and the papillary type. J Craniomaxillofac Surg 1987; 15:359–364.
12. Aberle AM, Abrams AM, Bowe R, Melrose RJ, Handlers JP: Lobular (polymorphous low-grade) carcinoma of minor salivary glands: A clinicopathologic study of 20 cases. Oral Surg Oral Med Oral Pathol 1985; 60:387–395.
13. Frierson HF Jr: Pathologic quiz case 1. Polymorphous low-grade adenocarcinoma (PMLGA) of minor salivary gland. Arch Otolaryngol Head Neck Surg 1986; 112:568–570.
14. Kennedy KS, Healy KM, Taylor RE, Strom CG: Polymorphous low-grade adenocarcinoma of the tongue. Laryngoscope 1987; 97:533–536.
15. Frierson HF, Covell JL, Mills SE: Fine-needle aspiration cytology of terminal duct carcinoma of minor salivary gland. Diagn Cytopathol 1987; 3:159–162.
16. Waldron CA, El-Mofty SK, Gnepp DR: Tumors of the intraoral minor salivary glands: A demographic and histologic study of 426 cases. Oral Surg Oral Med Oral Pathol 1988; 66:323–333.
17. Dardick I, Van Nostrand AWP: Polymorphous low-grade adenocarcinoma: A case report with ultrastructural findings. Oral Surg Oral Med Oral Pathol 1988; 66:459–465.
18. Nicolatou O, Kakarantza-Angelopoulou E, Angelopoulos AG, Anagnostopoulou S: Polymorphous low-grade adenocarcinoma of the palate: Report of a case with electron microscopy. J Oral Maxillofac Surg 1988; 46:1008–1013.
19. Scally CM, Irwin ST, Nirodi N: Low grade polymorphous adenocarcinoma of a minor salivary gland. J Laryngol Otol 1988; 102:284–287.
20. Whitt JC, Ellis GL, Koudelka BM: Case for diagnosis. Military Medicine 1988; 153:323–324.
21. Wenig BM, Harpaz N, DelBridge C: Polymorphous low-grade adenocarcinoma of seromucous glands of the nasopharynx: A report of a case and a discussion of the morphologic and immunohistochemical features. Am J Clin Pathol 1989; 92:104–109.
22. Mitchell DA, Eveson JW, Ord RA: Polymorphous low-grade adenocarcinoma of minor salivary glands: A report of three cases. Br J Oral Maxillofac Surg 1989; 27:494–500.
23. Anderson C, Krutchkoff D, Pedersen C, Cartun R, Berman M: Polymorphous low-grade adenocarcinoma of minor salivary gland: A clinicopathologic and comparative immunohistochemical study. Modern Pathol 1990; 3:76–82.
24. Tortoledo ME, Luna MA, Batsakis JG: Carcinoma ex pleomorphic adenoma and malignant mixed tumors. Histomorphologic indexes. Arch Otolaryngol 1984; 110:172–176.
25. Gnepp DR, Chen JC, Warren C: Polymorphous low-grade adenocarcinoma of minor salivary gland: An immunohistochemical and clinicopathologic study. Am J Surg Pathol 1988; 12:461–468.
26. Luna MA, Batsakis JG, Ordonez NG, Mackay B, Tortoledo E: Salivary gland adenocarcinomas: A clinicopathologic analysis of three distinctive types. Sem Diagn Pathol 1987; 4:117–135.
27. Zarbo RJ, Regezi JA, Batsakis JG: S-100 protein in salivary gland tumors: An immunohistochemical study of 129 cases. Head Neck Surg 1986; 8:268–275.
28. Zarbo RJ, Regezi JA, Hatfield JS, Maisel H, Trojanowski JQ, Batsakis JG, Crissman JD: Immunoreactive glial fibrillary acidic protein in normal and neoplastic salivary glands: A combined immunohistochemical and immunoblot study. Surg Pathol 1988; 1:55–63.
29. Nakazato Y, Ishida Y, Takahashi K, Suzuki K: Immunohistochemical distribution of S-100 protein and glial fibrillary acidic protein in normal and neoplastic salivary glands. Virchows Arch [A] 1985; 405:299–310.
30. Nakazato Y, Ishizeki J, Takahashi K, Yamaguchi H, Kamei T, Mori T: Localization of S-100 protein and glial fibrillary acidic protein-related antigen in pleomorphic adenoma of salivary glands. Lab Invest 1982; 46:621–626.

31. Regezi JA, Lloyd RV, Zarbo RJ, McClatchey KD: Minor salivary gland tumors: A histologic and immunohistochemical study. Cancer 1985; 55:108–115.
32. Batsakis JG, Ordonez NG, Ro J, Meis JM, Bruner JM: S-100 protein and myoepithelial neoplasms. J Laryngol Otol 1986; 100:687–698.
33. Stead RH, Qizilbash AH, Kontozoglou T, Daya AD, Riddel RH: An immunohistochemical study of pleomorphic adenomas of the salivary gland: Glial fibrillary acidic protein-like immunoreactivity identifies a major myoepithelial component. Hum Pathol 1988; 19:32–40.
34. Batsakis JG: Salivary gland neoplasia: An outcome of modified histogenesis and cytodifferentiation. Oral Surg Oral Med Oral Pathol 1980; 49:229–232.
35. Chen JC, Gnepp DR, Bedrossian CW: Adenoid cystic carcinoma of salivary glands: An immuno-histochemical analysis. Oral Surg Oral Med Oral Pathol 1988; 65:316–326.
36. Caselitz J, Schulze I, Seifert G: Adenoid cystic carcinoma of the salivary glands: An immunocyto-chemical study. J Oral Pathol 1986; 15:308–318.
37. Dardick I, Byard RW, Carnegie JA: A review of the proliferative capacity of major salivary glands and the relationship to current concepts of neoplasia in salivary glands. Oral Surg Oral Med Oral Pathol 1990; 69:53–67.
38. Dardick I, van Nostrand AWP: Morphogenesis of salivary gland tumors: A prerequisite to improving classification. Pathol Annu 1987; 22(pt 1):1–53.
39. Fliss DM, Zirkin H, Puterman M, Tovi F: Low-grade papillary adenocarcinoma of buccal mucosa salivary gland origin. Head Neck 1989; 11:237–241.
40. Whitaker JS, Turner EP: Papillary tumours of the minor salivary glands. J Clin Pathol 1976; 29:795–805.
41. Edwards EG: Tumors of the minor salivary glands. Am J Clin Pathol 1960; 34:455–463.
42. Cady B, Hutter RVP: Nonepidermoid cancer of the gum. Cancer 1969; 23:1318–1324.
43. Calhoun NR, Cerine FC, Mathews MJ: Papillary cystadenoma of the upper lip. Oral Surg Oral Med Oral Pathol 1965; 20:810–813.
44. Brooks HW, Hiebert AE, Pullman NK, Stofer BE: Papillary cystadenoma of the palate: A review of the literature and report of two cases. Oral Surg Oral Med Oral Pathol 1956; 9:1047–1050.
45. Chaudhry AP, Leifer C, Cutler LS, Satchidanand S, Labay GR, Yamane GM: Histogenesis of adenoid cystic carcinoma of the salivary glands: Light microscopic and electronmicroscopic study. Cancer 1986; 58:72–82.

24

EPITHELIAL-MYOEPITHELIAL CARCINOMA

Russell L. Corio

The epithelial-myoepithelial carcinoma (EMC) of intercalated duct origin is a rare biphasic type of low-grade salivary gland carcinoma that constitutes less than 1 percent of salivary gland neoplasms.[1] Donath and coworkers[1] reported eight cases in 1972 and introduced the term *epithelial-myoepithelial carcinoma of intercalated duct origin.* In their original description, these authors postulated that the tumor is composed of tubular structures that are limited on their outer border by a wide, hyalinized basal membrane. Two cellular forms were described in the ductlike arrangement of cells: an inner layer of darker cells that represents the intercalated duct epithelial component and an outer layer of cells with clear, glycogen-rich cytoplasm that represents the myoepithelial component. Rarely, the myoepithelial cells may be surfaced by individual spindle-shaped cells with little cytoplasm. Donath and coworkers indicated that the proportions of each of these two primary cell types are not constant in all tumors and may vary from one neoplasm to another and even within different fields of the same tumor. The authors examined the neoplasm ultrastructurally, and their observations confirmed their impression on light microscopy of the tumor as having a biphasic cellular composition. In spite of the tumor cells' exhibiting a high degree of differentiation, the neoplasm was classified as a carcinoma based on a locally infiltrative and destructive growth pattern, a frequent rate of local recurrence, and in a minority of cases, the potential for early metastasis to regional and distant lymphatics. Histologically, the presence of focal areas of necrosis and perineural involvement tended to further support the malignant nature of the tumor.

The literature describes under several different names biphasic salivary gland neoplasms with a clear cell composition that probably represent EMC. These neoplasms include tubular solid adenoma,[2] cystic adenoma,[3] adenomyoepithelioma,[4] and clear cell adenoma.[5-7] These neoplasms with a predominant clear cell myoepithelial component have been confused with so-called glycogen-rich clear cell adenoma.[6] Saksela and colleagues[7] reported a case involving a parotid tumor that they diagnosed as clear-cell adenoma of possible myoepithelial origin. Although they considered this tumor to be a rare variant of pleomorphic adenoma, the histomorphologic and electron microscopic features are highly suggestive of EMC. It is interesting that these authors also considered their tumor to be identical to the two cases of tubular solid adenoma reported earlier (1964) by Feyrter.[2]

The histogenesis of the clear cells in salivary gland neoplasms may be from a variety of cells, including myoepithelial cells, reserve cells, intercalated duct cells, mucous cells, sebaceous cells, and acinar cells.[8, 9] Accordingly, tumors with these cellular elements may contain clear cells in varying proportions. In numerous studies, investigators have analyzed the histochemical and ultrastructural features of these clear cells and have concluded that their appearance may be attributed to one of the following three causes: (1) a minimal degree of cellular differentiation with a deficiency of cytoplasmic organelles; (2) an increase in the degree of cellular differentiation with a marked accumulation of cytoplasmic glycogen, mucin, lipid, or clear secretory granules; or (3) tissue fixation and/or processing artifact.[1, 8, 9-13] Clear cells attributed to postsurgical fixation artifact are seen occasionally in oncocytic lesions and acinic cell adenocarcinomas.[9, 14] In regard to acinic cell adenocarcinoma, the clear cell features have also been attributed to the presence of clear secretory granules as a result of disordered protein synthesis or the presence of organelle-deficient intercalated duct cells.[9] Batsakis[9] observed that in tumors in which clear cells predominate, the cells either are indifferent duct cells with few organelles or are myoepithelial in origin. These cells are generally mucin-negative, and depending on the degree of differentiation and the processing procedures, the amount of cytoplasmic glycogen in these cells varies. When clear cells are a minor component of a salivary gland tumor, such as mucoepidermoid carcinoma and acinic cell adenocarcinoma, appropriate classification with its implied biologic potential can usually be determined by the predominant histopathologic features.[14]

The histomorphologic features of EMC vary, and this can be explained by the participation and varying expression patterns of both epithelial and myoepithelial cells. The multifaceted nature of the myoepithelial cell may be explained, in part, by its location within the terminal duct unit. Portions of this cell, namely, those areas directed toward the lumen, are deficient in cell organelles and appear as pale or clear projections with both light and electron microscopes. The opposite or stromal interface of these cells generally contains pinocytotic vesicles and glycogen granules.[15] The composition of the two cells described by Donath and colleagues[1] in EMC may be a reflection of the biphasic nature of the myoepithelial cells as seen ultrastructurally and with special stains.

CLINICAL FEATURES

Epithelial-myoepithelial carcinoma is most prevalent in older individuals, with approximately two thirds of the tumors occurring in the sixth and seventh decades of life. Analysis of 57 cases in the salivary gland registry of the AFIP since 1973, including the 16 previously reported cases by Corio and colleagues,[16] shows a mean age of 59.4

years, with the average age of female patients being nearly equal to that of males. Eight cases (14.4 percent) affected patients under 50 years of age, and eleven cases (19.7 percent) affected patients over 70 years of age (Fig. 24–1). A majority involving 37 cases (66.1 percent) occurred in patients between the ages of 50 and 70 years. The age range of all patients was 15.0 to 81.0 years. The age range in the AFIP material is greater than for the nine cases reported by Luna and colleagues[17] (52 to 77 years), and the mean age of patients in their study (64.2 years) was about 5 years older than in the AFIP series. In a histopathologic review of patients with salivary gland tumors that occurred during childhood, Lack and Upton[18] described two congenital parotid salivary gland tumors that resembled EMC.

In previous studies[1, 15, 16] the neoplasm has exhibited a predilection for female patients, with a peak incidence of occurrence in the seventh decade of life. The AFIP data indicate that among civilian patients, 55 percent were females. For those 29 patients whose race was recorded, 28 (96.6 percent) were white.

Epithelial-myoepithelial carcinoma may arise in any salivary tissue, but it has a predilection for the parotid gland.[1, 9, 15-17] Analysis of cases in the AFIP material confirms this observation, with 43 tumors (75.4 percent) arising in the parotid gland; 7 (12.3 percent) occurring in the submandibular gland; and 7 (12.3 percent) manifesting in minor salivary gland tissue, mainly in the palate and tongue (Table 24–1).

Clinically, most patients present with an asymptomatic or painful salivary gland swelling with a history of steady increase in size over an extended period of time.[1, 16, 17] Patients may also complain of facial paralysis.[15] Nasal obstruction and facial deformity may represent major complaints of patients with maxillary involvement.[17]

Studies of patients with salivary gland malignancies indicate that these patients may have an increased risk of a second primary tumor (see Chap-

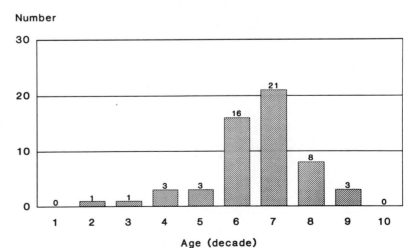

Figure 24–1. Age distribution of 56 patients with EMC in the AFIP registry of salivary gland pathology.

Table 24–1. Anatomic Distribution of 57 Patients with Epithelial-Myoepithelial Carcinoma from the AFIP Salivary Gland Registry

Anatomic Site	Number of Cases	Percentage
Major Glands		
Parotid	43	75.4
Submandibular	7	12.3
Minor Glands		
Palate (total)	4	7.0
Hard palate	(2)	(3.5)
Palate, not specified	(2)	(3.5)
Tongue	1	1.8
Other	2	3.5
*Total**	57	100.0

*Does not include numbers in parentheses

ter 9). Berg and colleagues[20] suggested that a special association existed between salivary gland neoplasms and breast carcinoma. Other studies[21, 22] have found this same relationship and have concluded that in addition to the association between salivary gland malignancies and breast cancer, other hormone-dependent sites may also be at risk. In a clinicopathologic study of 367 cases of mucoepidermoid carcinoma, Spiro and coworkers[23] reported that 46 (18 percent) of their patients had multiple primary neoplasms. Pogrel and

Hansen[19] reported a case of EMC in the parotid gland that occurred synchronously with a follicular cell carcinoma of the thyroid. They believed this to be the first report of such an association and the third report of a salivary gland tumor occurring in conjunction with a thyroid tumor. In a follow-up report, they stated that the patient died 2 months after palliative treatment, and postmortem examination disclosed the presence of metastatic tumor from the parotid gland to the ipsilateral temporal lobe of the brain.[24]

The association of EMC with another primary salivary gland tumor was made by Donath and coworkers[1] in their initial report of eight cases. In their first case, in addition to EMC in the left parotid gland, the patient developed a pleomorphic adenoma at the junction of the hard and soft palates.

One of the patients with an EMC reviewed at the AFIP (a 70-year-old man) had a 2.5-cm neoplasm in the right parotid gland that demonstrated a spectrum of histologic features that were compatible with three different types of salivary gland adenocarcinoma: EMC, adenoid cystic carcinoma, and basal cell adenocarcinoma (Fig. 24–2). Whether these represent variations in one neoplasm or multiple neoplasms is speculative; however, the gross pathology description and the microscopic anatomy suggested separate neoplasms.

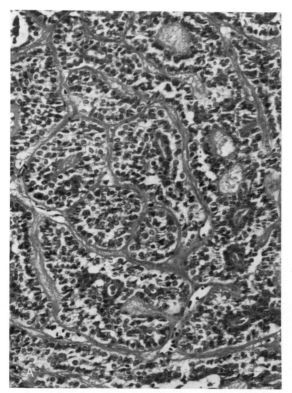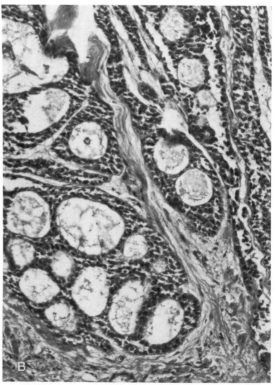

Figure 24–2. Parotid gland tumor in a 70-year-old male had a spectrum of histologic features including EMC *(A)* and adenoid cystic carcinoma *(B)* *(A* and *B,* × 150).

GROSS AND MICROSCOPIC PATHOLOGY

The majority of primary, untreated EMCs occur as single, well-circumscribed, firm, lobulated, neoplasms that usually range in size from 2 to 8 cm.[16, 17] They are typically bosselated neoplasms and on cross-sectional examination exhibit a multinodular growth pattern with irregular cystic spaces. It is not unusual for these tumors to have an infiltrative growth pattern. In addition, recurrent tumors may exhibit superficial lobulation or multicentric growth with irregular tumor borders and central areas of necrosis (Fig. 24–3).

The histomorphologic features of EMC may vary greatly. Most show a multinodular growth pattern with islands of tumor cells separated by dense bands of fibrous connective tissue (Fig. 24–4). The islands of tumor cells are composed of small ducts lined with cuboidal epithelium that is surrounded by clear cells that interface with a thickened, hyalinelike basement membrane (Fig. 24–5). The inner, luminal cuboidal cells have finely granular, dense, eosinophilic cytoplasm and central or basally located round nuclei. Columnar cells and squamous foci may also be seen proliferating within cystic and microcystic spaces that often contain material that reacts positively to periodic acid–Schiff (PAS) stain. The outer, clear myoepithelial cells vary in shape from columnar to ovoid and have well-defined cell borders and eccentrically located vesicular nuclei located toward the basement membrane. Generally, the clear myoepithelial cell component predominates, and the biphasic character of the neoplasm may

not be readily apparent. The tumors' growth patterns may vary from solid lobules that are separated by bands of hyalinized, vascular, fibrous connective tissue to irregular, papillary cystic arrangements with tumor cells that partially or completely fill cystlike spaces. Although mitotic figures are rarely seen, it is not unusual for tumor cells to exhibit vascular invasion and neurotropism (Fig. 24–6). Generally, if a fibrous capsule is present, it is infiltrated by tumor cells, which results in satellitosis of the tumor element.

The cytoplasm of the clear cells shows a positive reaction to PAS stain, but this positive reaction is susceptible to diastase digestion before staining, which indicates the presence of glycogen. Although the ductal lumina may exhibit mucicarminophilic material and positive staining with Alcian blue, intracytoplasmic mucin is not present in either the clear or the ductal epithelial cells. The dense, hyaline, basement-membranelike material that separates islands of tumor cells stains strongly with PAS and periodic acid–methenamine silver stains[17] (Fig. 24–7).

Using immunohistochemical staining, Luna and colleagues[17] investigated eight EMCs. All neoplasms showed cytoplasmic and intranuclear immunoreactivity of clear cells for S-100 protein (Fig. 24–8). The staining pattern tends to be diffuse in tumors with a solid clear cell composition but limited to the peripheral cells in the biphasic areas. Occasionally, these same cells show immunoreactivity for myosin, with intense staining in areas adjacent to the basement membrane. The ductal cells generally show strong immunoreactivity for keratin. Four EMCs contained focal ductal cells

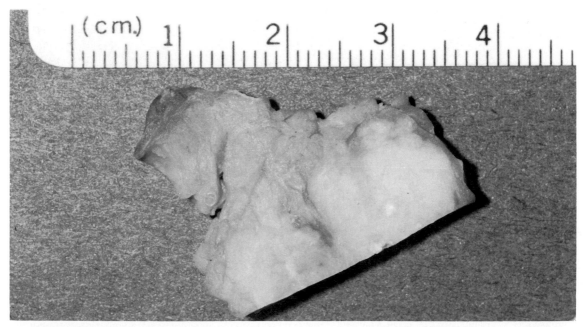

Figure 24–3. EMC is shown with a multinodular growth pattern and irregular borders (Courtesy AFIP).

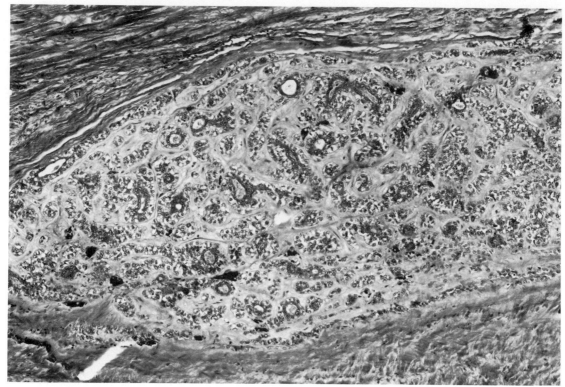

Figure 24–4. Nodule of EMC is surrounded by dense fibrous connective tissue (× 75).

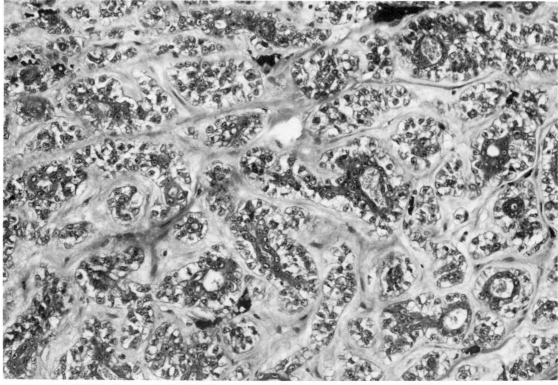

Figure 24–5. Tumor is composed of small ducts that are lined with cuboidal epithelium and are surrounded by clear cells interfacing a thickened, hyalinelike basement membrane (× 150).

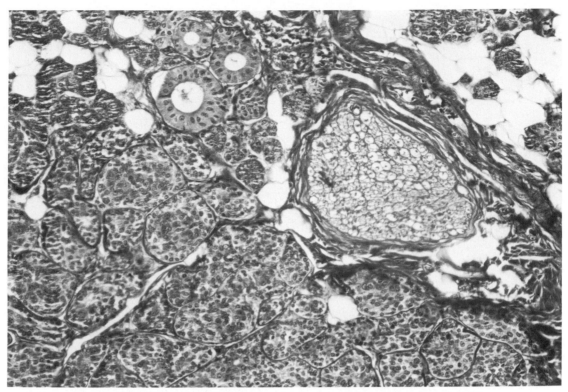

Figure 24–6. EMC shows infiltrative growth pattern and surrounds a nerve (× 150).

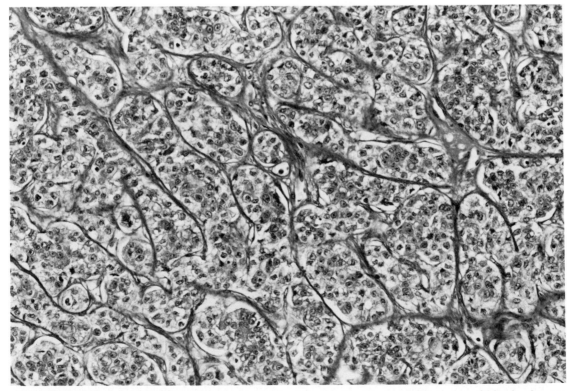

Figure 24–7. Periodic acid–Schiff stain depicts a prominent hyaline basement membrane around islands of tumor cells forming an organoid pattern (× 150).

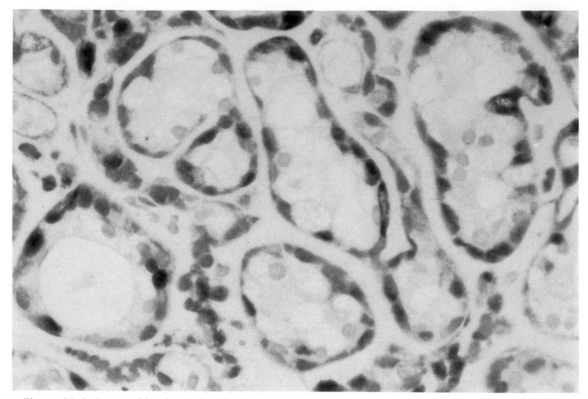

Figure 24–8. Immunohistochemical stain shows presence of S-100 protein in the peripheral epithelial cell component but not in the luminal cells of the neoplasm (× 400).

that were immunoreactive for amylase, which was mainly concentrated in the apical cytoplasm. Myoepithelial type cells were negative.

ELECTRON MICROSCOPIC FEATURES

Electron microscopic studies confirm the dual cell population in this neoplasm.[16, 17] The ductal epithelial cells adjacent to the lumen contain intracytoplasmic tonofilament bundles, well-formed desmosomes, and atypical microvilli along the luminal border. These cells also contain varying numbers of mitochondria; dilated, granular endoplasmic reticulum cisternae; and Golgi complexes. Nuclei are usually oval, with dispersed chromatin and inconspicuous nucleoli. The outer myoepithelial cells lie within the external lamina and contain abundant glycogen and a peripheral array of fine filaments with electron-dense areas typical for cells with smooth muscle differentiation. The basal lamina at the stromal-epithelial interface may display an elaborate replication pattern (Figs. 24–9 and 24–10).

DIFFERENTIAL DIAGNOSIS

The intercalated duct and myoepithelial cells are capable of manifesting numerous patterns of differentiation. The presence of clear cells in varying proportions leads to consideration of other salivary gland neoplasms in the histologic differential diagnosis. As stated previously, the clarity of the cytoplasm by light microscopy may be the result of minimal cellular differentiation with few cytoplasmic organelles; the result of the storage or accumulation of glycogen, mucus, or lipid; or the result of fixation or processing artifact. Accordingly, neoplasms that would have to be considered in a histologic differential diagnosis include pleomorphic adenoma, acinic cell adenocarcinoma, adenoid cystic carcinoma, mucoepidermoid carcinoma, sebaceous carcinoma, and oncocytoma.

Pleomorphic adenomas contain both intercalated duct cells and myoepithelial cells. However, the varying growth patterns and chondromyxoid areas are not seen in EMC. On the other hand, benign and malignant mixed tumors may demonstrate focal EMC-like histologic features. These histomorphologic features are not known to influence the biologic behavior of an otherwise benign mixed tumor.

Acinic cell adenocarcinomas may occasionally contain clear cells. These cells generally show a negative reaction to PAS stain, unlike the glycogen-rich, myoepithelial portion of the EMC. Echevarria[11] believes there is no biologic clear cell variant of acinic cell adenocarcinoma and that the

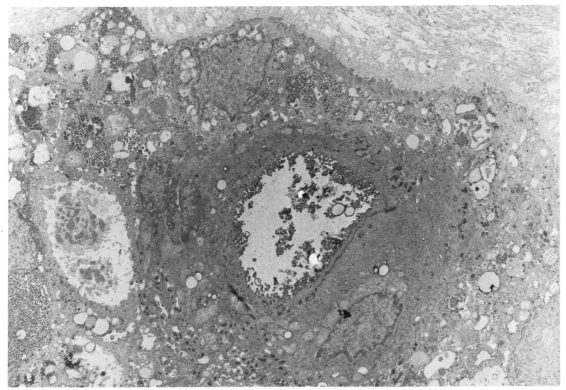

Figure 24–9. Electron micrograph of formalin-fixed material shows a centrally located cystic lumen that contains cellular debris. A smaller lumen that contains amorphous material is also seen. These lumina are surrounded by ductal epithelial cells, whereas more peripheral cells demonstrate differentiation toward myoepithelial cells. Clusters of glycogen particles are scattered within the cytoplasm of the peripheral cells (× 6,000).

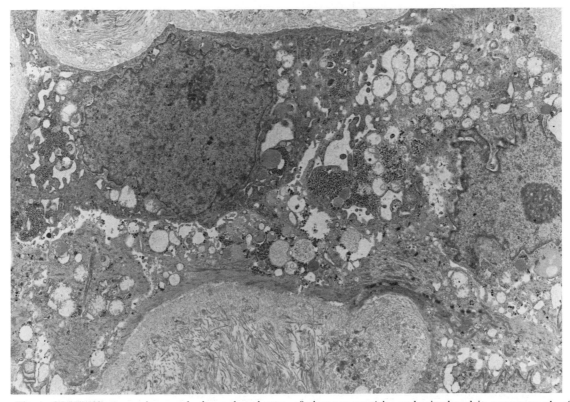

Figure 24–10. Electron micrograph shows that clusters of glycogen particles and mitochondria occupy much of the cytoplasm of the cells that border the supportive stromal tissue. Filamentous material arranged parallel to the cell surface is seen in a subplasmalemmal location (× 6,700).

419

clear cells in this tumor, as in some oncocytomas,[19] are the result of artifact encountered during tissue processing. Electron microscopic examination of the clear cells has shown varying degrees of cytoplasmic degeneration.

The adenoid cystic carcinoma is differentiated from EMC by its more isomorphic cytologic features, paucity of large clear cells, and characteristic formation of small cystlike structures that contain basal membranelike intercellular substance. Although mucoepidermoid carcinomas may have significant numbers of clear cells, unlike EMC, these tumors also contain mucous and epidermoid cells. In addition, this tumor lacks a visible myoepithelial cell component. In contrast to EMC, the clear cells in sebaceous carcinoma are negative for glycogen but stain positively for lipid. Rarely, carcinomas with a clear cell component may metastasize to the regions of the salivary glands from distant primary sites, such as the kidney, thyroid, and parathyroid glands. Differentiation from EMC is usually facilitated by clinical (medical) history and special stains.

PROGNOSIS AND TREATMENT

The duration of clinical signs and symptoms varies from several months to years. Local recurrences, sometimes multiple, are not unusual. Donath and colleagues[1] reported three tumors that recurred. One recurred multiple times. Corio and colleagues[16] obtained follow-up information on 8 of 16 patients and found recurrences in 5 cases. One of these patients had 6 recurrences over a 28-year-period with eventual metastasis to the kidney, and 2 other patients had 2 recurrences ranging from 1 to 14 years after initial diagnosis. Five of nine patients reported by Luna and coworkers[17] experienced local recurrence of tumor between 1 and 6 years after initial treatment. Two of these patients had two recurrences each, and one patient had three recurrences. One of these patients eventually died after widespread metastases. These same authors summarized 33 cases of EMC from the literature and from cases compiled at M.D. Anderson Hospital, and they reported 13 patients (39 percent) with local recurrences and 2 patients whose deaths were attributed directly to the neoplasms.

Little, if any, precise information exists in regard to the effectiveness of the various types of treatment for EMC. Currently, surgery is considered the primary mode of treatment. Total parotidectomy is advocated for tumors in the parotid gland, and the facial nerve branches should be resected if they are involved by tumor.[25] Simple enucleation or shelling out of the tumor should be discouraged, because this is a cause of local recurrence and, in some instances, may result in metastasis. Even with complete surgical resection, recurrences and distant metastasis remain a concern and may occur from a few months to years after the initial surgery.[25] At present, data and experience with this neoplasm are insufficient to determine the efficacy of adjuvant postoperative radiotherapy.

REFERENCES

1. Donath K, Seifert G, Schmitz R: Zur Diagnose und Ultrastruktur des tubulären Speichelgangcarcinoms: Epithelial-myoepitheliales Schaltstückcarcinom. Virchows Arch [A] 1972; 356:16–31.
2. Feyrter F: Cher das solide (tubular-solide) adeno de schlerm und speicheldrusen. Frankfurt Z Pathol 1964; 71:300–326.
3. Snellman A: Ein fall von adenoma-cysticum. Arb Pathol Inst Hesingfors 1933; 7:42–50.
4. Bauer WH, Fox RA: Adenomyoepithelioma (cylindroma) of palatal mucous glands. Arch Pathol 1945; 39:96–102.
5. Evans RW, Cruickshank AH: Epithelial Tumours of the Salivary Glands. Philadelphia, WB Saunders Co, 1970; 269–275.
6. Corrdon M: Glycogen-rich clear cell adenoma of the parotid gland. J Pathol Bact 1956; 72:623–626.
7. Saksela E, Tarkkanen J, Wartiovaara J: Parotid clear-cell adenoma of possible myoepithelial origin. Cancer 1972; 30:742–748.
8. Regezi JA, Sciubba JJ: Oral Pathology, Clinical-Pathologic Correlations. Philadelphia, WB Saunders Co, 1989; 274.
9. Batsakis JG: Clear cell tumors of salivary glands. Ann Otol Rhinol Laryngol 1980; 89:196–197.
10. Hamperl H: The myothelia (myoepithelial cells): Normal state; regressive changes; hyperplasia; tumors. Curr Top Pathol 1970; 53:161–220.
11. Echevarria RA: Ultrastructure of the acinic cell carcinoma and clear cell carcinoma of the parotid gland. Cancer 1967; 20:563–571.
12. Mohamed AH, Cherrick HM: Glycogen-rich adenocarcinoma of minor salivary glands: A light and electron microscopic study. Cancer 1975; 36:1057–1066.
13. Goldman RL, Klein HZ: Glycogen-rich adenoma of the parotid gland: An uncommon benign clear-cell tumor resembling certain clear-cell carcinomas of salivary origin. Cancer 1972; 30:749–754.
14. Ellis GL: "Clear cell" oncocytoma of salivary gland. Hum Pathol 1988; 19:862–867.
15. Batsakis JG: Tumors of the Head and Neck. Clinical and Pathological Considerations, 2nd Ed. Baltimore, Williams & Wilkins Co, 1979; 47.
16. Corio RL, Sciubba JJ, Brannon RB, Batsakis JG: Epithelial-myoepithelial carcinoma of intercalated duct origin. Oral Surg Oral Med Oral Pathol 1982; 53:280–287.
17. Luna MA, Ordonez NG, Mackay B, Batsakis JG, Guillamondegui O: Salivary epithelial-myoepithelial carcinoma of intercalated ducts: A clinical, electron microscopic, and immunocytochemical study. Oral Surg Oral Med Oral Pathol 1985; 59:482–490.

18. Lack EE, Upton MP: Histopathologic review of salivary gland tumors in childhood. Arch Otolaryngol Head Neck Surg 1988; 114:898–906.

19. Pogrel MA, Hansen LS: Second primary tumor associated with salivary gland cancer. Oral Surg Oral Med Oral Pathol 1984; 58:71–72.

20. Berg JW, Hunter RVP Jr: The unique association between salivary gland cancer and breast cancer. JAMA 1968; 204:771–774.

21. Dunn JE Jr, Bragg KU, Sautter C, Gardipee C: Breast cancer risk following a major salivary gland carcinoma. Cancer 1972; 29:1343–1346.

22. Prior P, Waterhouse JAH: Second primary cancers in patients with tumors of the salivary glands. Br J Cancer 1977; 36:263–268.

23. Spiro RH, Huvos AG, Berk R, Strong EW: Mucoepidermoid carcinoma of salivary gland origin: A clinicopathologic study of 367 cases. Am J Surg 1978; 136:461–468.

24. Pogrel MA, Hansen LS: Follow-up report on epithelial-myoepithelial carcinoma of intercalated duct origin. Oral Surg Oral Med Oral Pathol 1984; 59:172–173.

25. Stiernberg CM, Batsakis JG, Bailey BJ, Clark WD: Epithelial-myoepithelial carcinoma of the parotid gland. Otolaryngol Head Neck Surg 1986; 94:240–242.

25

UNDIFFERENTIATED CARCINOMA

Lewis R. Eversole, Douglas R. Gnepp,
and Galen M. Eversole

Epithelial tumors that for the most part lack microscopic features of differentiation are uncommonly encountered in the salivary gland. When they originate from salivary epithelium, these tumors are usually located in the parotid gland, although a few have been reported to arise in the submandibular gland. Minor gland origin is extremely rare. This discussion focuses on three distinct entities: (1) lymphoepithelial carcinomas (so-called malignant lymphoepithelial lesion), (2) undifferentiated large cell carcinomas, and (3) undifferentiated small cell carcinomas. The small cell types bear a resemblance to oat cell carcinomas arising in other sites, whereas the large cell tumors are more akin to undifferentiated carcinomas of the nasopharynx. Lymphoepithelial carcinomas exhibit architectural features and histomorphologic growth patterns similar to those of the benign lymphoepithelial lesion.[1–12] Although some authors have indicated that as many as 30 percent of all malignant salivary gland tumors are undifferentiated, Blanck and colleagues[1] indicated that 4.5 percent of 1,678 parotid gland tumors were undifferentiated, and Donath and others[5] classified 6.5 percent of all malignant tumors from their series as undifferentiated. From over 15,000 salivary gland tumors accessioned by the Armed Forces Institute of Pathology (AFIP), about 0.4 percent were diagnosed as undifferentiated carcinomas.

It is difficult to procure reliable data from the literature for these three variants of undifferentiated carcinomas of salivary gland origin, since the small and large cell tumors are often grouped as a single entity in many large series reports. Furthermore, some cases subsumed under the lymphoepithelial carcinoma category are probably simple large cell carcinomas, which lack the char-acteristic architectural features of benign lymphoepithelial lesion. Last, a few cases that were accepted as examples of malignant lymphoepithelial lesion are most likely adenocarcinomas arising in a preexisting benign lymphoepithelial lesion. In this chapter, we have outlined rigid criteria for inclusion of cases under the three specific variants of undifferentiated carcinoma.

LYMPHOEPITHELIAL CARCINOMA

In 1952, Godwin[13] condensed a group of inflammatory lesions of the salivary glands under the appellation *benign lymphoepithelial lesion*. These lesions, previously referred to as *adenolymphoma, lymphoepithelioma, lymphocytoid tumor,* and *Mikulicz's disease,* all shared histopathologic features consisting of diffuse lymphocytic infiltration with salivary parenchymal degeneration and persistent ductal remnants. Morgan and Castleman,[14] in 1953, promulgated the thesis that the epithelial foci encountered in the benign lymphoepithelial lesion were ductal remnants undergoing reactive myoepithelial proliferation. They introduced the term *epimyoepithelial islands* to describe these structures and further proposed that their presence was pathognomonic for Mikulicz's disease. Subsequently, Sjögren's syndrome was included as a disease exhibiting the features of benign lymphoepithelial lesion (see Chapter 6).[15]

Since bilateral parotid gland and lacrimal gland enlargement characterized microscopically by parenchymal degeneration with lymphocytic infiltration was first described in 1888 by Johann von Mikulicz-Radecki, numerous publications have reported both benign and malignant courses for the condition.[16, 17] Whereas Mikulicz's case was probably a benign lymphoepithelial lesion, subsequent studies indicated that a similar clinical presentation could be encountered in other disease processes, including malignant lymphoma involving the salivary glands.[18–20] By current definition, Mikulicz's disease is characterized by the presence of the benign lymphoepithelial lesion, whereas Mikulicz's syndrome is alleged to be any other disease manifesting with bilateral parotid gland involvement, including granulomatous (e.g., sarcoidosis, Heerfordt's syndrome) and neoplastic processes (e.g., intraparotid lymphoma). Lymphoma of the major salivary glands has been recognized since the first decade of the twentieth century. Although the vast majority arise within lymph nodes of the parotid gland region, rarely lesions may arise within a preexisting benign lymphoepithelial lesion (see Chapter 30).[21, 22]

In 1962, Hilderman and others[9] described an epithelial malignancy of the parotid gland that to some degree emulated benign lymphoepithelial lesion. Since this initial report, the malignant lymphoepithelial lesion has become recognized as a distinct entity with well-defined histopathologic features.[10–12] The term *malignant lymphoepithelial lesion* is obfuscatory, since it does not imply which cell type (lymphoid or epithelial) is malignant; therefore, we prefer the term *lymphoepithelial carcinoma* to clarify that the epithelial component rather than the lymphoid element is malignant.

Clinical and Epidemiologic Features

There have been over 100 instances of lymphoepithelial carcinoma reported in the world literature. The vast majority have occurred among North American and Greenland Eskimos and among Asian Orientals. Less commonly, cases that involved whites and Alaskan or Canadian Native Americans have been published, although no cases reported have involved Native Americans of the contiguous United States. Steiner[23] has surveyed salivary gland tumor prevalence in the United States and has estimated that 0.25 to 0.43 percent of all cancers are of salivary gland origin. Schaefer[24, 25] was probably the first to witness an increased incidence of salivary gland cancer among people of the Arctic regions, and subsequent to the initial description of the so-called malignant lymphoepithelial lesion by Hilderman and colleagues,[9] Wallace and coworkers[26] published the first report on a series of lymphoepithelial carcinomas occurring among Eskimos. In their series of 14 salivary tumors, 9 cases were classified as undifferentiated carcinomas, and a microscopic resemblance to the benign lymphoepithelial lesion was noted by these authors. Indeed, Wallace and others[26] reported that this group of nine tumors constituted 28 percent of all cancers that occur among this Eskimo population. Krishnamurthy and others[27] found 12 in-

stances of lymphoepithelial carcinoma among 16 cases of salivary gland tumors that involved Eskimo and Native American patients residing in Alaska. Arthaud[28] found seven instances of undifferentiated carcinoma among nineteen Eskimos and Aleut Indians with salivary gland tumors. Whereas Merrick and others[29] estimated a 4.5-fold increase in the occurrence of salivary gland tumors among Eskimo males and a 9.0-fold increase among Eskimo females in comparison with the occurrence of these tumors in white Europeans, Lanier and others[30, 31] have estimated that the affliction rate among Eskimos for lymphoepithelial carcinoma, in particular, is 15 times that among whites.

Clinically, the overall female to male ratio for 106 patients, including the AFIP series and the cases reported in the literature (regardless of ethnic background) is slightly less than 2 to 1. Gender predilections for these tumors vary according to race and ethnicity. Among Eskimos, a preponderance of female patients is notable, whereas lymphoepithelial carcinoma occurring among Chinese patients manifests a slight male predilection.[26–29, 32–34] Merrick and others[29] have identified a tendency for familial clustering; they reported two Eskimo kindreds with a total of five affected females. The mean age for patients with lymphoepithelial carcinoma at the time of diagnosis is 44 years for males and 36 years for females.[27] Among the 106 tabulated cases, over 50 percent were detected in the fourth and fifth decades (Fig. 25–1).

The parotid gland is involved in over 90 percent of Eskimo and white patients with lymphoepithelial carcinoma, whereas a submandibular localization is encountered among one third to one half of the Oriental patients. The average duration of signs or symptoms is 1.5 years. The primary physical finding is an indurated mass in the parotid region; pain or discomfort is a complaint among about one half of the patients, and drainage may be observed. Facial paralysis is observed in less than 20 percent.[9–12, 26–29, 32–45] Unfortunately, no data are available that related sialographic or other imaging features of these tumors.

Of major significance in the cases of lymphoepithelial carcinoma is the issue regarding any relationship with preexisting benign lymphoepithelial lesion or any association with Sjögren's syndrome. Many authors have implied that lymphoepithelial carcinoma arises from a preexisting benign lymphoepithelial lesion (BLEL); however, a critical evaluation of these publications discloses that such conclusions are usually based on the observation that BLEL-like foci lie adjacent to the carcinomatous element.[34, 36, 38] It is axiomatic that such a finding should be interpreted with caution, since BLEL-like areas may represent low-grade carcinomatous foci or a reactive phenomenon that is secondary to the coexistent malignant lesion. A BLEL preceding the emergence of lymphoepithelial carcinoma by many years has been reported,

No. of patients

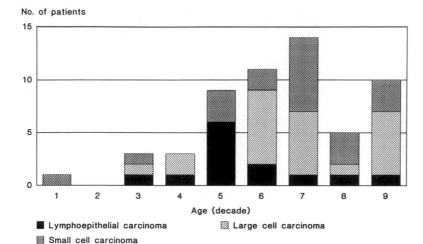

Figure 25–1. Age distribution for 56 patients with undifferentiated carcinomas from the AFIP registry of salivary gland pathology.

and most instances of this nature are encountered among whites.[10, 39] Among the Arctic region cases, no association with Sjögren's syndrome has been made, and none of the affected patients have presented with any of the stigmata characteristic for the syndrome.[12, 32] Furthermore, serologic studies for autoantibodies performed on a population of Eskimo patients failed to disclose any associations with autoimmune diseases. Specifically, serologic tests of anti-SS-A and anti-SS-B, Sjögren's antibodies, were negative in ten patients; other antinuclear antibodies were not detectable either.[27]

Considering the histopathologic features of anaplasia that simulate, to some extent, nasopharyngeal carcinomas and heeding the occurrence of this tumor among Orientals, investigators have studied the Epstein-Barr virus (EBV) as a potential etiologic agent.[46] Saw and others[33] noted elevated titers of antibodies to EBV antigens in six of eight Chinese patients with lymphoepithelial carcinoma; however, Krishnamurthy and colleagues,[27] although finding serologic evidence for past EBV exposure, could not correlate high titers of antibody with extent of disease as observed with nasopharyngeal carcinoma. These latter authors did, however, identify EBV genomes in two cases of lymphoepithelial carcinoma using DNA in situ hybridization methods. Sehested and colleagues[47] were unable to see any viral particles in their ultrastructural investigation of 19 cases of tumors occurring in Greenland Eskimos. Using in situ hybridization, Weiss and others[48] analyzed a variety of lymphoepitheliomalike lesions (none were salivary gland lesions) and were able to identify EBV genomes in all of six nasopharyngeal carcinomas; however, they found only one genome positive reaction from among fourteen non-nasopharyngeal undifferentiated carcinomas. As discussed later in this chapter, we were unable to detect EBV DNA in four cases tested from the AFIP series.

Gross and Microscopic Pathology

Typically, the tumor is solid and measures 2 to 3 cm, although massive lesions have been reported. In the parotid gland, the tumor is firm and fixed yet usually circumscribed; nevertheless, tumors have been variably described as grossly encapsulated, partially circumscribed, multinodular, and infiltrative.[12, 27, 28, 33, 35] Sections of tumor tissue vary from gray-tan to yellow-gray. Zonal necrosis and hemorrhage are not typical features.

Microscopically, at lower magnifications, lymphoepithelial carcinoma resembles benign lymphoepithelial lesion with oval and irregular elongated epithelial islands that occasionally anastomose and that are isolated by a benign lymphoid stroma (Fig. 25–2A, B). Acini and ducts may also be seen, particularly at the periphery, effaced by lymphoid infiltrates. Germinal centers and fibrosis may be evident. At higher magnification, the epithelial cells appear polygonal to spindled, without keratinization or formation of lumina. The nuclei are large and somewhat vesicular (Fig. 25–2C).[34, 35, 37] Mitoses are easily seen, but anaplasia is usually not a prominent finding. Importantly, within the tumor proper, as opposed to the margins that are confluent with the normal gland, cuboidal epithelium-lined ducts with true epimyoepithelial islands are rare. Rather, the epithelial element is solid, lacking any orientation around residual ducts. The lymphoid stroma includes plasma cells and immunoblasts as well as occasional epithelioid histiocytes, the latter of which may palisade about foci of fibrinous material, yielding a granulomatous appearance. The small lymphocytes are mature with regular nuclear membranes. Areas of fibrosis and hyalinization are not uncommon; indeed, in many cases, foci of neoplastic epithelial cells that are located in a fibrous stroma devoid of any prominent lymphoid infiltration are present (Fig. 25–2D). Perineural invasion is frequently appreciated.[33]

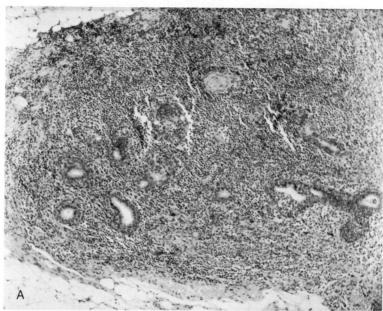

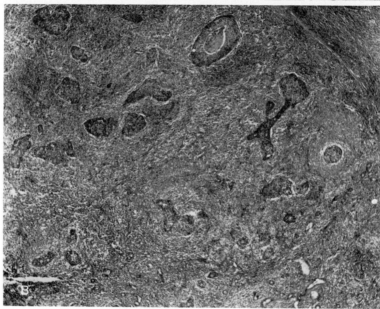

Figure 25–2. *A,* Benign lymphoepithelial lesion shows epimyoepithelial islands with ductal lumina and surrounding lymphoid tissue (× 40). *B,* Lymphoepithelial carcinoma has similar architecture to the benign lymphoepithelial lesion (× 40).

Illustration continued on following page

A spectrum of cases showing low- to high-grade histology have been reported. The lower grade lesion tends to resemble BLEL more closely, with germinal centers and circumscription, but unlike BLEL these lesions are more disorderly, with syncytial epithelium tending to form distinct trabeculae, sheets, and anastomosing islands. The cells tend to have vesicular nuclei with single nucleoli and easily recognized mitoses but no anaplasia.[27, 34] Atypical acini and ducts may be enveloped by the neoplastic islands; however, true epimyoepithelial islands are not seen in the central regions of the tumor.[28] A higher grade lesion shows more diffuse infiltration of the epithelial islands by lymphoid cells, and germinal center formation is much less noticeable. The individual carcinoma cells are highly pleomorphic. In some cases, as mentioned previously, regions of the tumor that lack lymphoid stroma are evident, and in other tumors, comedolike islands with central necrosis may be present. It is noteworthy that the neoplastic islands in lymphoepithelial carcinoma may show significant degrees of anaplasia from one nest to the next; some nests appear quite cytologically benign, whereas others are decidedly malignant.[27, 32]

Some of the reported cases occurring among whites manifest histopathologic features that vary from those documented among the Eskimo and Oriental groups. We believe that some of the

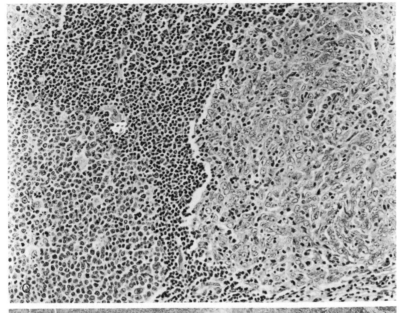

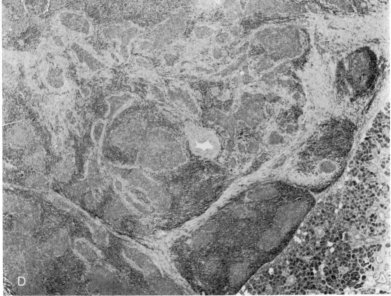

Figure 25–2 *Continued C,* Lymphoepithelial carcinoma demonstrates neoplastic epithelium with large vesicular nuclei and eosinophilic cytoplasm arranged in syncytial sheets; no ductal structures are evident (× 200). *D,* Lymphoepithelial carcinoma. Foci of fibrosis are commonly seen (× 40).

lesions in white patients are not truly lymphoepithelial carcinoma; however, it is difficult to make diagnostic judgments of reported cases when glass slides of tissue from these cases are not available. Nevertheless, from the published data, it appears that a few cases may represent adenocarcinomas or differentiating squamous carcinomas that arose from a preexisting BLEL, since the carcinoma cells in these cases showed some degree of adenoid or squamous cell differentiation.[39, 49]

Histochemical and Ultrastructural Findings

The histologic pattern of lymphoepithelial carcinoma is not unique to the salivary gland; a similar picture may be seen with nasopharyngeal carcinoma. In addition, carcinoma with lymphoid stroma has been reported in the esophagus, breast, stomach, and cervix.[50–53] In the esophagus, the epithelium appears to be squamous; however, cells testing positively for S-100 protein are present and are associated with a better prognosis for the patient.[52] Salivary duct cells may also test positively for S-100 protein, but the expression of this protein has not yet been reported in lymphoepithelial carcinoma of salivary gland origin. Cytokeratin reactivity has been demonstrated in this tumor, which indicates the presence of either an epithelial or myoepithelial phenotype. Cases from the AFIP series were evaluated for the presence of cytokeratin, S-100 protein, and muscle-specific actin using the peroxidase-antiperoxidase method, and all protein species were found to be present in the epithelial component of lymphoepithelial carcinoma.

Although an association of positive serologic testing for EBV has been found with some cases of lymphoepithelial carcinoma and has been firmly established with regard to nasopharyngeal carcinoma, the chapter authors' unpublished experience with in situ hybridization for EBV in four cases from the AFIP series is that at the limit of the technique's sensitivity, no viral genomes were detected. Such findings do not negate the presence of EBV in these tumors because single integrated copies of virus are not detectable with the in situ procedure. Southern blot or polymerase chain reaction technology detects a single copy of virus per cell, and investigations of this nature could be informative for this unique tumor.

Diagnostic electron microscopy has shown round nuclei with prominent nucleoli, marginated chromatin, and a paucity of cytoplasmic organelles.[11, 37, 38] Basement membrane, adenomatous differentiation, and viral particles have not been identified. Sehested and coworkers[47] were able to demonstrate desmosomes in 18 of 19 cases and tonofilaments in 16 cases.

Differential Diagnosis

The differential diagnosis of lymphoepithelial carcinoma includes squamous carcinoma and high-grade mucoepidermoid carcinoma in which a significant degree of lymphoid infiltration is an accompaniment, poorly differentiated large cell carcinoma of salivary origin, and nasopharyngeal carcinoma with parotid extension or metastasis to lymph nodes of the parotid region. The background lymphoid infiltrate and the typical architecture simulating BLEL should help eliminate the first three lesions from consideration; also, a lack of any adenomatous features, particularly mucus-secreting cells, should remove any likelihood of mucoepidermoid carcinoma. In the absence of the typical lymphoepithelial pattern, it is paramount to consider nasopharyngeal carcinoma. In such instances, the pathologist should consult with the clinician and recommend a thorough nasopharyngeal examination. Anaplastic epithelioid and spindled cell tumors without the typical lymphoid background and lymphoepithelial pattern should be classified as undifferentiated large cell carcinomas rather than as lymphoepithelial carcinomas.

Another entity that should be mentioned in the context of differential diagnosis of lymphoepithelial carcinoma is papillary cystadenoma lymphomatosum that has undergone malignant transformation. Carcinoma arising in papillary cystadenoma lymphomatosum is extremely rare; however, it should not be confused with lymphoepithelial carcinoma. The characteristic morphology of Warthin's tumor is retained, and within the benign tumor mass, a focus of adenocarcinoma is present.[53, 54] We have also seen papillary carcinoma of the thyroid associated with a pronounced mononuclear cell stromal component that metastasized to the periparotid gland region and mimicked papillary cystadenoma lymphomatosum except for the absence of germinal centers and a uniform nuclear bilayer in the epithelium. These entities, although composed of both epithelial and lymphoid elements, are easily differentiated from lymphoepithelial carcinoma.

Behavior and Treatment

Attempts to collate all reported cases of lymphoepithelial carcinoma to assess behavior, natural history, and response to therapy are problematic because of the variety of ways in which follow-up data have been expressed. Late disease and large tumor masses were seen in many of the Arctic region patients. When case series are analyzed, it appears that regional metastases occur among 30 to 50 percent of the Eskimo patients; however, the incidence of regional spread among Oriental patients is far lower, occurring in less than 10 percent. Distant metastases are also more prevalent among Eskimos than among Orientals. Akin to regional lymph node metastasis, distant spread occurs among 30 to 40 percent of Eskimo patients, and such metastases are often widespread, involving visceral organs as well as bone.[10, 12, 29, 32–34] It is noteworthy that distant foci are characterized microscopically by sheets of undifferentiated carcinoma cells without a lymphoid component.[9, 32] Both Krishnamurthy and coworkers[27] and Povah and others[32] segregated their cases into low-grade and high-grade varieties based on histomorphologic and cytologic features of malignancy (i.e., mitotic activity and cellular pleomorphism). Patients with low-grade tumors fared extremely well, with almost all being alive and well without distant spread. Patients with high-grade tumors had a very dire prognosis, with local recurrence and regional as well as distant metastatic disease developing in most patients. Indeed, local recurrence proved to be a major problem in almost all of the high-grade tumors, and most patients died within 2 years of diagnosis.

Treatment for lymphoepithelial carcinoma has consisted of surgery alone or of surgery in combination with radiotherapy. Surgical therapy has varied from local excision to radical excision with node dissection, and in a significant number of those with massive tumors, complete excision was not possible. Combined radiation therapy has included fractionated dosage from 2000 to 6000 rad. For those patients with a high-grade tumor, the prognosis was poor, with death being inevitable regardless of the mode of therapy. None of the cases were treated by radiation therapy alone; therefore, at present, radioresponsiveness, as seen in nasopharyngeal carcinoma, cannot be assessed. At the least, these tumors should be treated by wide excision, preferably sialectomy, and in light of the moderately high rate of nodal spread, particularly in high-grade tumors, ipsilateral prophylactic neck dissection should be considered.

UNDIFFERENTIATED CARCINOMA, LARGE CELL TYPE

A review of the literature on large cell undifferentiated carcinomas arising from salivary tissue reveals a dearth of information, since most papers dealing with undifferentiated carcinomas include both large and small cell variants. Consequently, the large cell cases are not easily culled from the small cell types. Koss and coworkers[6] were the first to publish a series of cases that they referred to as small or "oat" cell carcinomas of salivary gland origin; Gnepp and others[8] later reviewed the literature and published a series of 12 small cell undifferentiated carcinomas from the AFIP files. Thus, the small cell variant has been recognized as a specific histopathologic entity, whereas no publications have examined the clinicopathologic features of only the large cell lesions. Recently Hui and coworkers[55] reported 12 cases of undifferentiated carcinomas and noted that 4 of the cases were of the large cell variety. Two of these patients died of disease. Donath and colleagues[5] indicated that seven of eleven undifferentiated salivary carcinomas were represented by epidermoid cells or undifferentiated appearing ductal cells, whereas the remaining four tumors consisted of a combination of poorly differentiated myoepithelial cells, epidermoid cells, and ductal cells. One of the cases reported by Yaku and coworkers[56] was classified as a large cell type of undifferentiated carcinoma, and on electron microscopic examination, the cells were found to contain secretory granules with features of ductal epithelium.

Blanck and others[1] pointed out that well-defined salivary tumor entities, such as adenoid cystic carcinoma, mixed tumors with adenocarcinomatous transformation, and high-grade adenocarcinomas that are not otherwise specified, harbor foci of highly anaplastic, undifferentiated epithelial cells. From a series of 1,678 parotid gland tumors (299 of which were classified as malignant), the authors identified 75 cases that they considered poorly differentiated. All of these tumors consisted of solid sheets of cells, and only 18 tumors exhibited any microscopic tendencies for differentiation. Twelve had an indication of adenomatous structures, and the remaining six tumors contained mucus-secreting cells. Although classified according to the degree of pleomorphism, these cases were not grouped according to cell size. Many of the cases illustrated in Blanck and coworkers'[1] article showed large and pleomorphic undifferentiated cell types growing in solid sheets. Nagao and coworkers[2] found 18 cases of undifferentiated carcinomas among 555 Japanese patients with parotid tumors, and they subclassified these lesions into small and large cell types. The latter constituted 33 percent of the total. The large cell type was more common among females (83 percent), with 67 percent occurring in the 30- to 49-year age group.

Because of a paucity of data (with the exception of Nagao and coworkers'[2] series), our analysis of data on undifferentiated large cell tumors is gleaned from the 23 cases on file at the AFIP. From the foregoing, it is evident that the microscopic criteria for the diagnosis of undifferentiated carcinoma with a large cell element are somewhat equivocal and that they vary from one group of authors to the next. Herein, we define undifferentiated large cell carcinoma as any tumor of salivary gland origin that exhibits a predominant poorly differentiated large cell component that occurs in islands or sheets, although minor foci within the tumor that exhibit some degree of adenoid or squamoid tendencies for differentiation may be present.

Clinical Features

From a total of 23 patients in the AFIP series, there were 15 males (68.2 percent) and 8 females (34.8 percent). Race was specified in 11 cases, and all were white. These patients ranged in age from 21 to 86 years with a mean age of 62.7 years. No significant difference in mean age was found according to sex. There was a bimodal age distribution, with 56 percent of the patients in the 6th to 7th decades of life and 26 percent in the 9th decade of life (Fig. 25–1). Thus, the undifferentiated large cell lesions affect an older population.

Fifteen of the twenty-three tumors arose in the parotid gland (65 percent), and three arose in the submandibular gland (13 percent). The remaining six arose in accessory salivary glands (22 percent), including one each in the palate, soft palate, oral floor, pharynx, and tongue.

Gross and Microscopic Pathology

Most of the large cell lesions lack encapsulation and are represented by grayish white infiltrative solid masses that are frequently found to extend into adjacent fascial and muscular tissues. Fixation to skin is commonly encountered, as is invasion of craniomaxillary osseous tissue and associated foramina. In tissue sections, the tumors are solid, cystic, and necrotic; hemorrhagic foci are unusual.

As stated by Thackray and Lucas,[57] undifferentiated carcinoma is a malignant tumor of epithelial structure that is too poorly differentiated to be placed in any of the other groups of carcinomas. Tubules, ductules, acinar structures, and keratin are not seen; however, if the malignancy arises out of preexisting mixed tumor, adenoid cystic carcinoma, squamous cell carcinoma, or adenocarcinoma, morphologic remnants may be admixed. As stated at the onset, other authors contend that undifferentiated carcinomas may have minor foci of differentiation within them; however, the primary tumor element is poorly differentiated or undifferentiated.[1, 5]

Among the AFIP cases, the tumor cells are usually polygonal or spindled, and they infiltrate in sheets or as thin trabeculae or cords separated by fibrovascular stroma. It has been speculated that the large polygonal cells that make up these tumors are of ductal origin, whereas the spindle cells may be derived from myoepithelial precursors.[1, 5, 57] Nevertheless, cell phenotype should not be viewed as an indicator of histogenesis. Zonal necrosis and hemorrhage may be evident, along with a high mitotic rate.

Although this chapter divides the undifferentiated tumors into large and small cell variants, we have seen some tumors that harbor mixtures of large vesicular cells and small hyperchromatic round cells that are arranged in a lobular pattern with trabecular infiltration (Fig. 25–3A, B, C). Occasional foci with ductal differentiation may be observed. Any attempt to identify distinct patterns of specific tumor types is complicated by their association with other neoplasms from which they may arise. When focal areas within the tumor show differentiated features or, indeed, show the histomorphology of well-recognized salivary tumor types, one may speculate that the poorly differentiated element arose from a preexisting adenoma or adenocarcinoma. Alternatively, it may be that both patterns evolved simultaneously. Although all cases in the AFIP series involved undifferentiated tumors, five cases showed some evidence of ductal differentiation, one case exhibited foci of both ductal and squamous differentiation, one harbored a spindle cell element, and another contained occasional mucus-secreting cells. Of significant interest is the fact that the undifferentiated large cell component coexisted with other well-recognized salivary gland tumor entities in five cases. Two of these cases showed foci reminiscent of adenoid cystic carcinoma. A third exhibited acinic cell-like areas, and in another, regions that simulated epithelial-myoepithelial carcinoma were apparent. The fifth case showed clear evidence of mixed tumor and should be classified as undifferentiated carcinoma ex pleomorphic adenoma. Another case of undifferentiated carcinoma was accompanied by a contralateral papillary cystadenoma lymphomatosum. Seven cases involved large cell undifferentiated tumors with no evidence of glandular, squamoid,

or myoepithelial origin, and they were not associated with any other type of salivary tumor.

From the foregoing, it should be obvious that the majority of undifferentiated carcinomas do indeed harbor foci with some degree of differentiation, and some are associated with microscopic fields typical of well-recognized salivary tumor entities. Although the premise is teleologically probable, it is difficult to prove that these defined entities preceded the anaplastic changes.

Histochemical and Ultrastructural Findings

Some of the small cell carcinomas may show ultrastructural evidence of neuroendocrine differentiation.[8] Recently, Hui and coworkers[55] evaluated a series of both small and large cell undifferentiated salivary tumors; immunohistochemical and ultrastructural analyses disclosed that the tumors showed evidence of neuroendocrine, ductal, acinar, epidermoid, or no distinguishing features. Nagao and colleagues[2] identified both desmosomes and tonofilaments, with no evidence of neurosecretory granules in the large cell variant of undifferentiated carcinoma, whereas Hui and coworkers[55] identified such granules in one large cell tumor.

Behavior and Natural History

Very few data are available concerning the behavior of these rare tumors. No follow-up data on the AFIP series are available, and most of the series in the literature do not give adequate attention to the large cell tumors. Hui and colleagues,[55] in their evaluation of both large and small cell lesions, observed that 53 percent of their subjects had recurrences, regional node metastases developed in 53 percent, distant metastases developed in 63 percent, and 63 percent died because of tumor. The most significant harbinger of a poor prognosis was found to be tumor size. Patients with lesions smaller than 4 cm had a mean survival time of 46 months, with 50 percent dying because of disease. When the tumors exceeded 4 cm, the mean patient survival time was 7.7 months, and 100 percent died from disease. Other indicators of poor prognosis were invasion of nerves larger than 0.25 mm and lymph node and distant metastases.

Differential Diagnosis

The differential diagnosis should include nasopharyngeal carcinoma with extension or metastasis to the parotid region; amelanotic melanoma (Fig.

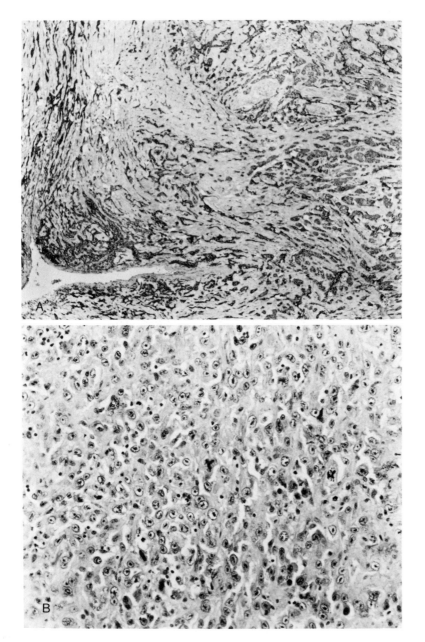

Figure 25–3. *A*, Salivary undifferentiated carcinoma, large cell type, showing infiltrative pattern (× 40). *B*, Large cell undifferentiated carcinoma with microscopic features akin to those of nasopharyngeal carcinoma (× 200).

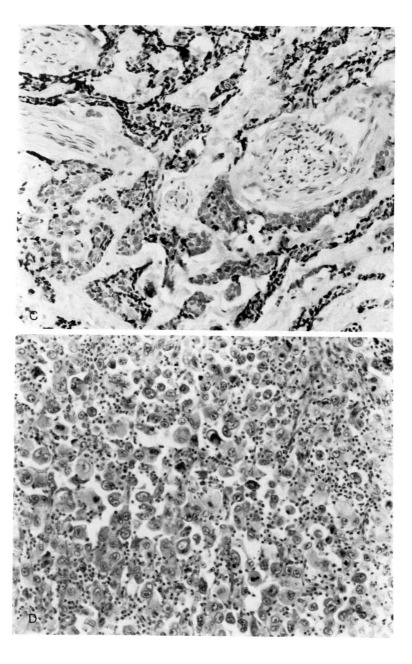

Figure 25–3 *Continued C,* Salivary undifferentiated carcinoma with large cells mixed with small hyperchromatic cells (× 100). *D,* Amelanotic melanoma, as depicted here, may show similar cytologic features, but the cells tend to have larger and more pleomorphic nuclei with prominent eosinophilic nucleoli (× 200).

25–3*D*); non-Hodgkin's lymphoma; lymphoepithelial carcinoma (malignant lymphoepithelial lesion); olfactory neuroblastoma; and sarcomas, including rhabdomyosarcoma, synovial sarcoma, malignant epithelioid schwannoma, and malignant fibrous histiocytoma. A variety of metastatic large cell undifferentiated carcinomas must be ruled out as well.

It is singularly important to seek out a primary lesion outside the salivary gland prior to establishing a definitive diagnosis of a primary undifferentiated carcinoma of salivary origin. Clinical and imaging studies should focus on the nasopharynx, Waldeyer's ring, the larynx, and other sites outside the head and neck area. Immunohistochemical marker studies may be employed to exclude melanoma (e.g., S-100 protein, HMB45), lymphoma (LCA, Kappa, Lambda, UCHL-1, L26), and sarcoma (ruled out with a positive cytokeratin test, excluding synovial sarcoma). However, it is important to be aware of the S-100 and muscle-specific actin reactivity of normal myoepithelium as well as of certain ductal cells when interpreting immunohistochemical stains.

SMALL CELL CARCINOMA

One form of undifferentiated carcinoma that can be distinguished from others in this group on the basis of morphology and immunohistochemical studies is small cell carcinoma. Small cell carcinoma, a common pulmonary neoplasm, rarely arises in the region of the head and neck. The most common site of involvement in this region is the larynx,[58] but small cell carcinoma has also been reported to arise in the paranasal sinuses,[6] oral cavity,[6, 59–60] nose,[6] pharynx,[6, 16] and cervical esophagus.[62] Small cell carcinoma is a rare salivary gland tumor. Its exact incidence is difficult to ascertain.

Undifferentiated carcinomas account for 0.3 to 3.2 percent of salivary gland tumors in several large series,[2, 63–65] and 0.4 percent of the more than 15,000 tumors in the AFIP salivary gland registry. Several investigators have classified undifferentiated carcinoma on the basis of cell size, and they include all tumors with cells as large as or slightly larger than lymphocytes,[2] or with cells less than 30 μm in diameter,[55] under the designation of small cell carcinoma. Some of these latter tumors have prominent nucleoli[2] and therefore would not be included under the World Health Organization's definition of small cell carcinoma,[66] which we prefer to use. Twenty (36 percent) of the 56 undifferentiated carcinomas in the AFIP registry were classified as small cell carcinomas, an incidence of slightly over 0.1 percent. In our experience, salivary small cell carcinomas are extremely rare and account for less than 1 percent of major salivary gland tumors.[8] However, there may be a greater incidence of these tumors in the minor salivary glands, where they accounted for 2.8

percent of 492 minor salivary gland tumors in one report.[6] This increased incidence was not seen in a more recent series[67] of minor salivary gland tumors. Part of this higher incidence might be explained by the greater percentage of malignant tumors arising in minor salivary glands;[68] however, it also may be due to referral bias.

Clinical Features

Approximately 54 small cell carcinomas of the major salivary glands, including 12 of the 20 AFIP cases, have been previously described in the literature.[2, 5, 7, 8, 55, 56, 69–78] Patients with small cell carcinomas of the major glands present most commonly during the fifth to seventh decades of life (range 5 to 84 years of age) (Fig. 25–1). There appears to be a slight male predominance, with 1.6 times as many tumors occurring in men than in women.[8, 74] Just over 85 percent of the small cell carcinomas arise in the parotid gland, and the remainder involve the submandibular gland. Patients present with nontender to painful masses, many of which are rapidly growing, measuring up to 8 cm in greatest dimension.[7, 8] The masses are usually present for less than 3 months; however, occasional patients have had symptoms related to the tumor for periods of up to 1 year.[8]

Pathologic Findings

Tumor margins are usually poorly demarcated with infiltrating edges; a rare tumor may be well circumscribed. Tumor consistency has been described as firm to hard, whereas color varies, including gray, gray-white, pink-gray to yellow-white, tan, and yellow.[8]

Histologically, the tumors fulfill criteria outlined by the World Health Organization[66] for the "oat cell" and "intermediate cell" categories of small cell carcinoma. The tumors are composed of infiltrating large sheets, ribbons, cords, or nests of anaplastic round-to-oval cells with minimal cytoplasm and hyperchromatic nuclei containing finely dispersed chromatin and inconspicuous nucleoli (Fig. 25–4). Mitoses are frequent, and tumor necrosis is usually prominent. Vascular invasion, a common characteristic of small cell carcinomas at other sites, is only occasionally observed. Perineural invasion and rosette formation are occasionally found (Fig. 25–5*A*). Small foci of ductal differentiation have been observed in a few tumors (Fig. 25–5*B*), and in focal areas, tumors have appeared to arise from basilar ductal epithelium (see Fig. 25–5).[8] A hybrid tumor with both a well-developed ductal component and small cell component has been described (Fig. 25–6).[74, 79] Well-developed squamous areas have not been found in any of the tumors, although tiny foci suggestive of early squamous differentiation have been de-

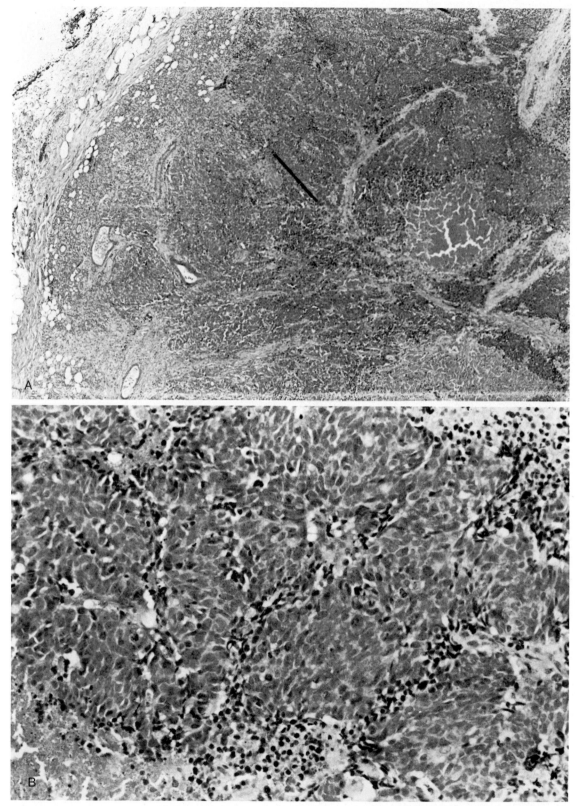

Figure 25–4. *A*, Small cell carcinoma infiltrates parotid gland (× 40). *B*, Higher magnification demonstrates a sheet of uniform round to oval hyperchromatic tumor cells with minimal cytoplasm and focal necrosis (× 100).

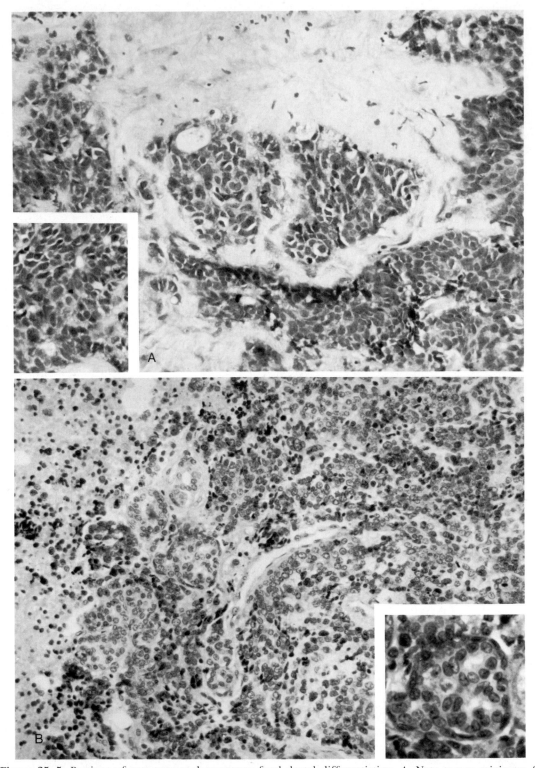

Figure 25–5. Portions of two tumors demonstrate focal ductal differentiation. *A,* Note tumor originates from basilar ductal epithelium (× 160). *Inset,* Detail of several rosettelike structures (× 160). *B,* A sheet of poorly differentiated tumor cells has an area of necrosis (left) and focal ductal differentiation (× 160). *Inset,* Detail of ductal differentiation (× 320). (With permission Gnepp DR, Corio RL, Brannon RB: Small cell carcinoma of the major salivary glands. Cancer 1986; 58:705–714.)

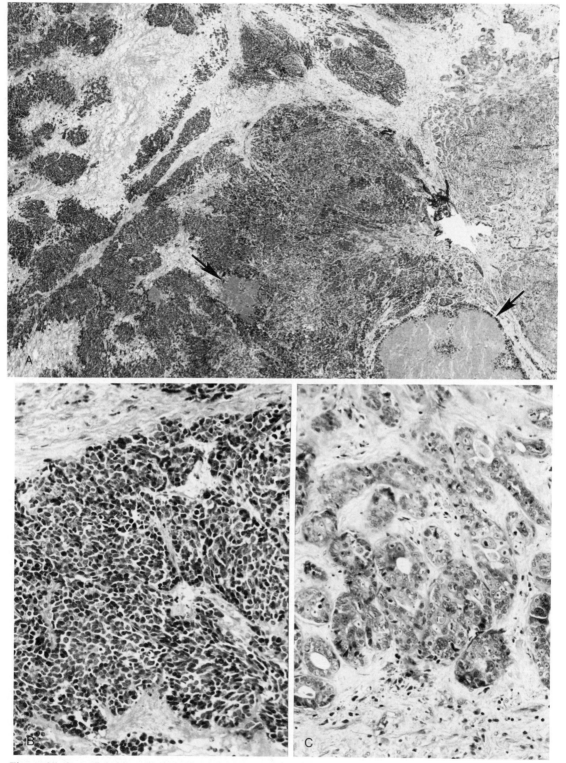

Figure 25–6. *A*, Hybrid small cell carcinoma has a small cell component (left and center) and a ductal component (right); prominent necrosis is indicated by arrow (× 40). *B*, Detail of small cell component shows uniform oval tumor cells, minimal cytoplasm, and hyperchromatic nuclei (× 200). *C*, Detail of ductal component shows ductal cells that are larger and more pleomorphic than the small cell component and have abundant cytoplasm with prominent nucleoli (× 200). (With permission Gnepp DR, Wick MR: Small cell carcinoma of the major salivary glands: An immunohistochemical study. Cancer 1990; 66:185–192.)

scribed.[7] Areas with crush artifact, typical of pulmonary small cell carcinoma, are also seen in many of the salivary gland tumors but usually to a lesser degree.

Histochemical and Ultrastructural Findings

Fifteen of thirty-two tumors (47 percent) studied ultrastructurally contained membrane-bound neuroendocrine granules with diameters in the range of 80 to 240 nm (Fig. 25–7).[2, 5, 7, 8, 55, 56, 69, 71, 72, 74–78] Ultrastructurally, sheets or cords of closely apposed, somewhat uniform, round to polygonal tumor cells have well to poorly developed junctional complexes, which include desmosomes. The plasma membranes are closely apposed with a few interlacing processes. The cytoplasm is scant and contains limited numbers of organelles, including scattered mitochondria, glycogen, microfilaments, and rough endoplasmic reticulum. Rare tonofilaments are also noted, almost always in cells without neuroendocrine granules. Neurosecretory gran-

ules, when present, are most commonly found in cytoplasmic processes. Occasional tumors have cell nests surrounded by well-defined basal lamina and, focally, myoepithelial-like cells, mimicking the normal intercalated duct.[72] Rarely, two cell populations are observed: one differentiated toward cells with myoepithelial characteristics and the other toward cells with epithelial characteristics.[77] Neuroendocrine granules have not been found in those tumors differentiated toward epithelial cells.

From the preceding, it appears that salivary gland small cell carcinoma contains two types of tumors: one type that has neuroendocrine characteristics (i.e., neurosecretory granules) and another that is more characteristic ultrastructurally of the intercalated duct.

A recent immunohistochemical study examined 11 primary salivary gland small cell carcinomas to determine whether the previously mentioned variants of small cell carcinoma were, in fact, similar and neuroendocrine in nature.[79] All cases were studied ultrastructurally, and four contained neurosecretory granules. The tumors were evaluated for the presence of cytokeratin, Leu-7, neuron-

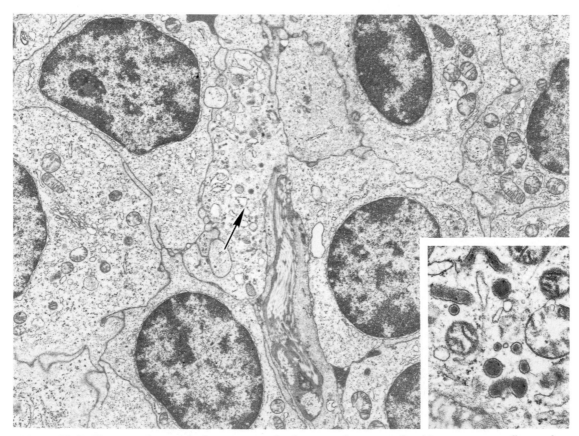

Figure 25–7. Electron micrograph demonstrates closely apposed tumor cells with sparse organelles, and two electron dense neurosecretory granules are indicated by arrow (× 7,500). *Inset,* Detail of granules from an adjacent region (× 25,000). (With permission Gnepp DR, Corio RL, Brannon RB: Small cell carcinoma of the major salivary glands. Cancer 1986; 58:705–714.)

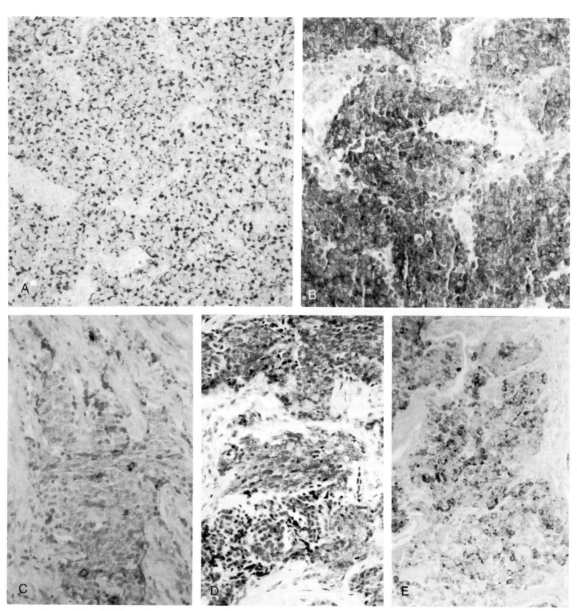

Figure 25–8. Immunoperoxidase stains for the following: *A,* cytokeratin with paranuclear staining typical of neuroendocrine tumors; *B,* neuron-specific enolase with diffuse cytoplasmic positivity; *C,* Leu-7 with focal positive staining of cytoplasm; *D,* synaptophysin with diffuse positive staining; and *E,* chromogranin with positive cytoplasmic and paranuclear staining in the majority of tumor cells (× 160). (With permission Gnepp DR, Wick MR: Small cell carcinoma of the major salivary glands: An immunohistochemical study. Cancer 1990; 66:185–192.)

thelioma-like carcinomas for Epstein-Barr viral genomes by in situ hybridization. Am J Surg Pathol 1989; 13:625–631.

49. Delaney WE Balogh K: Carcinoma of the parotid gland associated with benign lymphoepithelial lesion (Mikulicz's disease) in Sjögren's syndrome. Cancer 1966; 19:853–860.

50. Watanabe H, Enjoji M, Imai T: Gastric carcinoma with lymphoid stroma: Its morphologic characteristics and prognostic correlations. Cancer 1976; 38:232–243.

51. Hasumi K, Sakamoto G, Sugano H, et al: Medullary carcinoma with marked lymphoid infiltration of the uterine cervix. Jpn J Cancer Clin 1974; 20:207–210.

52. Mori M, Matsuda H, Kuwano H, Matsuura H, Sugimachi K: Oesophageal squamous cell carcinoma with lymphoid stroma. A case report. Virchows Arch [A] 1989; 415:473–479.

53. Ruebner B, Bramhall JL: Malignant papillary cystadenoma lymphomatosum: Report of case with brief review of literature. Arch Pathol 1960; 69:110–117.

54. Seifert G, Heckmayr M, Donath K: Carcinome in Papillaren Cystadenolymphomen der Parotis. Definition und Differentialdiagnose. Z Krebsforsch 1977; 90:25–36.

55. Hui KK, Luna MA, Batsakis JG, Ordonez NG, Weber R: Undifferentiated carcinomas of the major salivary glands. Oral Surg Oral Med Oral Pathol 1990; 69:76–83.

56. Yaku Y, Kanda T, Yoshihara T, Kanekot T, Nagao K: Undifferentiated carcinoma of the parotid gland. Case report with electron microscopic findings. Virchows Arch [A] 1983; 401:89–97.

57. Thackray AC, Lucas RB: Tumors of the Major Salivary Glands, Fascicle 10, 2nd series. Atlas of Tumor Pathology. Washington DC, Armed Forces Institute of Pathology, 1974.

58. Gnepp DR, Ferlito A, Hyams V: Primary anaplastic small cell (oat cell) carcinoma of the larynx: Review of the literature and report of 18 cases. Cancer 1983; 51:1731–1745.

59. Hull MT, Eble JN, Warfel KA: Extrapulmonary oat-cell carcinoma of the tongue: An electron-microscopic study. J Oral Pathol 1984; 13:489–496.

60. Hayashi Y, Nagamine S, Yanagawa T, Yoshida H, Yura Y, Azuma M, Sato M: Small cell undifferentiated carcinoma of the minor salivary gland containing exocrine, neuroendocrine, and squamous cells. Cancer 1987; 60:1583–1588.

61. Heimann R, Dehou MF, Lentrebec QB, Faverly D, Simonet ML, Dor P, Chanoine F: Anaplastic small cell (oat cell) carcinoma of the tonsils: Report of two cases. Histopathology 1989; 14:67–74.

62. Ibrahim NBN, Briggs JC, Corbishley CM: Extrapulmonary oat cell carcinoma. Cancer 1984; 54:1645–1661.

63. Eneroth CM: Histological and clinical aspects of

parotid tumors. Acta Otolaryngol (Stockh) (Suppl) 1964; 191:1–99.

64. Sharkey FE: Systematic evaluation of the World Health Organization classification of salivary gland tumors: A clinicopathologic study of 366 cases. Am J Clin Pathol 1977; 67:272–278.

65. Woods JE, Chong GC, Beahr OH: Experience with 1360 primary parotid tumors. Am J Surg 1975; 130:460–462.

66. The World Health Organization histological typing of lung tumours. 2nd ed. Am J Clin Pathol 1982; 77:123–136.

67. Waldron CA, El-Mofty SK, Gnepp DR: Tumors of the intraoral minor salivary glands: A demographic and histologic study of 426 cases. Oral Surg Oral Med Oral Pathol 1988; 66:323–333.

68. Batsakis JG: Tumors of the Head and Neck: Clinical and Pathological Considerations, 2nd Ed. Baltimore, Williams & Wilkins, 1979; 77.

69. Dardick I: Diagnostic electron microscopy. In Gnepp DR (ed.): Pathology of the Head and Neck. New York, Churchill Livingstone, 1988; 101–190.

70. Dubois PJ, Orr DP, Meyers EN, Barnes LE: Undifferentiated parotid carcinoma with osteoblastic metastases. Am J Roentgenol 1977; 129:744–746.

71. Huntrakoon M: Neuroendocrine carcinoma of the parotid gland: A report of two cases with ultrastructural and immunohistochemical studies. Hum Pathol 1987; 18:1212–1217.

72. Kraemer BB, Mackay B, Batsakis JG: Small cell carcinomas of the parotid gland: A clinicopathologic study of three cases. Cancer 1983; 52:2115–2121.

73. Levenson RM Jr, Ihde DC, Matthews MJ, Cohen MH, Gazdar AF, Bunn PA, Minna JD: Small cell carcinoma presenting as an extrapulmonary neoplasm: Sites of origin and response to chemotherapy. J Natl Cancer Inst 1981; 67:607–612.

74. Patterson SD: Oat-cell carcinoma, primary in parotid gland. Ultrastruct Pathol 1985; 9:77–82.

75. Recant L, Lacy P: Clinicopathological conference: Cushing's syndrome associated with a parotid gland tumor. Am J Med 1963; 34:394–406.

76. Scher RL, Feldman PS, Levine PA: Small-cell carcinoma of the parotid gland with neuroendocrine features. Arch Otolaryngol Head Neck Surg 1988; 114:319–321.

77. Wirman JA, Battifora HA: Small cell undifferentiated carcinoma of salivary gland origin: An ultrastructural study. Cancer 1976; 37:1840–1848.

78. Mair S, Phillips JI, Cohen R: Small cell undifferentiated carcinoma of the parotid. Cytologic, histologic, immunohistochemical, and ultrastructural features of a neuroendocrine variant. Acta Cytol 1989; 33:164–168.

79. Gnepp DR, Wick MR: Small cell carcinoma of the major salivary glands: An immunohistochemical study. Cancer 1990; 66:185–192.

26

BASAL CELL ADENOCARCINOMA

Gary L. Ellis and Paul L. Auclair

It is well known that benign salivary gland neoplasms may have malignant counterparts or may undergo malignant transformations. Certainly, malignant transformation in mixed tumor is the most common type of transformation, and malignant mixed tumors make up a large percentage of malignant epithelial salivary gland neoplasms (see Chapter 20). However, malignant counterparts or transformations of other adenomas are relatively rare. Of these other malignant adenomas, the malignant oncocytoma (oncocytic carcinoma) has been reported most frequently.[1] Reports of malignant basaloid salivary gland tumors are extremely rare. However, for a number of years pathologists at the Armed Forces Institute of Pathology (AFIP) have recognized a group of epithelial salivary gland neoplasms with cytologic characteristics of basal cell adenomas but morphologic growth patterns indicative of malignancy. Follow-up of a number of these patients has indicated that, indeed, these tumors have malignant potential. These neoplasms have been designated basal cell adenocarcinomas.[2]

The terminology that has been employed by various authors for monomorphic adenomas in general and for the group of basaloid salivary adenomas specifically has often been confounding. Terms such as *basal cell adenoma, trabecular adenoma, tubular adenoma, canalicular adenoma,* and *monomorphic adenoma* have, at different times, been used synonymously and exclusively.[3, 4] We subscribe to the use of the term monomorphic adenoma for a heterogeneous group of benign salivary adenomas to be distinguished from mixed tumors. Within this heterogeneous group, the basal cell adenomas are a distinct morphologic variant (see Chapter 12). Kleinsasser and Klein[5] first used the term *basal cell adenoma* to describe encapsulated, slow-growing, purely epithelial neoplasms composed of what appeared to be basal

cells arranged in solid, trabecular, and tubular patterns. Later, Evans and Cruickshank[6] also used the classification *basal cell adenoma* for a group of "purely" epithelial salivary gland tumors with patterns that were in accordance with those of Kleinsasser and Klein.[5] More recently, the membranous type of basal cell adenoma has been described.[7–11]

Some authors have speculated that the basal cell adenoma may be the benign counterpart of the adenoid cystic carcinoma.[6, 12–16] Indeed, rare reports of adenoid cystic carcinoma associated with basal cell adenoma or adenocarcinoma have been made. Evans and Cruickshank[6] mentioned a hybrid basal cell adenoma and adenoid cystic carcinoma in which both basal cell and adenoid cystic elements were widely infiltrating. Bernacki and colleagues[12] described a parotid tumor in which the central portion was a basal cell adenoma that blended into peripheral areas of invasive adenoid cystic carcinoma. Simpson and coworkers[17] reported a congenital hybrid basal cell adenoma-adenoid cystic carcinoma in the parotid gland with local metastatasis. We also have had experience with similar tumors that demonstrated features of both basal cell adenoma or adenocarcinoma and adenoid cystic carcinoma. Whether the few reports of adenoid cystic carcinoma in association with basal cell adenoma indicate an interrelationship between these tumors is uncertain. A similar relationship has been proposed for polymorphous low-grade adenocarcinoma and adenoid cystic carcinoma.[18] In addition, we have occasionally observed other salivary gland tumors with a combination of tumor types, including adenoid cystic carcinoma with epithelial-myoepithelial carcinoma and acinic cell adenocarcinoma with undifferentiated carcinoma. Warthin's tumor (papillary cystadenoma lymphomatosum) occurs more often synchronously with another salivary gland tumor than any other tumor type and has been associated with many different types of tumors (see Chapters 9 and 11).

Reports of malignant, purely basaloid salivary gland tumors are also extremely rare. In their textbook, Evans and Cruickshank[6] mentioned the existence of a "malignant basal cell tumour" and illustrated several photomicrographs but did not provide any details. Using criteria of infiltrative growth, abundant mitotic figures, hyalinized supporting connective tissue, and necrosis, Klima and coworkers[19] reported a case of a "basal cell carcinoma" of the parotid gland. These investigators did not discuss the patient's prognosis or the biologic behavior of this tumor. Pingitore and Campani[20] described a man with both dermal and salivary gland eccrine cylindroma type neoplasms who died with lung metastases; however, the metastases were presumed to be from a scalp tumor that had invaded the skull and dura. At the American Society of Clinical Pathologists' Annual Anatomic Pathology Slide Seminar, in 1983, Batsakis and colleagues[21] presented a case in which a carcinoma arose in a membranous type basal cell adenoma. Their criteria for malignancy were significant cellular atypia, destructive infiltrative growth, and signs of ductal adenocarcinoma. Likewise, Chen[22] described a case in which carcinoma arose in a membranous type adenoma of the parotid gland. Recently, Murty and colleagues[23] reported a basal cell adenocarcinoma in the parotid gland of a 55-year-old woman. Despite the histopathologic features of malignancy in these tumors, follow-up evidence of malignant biologic behavior of the lesion, i.e., the ability to metastasize and kill patients, has been lacking in these reports. The recent report of Ellis and Wiscovitch[2] was the first to document a series of these malignant-appearing basaloid cell salivary gland neoplasms and to provide follow-up evidence of their malignant biologic potential.

CLINICAL FINDINGS

At present, we have accumulated 43 cases of basal cell adenocarcinoma within the files of the AFIP (Table 26–1). Although this amount is approximately 1 percent of all malignant epithelial salivary gland tumors in the registry, this figure is deceptively low. The pathologists at the AFIP have been distinguishing basal cell adenocarcinoma from other types of salivary gland neoplasms for only approximately 10 years. Only as we have accumulated experience have we become confident in establishing the diagnosis. Over the last 10 years, basal cell adenocarcinomas have composed about 2 percent of malignant epithelial salivary gland tumors. As yet, we have not confidently identified this tumor in minor salivary glands. Thirty-nine and four tumors occurred in the parotid gland and submandibular gland, re-

Table 26–1. Anatomic Distribution of 43 Patients with Basal Cell Adenocarcinoma from the AFIP Registry

Anatomic Site	Number of Cases	Percentage
Parotid gland	39	90.7
Submandibular gland	4	9.3
Total	43	100.0

spectively. Two tumors were stated by the clinicians to be present in the cheek or buccal mucosa, but no nontumor salivary gland tissue was present in the tissue specimens. It seems likely that these two tumors either grew adjacent to the parotid gland or arose in ectopic parotid tissue, which occurs frequently along the course of Stensen's duct. Therefore, basal cell adenocarcinomas have composed about 4.5 percent of all primary parotid carcinomas over this 10-year period.

No predilection for occurrence of basal cell adenocarcinoma in either men or women is apparent. We have not found this tumor in children; all of the patients have been adults who ranged in age from 27 to 92 years. Eighty percent of the patients are over 50 years, with the average age being 60 years (Fig. 26–1). Although the total number of cases is still relatively low, we have documented only one tumor in a black person.

Like most salivary gland tumors, swelling is the principal symptom, but pain or tenderness occasionally may be an associated complaint. The tumors have grown to sizes as great as 4 cm in diameter and, on average, are discovered in the parotid or submandibular gland when they are approximately 2 cm in diameter. Occasionally, the swelling has been described as rapid in onset, but this has not had any prognostic significance. The patients have reported being aware of their tumors before diagnosis for from several weeks to 7 years, but on average, it has been just over 1.5 years.

MICROSCOPIC FINDINGS

The cytologic features of individual cells and the general morphologic features of basal cell adenocarcinoma are markedly similar to those of basal cell adenoma. In fact, aside from those few cases with a mitotic index so high that a malignant diagnosis can be considered on the basis of this feature alone, it may be impossible to differentiate basal cell adenoma from basal cell adenocarcinoma on a cytomorphologic basis. The growth of the tumor in relation to the surrounding tissues is the key feature used to distinguish adenoma from carcinoma for basaloid salivary gland neoplasms. Sometimes, the surgeon fails to appreciate the

No. of patients

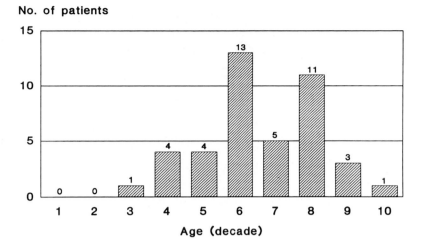

Figure 26–1. Age distribution of 42 patients with basal cell adenocarcinoma from the AFIP registry of salivary gland pathology.

difficult or irresolvable situation that is created for the pathologist when he or she judicously removes only salivary gland tumor tissue without some adjacent normal tissue.

Using low-magnification microscopy, basal cell adenocarcinomas have a uniform, monomorphic appearance that resembles basal cell epitheliomas or eccrine cylindromas of the skin (Fig. 26–2). This is not to say, however, that they are iso-

morphic in cytologic appearance. Just as in basal cell adenoma, two forms of epithelial cell are observed and are usually intermingled with one another (Fig. 26–3). Either cell form may predominate in one specific tumor or in an individual tumor nest. One form is a small, round cell, with scant cytoplasm and a dark basophilic nucleus. The other form is a larger polygonal-to-elongated cell with eosinophilic or amphophilic cytoplasm

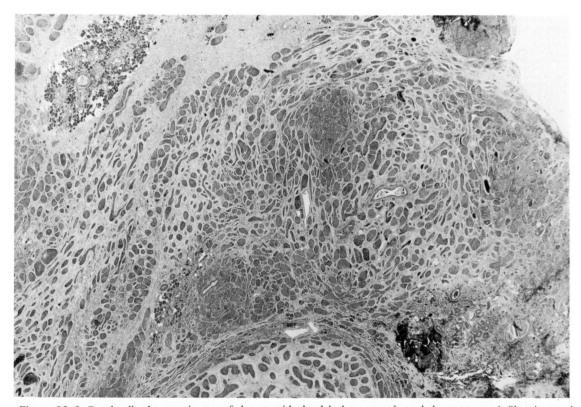

Figure 26–2. Basal cell adenocarcinoma of the parotid gland lacks a capsule and demonstrates infiltration and destruction of parotid parenchyma by tumor cells arranged in discrete islands (× 15).

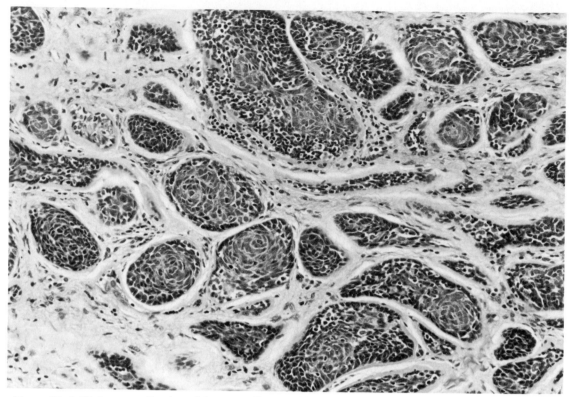

Figure 26–3. Higher magnification of the tumor illustrated in Figure 26–2 reveals that many of the tumor islands are composed of cells with two morphologic forms. Small cells with little cytoplasm and round dark nuclei are frequently located peripheral to larger cells with more cytoplasm and larger, paler nuclei. This morphologic character is very similar to that of basal cell carcinoma of the skin (× 150).

and a larger, pale, basophilic nucleus. In both types of cells, the cell-to-cell boundaries are indistinct. Frequently, the small dark cells are located peripherally to the larger pale cells and may produce palisading of the nuclei of the cells along the epithelial-stromal interface. This palisading of nuclei is usually less conspicuous than that seen in basal cell adenomas. The larger, pale cells sometimes appear to form swirls or eddies within the islands of tumor. These eddies have a squamoid appearance and occasionally keratinize in a process similar to keratinization of basal cell epitheliomas of the skin (Fig. 26–4). Some tumors demonstrate these squamous eddies more than others.

Small tubules or lumina can be seen in many of the epithelial islands and may be prominent in focal areas, suggesting a slight resemblance to eccrine spiradenoma (Fig. 26–5). Eosinophilic and periodic acid–Schiff (PAS)-positive hyaline material may be seen as coalescing, intercellular droplets and membranes that surround individual tumor islands (Fig. 26–6). This latter feature may produce a marked resemblance to dermal cylindromas, especially in those tumors categorized as the membranous type basal cell adenocarcinomas (see later). Ultrastructural examination shows that this hyaline material is a reduplicated basal lamina.

The amount of this hyalinized basal lamina varies from tumor to tumor but is most conspicuous in membranous basal cell adenocarcinomas.

Cytologic indices of malignancy are generally low or absent. Cellular and nuclear pleomorphism in most cases are not overtly remarkable. We have seen the mitotic figure count vary in these tumors from zero to nine per ten high-power (× 400) fields, but the average count is typically two or less. Tumor cell necrosis has been notable in only a small number of these tumors, and hemorrhage has occurred within a few lesions. To repeat, cytologic features are unreliable indicators of the malignant potential of these tumors.

In accordance with the histomorphologic patterns described for basal cell adenomas, basal cell adenocarcinomas can be divided into four subtypes: solid, trabecular, tubular, and membranous. Although one of these patterns is usually dominant in any specific tumor, transitions from one pattern to another occasionally occur. The solid type is characterized by contiguous tumor cells arranged in islands and masses within the fibrous connective tissue stroma. In some lesions these basaloid epithelial cells form numerous, small tumor islands that tend to be round to oval (Figs. 26–2 and 26–6). In other tumors of the solid type,

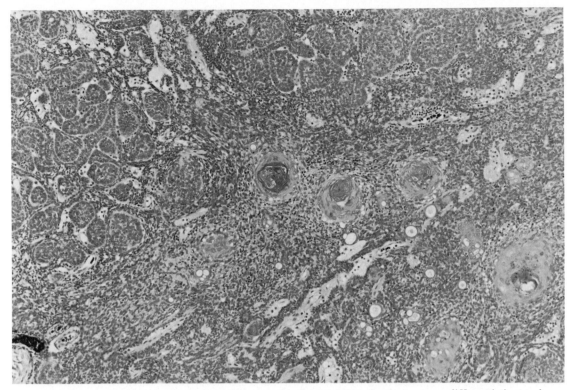

Figure 26–4. Basal cell adenocarcinoma of the parotid gland exhibits focal squamous differentiation and even some keratinization. Squamous differentiation is only an occasional finding, and many basal cell adenocarcinomas do not have these so-called squamous eddies (× 75).

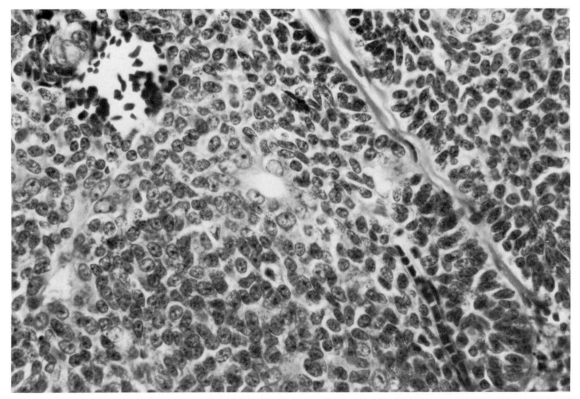

Figure 26–5. A small lumen or tubule is evident in this area of a basal cell adenocarcinoma. In a few cases, small ducts or tubules are a conspicuous feature (× 400).

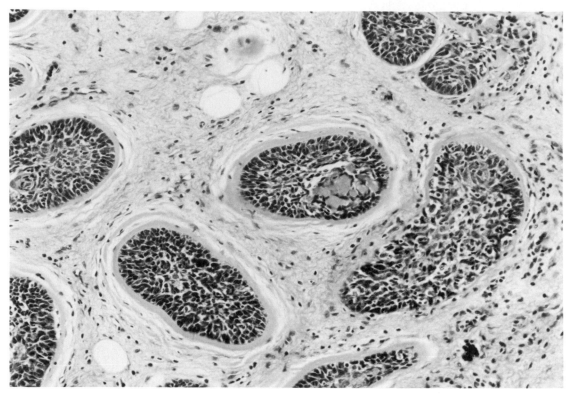

Figure 26–6. Eosinophilic hyaline material, probably representing basal laminae, can be seen as intercellular droplets and perinodular membranes in a parotid gland basal cell adenocarcinoma. This feature invokes a resemblance to dermal cylindromas (× 150).

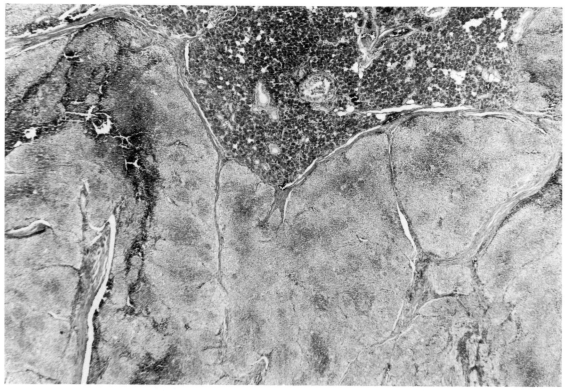

Figure 26–7. In contrast to the small tumor islands seen in Figure 26–2, the basaloid cells in this tumor are arranged in large nodules and broad sheets (× 25).

the epithelium forms large irregular masses (Fig. 26–7). Eosinophilic hyaline material is often present within these tumor nests, and some epithelial islands may have thin peripheral membranes (Fig. 26–3). However, the thick hyaline membranes characteristic of the membranous type basal cell adenocarcinoma are distinctly less evident. The membranous type is distinguished by thick eosinophilic, PAS-positive hyaline laminae that surround and separate one tumor nest from another and may create a jigsaw puzzle image in portions of the tumor (Fig. 26–8). Anastomosing cords and bands of basaloid epithelial cells characterize the trabecular type of basal cell adenocarcinoma (Fig. 26–9). These interconnecting cords may be likened to the configurations shaped like Chinese characters that are formed by bone trabeculae in fibrous dysplasia of bone. Conspicuous small lumina or pseudolumina characterize the tubular type of basal cell adenocarcinoma (Fig. 26–10). These lumina are not surrounded by intralobular or interlobular type ductal cells but by basal cells that blend indistinctly with adjacent basal cells that do not bound lumina. The lumina appear to resemble tiny cystic spaces more than true duct lumina. A solid morphologic pattern is predominant in about two thirds of the tumors. The membranous type is the second most frequent and

composes about 20 percent of these tumors. The trabecular and tubular types, in that order, are only occasionally the dominant patterns.

Salivary gland mucin, as demonstrated by mucicarminophilia, is absent or insignificant within all of these basal cell adenocarcinomas. Periodic acid–Schiff stain nicely highlights the basal lamina material in and around the tumor cell nests. Cellular glycogen content, as demonstrated by a decrease in the cellular reactivity to PAS after digestion of the tissue with diastase, is insignificant.

The distinctive diagnostic feature that separates these adenocarcinomas from typical benign basal cell adenomas is invasive growth. Basal cell adenomas in the major salivary glands are generally well circumscribed, encapsulated mononodular tumors that appear to grow by expansion, with compression and atrophy of the surrounding salivary gland parenchyma. The exceptions are some membranous type basal cell adenomas that may be multifocal or multinodular without distinct encapsulation. However, the invasive growth pattern of basal cell adenocarcinomas is distinct from a multifocal growth pattern. Nests and strands of tumor cells insinuate into the salivary gland lobules between the acini and/or into the adjacent structures, such as skeletal muscle, fat, and dermis (Figs. 26–11, 26–12). About one third of the

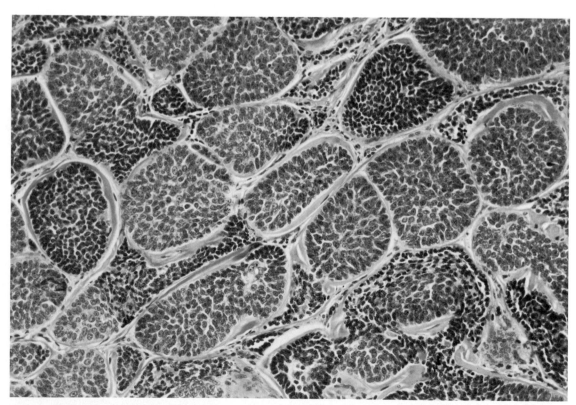

Figure 26–8. Prominent hyaline membranes surround closely apposed nests of basaloid cells and impart a "jigsaw puzzle" appearance to this so-called membranous type basal cell adenocarcinoma (× 160).

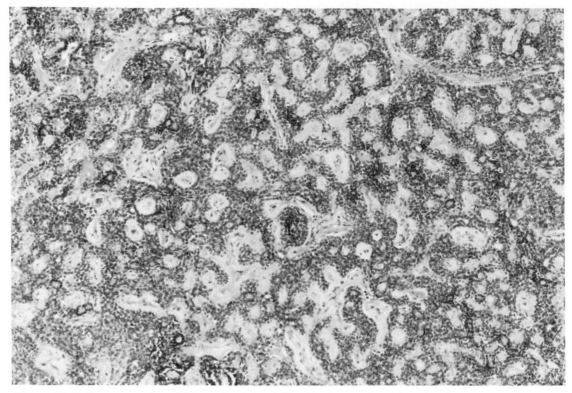

Figure 26–9. Interconnecting, thick cords of basaloid cells characterize this trabecular pattern of basal cell adenocarcinoma. The tumor cells are virtually identical to those seen in the discrete islands and sheets of cells in the solid pattern (× 75).

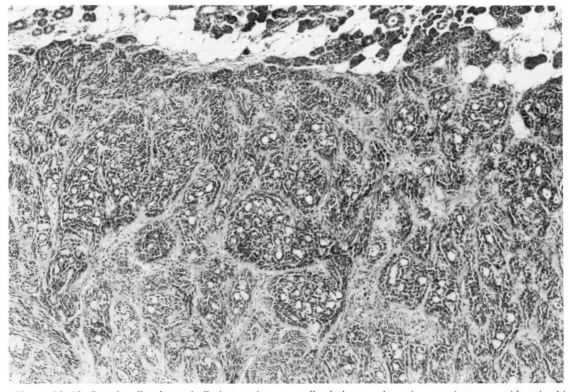

Figure 26–10. Occasionally, the typically inconspicuous small tubules may be quite prominent, as evident in this tubular pattern of basal cell adenocarcinoma (× 75).

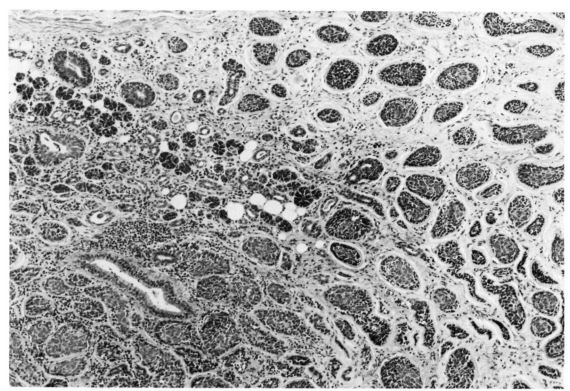

Figure 26–11. Islands of basaloid tumor cells infiltrate through a lobule of parotid gland parenchyma. A residual duct is present in the lower left, and residual serous acini are evident in the middle to upper left (× 75).

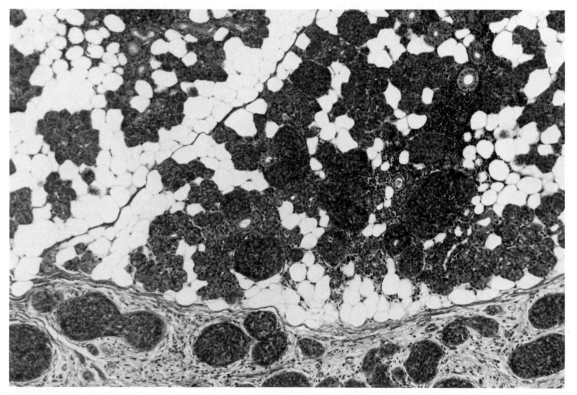

Figure 26–12. Although a distinct interface between tumor and parotid parenchyma extends across the bottom of the photomicrograph, islands of tumor cells that have infiltrated into the acinar lobules can be seen above the interface (× 75).

tumors we have examined have displayed perineural growth (Fig. 26–13), and nearly one fourth have exhibited intravascular invasion (Fig. 26–14). Although the majority of basal cell adenocarcinomas are the solid type, this type seems to have a disproportionate propensity for perineural and intravascular growth.

The amount of supporting collagenous stroma can vary from inconspicuous to extensive. This is not an encapsulating stroma but a supporting stroma that proliferates concomitantly with the infiltrating epithelial tumor. In particular, those solid type tumors that are composed of numerous small tumor nests can have a substantial amount of collagenous stroma. We have also found that more than half of the basal cell adenocarcinomas have an associated inflammatory cell infiltrate. This is nearly always a lymphocytic infiltrate and can be mild to moderately intense. At this time, we have found no prognostic significance attached to the presence, absence, or degree of this infiltrate.

Similar to the diathesis of dermal cylindromas and membranous basal cell adenomas that has been reported,[7–9] we are aware that at least three patients with basal cell adenocarcinomas also had dermal cylindromas of the scalp. Two of these patients had solid type basal cell adenocarcinomas, and one patient had a membranous type basal cell adenocarcinoma.

Currently, little information is available on the ultrastructural and immunohistochemical features of these tumors. Dardick (personal communication) has performed some limited electron microscopic study, which reveals irregular nuclear profiles; a few cytoplasmic mitochondria; and limited endoplasmic reticulum, intercellular junctions, and basal lamina formation (Fig. 26–15).

BEHAVIOR AND TREATMENT

Follow-up information has been obtained on 25 cases of basal cell adenocarcinoma in the AFIP files.[2] Because most basal cell adenocarcinomas in our files have been diagnosed within the last 10 years, the follow-up period was on average only 4.5 years, although it extended to just over 10 years for some patients. Recurrence is not necessarily an indicator of malignancy; however, recurrence after therapy is a common feature of malignant tumors. Among the 25 patients, 7 experienced at least one incidence of tumor recurrence. More significantly, three patients had tumors that metastasized to cervical lymph nodes, and one of these patients also had a metastasis to the lung. One patient died from local spread of tumor. Interestingly, the patient with pulmonary metastasis was free of disease 6 years after his pneumonectomy and 7 years after his parotidectomy. On the basis of this limited follow-up data, it is clear that these neoplasms do have a malignant potential to metastasize and kill patients. However, at present, we believe these to be low-grade adenocarcinomas, with a relatively good prognosis. Therapy should be comparable to that given for other low-grade salivary gland carcinomas, such as acinic cell adenocarcinoma and low-grade mucoepidermoid carcinoma. Surgical excision with a wide enough margin to ensure complete removal of the tumor is the primary treatment. Regional lymph node dissection is recommended only if there is evidence of metastatic disease. For parotid tumors, this would mean partial or complete parotidectomy, and for submandibular gland tumors, complete glandectomy is required.

At this time, we have not found any prognostic significance in the duration of the tumor, size of the tumor, or symptoms. In fact, on average, those patients with tumors that either recurred or metastasized were younger than the other patients in the study, and their tumors were smaller than the other tumors reported on. The parotid gland has been the primary site for those tumors that recurred or metastasized. A solid growth pattern has been evident in all but two recurrent tumors. Paradoxically, none of the tumors that recurred or metastasized manifested vascular invasion. No specific histopathologic parameters have been found to be predictors of biologic behavior, although the mean mitotic index has been slightly higher in the recurrent and metastatic tumor cases. However, there has been great variability in the mitotic rate from tumor to tumor.

We have not been able to confidently document the transformation of a benign basal cell adenoma into basal cell adenocarcinoma, such as occurs in the evolution of mixed tumor to carcinoma ex mixed tumor. We suspect that most basal cell adenocarcinomas arise de novo. This concept is supported by the fact that the average age of occurrence is similar for basal cell adenoma and basal cell adenocarcinoma, unlike carcinoma ex mixed tumor, for which the mean age of occurrence is about 10 years older than that of benign mixed tumor.

Only tumors with a solid growth pattern are known to have metastasized, and whether all of the tumor patterns, trabecular, tubular, and membranous, have true malignant potential remains to be determined by further reports and by long-term follow-up studies.

DIFFERENTIAL DIAGNOSIS

Indicative of the diagnostic dilemma created by the bland cytologic features and the infiltrative growth of these tumors is the observation that about one half of the pathologists who contributed these cases to the AFIP designated their cases as carcinomas, whereas the other half classified them

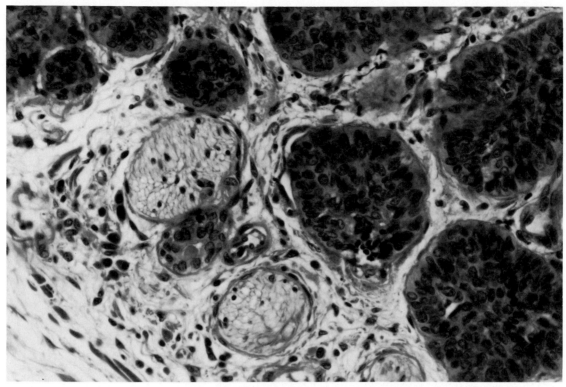

Figure 26–13. Small nests of basaloid tumor cells extend around and between branches of the facial nerve (× 300).

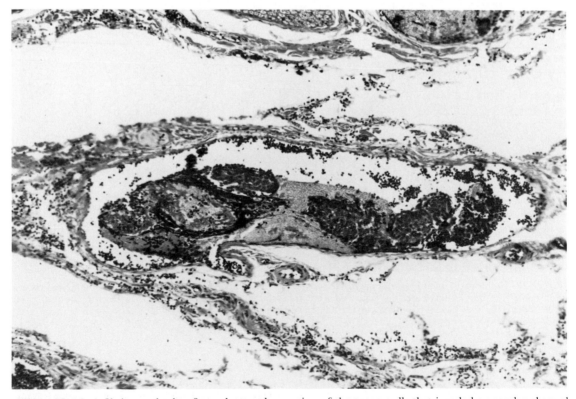

Figure 26–14. A fibrinous clot has formed around a portion of the tumor cells that invaded a vascular channel. This tumor embolus was associated with the large, solid, basal cell adenocarcinoma seen in Figure 26–7 (× 100).

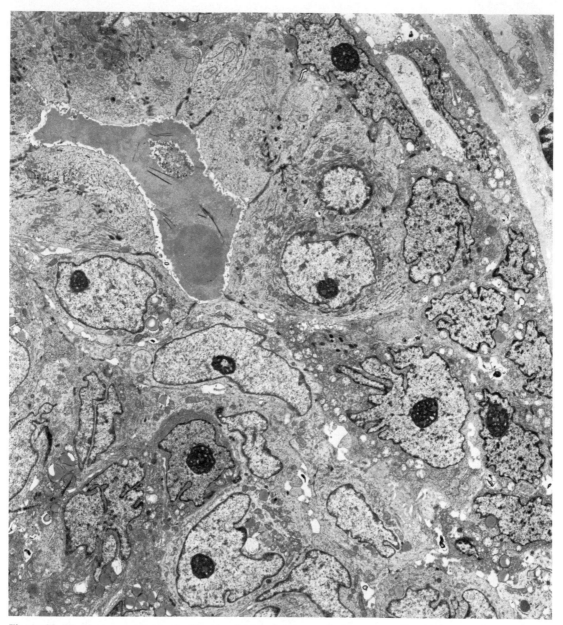

Figure 26–15. Electron micrograph of basal cell adenocarcinoma demonstrates cells with limited mitochondria and endoplasmic reticulum, intercellular junctions, and irregular nuclear outlines. A lumen is evident in the upper left, and the bordering cells have a few microvilli (× 3,700). (Courtesy of Irving Dardick, University of Toronto.)

as adenomas. Of course, basal cell adenoma is the principal consideration in the differential diagnosis, but adenoid cystic carcinoma and polymorphous low-grade adenocarcinoma may also be considered.

As we have already stated, the fundamental distinction between basal cell adenoma and basal cell adenocarcinoma is the invasive growth demonstrated by basal cell adenocarcinoma. Cytologic features alone are usually inadequate for differentiating benign from malignant basaloid tumors. When evident, a mitotic count greater than four or five per ten high-power fields is indicative of malignancy. The membranous basal cell adenoma may be the most difficult to differentiate from basal cell adenocarcinoma because of its lack of encapsulation and its multifocal pattern. However, intravascular and perineural invasion and penetrating growth into acinar lobules denote malignancy.

Adenoid cystic carcinoma, especially so-called solid or basaloid types, can be confused with basal cell adenocarcinoma, and we suspect that some basal cell adenocarcinomas have been diagnosed as adenoid cystic carcinoma. The cribriform pattern, which is seen commonly in adenoid cystic carcinoma, is distinctive and not found in basal cell adenocarcinoma. The amorphous, pale basophilic material located in the pseudocysts of adenoid cystic carcinoma is not encountered in basal cell adenocarcinoma. Despite the fact that both ductal and myoepithelial cells are cellular components of adenoid cystic carcinoma, the cytologic features are more uniform in adenoid cystic carcinoma than basal cell adenocarcinoma. The intermingling of small dark and large pale cells is not typical of adenoid cystic carcinoma. In addition, the nuclei in adenoid cystic carcinoma tend to be more hyperchromatic and angular than the round and ovoid nuclei of basal cell adenocarcinoma. The cytoplasm of the tumor cells in adenoid cystic carcinoma often tends to be very pale or even clear with standard hematoxylin and eosin staining, which causes the nuclei to stand out against this poorly staining cytoplasmic background. Both adenoid cystic carcinoma and basal cell adenocarcinoma may produce an eosinophilic, hyalinized basal lamina. However, this basal lamina material is not usually found in intercellular droplets in adenoid cystic carcinoma as it may be in basal cell adenocarcinoma. Of course, perineural invasion may be seen in both tumors.

Bland cytologic features, infiltrative growth, and low-grade malignant behavior are common to both basal cell adenocarcinoma and polymorphous low-grade adenocarcinoma. Thus far, we have not diagnosed polymorphous low-grade adenocarcinoma in the parotid or submandibular glands or basal cell adenocarcinoma in the minor salivary glands. One might speculate that these are the same neoplasms manifesting in different sites. However, basal cell adenocarcinoma does not manifest the plethora of morphologic patterns exhibited by polymorphous low-grade adenocarcinoma, both from tumor to tumor and within the same tumor (see Chapter 23). In particular, the single-file formations, cystic structures, and swirling tumor formations frequently seen in polymorphous low-grade adenocarcinoma are not observed in basal cell adenocarcinoma.

REFERENCES

1. Goode RK, Corio RL: Oncocytic adenocarcinoma of salivary glands. Oral Surg Oral Med Oral Pathol 1988; 65:61–66.
2. Ellis GL, Wiscovitch JG: Basal cell adenocarcinomas of the major salivary glands. Oral Surg Oral Med Oral Pathol 1990; 69:461–469.
3. Crumpler C, Scharfenberg JC, Reed RJ: Monomorphic adenomas of salivary glands: Trabecular-tubular, canalicular, and basaloid variants. Cancer 1976; 38:193–200.
4. Nagao K, Matsuzaki O, Saiga H, Suyano, I, Shigematsu H, Kaneko T, Katoh T, Kitamura T: Histopathologic studies of basal cell adenoma of the parotid gland. Cancer 1982; 50:736–745.
5. Kleinsasser O, Klein HJ. Basalzelladenome der Speicheldrüsen. Arch Klin Exp Ohr Nas Kehlkopf heilk 1967; 189:302–316.
6. Evans RW, Cruickshank AH: Epithelial Tumours of the Salivary Glands. Philadelphia, WB Saunders Co, 1970; 58–76.
7. Headington JT, Batsakis JG, Beals TF, Campbell TE, Simmons JL, Stone WD: Membranous basal cell adenoma of parotid gland, dermal cylindromas, and trichoepitheliomas: Comparative histochemistry and ultrastructure. Cancer 1977; 39:2460–2469.
8. Reingold I, Keasbey LE, Graham JH: Multicentric dermal-type cylindromas of the parotid glands in a patient with florid turban tumor. Cancer 1977; 40;1702–1710.
9. Batsakis JG, Brannon RB: Dermal analogue tumors of major salivary glands. J Laryngol Otol 1981; 95:155–164.
10. Ferrandiz C, Campo E, Baumann E: Dermal cylindromas (turban tumour) and eccrine spiradenomas in a patient with membranous basal cell adenoma of the parotid gland. J Cutan Pathol 1985; 12:72–79.
11. Herbst EV, Utz W: Multifocal dermal-type basal cell adenomas of parotid glands with co-existing dermal cylindromas. Virchows Arch [A] 1984; 403:95–102.
12. Bernacki EG, Batsakis JG, Johns ME: Basal cell adenoma: Distinctive tumor of salivary glands. Arch Otolaryngol 1974; 99:84–87.
13. Thawley SE, Ward SP, Ogura JH: Basal cell adenoma of the salivary glands. Laryngoscope 1974; 84:1756–1766.
14. Luna VA, MacKay B: Basal cell adenoma of the parotid gland: Case report with ultrastructural observations. Cancer 1976; 37:1615–1621.
15. Gyorkey F, Min KW, Sirbasku D, Gyorkey P: Ultrastructure of basal cell adenoma of the parotid gland (abst). Lab Invest 1975; 32:448.

16. Jao W, Keh PC, Swerdlow MA: Ultrastructure of the basal cell adenoma of parotid gland. Cancer 1976; 37:1322–1333.

17. Simpson PR, Rutledge JC, Schaefer SD, Anderson RC: Congenital hybrid basal cell adenoma-adenoid cystic carcinoma of the salivary gland. Pediatr Pathol 1986; 6:199–208.

18. Aberle AM, Abrams AM, Bowe R, Melrose RJ, Handlers JP: Lobular (polymorphous low-grade) carcinoma of minor salivary glands: A clinicopathologic study of twenty cases. Oral Surg Oral Med Oral Pathol 1985; 60:387–395.

19. Klima M, Wolfe SK, Johnson PE: Basal cell tumors of the parotid gland. Arch Otolaryngol 1978; 104:111–116.

20. Pingitore R, Campani D: Salivary gland involvement in a case of dermal eccrine cylindroma of the scalp (turban tumor): Report of a case with lung metastases. Tumori 1984; 70:385–388.

21. Batsakis JG, Hyams VJ, Morales AR: Proceedings of the Forty-eighth Annual Anatomic Pathology Slide Seminar of the American Society of Clinical Pathologists: Special Tumors of the Head and Neck. Chicago, American Society of Clinical Pathologists, 1983; 49–54.

22. Chen KTK: Carcinoma arising in monomorphic adenoma of the salivary gland. Am J Otolaryngol 1985; 6:39–41.

23. Murty GE, Welch AR, Soames JV: Basal cell adenocarcinoma of the parotid gland. J Laryngol Otol 1990; 104:150–151.

27

OTHER MALIGNANT EPITHELIAL NEOPLASMS

Gary L. Ellis, Paul L. Auclair, Douglas R. Gnepp, and Robert K. Goode

This chapter describes other types of malignant epithelial tumors that have not already been discussed. The lesions to be considered include adenosquamous carcinoma; oncocytic carcinoma; cystadenocarcinoma; malignant sebaceous neoplasms, including sebaceous carcinoma and sebaceous lymphadenocarcinoma; salivary duct carcinoma; mucinous adenocarcinoma; and myoepithelial carcinoma.

ADENOSQUAMOUS CARCINOMA

Adenosquamous carcinoma of the salivary gland is a controversial neoplasm that is not included in many classifications of salivary gland tumors.[1-4] Evans and Cruickshank[5] included a possibly analogous entity called *adenoacanthoma* within their classification of salivary gland carcinomas, but they provided no information about this tumor. Although adenosquamous carcinoma has been described in numerous epithelial tissues throughout the body, including the colon,[6] ileum,[7] skin,[8] lung,[9] gallbladder,[10] ovary,[11] liver,[12] prostate,[13] stomach,[14] kidney,[15] endometrium,[16] urethra,[17] fallopian tube,[18] pancreas,[19] thyroid gland,[20] larynx,[21] and nasal cavity,[22] it has rarely been reported in the oral cavity. Gerughty and colleagues[22] reported ten adenosquamous carcinomas of the nasal, oral, and laryngeal cavities that included five oral lesions. Siar and Ng[23] described an adenosquamous carcinoma of the floor of the mouth that occurred 8 years after radiation therapy for a squamous cell carcinoma in the same site. Sanner[24] reported a combined adenosquamous carcinoma and ductal adenoma of the hard and soft palates, but the adenosquamous carcinoma was described as aris-

ing in the maxillary sinus. The lack of appreciation for adenosquamous carcinoma may result from the combined factors of the rarity of this tumor in the oral cavity and the fact that some pathologists may conceptually consider it to be of surface mucosal epithelial origin rather than glandular origin. Although by our definition of this entity (see later) the mucosal surface epithelium is certainly involved in this neoplasm, glandular differentiation within the tumor justifies its discussion within this text and, at least, some consideration for its inclusion in the classification of salivary gland tumors.

Adenosquamous carcinoma is a malignant epithelial neoplasm that has histomorphologic features of both adenocarcinoma and squamous cell carcinoma. Without some further qualification, mucoepidermoid carcinoma could be considered to fall within the definition of adenosquamous carcinoma, since it has epidermoid and adenomatous differentiation. In fact, the demonstration of intracellular mucin was one of the criteria used by Gerughty and associates[22] for the diagnosis of adenosquamous carcinoma. Conversely, some might consider it appropriate to classify adenosquamous carcinoma as a high-grade mucoepidermoid carcinoma. We, however, believe that the histomorphologic features of adenosquamous carcinoma are different from those of mucoepidermoid carcinoma. In our interpretation of this lesion, a simultaneous carcinomatous change occurs in the mucosal surface epithelium and the ductal epithelium of the minor salivary gland excretory ducts that results in squamous cell carcinoma and adenocarcinoma, respectively. Since the report of Gerughty and colleagues,[22] 52 cases of oral adenosquamous carcinoma have been cataloged in the salivary gland registry at the Armed Forces Institute of Pathology (AFIP).

Clinical Features

The six cases reported by Gerughty and colleagues[22] and Siar and Ng[23] involved the tongue and the floor of the mouth. Similarly, in the AFIP experience, over 85 percent of the tumors have involved the tongue, floor of the mouth, and tonsillar-palatine region. The buccal mucosa, retromolar region, and lower lip are other sites of occurrence. In all of the cases reported in the literature, the patients are men. Although, among AFIP patients, men outnumber women by a two to one ratio, an even gender distribution is found when the male bias of the military/veterans cases is not considered. We are not aware of any children that have been affected, and the peak incidence of this tumor occurs among patients in the sixth and seventh decades of life.

Mucosal ulceration, pain, and swelling are common clinical signs and symptoms.

Histopathologic Features

According to our definition, adenosquamous carcinoma of the oral cavity manifests carcinomatous transformation of the mucosal surface epithelium and ductal adenocarcinoma of the underlying minor salivary gland excretory ducts (Figs. 27–1, 27–2). Carcinomatous changes in the surface mucosal squamous epithelium were noted but not emphasized by Gerughty and associates;[22] however, we consider this to be an important diagnostic feature. Carcinoma-in-situ is typically evident in the mucosal epithelium overlying or adjacent to the tumor and may be contiguous with similar changes in the minor salivary gland excretory ducts. Infiltrative, poorly to moderately well-differentiated squamous cell carcinoma is usually present in the lamina propria and submucosa, but occasionally, in cases that we suspect are in early development, only carcinoma-in-situ may be apparent. In the better-differentiated tumors, intercellular bridges, individual cell keratinization, and keratin pearls can be seen. In less well-differentiated neoplasms, tumor islands and cords of more basaloid cells are observed. Intermixed with the squamous cell carcinoma elements, but more conspicuous in the deeper portions of the tumor, a malignant glandular neoplastic proliferation that apparently arises from the excretory or interlobular salivary gland ducts is seen. This adenocarcinomatous portion is characterized by cuboidal or basaloid cells that form tubular or ductal structures with narrow to cystic lumina. Unlike Gerughty and coworkers,[22] we do not believe that mucous cell differentiation is requisite for the diagnosis. Most tumors demonstrate areas with distinct and separate adenocarcinoma and squamous cell carcinoma, but ostensible transitional areas between squamous carcinoma and adenocarcinoma can sometimes be found. These tumors, of course, are unencapsulated, infiltrative, and destructive. Perineural and vascular invasion are frequent (see Fig. 27–2C).

The extent of cytologic abnormalities, such as nuclear and cytoplasmic pleomorphism, nuclear hyperchromatism, and number of mitotic figures, is quite variable from tumor to tumor and, naturally, reflects the degree of differentiation of the tumor.

Prognosis and Therapy

Although follow-up data on the cases in the AFIP files are inadequate, five of the six patients reported in the literature died as a result of their tumor, and the sixth patient was alive with metastases. This poor prognosis may be as much attributable to the preferred sites of occurrence as to the inherent aggressiveness of these tumors. For example, survival rates for patients with squamous cell carcinomas of the posterior tongue, floor of the mouth, and tonsillar pillars are poorer than those for patients with squamous cell carcinomas of similar grades in other oral sites. Therapy should be comparable to that for squamous cell carcinoma or high-grade adenocarcinoma in these same sites (i.e., the posterior tongue, floor of the mouth, and tonsillar pillars), and consideration should be given to surgical excision, radical neck dissection, and radiotherapy because of the frequent early metastasis of carcinomas from these sites.

Differential Diagnosis

Two entities, mucoepidermoid carcinoma and adenoid squamous cell carcinoma, should be very carefully considered in the differential diagnosis for adenosquamous carcinoma. In comparing mucoepidermoid carcinoma and adenosquamous carcinoma, one sees that both tumors manifest epidermoid and glandular features. However, the configurations of these two tumors are different. Separate and definitive areas of adenocarcinoma and squamous cell carcinoma are not seen in mucoepidermoid carcinoma. Although mucicarminophilic cells may be found in adenosquamous cell carcinoma, they are not requisite, as in mucoepidermoid carcinoma, and, certainly, the distinct aggregates and/or cyst-lining rows of mucous cells typical of mucoepidermoid carcinoma are not present in adenosquamous carcinoma. More subtle differences include the infrequent occurrence of individual cell keratinization and keratin pearl formation in mucoepidermoid carcinoma as compared with adenosquamous carcinoma and the absence of carcinomatous changes in the surface mucosal epithelium in mucoepidermoid carcinoma.

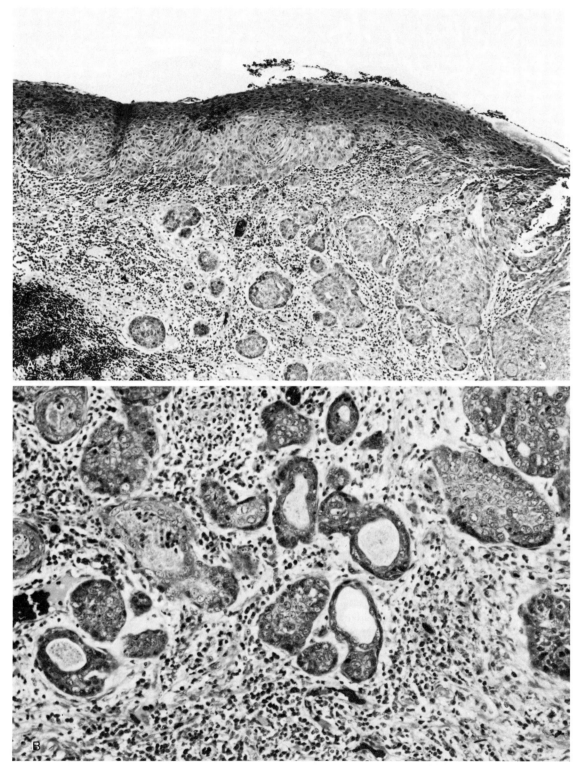

Figure 27–1. Adenosquamous carcinoma of the floor of the mouth exhibits *(A)* carcinoma-in-situ of the mucosal epithelium with subjacent invasive squamous cell carcinoma and *(B)* ductal differentiation in the deeper portion of the carcinoma. There appears to be formation of true lumina rather than formation of pseudolumina caused by acantholysis as in adenoid squamous cell carcinoma. *(A, × 75; B, × 150.)*

estimated to represent only 5 percent of oncocytic salivary gland tumors and 0.05 percent of all benign and malignant epithelial salivary gland neoplasms.[46]

At present, 32 acceptable cases of salivary gland oncocytic carcinoma have been reported in the literature. This total does not include five cases reported from glandular mucosa of the nasal cavity. Augmenting the nine cases previously reported by Goode and Corio,[46] sixteen additional oncocytic carcinomas have been added to the salivary gland registry at the AFIP, bringing our experience with this neoplasm to 25 cases. Oncocytic carcinomas represent 11 percent of all oncocytic salivary gland neoplasms, 0.5 percent of all epithelial salivary gland malignancies, and 0.18 percent of all epithelial salivary gland tumors in the AFIP registry of salivary gland pathology.

Clinical Features

Oncocytic carcinoma is a tumor predominantly found in the elderly population. Based on analysis of 25 cases in the salivary gland registry at AFIP, the average age of occurrence is 64 years. Ages ranged from 29 to 91 years, with 16 patients (64 percent) in the seventh and eighth decades of life. It appears that oncocytic carcinoma develops at an earlier age in females than in males, with average ages of occurrence of 56.7 and 70.0 years, respectively. In addition to those cases reported by Goode and Corio,[46] there are 20 reported cases in which patient age and gender are known. Generally, similar findings were observed with average ages for eight females and twelve males of 55.50 and 60.75 years, respectively.

AFIP data concerning racial characteristics of patients with oncocytic carcinoma proved insufficient to render any unequivocal conclusion. In 11 cases (44 percent of the total number of cases), race was not indicated. Among the other 14 patients, 13 were white; none were black; and 1 patient was Asian.

Oncocytic carcinoma appears to demonstrate a male predilection. In 24 AFIP cases for which gender was stated, 15 patients (62.5 percent) were male and 9 patients (37.5 percent) were female. This statistic was unaffected by any possible gender bias that might result from military cases, because all 24 cases were submitted from civilian institutions. Review of the literature before 1988 indicated a male predominance by a ratio of 3 to 2.

According to AFIP salivary gland registry data, 18 (72 percent) oncocytic carcinomas were observed in the parotid gland. An additional three tumors (12 percent) were in the submandibular gland, and two tumors (8 percent) were in the neck. Single cases were also observed in minor salivary glands of the palate and buccal mucosa. The literature conforms to the AFIP findings, with 21 tumors (91.3 percent) reported in the parotid gland. A single case each was observed in the submandibular gland and minor glands of the palate.

Oncocytic carcinoma cannot be clinically distinguished from other salivary gland tumors. It may result from transformation of a long-standing benign oncocytoma or may arise de novo. Eneroth[31] reported a tumor exhibiting sudden rapid growth after 19 years of quiescence, which may suggest malignant transformation because similar clinical characteristics are displayed by carcinoma ex mixed tumor. Tumor size has ranged from 0.5 to 8.0 cm. Infiltration by the tumor may produce facial nerve pain, paresthesia, or paralysis in some cases.

Flow cytometry has been used for evaluation of oncocytic neoplasms. Rainwater and colleagues[51] reported DNA ploidy studies using extracted nuclei of oncocytic cells from benign salivary gland oncocytoma and malignant oncocytic thyroid gland and kidney tumors. In tumors of all three organs, those patients with tumors displaying a normal histogram experienced a favorable outcome with no recurrences or metastases and long survival times. Approximately 60 percent of patients with oncocytic thyroid malignancies in which an aneuploid DNA peak was noted succumbed to their disease. Further studies with salivary gland oncocytic carcinoma may prove useful in predicting biologic behavior.

Microscopic Features

The diagnosis of oncocytic carcinoma can be exceedingly difficult to render. The first criterion requires the histomorphologic recognition of an oncocytic neoplasm, which is characterized by large polyhedral or round cells that exhibit eosinophilic granular cytoplasm and that are arranged in an alveolar or syncytial pattern. As in benign oncocytoma, examination of special stains or use of electron microscopy is often necessary to confirm oncocytic differentiation. The second criterion that must be fulfilled for the diagnosis of oncocytic carcinoma is observation of malignant clinical and/or histopathologic behavior. Determination of malignancy based on cellular histomorphology is highly subjective, since benign oncocytes may exhibit varying degrees of cellular atypia and nuclear pleomorphism. Overwhelming evidence of nuclear and cellular pleomorphism and markedly increased or abnormal mitotic figures are indicative of malignancy (Figs. 27–3 and 27–4). Lack of encapsulation is an important criterion in assessing malignancy in major salivary gland oncocytic tumors. However, care must be taken to avoid misinterpretation of oncocytosis as infiltration into glandular parenchyma. Other malignant histopathologic features include invasion and replacement of the salivary gland by tumor (Fig. 27–5), perineural infiltration (Fig. 27–6), vascular

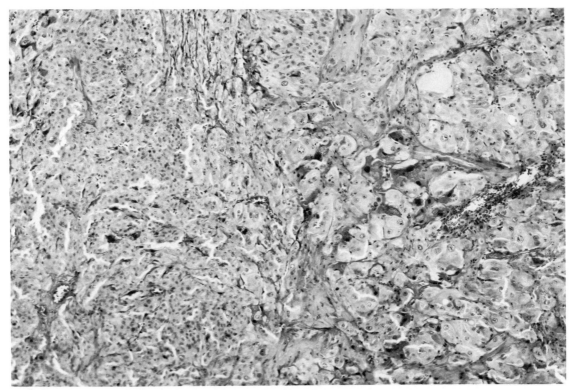

Figure 27–3. Oncocytic carcinoma exhibits transition between an area of typical oncocytes and larger, pleomorphic oncocytes with hyperchromatic and vesiculated nuclei (× 150).

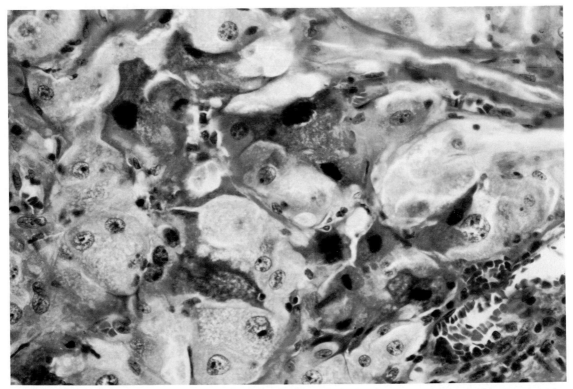

Figure 27–4. Oncocytic carcinoma demonstrates cells with cytoplasmic granularity, pleomorphism, and nuclear hyperchromatism (× 300).

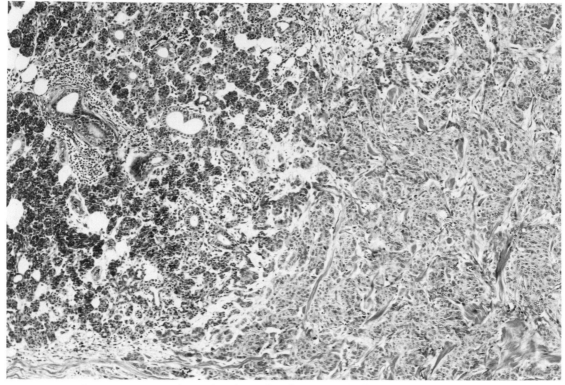

Figure 27–5. Oncocytic carcinoma invades and replaces normal salivary gland parenchyma (× 150).

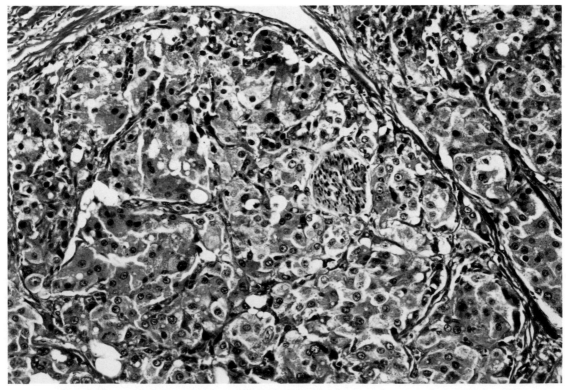

Figure 27–6. Oncocytic carcinoma exhibits an alveolar pattern and surrounds a nerve (× 160).

or lymphatic channel invasion (Fig. 27–7), infiltration of surrounding connective tissues, and regional lymph node metastasis.

Lee and Roth[39] as well as Johns and coworkers[42] compared the ultrastructural features of benign oncocytomas and oncocytic carcinomas. They observed that oncocytic carcinoma tumor cells fail to demonstrate basal laminae or intracytoplasmic glycogen but do exhibit a wider intercellular space than benign oncocytes. These subtle differences were insufficient, however, to provide a basis for determination of biologic behavior. They recommended that evaluation of malignancy be accomplished at the light-microscopic and clinical levels.

The histopathologic differential diagnosis for oncocytic carcinoma includes incompletely excised or recurrent benign oncocytoma, atypical oncocytoma, salivary duct carcinoma, well-differentiated acinic cell carcinoma, mucoepidermoid carcinoma, and carcinoma ex mixed tumor demonstrating oncocytic differentiation. A documented history of prior local excision is important in separating some cases of persistent or recurrent benign oncocytoma from its malignant counterpart. The diagnosis of atypical oncocytoma is highly subjective and, in our opinion, represents a midpoint in the spectrum of biologic behavior for oncocytic salivary gland tumors. Atypical on-

cocytoma may exhibit a singular ominous histopathologic feature, such as loss of encapsulation with islands of tumor that focally extend into parotid gland parenchyma, but sufficient additional evidence may not be present to warrant a malignant interpretation. Special staining procedures and electron microscopic examination for mitochondria may be helpful in differentiating oncocytic carcinoma from other adenocarcinomas. Salivary duct carcinoma may exhibit similar large pleomorphic cells with granular cytoplasm and focal areas of necrosis, but it does not stain with phosphotungstic acid–hematoxylin and lacks consistent electron microscopic findings of mitochondrial hyperplasia. Similarly, although oncocytic carcinoma may contain glycogen or sialomucin or both, observation of prominent zymogen granularity with periodic acid–Schiff reagent or intracytoplasmic mucin with mucicarmine or Alcian blue stains would, instead, favor diagnoses of acinic cell or mucoepidermoid carcinoma, respectively. Oncocytic carcinoma should not exhibit histopathologic features of mixed tumor. When evidence of myoepithelial, chondroid, osseous, or myxomatous features is observed in conjunction with areas of oncocytic differentiation, the diagnosis of carcinoma ex mixed tumor is preferred over oncocytic carcinoma.

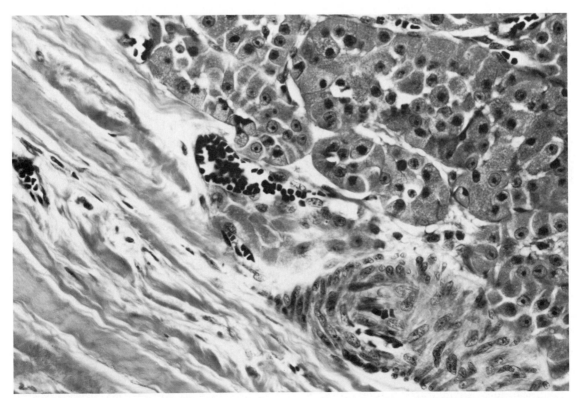

Figure 27–7. Oncocytic carcinoma erodes the wall of a vascular channel. Note the benign appearance of tumor cells immediately adjacent to the vessel wall (× 300).

Behavior and Treatment

Analysis of the literature revealed that oncocytic carcinomas exhibited metastases to regional lymph nodes or distant organs in 19 of 32 reported cases (60 percent). Of those patients with metastases, at least nine (47 percent) are known to have died of their disease, with one patient alive with persistent disease at the time of the report. Another patient with metastasis was lost to follow-up. The time interval from initial surgery to metastatic presentation ranged from 0.25 to 7.0 years, averaging 2.9 years. Patient survival from the time of initial treatment ranged from 0.25 to 11.0 years and averaged 3.6 years. Patient survival time after discovery of metastasis ranged from only days to 4 years and averaged approximately 1 year. The recurrence rate was approximately 33 percent, and multiple recurrences were noted in several cases.[28, 38, 39, 42, 46] Goode and Corio[46] reported that in five of their nine patients, tumors recurred, with an incidence of metastasis after recurrence of 80 percent. Of their four patients with metastasis that followed local recurrence, three patients died of their disease, and one was alive with persistent tumor.

Few investigators of oncocytic carcinoma have reported follow-up data with treatment information.[38, 40–43] It is therefore difficult to make unequivocal survival predictions based on any given course of therapy. Batsakis[2] suggested that patients with oncocytic carcinoma appear to have good short-term survival, but he warned that long-term biologic behavior was likely to parallel that of low-grade salivary gland malignant tumors, such as acinic cell adenocarcinoma. Goode and Corio[46] attempted clinicopathologic correlation of their nine cases of oncocytic carcinoma and offered some preliminary conclusions while recommending further study. They reported that patients with oncocytic carcinoma of the salivary gland did not exhibit favorable short-term prognosis if initial surgical treatment was conservative. In this study, four of the five tumors that recurred followed initial therapies of either local excision or partial parotidectomy of tumors 2 to 4 cm in diameter, rather than treatments that involved more aggressive surgical intervention. Subsequently, metastases developed in three of these patients and in another patient initially treated by partial parotidectomy, and all four died of their disease, in spite of measures combining radical surgery, radiation therapy, and chemotherapy. Laurian and coinvestigators[43] reported a similar case in which the patient succumbed to recurrent and metastatic disease after superficial parotidectomy, despite subsequent heroic salvage attempts. Johns and coworkers[42] reported one patient with recurrence after local excision.

Radiation therapy as a primary treatment does not appear to favorably affect patient survival. Ross[41] reported a case treated by radiation therapy in which the patient succumbed to disease within 3 months. Goode and Corio[46] concluded that total parotidectomy as the initial therapeutic procedure offers the patient the best chance for prolonged survival.

Correlation of histopathologic features and patient survivals offer inconclusive evidence on which to predict biologic behavior. Goode and Corio[46] reported an association between tumors with either excessive pleomorphism (100 percent) or neural, vascular, or lymphatic involvement (75 percent) and patients who subsequently died of their disease. However, tumors from several well patients exhibited histopathologic features similar to tumors from those who failed to survive. They suggested that it may be premature to conclude that the surviving patients who had tumors with ominous histopathologic features will continue to remain free from disease for a prolonged interval.

It has been suggested that local recurrence is an indicator of metastatic potential, and once regional lymph node metastasis occurs, it carries a grave prognosis. Therefore, even for lesions smaller than 2 cm, total parotidectomy, (with preservation of the facial nerve, whenever possible) would appear warranted. Prophylactic neck dissection may also be indicated if the histopathologic finding of lymphatic channel infiltration suggests that the tumor is likely to spread to regional lymph nodes.

CYSTADENOCARCINOMA

Salivary gland cystadenocarcinomas are those adenocarcinomas that are histopathologically dominated by large cystic structures with epithelial linings that may or may not have a papillary growth pattern. Furthermore, except in focally limited areas of rare cases, these tumors do not possess features of other types of malignant salivary gland tumors that also may form large cystic structures, such as acinic cell adenocarcinoma and mucoepidermoid carcinoma. Conceptually, these tumors are the malignant counterparts of benign cystadenomas.

We are not aware of any report that clearly defines and illustrates these tumors. Cystadenocarcinomas were not included as separate salivary gland tumors in the classification schemes proposed by Foote and Frazell,[54] Evans and Cruickshank,[55] Thackray and Lucas,[56] or by the World Health Organization in 1972[57] (see Chapter 8). Nonetheless, several investigators have used the term *cystadenocarcinoma*, at least descriptively, for a small number of salivary gland tumors in their series, which also included most of the more common types.[58–62] Based either on their descriptions or photomicrographs, we believe other investigators have reported tumors that may also represent cystadenocarcinomas under the terms *malignant papillary cystadenoma*,[63] *mucus-producing adenopapillary (nonepidermoid) carcinoma*,[64–67] and *papillary adenocarcinoma*.[27, 59, 68–70]

One morphologically relatively homogeneous group of cystic minor salivary gland tumors has been reported under the term "low-grade papillary adenocarcinoma."[71–75] In 1984, Mills and colleagues[74] discussed 12 cases, including 7 from the literature, which, in our opinion, share some features with papillary cystadenocarcinoma. These tumors were considered to represent examples of a purely papillary variant of polymorphous low-grade adenocarcinoma.[74, 76] The investigators observed more aggressive behavior among tumors of the papillary variant compared with those of the nonpapillary type and, consequently, argued for segregation of the two types. In 1987, Slootweg and Müller[75] also reported papillary and nonpapillary forms of polymorphous low-grade adenocarcinoma and noted that both forms were prone to local recurrence and that the papillary type gave rise to local and distant metastatic disease. The papillary cystic morphology and the more aggressive behavior of the papillary variant raise the question of whether it is more appropriate to label these tumors *papillary cystadenocarcinomas* (see Chapter 23 and the discussion of differential diagnosis for cystadenocarcinoma later in this section).

In many instances, other previously published series that may have included cystadenocarcinomas under other terminology have been inadequately illustrated to verify the diagnosis. For example, in a study of 405 cases of salivary gland carcinoma, 58 cases (14.3 percent) were reported as papillary adenocarcinomas, but none were illustrated.[61] Spiro and colleagues[70] reported 24 salivary gland tumors as papillary adenocarcinomas, and photomicrographs of some of these cases suggest that they were cystadenocarcinomas. We interpret another case in this series, reported as low-grade mucin-producing adenocarcinoma, similarly. Blanck and colleagues[65] reported 47 cases of tumors that they labeled mucus-producing adenopapillary (nonepidermoid) carcinoma. Although we interpret several of their illustrated cases as epithelial-myoepithelial carcinoma and acinic cell adenocarcinoma, it appears that at least one cystadenocarcinoma is also illustrated.

Clinical Features

As with other types of salivary gland tumors, clinical signs and symptoms largely depend on the site of involvement. These tumors usually occur as asymptomatic masses and have protracted clinical courses. In the parotid gland, pain and facial nerve weakness may be evident, but fixation to overlying structures is unusual. Intraoral cystadenocarcinomas most often present as painless masses with intact overlying mucosa.

At the AFIP, the diagnostic term *cystadenocarcinoma* was first applied to salivary gland tumors in 1978, and between then and the end of 1988, the diagnosis has been made in 23 cases. Twelve

tumors occurred in the parotid glands, four in the submandibular glands and one in the sublingual gland. Of the six tumors that arose in the minor glands, three occurred in the palate, two in the upper lip, and one in the buccal mucosa.

The ages of the patients with cystadenocarcinoma in the AFIP registry range from 20 to 86 years, and the average age is 54.7 years. Over 90 percent of these tumors have occurred in patients in the fourth through the eighth decades of life. Of seventeen patients from civilian institutions, ten were female, and seven were male.

Pathologic Features

Although this group of tumors shows a moderate degree of histomorphologic diversity, the common denominator for diagnosis is numerous cystic spaces. A cystic growth pattern must dominate the histologic appearance for the diagnosis to be considered. These cystic spaces vary in size both from one tumor to the next and within the same tumor. These neoplasms may appear circumscribed or reveal haphazard growth throughout a salivary gland (Fig. 27–8). Occasionally, uniform, medium to large, round to ovoid "cysts" form the vast majority of the tumor, but more often, large cystic spaces are accompanied by intervening, irregularly shaped, ramifying and anastomosing smaller cystic channels (Fig. 27–9). The lumina often are filled with mucus, and hemorrhage and dystrophic calcifications are sometimes evident focally.

The cyst lining epithelium shows a wide range of morphologic appearances and proliferative capacity. In our experience, the epithelial lining in about 80 percent of all cystadenocarcinomas demonstrates papillary growth at least focally. The papillae vary from single, large peninsular structures that have central cores of vascular fibrous connective tissue to multiple, small, compact papillations composed of two rows of closely apposed epithelial cells (Fig. 27–10).

The lining cells vary from cuboidal to tall columnar, and often a single tumor contains basaloid, oncocytic, clear, and, occasionally, mucous cells that form adenomatous or nodular, solid epithelial areas. These solid areas usually occupy the space between the cystic structures. In most cases, nuclear hyperchromatism and nuclear variability are subtle, and only rare mitotic figures are present. Nucleoli may be obvious. However, encapsulation is incomplete, and infiltration into either salivary gland parenchyma or fibrous or adipose tissue is indisputable (Fig. 27–11). The tumor may infiltrate either as cystlike structures or as solid islands.

Although the vast majority of cystadenocarcinomas are low-grade lesions, we have reviewed several cases that showed moderate nuclear pleomorphism (Fig. 27–12) in addition to the infiltrative growth pattern. We have interpreted these lesions as intermediate grade neoplasms. Other

Text continued on page 470

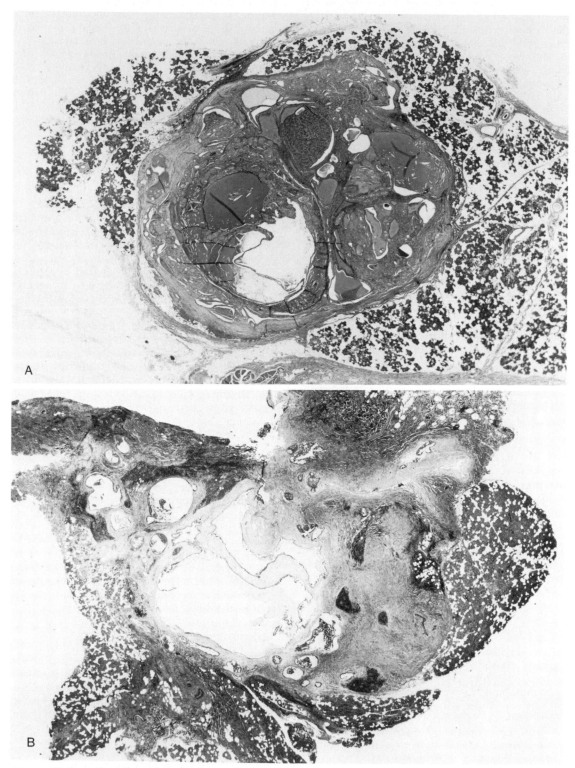

Figure 27–8. *A*, Cystadenocarcinoma from a 61 year old man is relatively well circumscribed (× 2.5). *B*, In contrast to *A*, this cystadenocarcinoma is infiltrating haphazardly throughout the parotid gland (× 9.9).

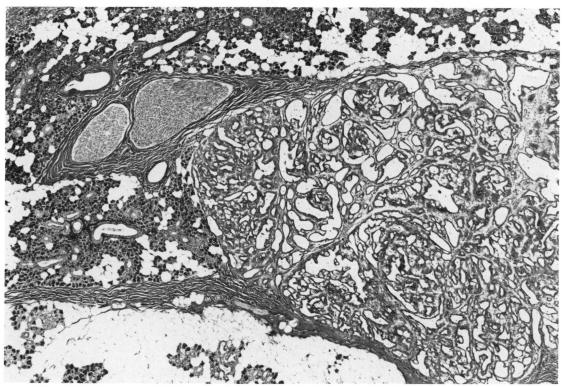

Figure 27–9. Cystadenocarcinoma in a 68 year old woman is characterized by cystic structures of uniform size. Infiltration of parotid parenchyma is evident, and the tumor is approaching a peripheral nerve ($\times$ 30).

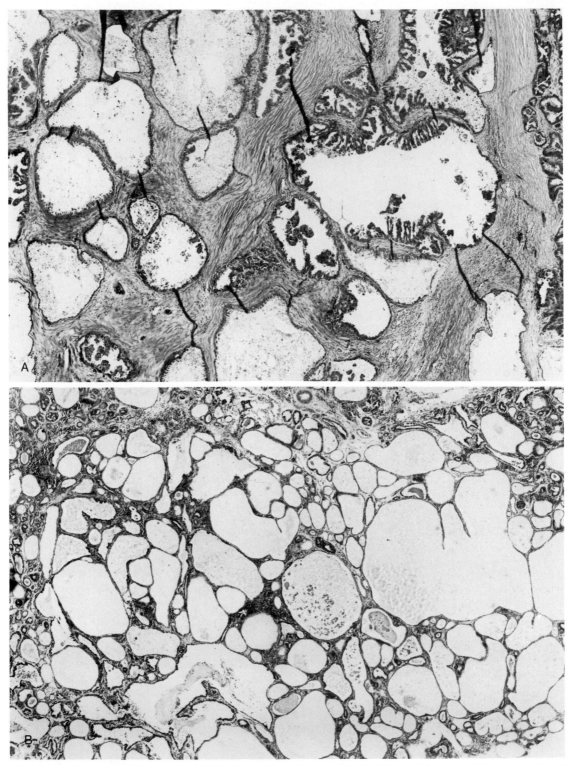

Figure 27–10. Two different cystadenocarcinomas are shown. *(A),* Papillary epithelial proliferation is focally prominent (× 30). *B,* Papillary growth is not seen in this tumor (× 30).

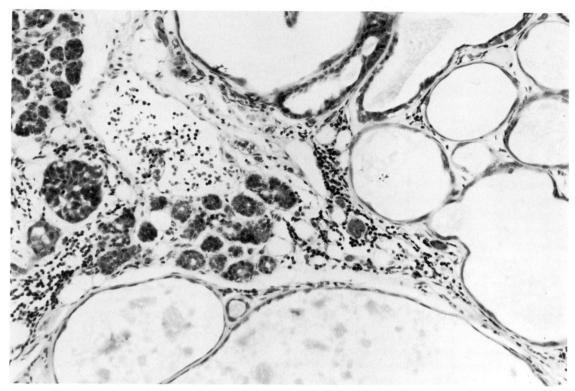

Figure 27–11. Despite morphologically bland, flattened to cuboidal epithelium lining the cystic spaces in this low-grade cystadenocarcinoma from a 32 year old woman, tumor has infiltrated and destroyed a large portion of the parotid gland (× 150).

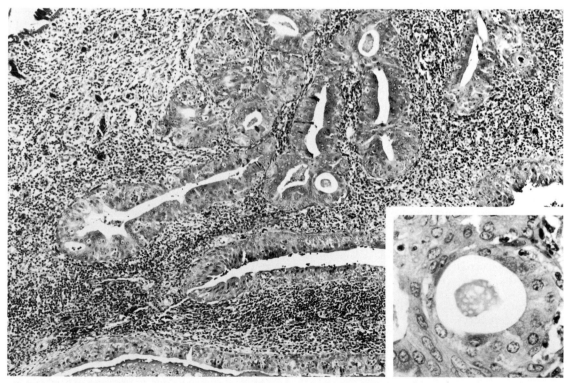

Figure 27–12. The epithelium in this cystadenocarcinoma reveals enlarged nuclei and prominent nucleoli. This is one of several cases considered to be of an intermediate grade (× 75; *inset* × 300).

investigators have also reported intermediate grade cystadenocarcinomas.[65, 70] Our cytomorphologic basis for grading contrasts with the criteria used by these other investigators,[65, 70] who have instead relied on the presence or absence of stromal infiltration.

We have occasionally reviewed cystadenocarcinomas that, in addition to the papillary cystic structures, focally showed features common to acinic cell adenocarcinoma, epithelial-myoepithelial carcinoma, or mucoepidermoid carcinoma. We stress that these areas were extremely limited and constituted a small proportion of the entire tumor (less than 5 percent of the total tumor in our estimation).

Differential Diagnosis

As one might expect, the differential diagnosis for cystadenocarcinomas includes any salivary gland tumor that exhibits a cystic or papillary growth pattern. Adenocarcinomas, not otherwise specified, have only rare or small cystic or papillary-cystic structures and show no features characteristic of another specific type of salivary gland tumor (see Chapter 18). Lesions such as intraductal papillomas, Warthin's tumors, and mucoepidermoid carcinomas rarely cause diagnostic problems, because they possess features that are sufficiently characteristic to readily permit accurate identification. The tumors that usually cause the greatest difficulties in separation from cystadenocarcinomas are cystadenomas, polymorphous low-grade adenocarcinomas, and papillary-cystic variants of acinic cell adenocarcinoma.

Distinction of cystadenocarcinoma from cystadenoma may occasionally be challenging. Both neoplasms usually reveal papillary proliferation of the epithelial lining and are composed of cells that possess bland cytomorphologic features. Furthermore, cystadenomas are often not well encapsulated, and some cystic structures may appear to be separated from the main portion of the tumor, suggesting infiltration. Differentiation of tumor types depends largely on the identification of actual infiltration of salivary gland parenchyma or surrounding connective tissue by either cystic or solid epithelium in cystadenocarcinomas. Step sections of a borderline tumor may yield unequivocal evidence of invasion.

Polymorphous low-grade adenocarcinomas (see Chapter 23) nearly always arise in the minor glands, unlike cystadenocarcinomas, and possess some relatively distinctive morphologic features. Common to both are papillary and cystic components, bland cytomorphology, few mitotic figures, and infiltrative growth. Different from cystadenocarcinoma, polymorphous low-grade adenocarcinoma infiltrates in islands, cords, tubules, and linearly arranged concentric whorling fascicles of cells that encircle tumor islands. Furthermore, in polymorphous low-grade adenocarcinoma, mucinous or hyalinized stroma is often focally promi-

nent; a cribriform growth pattern may be present in some areas of the tumor; and, when present, the papillary component is not a dominant feature. In contradistinction to cystadenocarcinomas, polymorphous low-grade adenocarcinomas frequently show perineural growth.

Review of most salivary gland tumors that have a prominent papillary-cystic component necessitates consideration of papillary-cystic acinic cell adenocarcinoma. Ellis and Corio[77] have noted that 25 percent of acinic cell adenocarcinomas show a papillary cystic growth pattern and that 45 percent manifest multiple growth patterns, including microcystic and solid acinar cell areas. This knowledge highlights the importance of searching thoroughly for areas possessing a microcystic growth pattern, a feature not seen in cystadenocarcinomas. Additionally, identification of large, round cells with deeply basophilic, granular cytoplasm that contains diastase-resistant material that stains positively for periodic acid–Schiff stain supports a diagnosis of acinic cell adenocarcinoma.

Prognosis and Treatment

Essentially no information is currently available that pertains specifically to the prognosis of salivary gland cystadenocarcinomas. Consequently, estimates of survival have to be extracted from large series that include many other tumor types. Spiro and coworkers[70] have noted that a determinate cure at 5 years was achieved for 69 percent of low-grade tumors as a group, including papillary adenocarcinomas. They also pointed out that, in general, better salvage was achieved in patients with oral or parotid tumors, with tumors that had papillary histology, and with stage I clinical disease. It may be important that the malignant tumors with the greatest morphologic similarity to cystadenocarcinoma, namely, acinic cell adenocarcinoma and polymorphous low-grade adenocarcinoma, behave in a manner similar to that of other low-grade tumors, although delayed recurrences and even metastases are possible. The need for study of a large series of these tumors that includes correlation of prognosis with treatment is obvious. Currently, it would seem reasonable to use the same treatment principles for low-grade cystadenocarcinoma as those used for other low-grade salivary gland adenocarcinomas.[78] These include consideration of the site, the clinical extent of the disease, and the histologic grade prior to institution of therapy. Facial nerve branches should be sacrificed only when involved by tumor and radical neck dissection performed only to resect obvious metastases.

MALIGNANT SEBACEOUS NEOPLASMS

Malignant sebaceous neoplasms of the salivary glands are very uncommon tumors, accounting for less than 0.05 percent of all salivary gland tumors in the AFIP salivary gland registry. They may be classified into two categories: sebaceous carcinoma and sebaceous lymphadenocarcinoma.

Sebaceous Carcinoma

Sebaceous carcinoma is a malignant tumor composed predominantly of sebaceous cells of varying maturity that are arranged in sheets and/or nests with different degrees of pleomorphism, nuclear atypia, and invasiveness (Figs. 27–13, 27–14).

When considered together, there is a biphasic age distribution evident among the 23 patients reported in the literature[79–97] and the six cases in the AFIP registry of salivary gland disease. Peak incidences of tumor occurrence are found in the third decade and seventh and eighth decades of life (range 17 to 93 years). The male and female incidence of occurrence is almost equal. Twenty-seven tumors have arisen in the parotid gland, one in the oral cavity, and one in the vallecula. Patients commonly are affected by painful masses, with varying degrees of facial nerve paralysis, and occasionally, fixation of the skin is present. Tumors have ranged in size from 0.6 to 8.5 cm in greatest dimension.

The color of tumor tissue varies among yellow, tan-white, grayish-white, white, and pale pink. Tumors are well circumscribed or partially encapsulated, with pushing or locally infiltrating margins. Cellular pleomorphism and cytologic atypia are uniformly present and are more prevalent than in sebaceous adenomas. Tumor cells may be arranged in multiple large foci or in sheets of cells and have hyperchromatic nuclei surrounded by abundant clear to eosinophilic cytoplasm. Areas of cellular necrosis and fibrosis are commonly found. Perineural invasion has been observed in more than 20 percent of tumors. Vascular invasion is extremely unusual. Rare oncocytes and foreign body giant cells with histiocytes may be observed, but lymphoid tissue with follicles or subcapsular sinuses is not seen.

Treatment varies from local excision and parotidectomy to preoperative and postoperative radiotherapy, with or without chemotherapy. Follow-up information was available in 20 cases. Patient survival ranged from 8 months to 13 years (mean 4.5 years). Six patients (26 percent) died of causes secondary to their disease; all died within 5 years after diagnosis. Eleven patients were alive and well with no evidence of recurrent disease. One patient expired from unrelated causes, after being successfully treated for two recurrences, with no evidence of carcinoma 5 years after initial surgery, and two patients were alive with evidence of disease 8 months after diagnosis. The longest period of survival, 13 years, involved a 22 year old patient. However, insufficient data are available to predict whether or not a difference exists

between the survival rates for the younger versus the older patient groups.

Sebaceous Lymphadenocarcinoma

Sebaceous lymphadenocarcinoma is the malignant counterpart of sebaceous lymphadenoma and represents carcinoma arising in sebaceous lymphadenoma. It is the rarest sebaceous tumor in the salivary glands. To date, only three of these tumors have been reported.[79, 80, 98] All three patients were in their seventh decade of life. Two patients were males, and one was female. The tumors arose within the parotid gland or in a periparotid lymph node. Two of the patients had histories of masses present for more than 20 years, while in the third patient, the mass was asymptomatic.

Tumor color varies from yellow-tan to gray. Tumors are focally encapsulated and locally invasive. They are composed of areas of sebaceous lymphadenoma that are intermixed with or adjacent to regions of pleomorphic carcinoma cells that exhibit varying degrees of invasiveness (Fig. 27–15). The malignant portion of the tumors has ranged from sebaceous carcinoma[98] to sheets of poorly differentiated carcinoma, with areas of ductal differentiation or foci of dermal cylindroma, solid adenoid cystic carcinoma, or epithelial-myoepithelial carcinoma.[79, 80] Perineural invasion was present in one tumor. Collections of histiocytes were present in two cases, whereas a foreign body giant cell reaction was found in one tumor. Oncocytes are not observed. The sebaceous lymphadenoma portion of all tumors contains lymphoid follicles. One tumor had a subcapsular marginal sinus. Cellular atypia has not been observed in the sebaceous lymphadenoma portion of any tumor.

One patient, who was treated by a superficial parotidectomy, expired because of unrelated causes 1.5 years after initial surgery, with no evidence of tumor. The second patient, who was treated with an unspecified type of surgery and radiation, expired from unrelated causes, with a solitary lung metastasis 13.5 years later. The third patient, who was treated by "total excision," is free of disease 14 months after surgery.

Malignant sebaceous neoplasms of salivary gland origin are rare tumors that appear to be similar to their orbital and skin counterparts with only a few exceptions.[99] Patients' age distribution shows a bimodal peak incidence of occurrence for salivary gland sebaceous carcinomas, although those patients with carcinomas arising in the orbit, the most common location for sebaceous carcinoma, exhibit a single broad peak incidence of occurrence, with 81 percent of the tumors occurring in the fifth to eighth decades.[99] Also, sebaceous carcinoma of salivary gland origin appears to behave in a more aggressive fashion than se-

Text continued on page 476

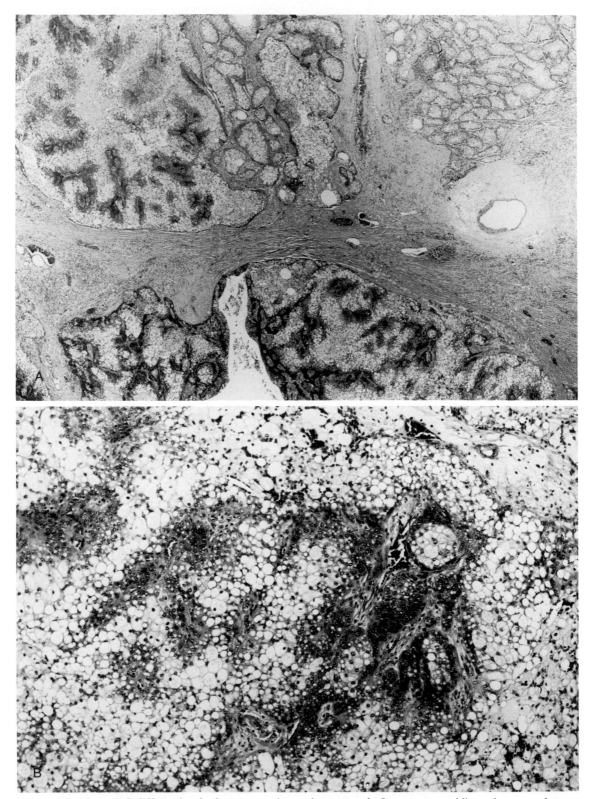

Figure 27–13. *A*, Well-differentiated sebaceous carcinoma is composed of an area resembling sebaceous adenoma (upper right) with adjacent regions containing sheets of carcinoma cells (× 20). *B*, Higher magnification of *A* shows a sheet of sebaceous carcinoma cells (× 100).

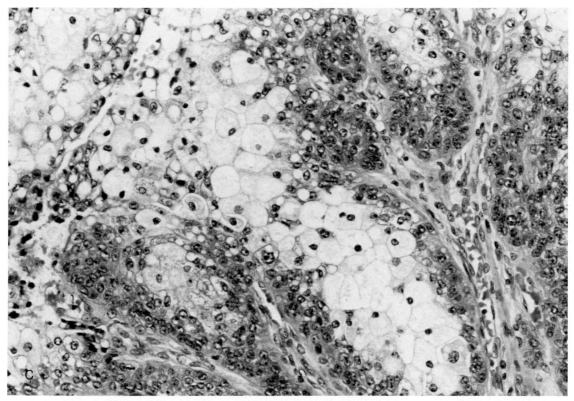

Figure 27–13 *Continued C,* Detail of tumor demonstrates areas of basaloid cells with minimal cytoplasm and prominent nucleoli maturing into cells with eccentric nuclei and abundant clear cytoplasm ($\times$ 200).

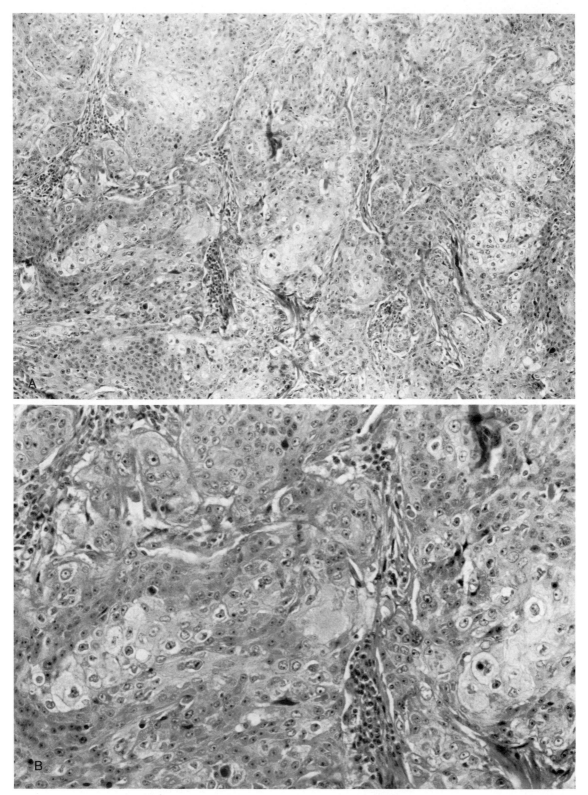

Figure 27–14. *A*, Poorly differentiated sebaceous carcinoma is composed of sheets containing pleomorphic, atypical tumor cells with prominent nucleoli and abundant cytoplasm (× 100). *B*, Higher magnification of *A* (× 200).

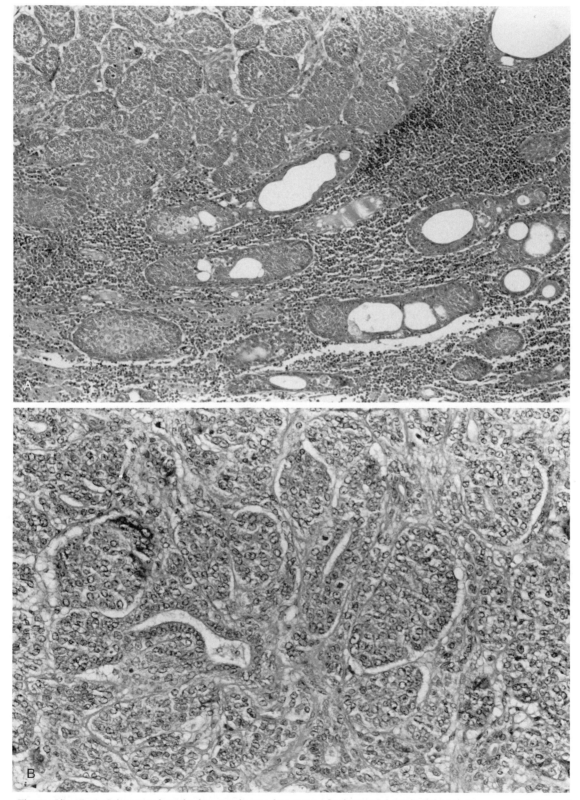

Figure 27–15. *A*, Sebaceous lymphadenocarcinoma has areas of sebaceous lymphadenoma (lower and right) and carcinoma (upper left). *B*, Higher magnification of the carcinoma portion of tumor shows coalescent nests of tumor cells with prominent nucleoli, minimal cytoplasm, focal ductal differentiation, and several mitoses (center).

Illustration continued on following page

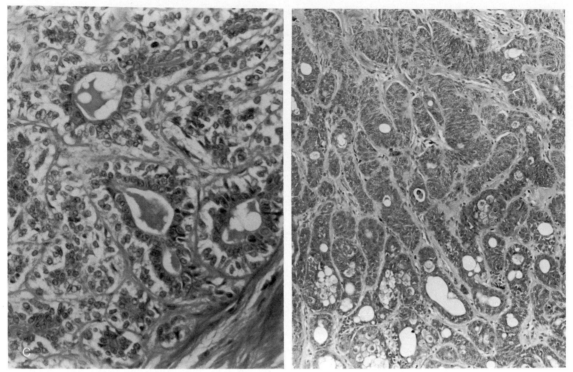

Figure 27–15 *Continued C,* An area of epimyoepithelial carcinoma (left) and of sebaceous carcinoma (right) (*A,* × 100; *B,* × 200; *C left,* × 200, *right,* × 100).

baceous carcinoma of the orbital region, with 5-year patient survival rates of 62.2 and 84.5 percent, respectively.[79, 80]

Sebaceous carcinoma and sebaceous lymphadenocarcinoma appear to be low-grade malignant tumors that have the ability to recur locally. Lymph node or distant metastases may develop late in the clinical evolution of these tumors.

SALIVARY DUCT CARCINOMA

The purpose of a classification system is to permit recognition of tumors with similar histopathologic features and to ascribe a predicted biologic behavior to the tumors in that group. Only recently has the tumor designated as *salivary duct carcinoma* begun to be generally recognized as a specific diagnostic category of salivary gland adenocarcinoma. Although Kleinsasser and colleagues[100] first described this entity and first used the term *salivary duct carcinoma* in 1968, reports of this uncommon tumor have accumulated slowly. In fact, it is now recognized that two of the five cases originally described by Kleinsasser and colleagues[100] are better classified as epithelial-myoepithelial carcinomas (see Chapter 24), which have a much better prognosis for the patient than salivary duct carcinoma.[101–103] At present, enough data have accrued to permit confident segregation

of this tumor from the other salivary gland adenocarcinomas. At the time of preparation of this text, we counted 50 cases that had been reported in the literature, and another 3 cases have been identified within the AFIP salivary gland registry.[100–108] It appears to us that the case reported by Gal and coworkers[109] was the same as *Case 2* reported by Zohar and colleagues.[108]

The term *salivary duct carcinoma* was selected because of the resemblance of these tumors to ductal carcinomas of the breast. Unfortunately, this term has the potential to create confusion for pathologists and clinicians, because nearly all carcinomas of the salivary glands arise from the duct system. Several older cases in the archives of the AFIP that were identified as *ductal* or *duct carcinomas* used these terms in a generic sense rather than for the specific entity now associated with the term *salivary duct carcinoma.* Review of some of these cases has shown that a few could be reclassified as epithelial-myoepithelial carcinomas or polymorphous low-grade adenocarcinomas, which are both entities that had not been defined when these cases were added to the registry. In fact, Seifert and others[110, 111] have used this term to identify what we believe are epithelial-myoepithelial carcinomas, just as Kleinsasser and colleagues[100] did in two cases. However, most reports in the literature have used the term *salivary duct carcinoma* to define a unique subset of carcinomas that is described in three of Kleinsasser and coworkers'[100] original cases and that is distinct from epithelial-myoepithelial carcinoma and other adenocarcinomas of the salivary glands.[37, 101–103, 106–108, 112] Although it is less than ideal, we have conformed to this established terminology and emphasize that even though nearly all salivary gland carcinomas arise from the duct system, salivary duct carcinoma is a specific clinicopathologic entity.

The incidence of salivary duct carcinoma is difficult to assess because most published surveys of salivary gland tumors do not include this specific category of tumor. It is likely that examples of this tumor have been included within a heterogenous group of tumors labeled *adenocarcinoma.* Judging by the limited reports in the literature and from our own experience, it is fair to say that these are uncommon salivary gland neoplasms.

Clinical Features

The parotid gland has been the site of occurrence in nearly 85 percent of the cases. Five tumors, which constituted one third of the cases reported by Hui and colleagues,[103] have been described in the submandibular gland. One of the tumors originally reported by Kleinsasser and colleagues[100] occurred in the hard palate. Garland and coinvestigators[102] did not accept this case because it did not demonstrate comedonecrosis, but Hui and colleagues[103] did accept it as a salivary duct carcinoma. Pesce and coworkers[105] described a tumor in the buccal mucosa, but it is difficult to determine from their very brief report whether this tumor was an example of salivary duct carcinoma. On the basis of the photomicrographs, we doubt that the tumor in the upper lip reported by Zohar and others[108] (their *Case 4*) was a salivary duct carcinoma. One of the tumors of Zohar and colleagues[108] arose in the sublingual gland.

These neoplasms have a definite predilection for older patients, since only one patient was less than 50 years old. Patients have ranged in age from 27 to 83 years old. There has been a decided male predominance, with male patients outnumbering female patients by 2.5 times.

In addition to the manifest swelling produced by these tumors, a number of patients have experienced facial nerve palsy or paralysis and/or pain. Onset and growth of the tumors has usually been rather rapid, with most patients seeking medical attention within 1 year of symptoms, but patients who have been aware of their tumors for up to 10 years have been noted.

Pathologic Features

Gross specimen examination has shown that these tumors vary in size from less than 1 cm to greater than 6 cm in diameter and are yellowish-gray to gray-white. They have sometimes been multinodular, but generally, they have been poorly demarcated and infiltrative, sometimes even diffusely distributed within and beyond the parotid or submandibular glands.

Nearly universally noted by all investigators has been the histopathologic resemblance of salivary duct carcinoma to that of ductal carcinoma of the breast. Characteristic of salivary duct carcinoma are intraductal or circumscribed nests of dysplastic ductal cells that grow in solid, cribriform, and papillary configurations. Central, comedo-type necrosis of the tumor nests is a distinctive feature (Fig. 27–16). Garland and coworkers[102] required comedonecrosis for the diagnosis of salivary duct carcinoma, but we and others[37, 101, 103, 106] regard comedonecrosis as characteristic but not requisite. Most tumors display a combination of solid, cribriform, and papillary patterns (Fig. 27–17). The circumscribed tumor nests or intraductal growths vary in size, and the larger tumor islands typically have large central cystic spaces. The tumor cells form a rim, several cells thick, around the cystic space (Fig. 27–18).

In addition to the intraductal and circumscribed tumor nests, infiltrative tumor elements are usually evident (Fig. 27–18). This component is typically composed of small clusters of tumor cells that may have small lumina or cribriform arrangements, but solid, irregularly shaped tumor cell aggregates are frequently present. The neoplastic epithelial cells are accompanied by a dense fibrous connective tissue stroma that may be hyalinized in some areas (see Figs. 27–17, 27–18). Invasion of nerves and blood vessels is frequently observed in addition to infiltration of salivary gland lobules and extrasalivary gland tissues, such as fat, muscle, and bone.

The tumor cells are cuboidal and polygonal with a moderate amount of eosinophilic cytoplasm (see Fig. 27–16). Some of the luminal cells have been described as apocrinelike, with prominent apical, eosinophilic cytoplasm;[112] however, we have not found this to be a consistent finding. Cellular and nuclear pleomorphism vary from mild to severe, even from one focus to another within a single tumor. Nucleoli may be noticeable in some of the more pleomorphic cells. Mitotic figures are nearly always evident and may be numerous in some tumors.

Mucicarmine and Alcian blue stains are generally negative, except, perhaps, for a small amount of luminal staining. Immunohistochemical and ultrastructural studies have identified ductal cells but no myoepithelial cells.[102, 103, 106, 112] These findings further emphasize the differences between salivary duct carcinoma and epithelial-myoepithelial carcinoma, which were apparently confused by Kleinsasser and others.[4, 100] Salivary duct carcinoma has been found to be immunoreactive for keratin, variably reactive for epithelial membrane antigen, and unreactive for S-100 protein and myosin.[112] Electron-microscopic investigations have described duct-like structures with basal lamina, luminal cells with microvilli, cuboidal and

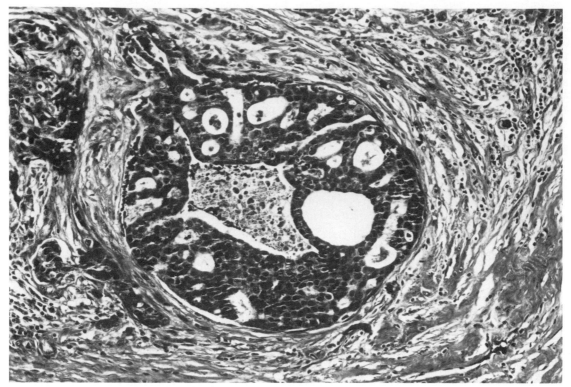

Figure 27–16. Intraductal growth in a cribriform pattern with central comedonecrosis is characteristic of salivary duct carcinoma, although comedonecrosis is not requisite. The tumor cells are cuboidal and polygonal ductal cells. Cytologic features of malignancy, such as cellular and nuclear pleomorphism, nuclear hyperchromatism, and mitotic figures, are usually evident (× 150).

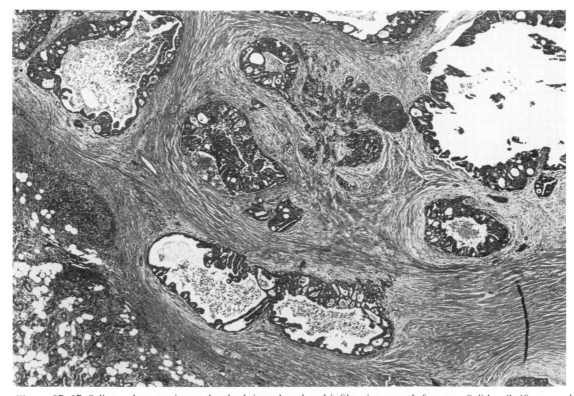

Figure 27–17. Salivary duct carcinoma has both intraductal and infiltrative growth features. Solid, cribriform, and papillary conformations are evident, with large and small cystic spaces and comedonecrosis. The tumor nests are surrounded by a dense fibrous stroma (× 30).

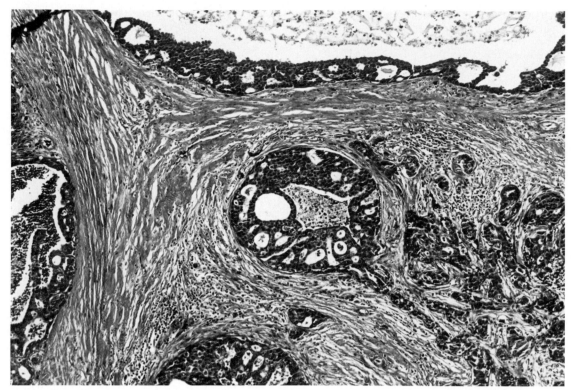

Figure 27–18. Salivary duct carcinoma with large cystic space at the top of the photograph, which is bound by a thin rim of tumor cells in a cribriform pattern. Beneath and to the right of the cystic space, small, solid islands of infiltrative tumor can be seen (× 75).

polygonal cells with slender cisternae of rough endoplasmic reticulum, and moderate numbers of mitochondria, some glycogen, and small desmosomes and tight junctions.[103, 112]

Prognosis and Treatment

Salivary duct carcinoma is a high-grade malignancy that must be treated aggressively. Of the 44 reported cases with at least some follow-up,[37, 100–103, 107, 108] 24 patients died of their tumors; 4 patients died of unrelated causes; 6 patients were alive with recurrent or metastatic tumor; and 10 patients were alive without disease. Only four of the sixteen patients who were living had been followed for longer than 5 years. Most patients died within 3 years of initial therapy. In a summary of the 30 cases reported by M.D. Anderson Hospital and the literature, Hui and colleagues[103] reported, in 1986, that 16 patients had died of tumor. In 1987, Luna and others[112] reviewed these same 30 cases and reported that 21 patients had died of tumor. The implication is that an additional five patients from the M.D. Anderson Hospital died during the interval between these reports. Of the total 44 reported cases with follow-up, distant metastases have developed in 26 patients, and regional lymph node metastatases have developed in 24 patients.

Lung and bone have been the most frequent sites for distant metastases.

Hui and coworkers[103] found that tumors greater than 3 cm in diameter were associated with significantly greater morbidity and mortality than tumors less than 3 cm in diameter.

Complete local excision with radical neck dissection and postoperative radiation therapy seems to offer the most potential for effective treatment of these highly malignant neoplasms.

Differential Diagnosis

Salivary gland carcinomas with ductal and papillary configurations and cells with eosinophilic cytoplasm are considered in the differential diagnosis of salivary duct carcinoma. Such tumors would include acinic cell adenocarcinoma, mucoepidermoid carcinoma, papillary cystadenocarcinoma, oncocytic carcinoma, and polymorphous low-grade adenocarcinoma.

In addition to a papillary cystic pattern, most acinic cell adenocarcinomas contain other tumor growth configurations, including microcystic, solid, and follicular patterns. Furthermore, a number of cell types, including acinar, intercalated duct, vacuolated, clear, and nonspecific glandular, are typically present in acinic cell adenocarcinoma, which contrasts with the one cell type observed in salivary duct carcinoma. Cytologically, the cells of salivary duct carcinoma are more pleomorphic and eosinophilic than those of acinic cell adenocarcinoma. Hyalinized fibrous stroma is characteristic of salivary duct carcinoma but not of acinic cell adenocarcinoma. In addition, an intraductal component is common in salivary duct carcinoma but is not a feature of acinic cell adenocarcinoma.

The presence of epidermoid and mucous cells distinguishes high-grade mucoepidermoid carcinoma from salivary duct carcinoma. Furthermore, high-grade mucoepidermoid carcinoma generally lacks cribriform and papillary growth patterns. Low-grade mucoepidermoid carcinoma does not usually pose a diagnostic problem.

Papillary cystadenocarcinoma, of course, shares papillary and cystic growth patterns with salivary duct carcinoma. However, unlike salivary duct carcinoma, it lacks the cribriform pattern, apocrinelike cells, and comedonecrosis, and it has many columnar cells that are often mucinous.

Oncocytic carcinoma generally lacks the comedonecrosis and papillary and cribriform growth patterns of salivary duct carcinoma. The cells of onocytic carcinoma are larger with more abundant and granular eosinophilic cytoplasm than that seen in the cells of salivary duct carcinoma.

Salivary duct carcinoma principally occurs in the major salivary glands, and polymorphous low-grade adenocarcinoma is a tumor of the minor salivary glands. Polymorphous low-grade adenocarcinoma is characterized by its uniform, bland cytologic features, whereas salivary duct carcinoma is cytologically pleomorphic, with conspicuous mitotic figures. Comedonecrosis is not a feature of polymorphous low-grade adenocarcinoma.

MUCINOUS ADENOCARCINOMA

Mucinous adenocarcinoma of the salivary gland is a rare tumor that has previously been poorly defined. In fact, most classifications of salivary gland tumors do not include this entity (see Chapter 8). Foote and Frazell[113] included a "mucous cell adenocarcinoma" in their classification in 1954. Their histopathologic description was quite limited, and although they stated that "there may be very abundant collections of mucus," we believe that this entity would be categorized as a cystadenocarcinoma in our classification. We consider the same to be true of the "mucous cell adenocarcinoma" of Vellios and Shafer.[114] Evans and Cruickshank[5] used the term *adenocystic carcinoma* in their classification. This may cause some confusion, because *adenocystic carcinoma* is a term that has been used synonymously with the term *mucinous carcinoma* of eccrine origin in the skin.[115] Evans and Cruickshank,[5] however, were referring to the salivary gland tumor that is better called

adenoid cystic carcinoma. The classification of Batsakis[116] contained a category called "mucus-producing adenopapillary and nonpapillary carcinoma;" however, on the basis of the brief histopathologic description provided, we would identify these tumors as cystadenocarcinomas also. Batsakis'[116] classification may have been partly based on the report of "mucus-producing adenopapillary carcinoma" by Blanck and colleagues.[65] However, by our interpretation, Blanck and colleagues[65] described a conglomeration of several tumor types, including acinic cell adenocarcinomas and cystadenocarcinomas. Their *Figure 5* may represent a mucinous adenocarcinoma, but the illustration is insufficient to make a definite identification. Spiro and others[68, 117] included "mucus adenocarcinoma" in their reviews of salivary gland tumors of the minor salivary glands and the parotid gland, but they provided no histologic descriptions. In a later study of 204 previously unclassified adenocarcinomas of the salivary gland, Spiro and coworkers[70] reported 25 "mucinous adenocarcinomas." The two photomicrographs demonstrated tumors that we would classify as cystadenocarcinomas. Main and colleagues[58] also included "mucinous adenocarcinoma" in their survey of 643 salivary gland tumors but provided no clinical or microscopic details.

We would like to make the point in this discussion that mucinous adenocarcinoma, as we define it, is a tumor histopathologically distinct from cystadenocarcinoma (see previous discussion in this chapter). Although the descriptions are sketchy, we believe that the labels *mucous cell adenocarcinoma, mucus-producing adenocarcinoma,* and *mucinous adenocarcinoma,* as they are used by previous authors, include a number of tumor types with the common feature of mucus-secreting cells. Most of these previously reported tumors are cystadenocarcinomas. In fact, Seifert and Schulz[118] found distinct mucus production in 40 percent of the salivary gland adenocarcinomas that they studied.

Mucinous adenocarcinoma has been reported in many sites other than the salivary glands, including the skin,[119] breast,[120] ovary,[121] cervix,[122] uterus,[123] rectum,[124] colon,[125] pancreas,[126] prostate gland,[127] urinary bladder,[128] trachea,[129] stomach,[130] appendix,[131] esophagus,[132] and lung.[133] Just as in salivary glands, however, many of these neoplasms have the same characteristics as those of mucus-secreting cystadenocarcinomas. However, the salivary gland tumors that we identify as mucinous adenocarcinomas have a marked resemblance to the mucinous carcinomas that have been described in the skin and breast. In fact, this similarity to the skin and breast tumors, as well as their unique histopathologic features, warrants their segregation from other salivary gland carcinomas, despite their rarity.

Only two cases of mucinous adenocarcinoma are on file in the registry of salivary gland pathology at the AFIP. We suspect a few more cases might be reclassifiable as such if all cases of adenocarcinoma were reevaluated today, since there has been no long-term consensus on the application of this diagnosis.

Clinical Features

As evident from the review of the literature above, it is impossible to derive any meaningful information on the clinical and biologic characteristics of this tumor. Both of the tumors in the AFIP files involved the submandibular gland. The patients, a man and a woman, were 41 and 68 years old, respectively. Clinically, these lesions are soft, spongy masses that may be thought to be cysts.

Pathologic Features

The gross specimens are very mucoid, with a slimy texture, and they may actually ooze mucoid material. Because of this lack of cohesiveness, piecemeal excision of this tumor runs the risk of seeding the surgical site with tumor. These tumors are circumscribed but not encapsulated.

Low-magnification microscopic examination reveals islands and cords of tumor cells that appear to be floating within pools of pale-staining mucin (Fig. 27–19). The pools of mucin may be divided into irregular lobules by fibrous connective tissue septa that course through the tumor. Microscopy confirms that the tumor is unencapsulated.

The tumor cells are moderately large, cuboidal, and polygonal cells, with eosinophilic to amphophilic cytoplasm. The nuclei are vesicular, and scattered mitotic figures may be found. Minimal to modest cellular and nuclear pleomorphism can be seen. The epithelial cells are arranged in irregular groups or cords that may anastomose (Fig. 27–20). The tumor islands are surrounded by a pale-staining mucoid substance. Pseudolumina may occur within many tumor nests, and in other areas, it can be seen that some "lumina" are only partially surrounded by epithelial cells and may communicate with the encasing mucoid substance.

The mucoid substance stains with mucicarmine, periodic acid–Schiff, and Alcian blue at pH 2.0. Mucicarmine stain also reveals that many, but not most, tumor cells contain intracytoplasmic mucin.

Differential Diagnosis

From the foregoing discussion, it is evident that cystadenocarcinoma, either papillary or nonpapillary, is the principal entity in the differential diagnosis of mucinous adenocarcinoma. By our definition, the distinctive histopathologic feature distinguishing mucinous adenocarcinoma from a

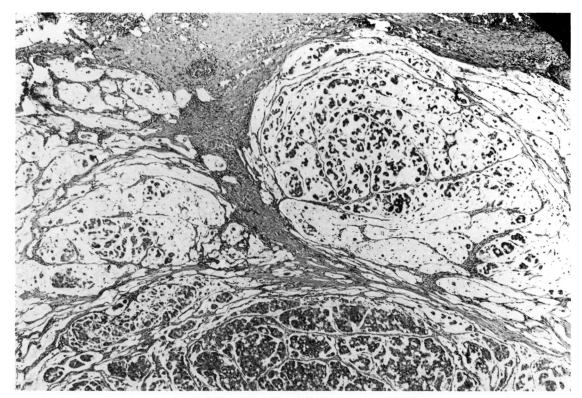

Figure 27–19. Mucinous adenocarcinoma of the submandibular gland is characterized by islands of tumor cells within pools of mucin. The mucin pools are traversed by fibrous connective tissue septa (× 30).

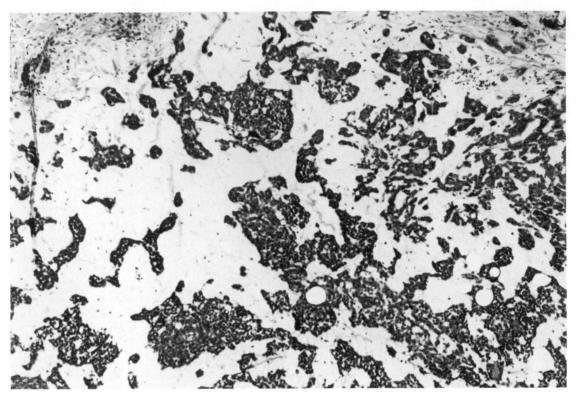

Figure 27–20. Anastomosing cords of epithelial cells in a mucinous adenocarcinoma are surrounded by mucoid substance. Occasional pseudolumina that are contiguous with the surrounding mucin pools in some areas can be seen (× 75).

mucus-producing cystadenocarcinoma is the relationship of the epithelial tumor cells to the mucoid product. In mucus-producing cystadenocarcinoma, the epithelial cells, for the most part, surround and confine the mucoid substance. The cystic structures are lined by epithelial cells and are supported by fibrous connective tissue. Occasionally, rupture of a cyst may occur with escape of mucin into the connective tissues, but this does not alter the overall architecture of the tumor. In contrast, the epithelial cells in mucinous adenocarcinoma are surrounded by the mucoid substance, which appears to be confined by the supporting fibrous tissue. Epithelium-lined cysts are minimal.

The marked similarity between mucinous carcinomas of eccrine and mucinous adenocarcinoma of salivary gland origin may make distinction between them impossible on a morphologic basis. A determination must be made as to whether the tumor appears to have arisen in the cutaneous tissues or in the salivary gland.

Prognosis and Treatment

No previous experience on which to determine a prognosis for patients with this tumor exists. Patients with similar tumors in the skin and breast seem to have a relatively better prognosis than patients with other types of carcinoma. The behavior of these tumors in the skin is characterized as frequently recurrent and sometimes regionally metastatic, but it rarely involves distant metastases. In the breast, they are slow growing, but a number of long-term survivors eventually die as a result of the tumors. Complete excision with care to avoid seeding the surgical site would seem to be a prudent course of treatment for these salivary gland tumors.

MYOEPITHELIAL CARCINOMA

Myoepithelial carcinoma is another rare salivary gland neoplasm that is not included in most classifications (see Chapter 8). Although not included within the first World Health Organization classification,[1] we understand that it is to be listed in the second World Health Organization classification of salivary gland neoplasms that was in preparation at the same time as this text. We define *myoepithelial carcinoma* as a malignant epithelial neoplasm whose tumor cells demonstrate cytologic differentiation toward myoepithelial cells and lack ductal or acinar differentiation.

Our review of the literature located only five possible cases of myoepithelial carcinoma.[134–138] One of these was inadequately documented, and

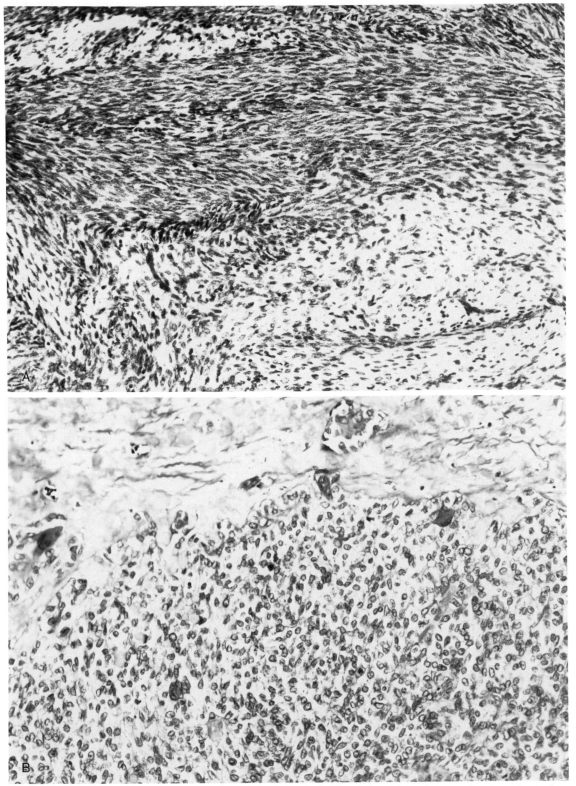

Figure 27–21. *A*, Cellular spindle cell area in malignant myoepithelioma is adjacent to myxoid zone (× 150). *B*, In this example cellular zones were composed of tumor cells with round to ovoid nuclei and indistinct cytoplasm (× 150).

the accuracy of the diagnosis is open to question.[134] In 1943, Sheldon[134] reported a series of 54 "so-called mixed tumors of the salivary glands." He defined a subgroup of these tumors that he labeled as myoepithelioma. On this subgroup he commented, "Only in one instance did the basket cells display evidence of low-grade cancer." In the other cases, myoepithelial differentiation was established by electron microscopy or immunohistochemistry or both. Among these four documented cases, three were in the parotid gland and one occurred in the maxillary gingiva and alveolar mucosa. Two patients were men, and two were women. They were 14, 66, 81, and 86 years of age. Five cases of myoepithelial carcinoma have also been accessed in the files of the AFIP. Three tumors occurred in the parotid gland, one in the submandibular gland, and one in the upper lip. The patients ranged in age from 40 to 85 years.

The cytologic features of individual cells and the general morphologic features resemble tumor cells in benign myoepithelioma and the myoepithelial cells of mixed tumor. The tumor cells may be spindle-shaped (Fig. 27–21A) or more rounded (Fig. 27–21B), sometimes with eosinophilic cytoplasm and eccentric nuclei, so-called hyaline or plasmacytoid cells. The cell types are often intermixed, but usually one or the other cell type predominates. The tumors may be quite cellular and more suggestive of sarcoma than carcinoma. The stroma in other areas of the tumors may be more conspicuous and myxoid. These tumors are distinguished from benign myoepithelial neoplasms by their infiltrative, destructive growth (Fig. 27–22). They usually demonstrate increased mitotic activity and cytologic pleomorphism.

Although reactions may be variable, immunohistochemistry can help identify the myoepithelial nature of these tumors. Some tumor cells should be immunoreactive for cytokeratin, S-100 protein, smooth muscle actin, and occasionally, glial fibrillary acidic protein. Ultrastructurally, the most prominent feature is the presence of bundles or loose arrays of actinlike microfilaments. Subplasmalemmal condensations may be found in some cells as well as pinocytotic vesicles, desmosomes, and basement membrane material.

Although local invasion and destruction characterize all of these tumors, metastasis, to an inguinal lymph node, has been reported in only one case.[136] Too few cases are available to make therapeutic judgments, but wide surgical excision seems to be preferred.

The tumor reported by Singh and Cawson[138] arose in a benign mixed tumor, but in the other cases, the tumors appeared to have arisen de novo.

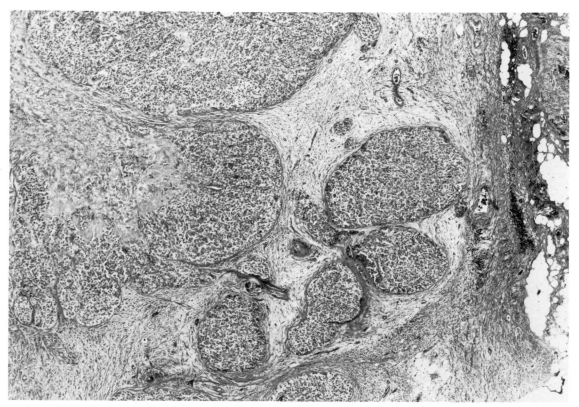

Figure 27–22. Low magnification of malignant myoepithelioma shows infiltration of connective tissue by tumor islands of various sizes that extend from the central tumor mass. Tumor necrosis is seen at left (× 30).

The absence of ductal, acinar, or squamous cell differentiation identifies myoepithelial carcinoma as distinct from carcinosarcoma and other salivary gland carcinomas. Differentiation from sarcoma is more problematic and may depend on the immunohistochemical markers noted previously.

REFERENCES

1. Thackray AC, Sobin LH: Histological Typing of Salivary Gland Tumours. Geneva, World Health Organization, 1972; 16.
2. Batsakis JG: Tumors of the Head and Neck: Clinical and Pathological Considerations, 2nd Ed. Baltimore, Williams & Wilkins Co, 1979; 9.
3. Thackray AC, Lucas RB: Tumors of the Major Salivary Glands, Fascicle 10. Atlas of Tumor Pathology, 2nd Series. Washington, DC, Armed Forces Institute of Pathology, 1974; 14.
4. Seifert G, Miehlke A, Haubrich J, Chilla R: Diseases of the Salivary Glands: Pathology-Diagnosis-Treatment-Facial Nerve Surgery. Stuttgart, Georg Thieme Verlag, 1986; 171.
5. Evans RW, Cruickshank AH: Epithelial Tumours of the Salivary Glands. Philadelphia, WB Saunders Co, 1970; 19.
6. Cerezo L, Alvarez M, Edwards O, Price G: Adenosquamous carcinoma of the colon. Dis Colon Rectum 1985; 28:597–603.
7. Griesser GH, Schumacher U, Elfeldt R, Horny HP: Adenosquamous carcinoma of the ileum: Report of a case and review of the literature. Virchows Arch [A] 1985; 406:483–487.
8. Weidner N, Foucar E: Adenosquamous carcinoma of the skin: An aggressive mucin- and gland-forming squamous carcinoma. Arch Dermatol 1985; 121:775–779.
9. Fitzgibbons PL, Kern WH: Adenosquamous carcinoma of the lung: A clinical and pathologic study of seven cases. Hum Pathol 1985; 16:463–466.
10. Larraza-Hernandez O, Henson DE, Albores-Saavedra J: The ultrastructure of gallbladder carcinoma. Acta Morphol Hung 1984; 32:279–293.
11. Tsukamoto N, Matsukuma K, Daimaru Y, Ota M: Cytologic presentation of ovarian adenosquamous carcinoma in ascitic fluid: A case report. Acta Cytol 1984; 28:703–705.
12. Moore S, Gold RP, Lebwohl O, Price JB, Lefkowitch JH: Adenosquamous carcinoma of the liver arising in biliary cystadenocarcinoma: Clinical, radiologic, and pathologic features with review of the literature. J Clin Gastroenterol 1984; 6:267–275.
13. Saito R, Davis BK, Ollapally EP: Adenosquamous carcinoma of the prostate. Hum Pathol 1984; 15:87–89.
14. Mingazzini PL, Barsotti P, Malchiodi Albedi F: Adenosquamous carcinoma of the stomach: Histological, histochemical and ultrastructural observations. Histopathology 1983; 7:433–443.
15. Howat AJ, Scott E, Mackie DB, Pinkerton JR: Adenosquamous carcinoma of the renal pelvis. Am J Clin Pathol 1983; 79:731–733.
16. Alberhasky RC, Connelly PJ, Christopherson WM: Carcinoma of the endometrium. IV. Mixed adenosquamous carcinoma: A clinical-pathological study of 68 cases with long-term follow-up. Am J Clin Pathol 1982; 77:655–664.
17. Saito R: An adenosquamous carcinoma of the male urethra with hypercalcemia. Hum Pathol 1981; 12:383–385.
18. Imm FC: Primary adenosquamous carcinoma of the fallopian tube. South Med J 1980; 73:678–680.
19. Ishikawa O, Matsui Y, Aoki I, Iwanaga T, Terasawa T, Wada A: Adenosquamous carcinoma of the pancreas: A clinicopathologic study and report of three cases. Cancer 1980; 46:1192–1196.
20. Shimaoka K, Tsukada Y: Squamous cell carcinomas and adenosquamous carcinomas originating from the thyroid gland. Cancer 1980; 46:1833–1842.
21. Damiani JM, Damiani KK, Hauck K, Hyams VJ: Mucoepidermoid-adenosquamous carcinoma of the larynx and hypopharynx: A report of 21 cases and a review of the literature. Otolaryngol Head Neck Surg 1981; 89:235–243.
22. Gerughty RM, Hennigar GR, Brown RM: Adenosquamous carcinoma of the nasal, oral and laryngeal cavities: A clinicopathologic survey of ten cases. Cancer 1968; 22:1140–1155.
23. Siar CH, Ng KH: Adenosquamous carcinoma of the floor of the mouth and lower alveolus: A radiation-induced lesion? Oral Surg Oral Med Oral Pathol 1987; 63:216–220.
24. Sanner JR: Combined adenosquamous carcinoma and ductal adenoma of the hard and soft palate: Report of case. J Oral Surg 1979; 37:331–334.
25. Shafer WG, Hine MK, Levy BM: A Textbook of Oral Pathology, 4th Ed. Philadelphia, WB Saunders Co, 1983; 131.
26. Langhans T: Uber die epithelialen Formen der malignen Struma. Virchows Arch [A] 1907; 189:69–188.
27. Bauer WH, Bauer JD: Classification of glandular tumors of salivary glands. Study of one hundred forty-three cases. Arch Pathol 1953; 55:328–346.
28. Sikorowa L: Oncocytoma malignum. Nowotwor 1957; 7:125–131.
29. Hamperl H: Benign and malignant oncocytoma. Cancer 1962; 15:1019–1027.
30. Marucci I, Fontana R, Mercado D: Gli oncocytomi della parotid. Arch Ital Otol 1962; 73:756–775.
31. Eneroth CM: Oncocytoma of major salivary glands. J Laryngol 1965; 79:1064–1072.
32. Briggs J, Evans JNG: Malignant oxyphilic granular-cell tumor (oncocytoma) of the palate: Review of the recent literature and report of a case. Oral Surg Oral Med Oral Pathol 1967; 23:796–802.
33. Loke YW: Salivary gland tumors in Malaya. Br J Cancer 1967; 21:665–674.
34. Baziz-Malik G, Gupta DN: Metastasizing (malignant) oncocytoma of the parotid gland. Z Krebsforch 1968; 70:193–197.
35. Abioye AA: Malignant oncocytoma (oxyphilic granular cell tumour) of the parotid gland. East Afr Med J 1972; 49:235–239.
36. Mair IWS, Johannessen TA: Benign and malignant oncocytoma of the parotid gland. Laryngoscope 1972; 82:638–642.
37. Fayemi AO, Toker C: Malignant oncocytoma of the parotid gland. Arch Otolaryngol 1974; 99:375–376.

38. Gray SR, Cornog JL, Seo IS: Oncocytic neoplasms of salivary glands: A report of 15 cases including 2 malignant oncocytomas. Cancer 1976; 38:1306–1317.

39. Lee SC, Roth LM: Malignant oncocytoma of the parotid gland: A light and electron microscopic study. Cancer 1976; 37:1607–1614.

40. Leventon G, Katz DR, Bell CD: Malignant oncocytic tumor of the parotid salivary gland. J Laryngol Otol 1976; 90:289–293.

41. Ross CF: Malignant oncocytoma (oxyphilic granular-cell tumour) of the parotid gland. Clin Oncol 1976; 2:253–260.

42. Johns ME, Regezi JA, Batsakis JG: Oncocytic neoplasms of salivary glands: An ultrastructural study. Laryngoscope 1977; 87:862–871.

43. Laurian N, Zohar Y, Kende L: Malignant oncocytoma. J Laryngol Otol 1977; 91:805–808.

44. Miyaguchi M, Ishida M, Ogino S, Tanaki H: Malignant oncocytoma of the parotid gland. Nippon Jibunkalsa Gakkai Kaiho 1981; 84:272–274.

45. Chu W, Strawitz JG: Oncocytoma of the parotid gland with malignant change. Arch Surg 1978; 113:318–319.

46. Goode RK, Corio RL: Oncocytic adenocarcinoma of salivary glands. Oral Surg Oral Med Oral Pathol 1988; 65:61–66.

47. Mahmoud N: Malignant oncocytoma of the nasal cavity. J Laryngol Otol 1979; 93:729–734.

48. DiMaio SJ, DiMaio VJM, DiMaio TM, Nicastri AD, Chen CK: Oncocytic carcinoma of the nasal cavity. South Med J 1980; 73:803–806.

49. Meijer SM, Hoitsma HFW: Malignant intrathoracic oncocytoma. Cancer 1982; 49:97–100.

50. Takeda A, Matsuyama M, Sugimoto Y, Suzumori K, Ishiwata T, Ishida S, Nakanishi Y: Oncocytic adenocarcinoma of the ovary. Virchows Arch [A] 1983; 399:345–353.

51. Rainwater LM, Farrow GM, Hay ID, Lieber MM: Oncocytic tumours of the salivary gland, kidney, and thyroid: Nuclear DNA patterns studied by flow cytometry. Br J Cancer 1986; 53:799–804.

52. Frazell EL, Duffy BJ: Hurthle cell cancer of the thyroid: A review of 40 cases. Cancer 1951; 41:952–956.

53. Batsakis JG: Tumors of the Head and Neck: Clinical and Pathologic Considerations, 2nd Ed. Baltimore, Williams & Wilkins Co, 1979; 57–62.

54. Foote FW Jr, Frazell EL: Tumors of the major salivary glands. Cancer 1953; 6:1065–1133.

55. Evans RW, Cruickshank AH: Epithelial Tumours of the Salivary Glands. Philadelphia, WB Saunders Co, 1970.

56. Thackray AC, Lucas RB: Tumors of the Major Salivary Glands, Fascicle 10. Atlas of Tumor Pathology, 2nd Series. Washington, DC, Armed Forces Institute of Pathology, 1974.

57. Thackray AC, Sobin LH: Histologic Typing of Salivary Gland Tumours. Geneva, World Health Organization, 1972.

58. Main JHP, Orr JA, McGurk FM, McComb RJ, Mock D: Salivary gland tumors: Review of 643 cases. J Oral Pathol 1976; 5:88–102.

59. Chaudhry AP, Vickers RA, Gorlin RJ: Intraoral minor salivary gland tumors: An analysis of 1,414 cases. Oral Surg Oral Med Oral Pathol 1961; 14:1194–1226.

60. Bhargava S, Sant MS, Arora MM: Histomorpho-

logic spectrum of tumours of minor salivary glands. Indian J Cancer 1982; 19:134–140.

61. Yu G-Y, Ma D-Q: Carcinoma of the salivary glands: A clinicopathologic study of 405 cases. Sem Surg Oncol 1987; 3:240–244.

62. Ma D-Q, Yu G-Y: Tumours of the minor salivary glands: A clinicopathologic study of 243 cases. Acta Otolaryngol (Stockh) 1987; 103:325–331.

63. Rawson AJ, Howard JM, Royster HP, Horn RC Jr: Tumors of the salivary glands: A clinicopathologic study of 160 cases. Cancer 1950; 3:225–458.

64. Eneroth C-M: Histological and clinical aspects of parotid tumors. Acta Otolaryngol (Suppl) 1964; 191:1–99.

65. Blanck C, Eneroth C-M, Jakobsson PA: Mucus-producing adenopapillary (non-epidermoid) carcinoma of the parotid gland. Cancer 1971; 28:676–685.

66. Eneroth C-M: Salivary gland tumors in the parotid gland, submandibular gland, and the palate region. Cancer 1971; 27:1415–1418.

67. Stene T, Koppang HS: Intraoral adenocarcinomas. J Oral Pathol 1981; 10:216–225.

68. Spiro RH, Koss LG, Hajdu SI, Strong EW: Tumors of minor salivary origin: A clinicopathologic study of 492 cases. Cancer 1973; 31:117–129.

69. Seifert G, Miehlke A, Haubrich J, Chilla R: Diseases of the Salivary Glands: Pathology-Diagnosis-Treatment-Facial Nerve Surgery. Stuttgart, Georg Thieme Verlag, 1986; 248–252.

70. Spiro RH, Huvos AG, Strong EW: Adenocarcinoma of salivary origin: Clinicopathologic study of 204 patients. Am J Surg 1982; 144:423–430.

71. Whittaker JS, Turner EP: Papillary tumours of the minor salivary glands. J Clin Pathol 1976; 29:795–805.

72. Allen MS Jr, Fitz-Hugh GS, March WL Jr: Low-grade papillary adenocarcinoma of the palate. Cancer 1974; 33:153–158.

73. Fliss DM, Zirkin H, Puterman M, Tovi F: Low-grade papillary adenocarcinoma of buccal mucosa salivary gland origin. Head Neck Surg 1989; 11:237–241.

74. Mills SE, Garland TA, Allen MS Jr: Low-grade papillary adenocarcinoma of palatal salivary gland origin. Am J Surg Pathol 1984; 8:367–374.

75. Slootweg PJ, Müller H: Low-grade adenocarcinoma of the oral cavity: A comparison between the terminal duct and the papillary type. J Craniomaxillofac Surg 1987; 15:359–364.

76. Frierson HF Jr, Mills SE, Garland TA: Terminal duct carcinoma of minor salivary glands. Am J Clin Pathol 1985; 84:8–14.

77. Ellis GE, Corio RL: Acinic cell adenocarcinoma: A clinicopathologic analysis of 294 cases. Cancer 1983; 52:542–549.

78. Spiro RH: Salivary neoplasms: Overview of 35-year experience with 2,807 patients. Head Neck Surg 1986; 8:177–184.

79. Gnepp DR, Brannon R: Sebaceous neoplasms of salivary gland origin: Report of 21 cases. Cancer 1984; 53:2155–2170.

80. Gnepp DR: Sebaceous neoplasms of salivary gland origin: A review. In Sommers S, Rosen PP (eds): Pathol Ann, Part 1. 1983; 18:71–102.

81. Pageaut G, Oppermann A, Carbillet JP: La meta-

plasie "sebacee" de la parotide normale, inflam-matorie et tumorale. Arch Anat Pathol (Paris) 1969; 17:101–105.

82. Batsakis JG, Littler ER, Leahy MS: Sebaceous cell lesions of the head and neck. Arch Otolaryngol 1972; 95:151–157.

83. Takashi T, Ogawa I, Nikai H: Sebaceous carcinoma of the parotid gland, an immunohistochemical and ultrastructural study. Virchows Arch [A] 1989; 414:459–464.

84. Granstrom G, Aldenborg F, Jeppsson P-H: Sebaceous carcinoma of the parotid gland: Report of a case and review of the literature. J Oral Maxillofac Surg 1987; 45:731–733.

85. Hayashi Y, Takemoto T, Tokuoka S, Tagashira N, Yazin K, Harada Y: Sebaceous carcinoma of the parotid gland: Report of a case. Byori To Rinsho 1985; 3:1135–41.

86. Miyamoto K, Yanagawa T, Azuma M, Aladib W, Yura Y, Kobayashi S, Yoshida H, Sato M: Establishment of a transformed human epithelial cell line with a sebaceous cell phenotype and effect of epidermal growth factor and dibutyryl cyclic adenosine 3':5'-mono-phosphate on the cellular phenotype. The Cancer Journal 1989; 3:414–422.

87. MacFarland JK, Vilori JB, Palmer JD: Sebaceous cell carcinoma of the parotid gland. Am J Surg 1975; 130:499–501.

88. Shulman J, Waisman J, Morledge D: Sebaceous carcinoma of the parotid gland. Arch Otolaryngol 1973; 98:417–421.

89. Akhtar M, Gosalbez TG, Brody H: Primary sebaceous carcinoma of the parotid gland. Arch Pathol 1973; 96:161–163.

90. Cheek R, Pitcock JA: Sebaceous lesions of the parotid: Report of two cases. Arch Pathol 1966; 82:147–150.

91. Schmid KO, Albrich W: Die Bedeutung von Talgzellen und Talgdrüsen für Parotisgeschwülste. Virchows Arch [A] 1973; 359:239–253.

92. Constant E, Leahy MS: Sebaceous cell carcinoma. Plast Reconst Surg 1968; 41:433–437.

93. Kleinsasser O, Hübner G, Klein HJ: Talgzellcarcinom der Parotis. Arch Klin Exp Ohren Nasen Kehlkopfheilk 1970; 197:59–71.

94. Silver H, Goldstein MA: Sebaceous cell carcinoma of the parotid region: A review of the literature and a case report. Cancer 1966; 19:1773–1779.

95. Mathis VH: Beitrag zur kenntnis der sialome. Dtsch Zahn-Mund Kiefer 1968; 50:205–208.

96. Assor D: Epidermoid carcinoma with sebaceous differentiation in the vallecula: Report of a case. Am J Clin Pathol 1975; 63:891–894.

97. Rauch S, Masshoff W: Die talgdrusenahnlichen sialome. Frank Zeit Pathol 1959; 69:513–525.

98. Linhartova A: Sebaceous glands in salivary gland tissue. Arch Pathol 1974; 98:320–324.

99. Boniuk M, Zimmerman LE: Sebaceous carcinoma of the eyelid, eyebrow, caruncle, and orbit. Trans Am Acad Ophthal Otolaryngol 1968; 72:619–642.

100. Kleinsasser O, Klein HJ, Hübner G: Speichelgangearcinom: Ein den Milchgangcarcinomen der Brustdrüse Analoge Gruppe von Speichldrüsentumoren. Arch Klin Exp Ohren Nasen Kehlkopfheilk 1968; 192:100–115.

101. Chen KTK, Hafez GR: Infiltrating salivary duct carcinoma: A clinicopathologic study of five cases. Arch Otolaryngol 1981; 107:37–39.

102. Garland TA, Innes DJ, Fechner RE: Salivary duct carcinoma: An analysis of four cases with review of literature. Am J Clin Pathol 1984; 81:436–441.

103. Hui KK, Batsakis JG, Luna MA, Mackay B, Byers RM: Salivary duct adenocarcinoma: A high grade malignancy. J Laryngol Otol 1986; 100:105–114.

104. Fayemi AO, Toker C: Salivary duct carcinoma. Arch Otolaryngol 1974; 99:366–368.

105. Pesce C, Colacino R, Buffa P: Duct carcinoma of the minor salivary glands: A case report. J Laryngol Otol 1986; 100:611–613.

106. de Araujo VC, de Souza SOM, Sesso A, Sotto MN, de Araujo NS: Salivary duct carcinoma: Ultrastructural and histogenetic considerations. Oral Surg Oral Med Oral Pathol 1987; 63:592–596.

107. Afzelius LE, Cameron WR, Svensson C: Salivary duct carcinoma—a clinicopathologic study of 12 cases. Head Neck Surg 1987; 9:151–156.

108. Zohar Y, Shem-Tov Y, Gal R: Salivary duct carcinoma in major and minor salivary glands: A clinicopathological analysis of four cases. J Craniomaxillofac Surg 1988; 16:320–323.

109. Gal R, Strauss M, Zohar Y, Kessler E: Salivary duct carcinoma of the parotid gland: Cytologic and histopathologic study. Acta Cytol 1985; 29:454–456.

110. Seifert G, Miehlke A, Haubrich J, Chilla R: Diseases of the Salivary Glands: Pathology-Diagnosis-Treatment-Facial Nerve Surgery. Stuttgart, Georg Thieme Verlag, 1986; 265–267.

111. Takata T, Caselitz J, Seifert G: Undifferentiated tumours of salivary glands: Immunocytochemical investigations and differential diagnosis of 22 cases. Pathol Res Pract 1987; 182:161–168.

112. Luna MA, Batsakis JG, Ordonez NG, Mackay B, Tortoledo ME: Salivary gland adenocarcinomas: A clinicopathologic analysis of three distinctive types. Semin Diagn Pathol 1987; 4:117–135.

113. Foote FW Jr, Frazell EL: Tumors of the Major Salivary Glands. Section IV, Fascicle 11. Atlas of Tumor Pathology. Washington, DC, Armed Forces Institute of Pathology, 1954; 114–115.

114. Vellios F, Shafer WG: Tumors of the intraoral accessory salivary glands. Surg Gynecol Obstet 1959; 198:450–456.

115. Mendoza S, Helwig EB: Mucinous (adenocystic) carcinoma of the skin. Arch Dermatol 1971; 103:68–78.

116. Batsakis JG: Tumors of the Head and Neck: Clinical and Pathological Considerations, 2nd Ed. Baltimore, Williams & Wilkins, 1979; 44–45.

117. Spiro RH, Huvos AG, Strong EW: Cancer of the parotid gland: A clinicopathologic study of 288 primary cases. Am J Surg 1975; 130:452–459.

118. Seifert G, Schulz JP: Das Adenokarzinom der Speicheldrüsen: Pathohistologie und Subklassifikation von 77 Fällen. HNO 1985; 33:433–442.

119. Balin AK, Fine RM, Golitz LE: Mucinous carcinoma. J Dermatol Surg Oncol 1988; 14:521–524.

120. Clayton F: Pure mucinous carcinomas of breast: Morphologic features and prognostic correlates. Hum Pathol 1986; 17:34–38.

121. Boyer M, Friedlander M, Bannatyne P, Atkinson K: Hypercalcemia in association with mucinous adenocarcinoma of the ovary: A case report. Gynecol Oncol 1989; 35:387–390.

122. Young RH, Scully RE: Mucinous ovarian tumors

associated with mucinous adenocarcinomas of the cervix: A clinicopathological analysis of 16 cases. Int J Gynecol Pathol 1988; 7:99–111.

123. Melhem MF, Tobon H: Mucinous adenocarcinoma of the endometrium: A clinico-pathological review of 18 cases. Int J Gynecol Pathol 1987; 6:347–355.

124. Sasaki M, Terada T, Nakanuma Y, Kono N, Kasahara Y, Watanabe K: Anorectal mucinous adenocarcinoma associated with latent perianal Paget's disease. Am J Gastroenterol 1990; 85:199–202.

125. Okuno M, Kehara T, Nagayama M, Kato Y, Yui S, Umeyama K: Mucinous colorectal carcinoma: Clinical pathology and prognosis. Am Surg 1988; 54:681–685.

126. Ordóñez NG, Balsaver AM, Mackay B: Mucinous islet cell (amphicrine) carcinoma of the pancreas associated with watery diarrhea and hypokalemia syndrome. Hum Pathol 1988; 19:1458–1461.

127. Odom DG, Donatucci CF, Deshon GE: Mucinous adenocarcinoma of the prostate. Hum Pathol 1986; 17:863–865.

128. Young RH, Parkhurst EC: Mucinous adenocarcinoma of bladder: Case associated with extensive intestinal metaplasia of urothelium in patient with nonfunctioning bladder for twelve years. Urology 1984; 24:192–195.

129. Reed DN Jr, Hassan AA, Wilson RF: Primary mucinous adenocarcinoma of the trachea: The case for complete surgical resection. J Surg Oncol 1985; 28:29–31.

130. Libson E, Bloom RA, Blank P, Emerson DS: Calcified mucinous adenocarcinoma of the stomach—the CT appearances. Comput Radiol 1985; 9:255–258.

131. Skaane P, Sauer T, Jerve F: Mucinous adenocarcinoma of the appendix presenting as an ovarian cystadenocarcinoma: Case report and review of appendiceal neoplasms with ovarian metastases. Eur J Surg Oncol 1986; 12:379–384.

132. Pope TL Jr: Mucinous adenocarcinoma of the esophagus metastatic to a spinal fusion. Semin Roentgenol 1987; 22:137–138.

133. Kish JK, Ro JY, Ayala AG, McMurtrey MJ: Primary mucinous adencarcinoma of the lung with signet-ring cells: A histochemical comparison with signet-ring cell carcinomas of other sites. Hum Pathol 1989; 20:1097–1102.

134. Sheldon WH: So-called mixed tumors of the salivary glands. Arch Pathol 1943; 35:1–20.

135. Stromeyer FW, Haggitt RC, Nelson JF, Hardman JM: Myoepithelioma of minor salivary gland origin: Light and electron microscopical study. Arch Pathol 1975; 99:242–245.

136. Crissman JD, Wirman JA, Harris A: Malignant myoepithelioma of the parotid gland. Cancer 1977; 40:3042–3049.

137. Dardick I: Malignant myoepithelioma of parotid salivary gland. Ultrastruct Pathol 1985; 9:163–168.

138. Singh R, Cawson RA: Malignant myoepithelial carcinoma (myoepithelioma) arising in a pleomorphic adenoma of the parotid gland: An immunohistochemical study and review of the literature. Oral Surg Oral Med Oral Pathol 1988; 66:65–70.

28

BENIGN MESENCHYMAL NEOPLASMS

R. Keith McDaniel

Benign neoplasms of mesenchymal origin that involve or encroach on the major salivary glands are often difficult to diagnose. Similar to a benign tumor arising from salivary gland parenchyma or ducts, a tumor of mesenchymal origin usually presents as an asymptomatic, slowly growing, well-circumscribed mass in the preauricular, submandibular, or—less frequently—submental region. The preoperative evaluation of such tumors often is perplexing if based primarily on the clinical features and medical history.

This chapter presents the pertinent features of those benign mesenchymal salivary gland tumors that have been recorded in the files of the Armed Forces Institute of Pathology (AFIP). The clinical and microscopic features, biologic behavior, and recommended treatment of tumors arising from tissues that include nerves, blood and lymphatic vessels, fibrous connective tissue, adipose tissue, and smooth muscle are discussed.

The 220 cases of benign mesenchymal tumors affecting major salivary glands in the AFIP files represent 1.4 percent of all salivary gland tumors accessioned. Of this group, 30.5 percent were neural tumors, 30.0 percent hemangiomas, 18.5 percent fibrous tumors, 9.0 percent lipomas, 7.0 percent lymphangiomas, and 5.0 percent other miscellaneous tumors (Table 28–1).

The parotid gland was the anatomic site for 87.5 percent of the benign mesenchymal tumors, whereas the submandibular gland accounted for 12.0 percent. Only one tumor (granular cell tumor) occurred in the sublingual gland. The specific major gland involved was not reported in five cases. Although mesenchymal tumors certainly involve the minor salivary glands of the oral and nasal regions, they were not included in this review because of the diffuse distribution of the glands and the lack of distinct boundaries. The striking predominance of mesenchymal tumors in the pa-

rotid gland, when compared with other major salivary glands, is attributed to anatomic differences; the parotid gland lacks a well-defined capsule and contains neurovascular structures.[1]

A 3 to 2 predominance of female patients was found among 143 civilian cases in the AFIP registry. Cases from military sources had a high male to female ratio. With the exception of lymphangiomas and hemangiomas, the occurrence of mesenchymal tumors was fairly even throughout the first 8 decades of life. Ninety-one percent of the lymphangiomas and 90 percent of the hemangiomas arose in patients during their first 3 decades of life (Fig. 28–1).

Valuable clinical information may be obtained through manual or bimanual palpation to check mobility of the mass, skin fixation, and the relationship of the mass to other structures.[2] Tumors in the parapharyngeal space, such as those arising in the deep lobe of the parotid gland, may not produce clinically obvious swelling until they are quite large in size. In those cases, the initial symptoms may be throat discomfort, swallowing problems, or airway obstruction.[2]

Because the histologic appearances of benign mesenchymal tumors are well described in other texts and because the main purpose of this chapter is to describe these entities as they occur in the salivary glands as well as to discuss their differential diagnoses, microscopic descriptions are brief.

TUMORS OF BLOOD AND LYMPHATIC VESSELS

Hemangioma

Of the various nonepithelial tumors affecting major salivary glands, hemangioma is one of the

Table 28–1. Benign Mesenchymal Tumors in the AFIP Salivary Gland Registry Listed According to the Histologic Type of Tumor and the Gender of the Patient

Type of Tumor	Males*	Females*	Sex Not Stated	Total	Percentage
Vascular/Lymphatic					
Hemangioma	17 (2)	35 (2)	11	67	30.0
Lymphangioma	4 (6)	2	4	16	7.0
Neural Tumors					
Neurilemoma	10 (10)	15	1	36	16.0
Neurofibroma	7 (5)	10	9	31	14.0
Meningioma	—	1	—	1	0.5
Adipose Tissue					
Lipoma	4 (10)	1	4	19	9.0
Fibrous Tissue					
Nodular fasciitis	10 (4)	3		17	8.0
Fibrous histiocytoma	3 (1)	5	2	11	5.0
Fibromatosis	3	4	1	8	3.5
Myxoma	(1)	1	1	3	1.5
Myofibromatosis	1	—	—	1	0.5
Smooth Muscle					
Angiomyoma	2	1	—	3	1.5
Other					
Granular cell tumor	1	1	1	3	1.5
Giant cell tumor	1	2	—	3	1.5
Glomangioma	—	—	1	1	0.5
Total				220	100.0

*Numbers in parentheses indicate military cases.

most common. In Seifert and coworkers'[1] study of 120 patients with nonepithelial tumors of the salivary glands, 32.5 percent of the lesions were pure hemangiomas. Of 220 cases recorded at the AFIP, hemangiomas make up 30.0 percent (see Table 28–1).

Clinical Findings

The vast majority of hemangiomas arise in the parotid gland (85.1 percent), and the remainder involve the submandibular gland. These tumors exhibit a marked predilection for occurring in female patients (2 to 1). The average age of patients with hemangiomas is 10 years, within a range of ages that spans from 2 months to 74 years. The propensity of these tumors to affect the parotid glands of infants and children is a consistent finding in previous case reports and retrospective studies.[1, 3–7] In Seifert and coworkers' report[1], 65 percent of the hemangiomas occurred during the first 2 decades of life.

The parotid hemangioma that occurs in infants (infantile or juvenile hemangioma) may be present at birth but is more frequently detected during

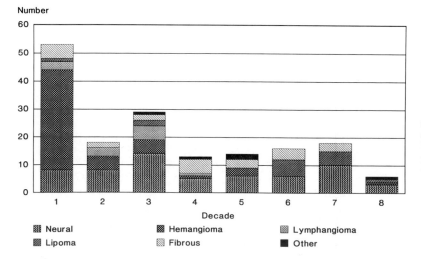

Figure 28–1. Distribution by age (in decades) and by histologic classification of 167 patients with benign mesenchymal tumors from the AFIP salivary gland registry.

the first 6 months of life. It appears as a nontender, soft mass near the ear lobe that may enlarge rapidly, often spreading over the entire gland (Fig. 28–2). In some cases, the overlying skin exhibits a red, reddish-blue, or blue discoloration that is accentuated when the head is inverted or the infant cries.[3, 4, 6] Some reports indicate a left-sided predominance.[3]

Intraparotid hemangiomas in adults are quite uncommon; an estimated 24 cases have been reported in the medical literature.[8] In the AFIP series, of the 59 hemangiomas known to be located in the parotid gland, 7 occurred in adults (older than 16 years).

Submandibular involvement by a vascular tumor is even less common. A search of the literature revealed only five cases, and one of those gave a history of a parotid hemangioma that first appeared at 5 years of age.[9, 10] In the cases at the AFIP, 14 percent (eight cases) were located in the submandibular gland, and four of those occurred in adults.

Microscopic Findings

In the classification of localized hemangioma outlined by Enzinger and Weiss,[11] two important types are capillary (including juvenile type) and cavernous. The capillary hemangioma is composed of a proliferation of capillary-sized vessels lined by flattened mature endothelium. The juvenile or infantile variant is an immature form of capillary hemangioma that in its early stages may be a diagnostic problem for the pathologist. Such lesions are composed of closely packed, plump endothelial cells that line inconspicuous vascular spaces (Fig. 28–3A). Occasional mitotic figures may be observed. As the lesions mature, endothelial cells become flattened, and the lumina of the capillary vessels become more apparent. The salivary gland lobules and ductal elements are preserved, but acinar parenchyma is replaced by angiomatous tissue. If the benign vascular nature of an early lesion is not clearly apparent, diagnostic aids may include (1) a special stain to demonstrate reticulin fibers at the periphery of the small indistinct blood vessels (Fig. 28–3B); (2) electron microscopy that will identify endothelial cells and pericytes; and (3) immunohistochemical techniques to identify Factor VIII–related antigen in neoplastic endothelial cells.[12] The cavernous type of hemangioma is characterized by large, thin-walled vascular spaces that are lined by markedly flattened endothelial cells.

In the AFIP salivary gland disease registry, 85 percent of the hemangiomas are the juvenile or capillary type. In those patients with the diagnosis of "juvenile" hemangioma, the average age of the patient was 9 months, and all but one of the lesions were located in the parotid gland.

Amorphous calcifications within the tumors are common, representing dystrophic calcification within organizing thrombi.[11] Phleboliths may be observed in the radiographs of such vascular lesions, occurring in perhaps 2 to 3 percent of angiomas in general.[13]

Discussion

Errors in the diagnosis of the juvenile hemangioma may be avoided if the clinician and pathologist are fully aware of the salient features of the entity. By means of careful clinical evaluation and noninvasive diagnostic techniques, the diagnosis of juvenile hemangioma is often possible without resorting to open biopsy, diagnostic angiography, or digital venous imaging. Computed tomography, especially dynamic computed tomographic scans, is reported to give an accurate picture of the degree of vascularity, and magnetic resonance imaging techniques may distinguish between hypervascular tumors (such as hemangioma, glomus tumor, or metastatic renal cell carcinoma) and hypovascular tumors (such as epithelial salivary gland tumors, neurogenic lesions, malignant lymphomas, and sarcomas).[14–16]

Rarely, an intramuscular hemangioma that occurs within the masseter muscle may be difficult to differentiate clinically from an intraparotid or submandibular tumor.[17] Microscopically, a plunging ranula with a prominent vascular stroma may be misinterpreted as a hemangioma in the sublingual or submandibular glands.[18]

The juvenile hemangioma may rapidly enlarge to reach its largest size over a period of several months and then begin a period of regression. It has been estimated that up to 90 percent of these lesions involute by the age of 7 years.[11] Seifert and colleagues[1] recommend avoiding surgical removal of such lesions from an infant patient, if possible, and postponing this treatment until after the patient has reached school age. Compression therapy using an acrylic splint and a head cap was suc-

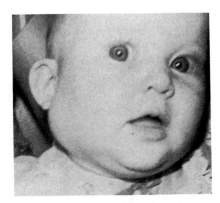

Figure 28–2. Hemangioma in parotid gland of infant. (With permission Snyderman NL, Johnson JT: Salivary gland tumors: Diagnostic characteristics of the common types. Postgrad Med 1987; 82:105–112.)

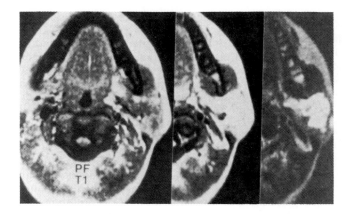

Figure 28–5. Magnetic resonance image of lymphangioma in left parotid area. (With permission Byrne MN, Spector JG, Garvin CF, Gado MH: Preoperative assessment of parotid masses: A comparative evaluation of radiologic techniques to histopathologic diagnosis. Laryngoscope 1989; 99:284–292.)

in significant morbidity because of poor circumscription, anatomic location, or a tendency to become secondarily infected.[11] Spontaneous regression is unlikely to occur. The treatment of choice for lymphangiomas and cystic hygromas is complete excision. Sclerosing agents and irradiation are not effective modes of therapy for cystic hygromas.[30, 42]

TUMORS OF PERIPHERAL NERVES

Neurilemoma (Schwannoma)

The neurilemoma arises within the Schwann cell sheath, pushing the nerve fascicles aside during growth.[11] Neurilemomas are the most common neurogenic tumors of the head and neck, occasionally arising from the sheath of the facial nerve. When a neurilemoma arises in the peripheral segment of the facial nerve, the resultant parotid mass is often thought clinically to represent an epithelial salivary gland tumor.[1, 45–52] An unusual case of multiple neurilemomas in the parotid gland has been reported.[51]

Clinical Findings

Neurilemomas constitute 16.0 percent of the 220 benign nonepithelial salivary gland tumors in the AFIP files (see Table 28–1). The vast majority (83 percent) occur in the parotid gland, and the remainder (17 percent) occur in the submandibular gland. A slight predilection for occurrence among female patients is apparent (1.5 to 1.0). The average age of patients with neurilemoma was 41.6 years, within a range from 7 to 77 years.

The neurilemoma is a slowly growing tumor that is often present for several years before diagnosis and, if small in size, does not cause pain or neurologic symptoms.[11] The consistency of the nodule or mass is usually described as "firm," "hard," or "stony hard."[47, 51]

Gross and Microscopic Findings

The sizes of neurilemomas arising in the parotid or submandibular glands range from 1.0 to 6.0 cm in diameter.[47–51] They may appear fusiform in shape along the nerve of origin or may occur as a well-defined eccentric nodule or mass.[11] Tissue sections of the tumor appear gray-white with fibrillary shiny areas, variably sized cystic spaces, or hemorrhagic foci.

Microscopically, most neurilemomas appear as encapsulated, well-defined, solitary nodules that are composed of Schwann cells in Antoni type-A or Antoni type-B configurations (Fig. 28–6). Certain cellular areas of a neurilemoma may resemble a sarcoma if Verocay bodies are absent and the nuclei are arranged in long fascicles. Degenerative changes, i.e., cystic areas, hyalinization, large blood vessels with hemorrhage and thrombi, and calcifications, may be observed in tumors of long duration (Figure 28–7). Tumors that exhibit severe degenerative changes have been termed "ancient" or "degenerated."[11]

One instance of melanocytic schwannoma in the parotid gland has been reported.[53] The presence of melanin pigment under light microscopy and of melanosomes under electron microscopy increases the possibility of an incorrect diagnosis of malignant melanoma. The reported recurrence rate of melanocytic schwannoma is 24 percent.[53]

Discussion

In diagnostically problematic cases, immunoperoxidase and ultrastructural studies should provide incontrovertible support. Immunohistochemical evaluation of neurilemomas for S-100 protein provides consistently positive results, especially in Antoni type-A areas. Electron micrographs show characteristic layers of electron-dense basal lamina and long-spacing collagen stacked between Schwann cells.[11]

Neurilemomas are nearly always solitary, are not associated with von Recklinghausen's disease,

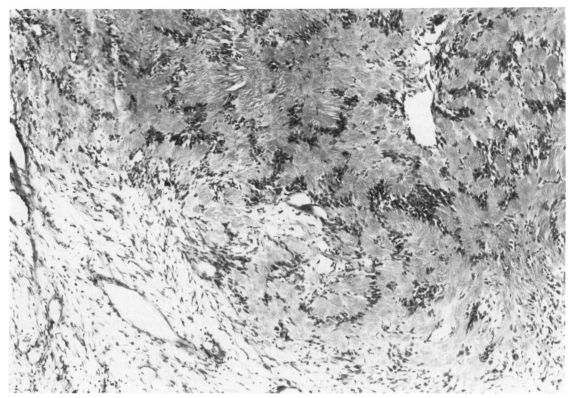

Figure 28–6. Neurilemoma exhibiting nuclear palisading in Antoni type-A area. Note myxoid Antoni type-B area (lower left) (× 75).

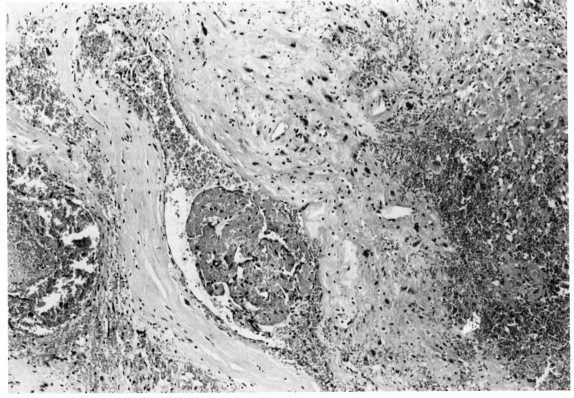

Figure 28–7. Ancient neurilemoma. Note large vessel with organizing thrombus and perivascular hyalinization (× 100).

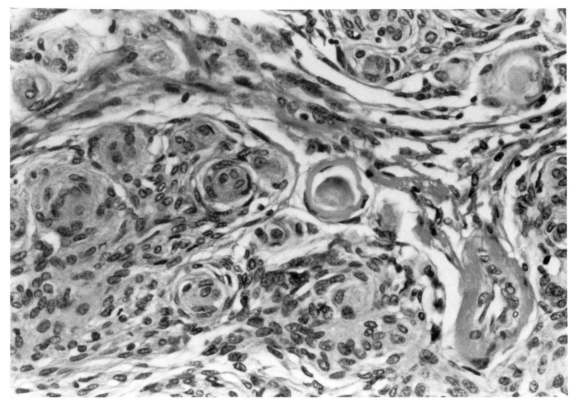

Figure 28–9. Characteristic whorling pattern of meningothelial cells in a transitional type of meningioma (× 400).

fibroblasts that may be arranged in various fascicular or storiform configurations. A notable example of such a nonneoplastic lesion that may cause diagnostic difficulty is nodular fasciitis.

Nodular Fasciitis

Nodular fasciitis is a benign, probably reactive, fibroblastic growth with pseudosarcomatous features. It is usually found in the upper or lower extremities or the trunk but may be found in the head and neck.[11, 64–67] Werning[65] reported 41 cases arising from the soft tissues of the orofacial region.

Clinical Findings

The AFIP files contain 17 cases of nodular fasciitis involving the parotid gland. A 4:1 predominance of occurrence in male patients was found. The average age of patients was 33 years, with an age range from 2 to 66 years. Nearly one third of the lesions affected individuals in the third decade of life. The usual presenting complaint is that of a painless or slightly tender mass that has developed in a relatively short period of time (2 weeks to 3 months).[65] On palpation, the lesions have been described as soft, elastic, firm, or hard. The usual size ranges from a few millimeters to 3 cm in diameter, with an average size

of about 1.5 cm.[67] Occasionally, the lesions may be tender or painful; however, the most disturbing clinical feature is rapid growth.

Microscopic Findings

When it arises from the parotid sheath, the lesion appears well circumscribed but unencapsulated and may infiltrate the parenchyma of the gland (Fig. 28–10). The nodule is composed of interlacing bundles of uniform, plump, apparently immature fibroblasts with bland, oval nuclei (Fig. 28–11). Some areas of the lesion are rich in mucopolysaccharides and contain only small amounts of collagen. Scattered foci of lymphocytes and erythrocytes may be observed, especially near the periphery of the lesion. Also prominent in the peripheral areas are capillaries, sometimes in a perpendicular configuration to the edge of the lesion. Mitotic figures are common but not atypical. Occasionally, lipid-laden macrophages or multinucleated giant cells are observed. Older lesions may exhibit hyaline fibrosis, small fluid-filled spaces, or a central cystic space.[11]

Discussion

The ultrastructure of nodular fasciitis was described by Wirman,[68] who concluded that nodular fasciitis is a lesion of myofibroblasts.

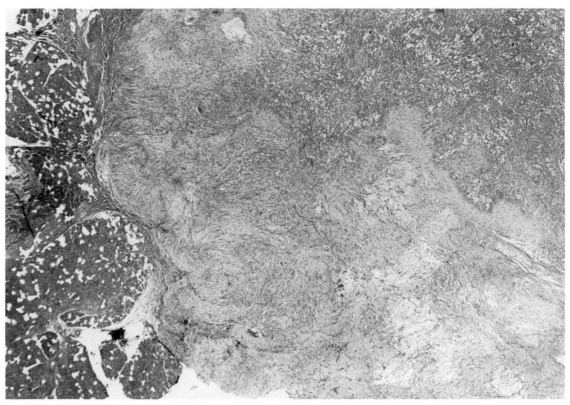

Figure 28–10. Nodular fasciitis in parotid gland. Note circumscription of lesion (× 30).

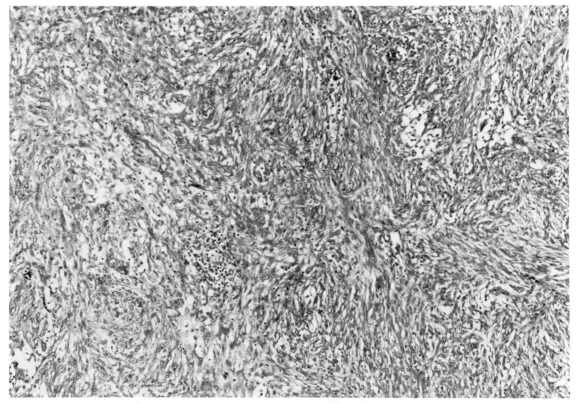

Figure 28–11. Nodular fasciitis showing random pattern of plump fibroblasts with scattered mucoid areas (× 75).

Nodular fasciitis behaves in a benign fashion, with rare recurrence after local excision (2 percent or less).[11, 67] Spontaneous regression has been known to occur.[11]

Fibrous Histiocytoma

Fibrous histiocytoma is considered to be a true neoplasm and is composed of an admixture of fibroblasts and histiocytelike cells that are often arranged in a cartwheel configuration with varying numbers of inflammatory cells, xanthoma cells, and hemosiderin-laden macrophages. It most commonly occurs in the dermis and subcutis, but it may arise in soft tissue or parenchymal organs.[11] Fibrous histiocytomas in the major salivary glands are rare; a search of the literature revealed only nine cases—seven in the parotid gland and two in the submandibular gland.[69–75]

Clinical Findings

The AFIP registry contains 11 cases of fibrous histiocytoma in major salivary glands. Ten of them occurred in the parotid gland, and the other case involved the submandibular gland. A female to male patient ratio of 3:1 was reported among the eight civilian cases. All of the patients with fibrous histiocytoma were white. The average patient age was 46 years, within a range from 21 to 68 years. No tumors occurred in patients under 20 years of age, and a fairly even distribution of cases was noted among patients in the third through seventh decades of life. Among the reported cases, those tumors involving the major salivary glands were all smaller than 5 cm in diameter, and the majority were between 2 and 4 cm in greatest dimension.[69–72, 74, 75] The presenting signs and symptoms, in those few cases providing such information, consisted of a firm, mobile, nontender mass.[69, 70]

Gross and Microscopic Findings

Grossly, a benign fibrous histiocytoma is a well-delineated but unencapsulated gray nodule with a homogenous, glistening gray-white surface. The nodules are firm to rubbery in consistency.[71, 74]

Microscopically, the periphery of the fibrous histiocytoma is well circumscribed but unencapsulated. The tumor is composed of compactly packed spindle cells arranged in whorls or storiform patterns with occasional fingerlike projections into gland parenchyma (Fig. 28–12). Scattered mononucleated and multinucleated. histiocytic cells that contain phagocytosed lipid and hemosiderin are sometimes present. The multinucleated cells may take the form of foreign body or Touton giant cells.[11] Variable numbers of chronic inflammatory cells and xanthoma cells may be seen occasionally. Mitotic figures are infrequent.

Discussion

The differential diagnosis of benign fibrous histiocytoma includes nodular fasciitis, neurofibroma, leiomyoma, myoepithelioma, and malignant fibrous histiocytoma. Immunohistochemistry may be helpful. Regezi and coworkers[76] used an avidin-biotin peroxidase technique to compare the immunoreactivity of benign fibrohistiocytic tumors with that of malignant fibrohistiocytic tumors. Both showed consistent immunoreactivity for alpha-1-antichymotrypsin and vimentin but negative reactivity for desmin, S-100, and keratin. Benign fibrous histiocytomas, in contrast to the malignant variety, exhibited fairly frequent (9 of 22) reactivity to leukocyte common antigen.

Electron microscopic studies have confirmed the presence of myofibroblasts and rounded cells resembling histiocytes.[77] The myofibroblasts have been ultrastructurally characterized by ruffled nuclear borders and actinlike filaments beneath the plasma membrane, whereas the rounded cells have shown numerous cell processes, mitochondria, and phagolysosomes.

Although relatively few cases of benign fibrous histiocytomas of the major salivary glands have been reported, complete surgical removal is the recommended treatment.[69–71] Recurrences are most likely caused by inadequate primary excision.[70] Of the nine cases reported in the literature, two of them recurred; one case involved the submandibular gland of a 62-year-old female patient (three recurrences in 41 months), and the other involved the parotid gland of a 50-year-old male patient (one recurrence in 8.5 years after initial treatment).[69, 70]

Fibromatosis

Fibromatosis, classified by Enzinger and Weiss as one of the deep (musculoaponeurotic) fibromatoses, is a deceptively benign-appearing tumor with the tendency to progressively enlarge, infiltrate adjacent tissues, and recur. Other terms that have been used to describe this entity are *aggressive fibromatosis*, *extra-abdominal desmoid*, *desmoid tumor*, and *fibrosarcoma grade 1 desmoid type*. For those lesions occurring in children younger than 16 years, some authors use the term *juvenile fibromatosis*.[78–83] Most of these lesions occur in the shoulder, thigh, or chest wall, but about 10 percent of the cases involve tissues of the head and neck.[11]

Clinical Findings

In most patients, the tumor occurs as a painless, sessile mass that may be partially fixed to adjacent and underlying tissues. The duration before treatment is sought is less than 1 year in most cases, but the rate of growth is typically slow and steady.[80] Three cases of fibromatosis in the parotid area have previously been reported.[83–85] The most

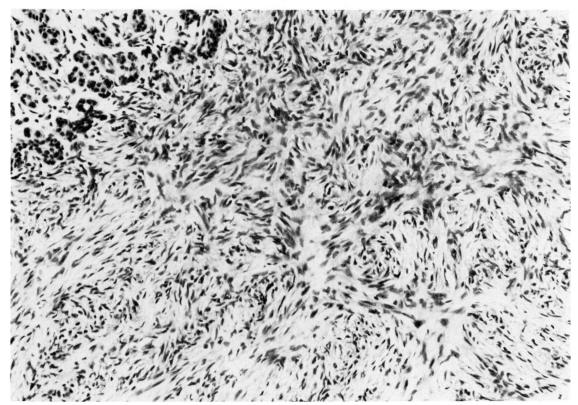

Figure 28–12. Fibrous histiocytoma of the parotid gland. Note the storiform pattern and absence of a peripheral capsule (upper left) (× 150).

common site in the head and neck region is the neck (45 to 85 percent of cases), followed by the face and scalp.[80, 83, 84]

Among the 220 benign mesenchymal tumors of salivary glands in the registry of the AFIP, 7 cases of fibromatosis (3.0 percent) were included. Four of the tumors involved the parotid gland, and three were located in the submandibular gland. Of the six cases in which gender was identified, males and females were equally affected. Patient age was 17.6 years on average and ranged from 2 months to 45 years.

Gross and Microscopic Findings

The gross appearance is typically one of an irregularly shaped mass of gray-white tissue that is unencapsulated and infiltrates the surrounding tissue. The tissue sections reveal interlacing bands of dense, gray-white connective tissue that resemble scar tissue.[11, 84]

Histopathologically, fibromatosis is characterized by a poorly circumscribed mass of collagenous fibrous connective tissue that infiltrates surrounding tissues. It is composed of spindle-shaped cells that are separated by abundant collagen arranged in ill-defined sweeping fascicles (Fig. 28–13). Although these tumors may exhibit a variable degree of cellularity, the nuclei are uniformly spaced and do not appear atypical or hyperchromatic. Mitotic figures are infrequent, and cytologic features of malignancy are absent.

Discussion

Enzinger and Weiss[11] list four lesions that may be confused with fibromatosis and should be considered in the differential diagnosis: fibrosarcoma, reactive fibrosis, myxoma, and nodular fasciitis. When contrasted with fibromatosis, a fibrosarcoma exhibits a marked degree of cellularity, distinct intersecting fascicles in a herringbone pattern, numerous mitotic figures, and greater variation in the size and staining characteristics of the nuclei. Reactive fibrosis typically shows variable growth patterns and contains focal areas of hemorrhage or hemosiderin deposits or both. Myxoma appears less cellular than fibromatosis and contains small amounts of collagen. Nodular fasciitis is composed of plump fibroblasts arranged in a loosely textured, feathery configuration, which contrasts with the fascicular pattern of uniform spindle cells characteristic of fibromatosis.

Aggressive fibromatoses are considered to have high postsurgical recurrence rates that range from 27 to 57 percent.[86] Tumors in the head and neck are considered serious because of the relatively restricted anatomic area and the close proximity

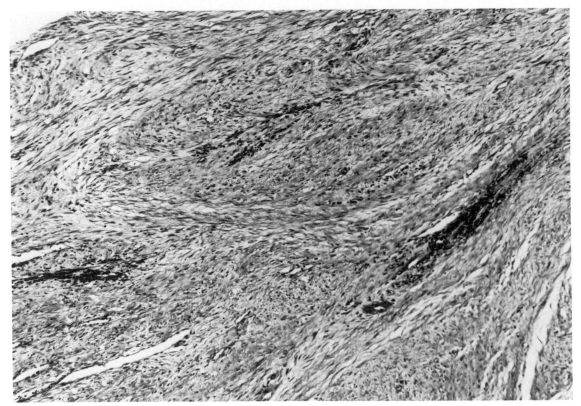

Figure 28–13. Fibromatosis composed of sweeping fascicles of mature-appearing fibroblasts (× 75).

of vital structures.[81] The most widely accepted treatment is a wide en bloc excision of the tumor.

Radiation therapy has been used as the sole treatment for fibromatosis or in combination with surgery.[86–88] Radiation therapy as the primary treatment modality for fibromatosis is still a controversial issue, and some authors recommend that its use be reserved for combination with surgery or for treating unresectable or recurrent tumors.[86] Induction chemotherapy followed by surgery was used by Goepfert and coworkers[89] in the treatment of six unresectable tumors. In all six patients, the tumors regressed, and five of them had no evidence of recurrence 3 to 72 months after surgery.

Myxoma

The soft tissue myxoma is a benign mesenchymal tumor composed of stringy, gelatinous tissue that microscopically resembles the core of the umbilical cord.[90] It usually occurs in the thigh, shoulder, or pelvic girdle and often infiltrates adjacent skeletal muscle.[90–92] Although myxoma in the soft tissues of the head and neck is rare, cases have been found in the skin and subcutaneous tissue, fascia, larynx, tonsils, ear, and parotid gland.[93–101] An estimated six cases have been reported in the parotid region.[96–101]

Clinical Findings

In most cases, the clinical manifestations resemble those of other benign mesenchymal tumors and consist of a painless palpable mass that may be firm, slightly movable, or fluctuant.[11] Of the reported cases of myxoma in the parotid region, two were associated with pain,[95, 97] and one caused facial paralysis.[95] Tumor size has ranged from 3.0 to 6.5 cm in greatest dimension. In the reported cases, patients have ranged in age from 1 to 56 years (average of 20 years).[96–101] Three cases of soft tissue myxoma in the parotid gland region are recorded in the files of AFIP, comprising 1.5 percent of the 220 benign mesenchymal tumors of salivary glands. The average age of affected patients was 44 years, with a range of 35 to 53 years.

Gross and Microscopic Findings

Gross specimen examination typically reveals an ovoid or globular mass of moderately firm, rubbery tissue that appears well circumscribed but unencapsulated. Tumor sections exhibit a striking exudation of slimy, gelatinous material from the surface of the snow-white or gray-white tissue, and occasional fluid-filled cystlike spaces may be apparent.

Microscopically, the myxoma is composed of an abundant mucoid stroma, sparse cells with small hyperchromatic nuclei and indistinct cytoplasm, and a meshwork of delicate reticular fibers (Fig. 28–14). The small nuclei often exhibit small vacuoles but are devoid of nucleoli or mitotic figures. Although a distinct fibrous capsule is not observed, a condensation of reticular fibers that are often frayed or fibrillated may be seen at the periphery of the tumor. Blood vessels are sparse and, when present, are of small caliber. Some of the larger oval cells may exhibit a vacuolated or ballooning cytoplasm. The mucoid material stains with Alcian blue stain at pH 2.6 and stains metachromatically with toluidine blue at pH 4.0. If the tissue sections are treated with testicular hyaluronidase, these reactions do not occur.[91, 102]

Discussion

Ultrastructural studies of ten cases of intramuscular myxoma by Feldman[103] indicated that the principal cells were fibroblasts. The abundant matrix consisted of finely granular material with scattered fibroblasts, collagen fibrils, infrequent macrophages, and rare capillaries. These findings support the concept that the cell of origin is an altered fibroblast that produces very little collagen but an excessive amount of mucopolysaccharides.[90–92]

Although intrabony myxomas of the maxilla and mandible are known to have a relatively high recurrence rate (approaching 25 percent),[100] the soft tissue myxomas apparently do not.[11, 91] However, one tumor in the parotid region of a 13-year-old female patient is reported to have recurred twice. In that case, a resection of the parotid gland—including the facial nerve and tissues of the subpharyngeal space—was necessary to control the tumor after previous surgery and irradiation failed.[95] Canalis and coworkers[100] emphasized that myxomas developing in or around the parotid gland may present special management problems and recommended a superficial parotidectomy as the initial treatment of choice.

Histologic distinction from prominently myxoid mixed tumors depends on the absence of any epithelial or myoepithelial elements. Immunohistochemical analysis for cytokeratin may be helpful in this regard.

NEOPLASMS OF ADIPOSE TISSUE

Lipoma

Lipoma is the most common mesenchymal neoplasm in the human body[11] and may occur in the major salivary glands. Parotid gland lipomas are

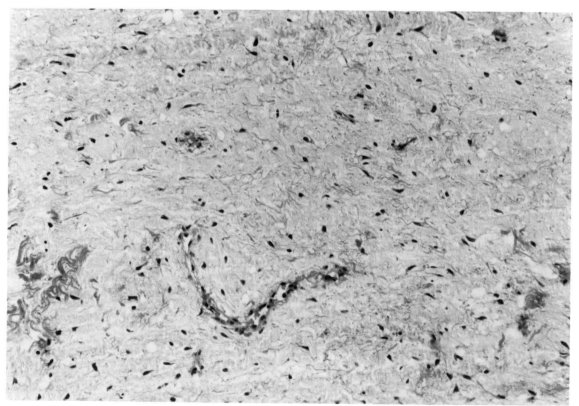

Figure 28–14. Myxoma of the parotid gland. Note the abundant mucoid stroma and small hyperchromatic nuclei (× 150).

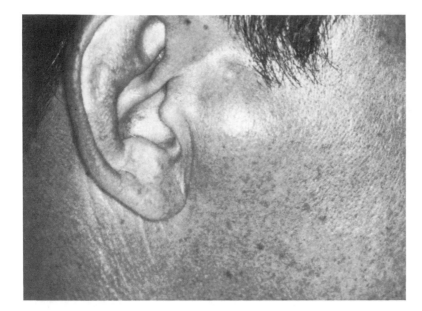

Figure 28–17. Angiomyoma in the parotid gland of a 50-year-old male patient. (With permission Kido T and Sekitani T: Vascular leiomyoma of the parotid gland. ORL J 1989; 51:187–191.)

Gross and Microscopic Findings

The gross appearance of an angiomyoma is usually described as a well-circumscribed ovoid nodule that is firm to palpation and is white or blue-gray.

Microscopically, the characteristic appearance is that of an encapsulated nodule of smooth muscle that contains thick-walled vessels and narrow lumina (Fig. 28–18). Smooth muscle cells are arranged tangentially from the periphery of the thick-walled vessels and blend with the intervascular smooth muscle fascicles.[135]

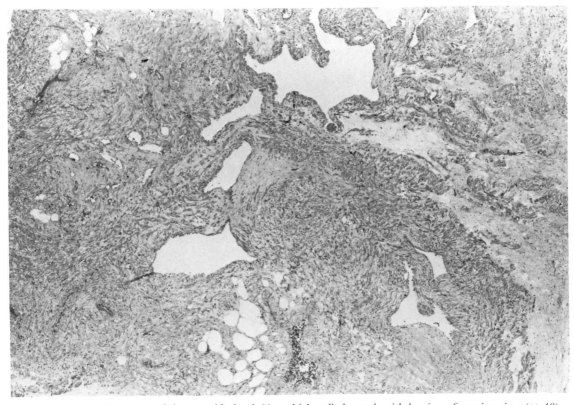

Figure 28–18. Angiomyoma of the parotid gland. Note thick-walled vessels with lumina of varying sizes ($\times$ 40).

Discussion

Diagnosis is rarely a problem. Special stains, such as Masson's trichrome or phosphotungstic acid–hematoxylin, may be employed to demonstrate myofibrils. Ultrastructural studies identify thin myofilaments (6 to 8 nm in diameter) that are oriented parallel to the long axis of the smooth muscle cells.[139] Angiomyomas are benign lesions that do not tend to recur.

OTHER BENIGN MESENCHYMAL LESIONS

Granular Cell Tumor (Granular Cell Myoblastoma)

Granular cell tumor is a fairly common soft tissue lesion. More than 1,200 cases have been reported in the medical literature.[11, 140–145] More than one half of the reported cases occur in the head and neck region, with the tongue being the most common site in this location.[142] At least three cases involving the parotid gland have been reported.[1, 146]

Since the first report of five cases by Abrikossoff[140] in 1926, the histogenesis of the tumor has been controversial. Investigators have suggested derivation from muscle fibers, fibroblasts, undifferentiated mesenchymal cells, and peripheral nerves.[112, 140, 144] Although support for neural origin is provided by reaction of tumor cells with anti–S-100 protein,[147] ultrastructural features favor derivation from undifferentiated mesenchymal cells.[145, 148]

Clinical Findings

Granular cell tumors usually present as asymptomatic, small (less than 2 cm) nonulcerated nodules. In a study of 95 cases, Strong and coworkers[149] calculated a 2:1 predilection for tumor occurrence in female patients and an average patient age of 38 years (range of 11 months to 68 years). Review of the AFIP cases on file (see Table 28–1) located three granular cell tumors in the major salivary glands, including one in the sublingual gland and two in the parotid gland. The average age of patients with the tumor was 34 years, with a range of 26 to 42 years. One patient was male and one was female; the sex of the third patient was unknown.

Gross and Microscopic Findings

The tumors are poorly circumscribed and unencapsulated. Tissue sections show a characteristic homogenous pale yellow-tan or yellow-gray appearance.[11]

Microscopically, the lesion is composed of medium to large, rounded or polyhedral cells, with small, centrally placed nuclei and distinctive granular, eosinophilic cytoplasm (Fig. 28–19). The cells are arranged in ribbons or nests that may be separated by bundles of collagen. The granular cells may infiltrate and replace gland parenchyma, and a close association with peripheral nerve fibers often is noted.

Ultrastructural studies of granular cells have revealed autophagic granules and variably sized vesicular bodies within the cytoplasm.[145, 148]

Discussion

Granular cell tumors usually do not recur after adequate local excision. The recurrence rate for 182 reported cases is about 5 percent, and several of the recurrences were attributed to incomplete removal.[141, 142, 144, 149] Rarely (approximately 2 percent) a granular cell tumor may exhibit malignant cytologic features and an aggressive biologic behavior.[11] Approximately 10 to 15 percent of patients with granular cell tumors have multiple lesions, usually located in subcutaneous tissue, submucosa, or viscera.[11, 146]

Giant Cell Neoplasm of Major Salivary Glands

In 1984, Eusebi and coworkers[150] reported on three adult patients with an unusual giant cell tumor located in the parotid gland. Among an additional four AFIP cases (see Table 28–1), one tumor was located in the submandibular gland of a 28-year-old woman, and three were found in the parotid glands (70-year-old female, 65-year-old male, and 73-year-old man).

Gross and Microscopic Findings

In the three cases reported by Eusebi and colleagues,[150] the tumors ranged from 1.0 to 2.5 cm in greatest diameter and were described as well-defined nodules composed of solid, homogenous red-brown tissue.

The histopathologic appearance of the tumor is distinctive; it is a well-vascularized cellular stroma composed of spindled and round mononuclear cells with scattered multinucleated giant cells. The multinucleated giant cells, characterized by acidophilic cytoplasm with 2 to 20 centrally located nuclei (Fig. 28–20), constitute about 10 to 20 percent of the whole cell population. Areas of osteoid formation, foci of hemorrhage and hemosiderin, and collections of inflammatory cells may be present. In one of the cases reported by Eusebi and colleagues,[150] the giant cell tumor was associated with a primary salivary gland tumor (carcinoma arising in pleomorphic adenoma). One of the AFIP cases was also associated with an adenocarcinoma in the submandibular region.

In some areas, the glomus cells may be arranged in solid sheets (Fig. 28–21B) and may show transition into elongated, mature smooth muscle cells. The glomus cell is characteristically small (8 to 12 nm), round or polygonal, with a round or ovoid centrally placed nucleus and amphophilic or eosinophilic cytoplasm. Ultrastructural studies confirm the presence of thin (8 nm) actinlike filaments in the cytoplasm. The periphery of the tumor may exhibit some collagen, with small nerves and vessels; however, it rarely shows a capsule.[11]

Discussion

In the parotid gland, the clinical differential diagnosis includes epithelial salivary gland tumors, neurofibroma, neurilemoma, lipoma, hemangioma, and other mesenchymal tumors. Special stains for epithelial mucin and reticulin fibers may be helpful in making the correct diagnosis.[11] Glomangiomas are considered to have a benign biologic behavior, and if adequately excised, they do not recur.

REFERENCES

1. Seifert G, Miehlke A, Haubrich J, Chilla R: Diseases of the Salivary Glands: Pathology-Diagnosis-Treatment-Facial Nerve Surgery. Stuttgart, Georg Thieme Verlag, 1986; 286–300.
2. Allison RS, Van Der Waal I, Snow GB: Parapharyngeal tumors: A review of 23 cases. Clin Otolaryngol 1989; 14:199–203.
3. Batsakis JG, Vascular tumors of the salivary glands. Ann Otol Rhinol Laryngol 1986; 95:649–650.
4. Tresserra L, Martinez-Mora J, Boix-Ochoa J: Hemangiomas of the parotid gland in children. J Maxillofac Surg 1977; 5:238–241.
5. Hilborne LH, Glasgow BJ, Layfield LJ: Fine-needle aspiration cytology of juvenile hemangioma of the parotid gland: a case report. Diagn Cytopathol 1987; 3:152–155.
6. Goldman RL, Perzik SL: Infantile hemangioma of the parotid gland: a clinicopathologic study of 15 cases. Arch Otolaryngol 1969; 90:89–92.
7. Kaban LB, Mulliken JB: Vascular anomalies of the maxillofacial region. J Oral Maxillofac Surg 1986; 44:203–213.
8. Chuong R, Donoff RB: Intraparotid hemangioma in an adult: Case report and review of the literature. Int J Oral Surg 1984; 13:346–351.
9. Stevenson EW: Hemangioma of the salivary gland: Review of the literature and report of a rare lesion in the submaxillary area. South Med J 1966; 59:1187–1190.
10. Stratiev A: Hemangioma of the submandibular gland. Stomatologia (Sofia) 1973; 55:464–467.
11. Enzinger FM, Weiss SW: Soft Tissue Tumors, 2nd Ed. St. Louis, CV Mosby Co, 1988.
12. Burgdorf WH, Mukai K, Rosai J: Immunohistochemical identification of Factor VIII—Related antigen in endothelial cells of cutaneous lesions of alleged vascular nature. Am J Clin Pathol 1981; 75:167–171.
13. Dempsey EF, Murley RS: Vascular malformations simulating salivary disease. Br J Plast Surg 1970; 23:77–84.
14. Som PM, Biller HF, Lawson W, Sacher M, Lanzieri CF: Parapharyngeal space masses: An updated protocol based upon 104 cases. Radiology 1984; 153:149–156.
15. Som PM, Braun IF, Shapiro, MD, Reede DL, Curtin HD, Zimmerman RA: Tumors of the parapharyngeal space and upper neck: MR imaging characteristics. Radiology 1987; 164:823–829.
16. Michael AS, Mafee F, Valvassori E, Tan WS: Dynamic computed tomography of the head and neck: Differential diagnosis value. Radiology 1985; 154:413–419.
17. Wolf GT, Daniel F, Krause CJ, Kaufman RS: Intramuscular hemangioma of the head and neck. Laryngoscope 1985; 95:210–213.
18. McClatchey KD, Appelblatt NH, Zarbo RJ, Merrel DM: Plunging ranula. Oral Surg Oral Med Oral Pathol 1984; 57:408–412.
19. Totsuka Y, Fukuda H, Tomita K: Compression therapy for parotid hemangioma in infants: A report of three cases. J Craniomaxillofac Surg 1988; 16:366–370.
20. Zarem HA, Edgerton MT: Induced resolution of cavernous hemangiomas following prednisolone therapy. Plast Reconstr Surg 1967; 39:76–83.
21. Schennemann H: Conservative parotidectomy in infancy and childhood. J Maxillofac Surg 1975; 3:37–40.
22. Williams HB: Hemangiomas of the parotid gland in children. Plast Reconstr Surg 1975; 56:29–34.
23. Popescu V: Intratumoral ligation in the management of orofacial cavernous hemangiomas. J Maxillofac Surg 1985; 13:99–107.
24. Bingham HG: Predicting the course of a congenital hemangioma. Plast Reconstr Surg 1979; 63:161–166.
25. Braun IF, Levy S, Hoffman JC: The use of trans-arterial embolization in the management of hemangiomas of the perioral region. J Oral Maxillofac Surg 1985; 43:239–248.
26. Redenbacher EAH: DeRanula sub lingua; speciali cum casu congenito. Monachii, Lindauer, 1828.
27. Wernher A: Die angeborenen kyten-hygrome und die ihnen verwandten geschwulste in Anatomischer, Diagnostesher und Theraputischer Beziehung Giessen. Vater G F Heyer, 1843; 76.
28. Sobol SM, Gogan RJ: Pathological Quiz Case 1: Parotid lymphangioma (cystic type). Arch Otolaryngol 1981; 107:320–323.
29. Bill AH Jr, Sumner DS: A unified concept of lymphangioma and cystic hygroma. Surg Gynecol Obstet 1975; 120:79–86.
30. Ninh TN, Ninh TX: Cystic hygroma in children: A report of 126 cases. J Pediatr Surg 1974; 9:191–195.
31. Noone RB, Brown HJ: Cystic hygroma of the parotid gland. Am J Surg 1970; 120:404–407.
32. Crawford AP: Lymphangioma of the parotid gland. Med J Aust 1981; 2:141–142.
33. Kennedy J, Briant T: Parotid lymphangioma. J Otolaryngol 1977; 6:23–27.
34. Lack EE, Upton MP: Histopathologic review of salivary gland tumors in childhood. Arch Otolaryngol Head Neck Surg 1988; 114:898–906.
35. Katz AD: Unusual lesions of the parotid gland. J Surg Oncol 1975; 7:219–235.

36. Zdichynec B: Lymphangioma of the parotid gland and diabetes mellitus. Cesk Otolaryngol 1977; 26:245–247.

37. Princ G, Brocheriou C, Crépy C: Les kystes de la parotide: A propos de 4 cas. Rev Stomatol Chir Maxillofac 1982; 83:317–320.

38. Landa LS, Montes GE, Ellauri AS: Congenital cystic lymphangioma of the parotid. Rev Esp Estomatol 1981; 29:293–296.

39. Baum RK, Perzik SL: Tumors of the parotid gland in children: Review of 40 cases. Am Surg 1965; 31:719–723.

40. Wright GL, Smith RJH, Katz CD, Atkins JH: Benign parotid diseases of childhood. Laryngoscope 1985; 95:915–920.

41. Takato T, Nakatsuka T, Ohhara Y: Lymphangioma of the parotid gland. Ann Plast Surg 1984; 13:353–356.

42. Stromberg BV, Weeks PM, Wray RC: Treatment of cystic hygroma. South Med J 1976; 69:1333–1335.

43. Goetsch E: Hygroma colli cysticum and hygroma axillare: Pathologic and clinical study and report of 12 cases. Arch Surg 1938; 36:394–480.

44. Schroeder BA, Czarnecki DJ, Wells RG, Sty JR: Salivary gland scintigraphy: Cystic hygroma of the parotid. Clin Nucl Med 1987; 12:485–486.

45. Kavanaugh KT, Panje WR: Neurogenic neoplasms of the seventh cranial nerve presenting as a parotid mass. Am J Otolaryngol 1982; 3:53–56.

46. Neely JG: Neoplastic involvement of the facial nerve. Otolaryngol Clin N Am 1974; 7:385–396.

47. Katz AD, Passy V, Kaplan L: Neurogenous neoplasms of major nerves of face and neck. Arch Surg 1971; 103:51–56.

48. Samet A, Podoshin L, Fradis M, Simon J, Lazarov N, Boss H: Unusual sites of schwannoma in the head and neck. J Laryngol Otol 1985; 99:523–528.

49. Roos DB, Byars LT, Ackerman LV: Neurilemomas of the facial nerve presenting as parotid gland tumors. Ann Surg 1956; 144:258–262.

50. Das Gupta TK, Brasfield RD, Strong EW, Hajdu SI: Benign solitary schwannomas (neurilemomas). Cancer 1969; 24:355–366.

51. Helidonis E, Dokianakis G, Pantazopoulos P: A schwannoma of the parotid gland—report of a case. J Laryngol Otol 1978; 92:833–838.

52. Conley JJ: Salivary Glands and the Facial Nerve. New York, Grune & Stratton, 1975; 103–105.

53. Bauserman SC: Melanocytic schwannoma. Cancer 1988; 62:174–183.

54. Zbaren P, Ducomman J-C: Diagnosis of salivary gland disease using ultrasound and sialography: A comparison. Clin Otolaryngol 1989; 14:189–197.

55. Seifert G, Oehne H: Die mesenchymalen (nichtepithelialen) Speicheldrüsentumoren: Analyse von 167 Tumorfällen des Speicheldrüsen-Registers. Laryngol Rhinol Otol 1986; 65:485–491.

56. Steffansson K, Wollmann R, Jerkovic M: S-100 protein in soft tissue tumors derived from schwann cells and melanocytes. Am J Pathol 1982; 106:261–268.

57. Krolls SO, Trodahl JN, Borgers RC: Salivary gland lesions in children: A survey of 430 cases. Cancer 1972; 30:459–469.

58. Weitzner S: Plexiform neurofibroma of major salivary glands in children. Oral Surg Oral Med Oral Pathol 1980; 50:53–57.

59. Mosso ML, Castello M, Bellani FF, Ditullio MT, Loiacano F, Paolucci G, Tamaro P, Terracini B, Pastore G: Neurofibromatosis and malignant childhood cancers: A survey in Italy, 1970–83. Tumori 1987; 73:209–212.

60. Nager GT, Heroy J, Hoeplinger M: Meningiomas invading the temporal bone with extension to the neck. Am J Otolaryngol 1983; 4:297–324.

61. Wolff M, Rankow RM: Meningioma of the parotid gland: An insight into the pathogenesis of extracranial meningiomas. Hum Pathol 1971; 2:453–459.

62. Farr HW, Gray GF, Vrana M, Pario M: Extracranial meningioma. J Surg Oncol 1973; 5:411–420.

63. Hoye SJ, Hoar CS Jr, Murray JE: Extracranial meningioma presenting as a tumor of the neck. Am J Surg 1960; 100:486–489.

64. Konwaler BE, Keasbey L, Kaplan L: Subcutaneous pseudosarcomatous fibromatosis (fasciitis). J Clin Pathol 1955; 25:241–252.

65. Werning JT: Nodular fasciitis of the orofacial region. Oral Surg Oral Med Oral Pathol 1979; 48:441–446.

66. Price EB Jr, Silliphant WM, Shuman R: Nodular fasciitis: A clinicopathologic analysis of 65 cases. Am J Clin Pathol 1961; 35:122–136.

67. Shimizu S, Hashimoto H, Enjoji M: Nodular fasciitis: An analysis of 250 patients. Pathology 1984; 16:161–166.

68. Wirman JA: Nodular fasciitis: A lesion of myofibroblasts. An ultrastructural study. Cancer 1976; 38:2378–2389.

69. Thompson SH, Shear M: Fibrous histiocytomas of the oral and maxillofacial regions. J Oral Pathol 1984; 13:282–294.

70. Hutchinson JC, Friedberg SA: Fibrous histiocytoma of the head and neck. Laryngoscope 1978; 88:1950–1955.

71. Fayemi PO, Ali M: Fibrous histiocytoma of the parotid gland. Mt Sinai J Med 1980, 47:290–292.

72. Shapshay SM, Wingert RH, Davis JS: Fibrous histiocytoma of the parotid gland. Laryngoscope 1979; 89:1808–1812.

73. Rice DH, Batsakis JG, Headington JT: Fibrous histiocytomas of the nose and paranasal sinuses. Arch Otolaryngol 1974; 100:398–401.

74. Nilsen R, Lind O: Benign fibrous xanthoma of the parotid gland: A case report. Br J Oral Surg 1978–1979; 16:111–114.

75. Ferrari PG, Viva E, Derada TG, Girardi E: Rare case of a fibrous histiocytoma located in the parotid. Minerva Stomatol 1982; 31:693–696.

76. Regezi JA, Zarbo RJ, Tomich CE, Lloyd RV, Crissman JD: Immunoprofile of benign and malignant fibrohistiocytic tumors. J Oral Pathol 1987; 16:260–265.

77. Fine G, Morales MD, Pardo V: Ultrastructure of histiocytomas (abst). Am J Clin Pathol 1977; 67:214.

78. Musgrove JE, McDonald JR: Extraabdominal desmoid tumors: Their differential diagnosis and treatment. Arch Pathol 1948; 45:513–546.

79. Stout AP: Juvenile fibromatoses. Cancer 1954; 7:953–978.

80. Conley J, Healey WV, Stout AP: Fibromatosis of the head and neck. Am J Surg 1966; 112:609–622.

81. Wilkins SA, Waldron CA, Matthews WH: Aggres-

sive fibromatosis of the head and neck. Am J Surg 1975; 130:412–415.

82. Brewster R, Ivins J: Extra-abdominal desmoid tumors. J Bone Joint Surg 1975; 57A:1026.

83. Fata JJ, Rabuzzi DD: Aggressive juvenile fibromatosis presenting as a parotid mass. Ear Nose Throat J. 1988; 67:678–684.

84. Masson JK, Soule EH: Desmoid tumors of the head and neck. Am J Surg 1966; 112:615–622.

85. Majmudar S, Winiarski N: Desmoid tumor presenting as a parotid mass. JAMA 1978; 239:337–339.

86. Wara WM, Phillips TL, Hill DR, Bovill E Jr, Luk KH, Lichter AS, Leibel SA: Desmoid tumors—treatment and prognosis. Radiology 1977; 124:225–226.

87. Benninghoff D, Robbins R: The nature and treatment of desmoid tumors. Am J Roentgenol 1964; 91:132–137.

88. Hill DR, Newman H, Phillips TG: Radiation therapy of desmoid tumors. Am J Roentgenol 1973; 117:84–89.

89. Goepfert H, Cangir A, Ayala AG, Eftekhari F: Chemotherapy of locally aggressive head and neck tumors: Desmoid fibromatosis and nasopharyngeal angiofibroma. Am J Surg 1982; 144:437–444.

90. Ireland DCR, Soule EH, Ivins JC: Myxoma of somatic soft tissues: Report of 58 patients, 3 with multiple tumors and fibrous dysplasia of bone. Mayo Clin Proc 1973; 48:401–410.

91. Enzinger FM: Intramuscular myxomas: A review and follow-up study of 34 cases. Am J Clin Pathol 1965; 43:104–113.

92. Wirth WA, Leavitt D, Enzinger FM: Multiple intramuscular myxomas: Another extraskeletal manifestation of fibrous dysplasia. Cancer 1971; 27:1167–1173.

93. Faccini JM, Williams JL: Myxoma involving the soft tissues of the face. J Laryngol Otol 1973; 87:817–822.

94. Rapidis AD, Trantafyllou AG: Myxoma of the oral soft tissues. J Oral Maxillofac Surg 1983; 41:188–192.

95. Dutz W, Stout AP: The myxoma in childhood. Cancer 1961; 14:629–635.

96. Bellinger CG: Preauricular myxoma: Case report. Plast Reconstr Surg 1970; 45:292–293.

97. Chaves E, Nobrega C, Oliveira AM, Cartaxo O: Congenital myxoma in childhood. Cancer 1971; 28:239–243.

98. Bertola VJ: Sobre un tumor mixomatoso de la region del corpusculo retrocarotideo. Bol Trab Acad Argent Cir 1942; 26:1102–1115.

99. Malfatti T: Considerations on a case of myxoma of the parotid. Clin Pediatr 1961; 43:747–752.

100. Canalis RF, Smith GA, Konrad HR: Myxomas of the head and neck. Arch Otolaryngol 1976; 102:300–305.

101. Smith GA, Konrad HR, Canalis RF: Childhood myxomas of the head and neck. J Otolaryngol 1977; 6:423–430.

102. Kindblom LG, Stener B, Angervall L: Intramuscular myxoma. Cancer 1974; 34:1737–1744.

103. Feldman PS: A comparative study including ultrastructure of intramuscular myxoma and myxoid liposarcoma. Cancer 1979; 43:512–525.

104. Baker SE, Jensen JL, Correll RW: Lipomas of the parotid gland. Oral Surg Oral Med Oral Pathol 1981; 52:167–171.

105. Watts AE, Perzik SL: Lipomatous lesions of the parotid area. Arch Otolaryngol 1976; 102:230–232.

106. Janecka IP, Conley J, Perzin KH, Pitman G: Lipomas presenting as parotid tumors. Laryngoscope 1977; 87:1007–1010.

107. Houston GD, Brannon RB: Lipoma of the parotid gland. Oral Surg Oral Med Oral Pathol 1985; 60:72–74.

108. Calhoun KH, Clark WD, Jones JD: Parotid lipoblastoma in an infant. Int J Pediatr Otorhinolaryngol. 1987; 14:41–44.

109. Adams G, Goycoolea MV, Foster C, Dehner L, Anderson RD: Parotid lipomatosis in a 2-month-old child. Otolaryngol Head Neck Surg 1981; 89:402–405.

110. Osguthorpe JD, Colman M, Rice DH, Canalis RF: Pathologic Quiz Case 2: Lipoma of the parotid gland. Arch Otolaryngol 1979; 105:742–745.

111. Cass KA, Whelan TJ: Simultaneous bilateral parotid papillary cystadenoma lymphomatosum. Arch Otolaryngol 1968; 87:618–619.

112. Catania CV, Galante E, Bandieramonte G, Salvadori B: Risultati delle terapia chirurgica di 622 casi di tumori della ghiandole salivari. Tumori 1974; 60:307–316.

113. Eddey HH: Parotid tumors: A review of 138 cases. Aust N Z J Surg 1970; 40:1–14.

114. Eneroth CM: Histological and clinical aspects of parotid tumors. Acta Otolaryngol Supp (Stockh.) 1964; 191:1–99.

115. Gaisford JC, Hanna DC, Richardson GS, Bindra RN: Parotid tumors. Plast Reconstr Surg. 1969; 43:504–510.

116. Grage TB, Lober PH, Shahon DB: Benign tumors of the major salivary glands. Surgery 1961; 50:625–633.

117. Kirklin JW, McDonald JR, Harrington SW, New GB: Parotid tumors. Surg Gynecol Obstet 1951; 92:721–733.

118. Lathrop FD: Benign tumors of the parotid gland: Twenty-five year review. Laryngoscope 1962; 72:992–1006.

119. Pricolo V, di Pietro S, Catania VC: I tumori della parotide e la loro terapia. Tumori 1954; 40:333–364.

120. Redon H, Belcour J: Enseignements à retirer d'une série de 455 tumeurs de la région parotidienne. Mem Acad Chir 1955; 81:991–998.

121. Nanavati SD: Lipoma of the parotid gland: A case report. J Indian Dent Assoc 1983; 55:441–443.

122. Favero L, Barbazza R, Calabro S: Lipoma of the parotid: Description of a case and review of the literature. G Stomatol Ortognatodonzia 1983; 2:117–118.

123. Reilly JS, Kelly DR, Royal SA: Angiolipoma of the parotid: Case report and review. Laryngoscope 1988; 98:818–821.

124. Boltri F, Cuzzupoli F: Lipoma of the parotid gland. Cancro 1969; 22:26–31.

125. Perilli M, Bagnariol V: Pure lipoma of the parotid (personal case). Arch Ital Otol 1969; 80:100–107.

126. Bucciarelli E: On a case of lipoma of the parotid gland (with references of salivary gland tumors observed in Perugia from 1941 to 1967). Lav Ist Anat Istol Patol Perugia 1967; 27:123–128.

127. Giardino C: A case of lipoma of the parotid. Arch Stomatol (Napoli) 1973; 14:3–10.

128. Gierek T, Majzel K, Myrcik H: A case of parotid fibrolipoma. Otolaryngol Pol 1980; 34:517–519.

129. Schmookler BM, Enzinger FM: Pleomorphic lipoma: A benign tumor simulating liposarcoma. A clinicopathologic analysis of 48 cases. Cancer 1981; 47:126–133.

130. Fischer HP, Stambolis C: Pleomorphes Lipom: Ein kasuistischer und differential diagnostischer Beitrag. Pathologe 1983; 4:103–106.

131. Korentager R, Noyek AM, Chapnik JS, Steinhardt M, Luk SC, Cooter N: Lipoma and liposarcoma of the parotid gland: High resolution preoperative imaging diagnosis. Laryngoscope 1988; 98:967–971.

132. Doyan D, Laudenbach P, Glon Y, Deboise A, Jabbour M: Magnetic resonance and salivary pathology: Identification of a lipoma of the parotid gland. Rev Stomatol Chir Maxillofac 1988; 89:117–118.

133. Stout AP: Leiomyoma of the oral cavity. Am J Cancer 1938; 34:31–36.

134. Duhig JT, Ayer JP: Vascular leiomyoma: A study of sixty-one cases. Arch Pathol 1959; 68:424–430.

135. Kido T, Sekitani T: Vascular leiomyoma of the parotid gland. ORL J 1989; 51:187–191.

136. Hagy DM, Halperin V, Wood C III: Leiomyoma of the oral cavity: Review of the literature and report of a case. Oral Surg Oral Med Oral Pathol 1964; 17:748–755.

137. Cherrick HM, Dunlap CL, King OH Jr: Leiomyomas of the oral cavity: Review of the literature and clinicopathologic study of seven new cases. Oral Surg Oral Med Oral Pathol 1973; 35:54–66.

138. Damm DD, Neville BW: Oral leiomyomas. Oral Surg Oral Med Oral Pathol 1979; 47:343–348.

139. Morales AR, Fine G, Pardo V, Horn RC Jr: The ultrastructure of smooth muscle tumors with a consideration of the possible relationship of glomangiomas, hemangiopericytomas, and cardiac myxomas. Pathol Ann 1975; 10:65–92.

140. Abrikossoff A: Über Myome ausgehened von der Quergestreiften willkuerlichen Muskulatur. Virchows Arch [A] 1926; 260:215–233.

141. Vance SF, Hudson RP Jr: Granular cell myoblastoma—clinicopathologic study of 42 patients. Am J Clin Pathol 1969; 52:208–211.

142. Thawley SE, Ogura JH: Granular cell myoblastoma of the head and neck. South Med J 1974; 67:1020–1024.

143. Bourdial J, Natali R, Mahé E: Un cas de tumeur bénigne sous-maxillaire à "cellules granuleuses". Ann Otolaryngol Chir Cervicofac 1966; 83:784–787.

144. Noonan JD, Horton CE, Old WL, Stokes TL: Granular cell myoblastoma of the head and neck—review of the literature and 10 year experience. Am J Surg 1979; 138:611–614.

145. Regezi JA, Batsakis JG, Courtney RM: Granular cell tumors of the head and neck. J Oral Maxillofac Surg 1979; 37:402–406.

146. Joner JK, Kuo TT, Griffiths CM, Itharat S: Multiple granular cell tumors. Laryngoscope 1980; 90:1646–1651.

147. Stefansson K, Wollmann RL: S-100 protein in granular cell tumors (granular cell myoblastoma). Cancer 1982; 49:1834–1838.

148. Sobel HJ, Schwartz R, Marquet E: Light and electron microscopic study of granular cell myoblastoma. J Pathol 1973; 109:101–111.

149. Strong EW, McDivitt RW, Brasfield RD: Granular cell myoblastoma. Cancer 1970; 25:415–422.

150. Eusebi V, Martin SA, Govoni F, Rosai J: Giant cell tumor of major salivary glands: Report of three cases, one occurring in association with a malignant mixed tumor. Am J Clin Pathol 1984; 81:666–675.

151. Salm R, Sisson HA: Giant cell tumors of soft tissues. J Pathol 1972; 107:27–39.

152. Aplfelberg DB, Teasley JL: Unusual locations and manifestations of glomus tumors (glomangiomas). Am J Surg 1968; 116:62–64.

153. Horton C, Maguire C, Georgiade N, Pickrell K: Glomus tumors: An analysis of twenty-five cases. Arch Surg 1955; 71:712–716.

29

NONLYMPHOID SARCOMAS OF THE MAJOR SALIVARY GLANDS

P. L. Auclair and G. L. Ellis

Primary, nonlymphoid sarcomas of the major salivary glands are extremely rare. These tumors represent only 0.6 percent of all salivary gland tumors in the Armed Forces Institute of Pathology (AFIP) salivary gland pathology registry, and a possible bias toward unusual tumors in these files may cause even this figure to exceed the true incidence. However, because of treatment considerations, it is important to recognize that malignant mesenchymal tumors may occur in these sites dominated by epithelial malignancies. The diagnosis of a primary sarcoma should be considered only if the patient has not had a previous sarcoma that may have metastasized to or secondarily involved the salivary gland. With rare exceptions, no histologic, ultrastructural, or immunohistochemical evidence of a neoplastic epithelial component should be apparent. We recognize that when a tumor is large, no unequivocal proof of the tumor's anatomic origin may be discernible.

Most reports in the literature regarding salivary gland sarcomas have been sporadic and limited to case reports or analysis of a few cases. These reports have included cases of rhabdomyosarcoma,[1–12] fibrosarcoma,[12–16] leiomyosarcoma,[10, 17, 18] malignant fibrous histiocytoma,[10, 19–22] malignant schwannoma (neurofibrosarcoma),[4, 10, 23–25] angiosarcoma,[26, 27] hemangiopericytoma,[28–43] malignant hemangioendothelioma,[10, 13] Kaposi's sarcoma,[44, 45] osteosarcoma,[46, 47] liposarcoma,[10, 48, 49] malignant paraganglioma,[50] and sarcomas that could not be further classified.[4, 23, 24, 27, 51] Many of these cases lacked detailed clinical or surgical information, and frequently only brief microscopic descriptions were provided.

Seifert and Oehne[10] reviewed 167 mesenchymal salivary gland tumors from the Salivary Gland Register at the University of Hamburg. Seventeen cases were sarcomas and that number represented 0.5 percent of all benign and malignant primary salivary gland tumors and about 2.1 percent of all primary malignant tumors in their registry. The specific types included five malignant fibrous histiocytomas, five malignant schwannomas, four rhabdomyosarcomas, one myxoid liposarcoma, one leiomyosarcoma, and one malignant hemangioendothelioma.

In 1984, Auclair and coworkers[52] reviewed 67 cases of sarcomas and sarcomatoid neoplasms of the major salivary gland regions reported in the files of the AFIP. All 67 cases clinically presented as primary salivary gland malignancies. In an attempt to more accurately determine the origin of the tumors, the cases were grouped into three divisions that were based on the relationship of the tumor with the surrounding tissue at the time of surgery. In nine cases, it was the surgeon's impression that the tumor probably arose from periglandular tissues and may have involved the gland secondarily. In 20 of the remaining 58 cases, the surgical findings indicated origin from the salivary gland proper; however, in the other 38 cases, the exact relationship to the gland could not be determined. Many of the patients had large tumors, which precluded a meaningful surgical assessment of their origin. Furthermore, based on immunohistochemical study of 27 of the 67 tumors, 5 tumors were reclassified as anaplastic carcinomas, 4 as conventional or spindled malignant melanoma, and 1 as neurotropic melanoma. These findings demonstrate the difficult, sometimes impossible, task of identifying the specific anatomic site of origin and the wide differential diagnosis that must be considered when sarcomatoid neoplasms are encountered in the region of the major salivary glands. These findings also emphasize the value of performing immunohistochemical evaluation of the spindle cell malignancies that occur in these sites.

HISTOGENESIS

Debate about the histogenesis of these tumors focuses on two diametrically opposed hypotheses. The first states that sarcomas of salivary glands are derived from myoepithelial cells that are capable of multidirectional differentiation. This concept is supported by the immunohistochemical evidence that both the epithelial and mesenchymal-like elements in mixed tumors are of epithelial origin.[53–57] These studies suggest that the myoepithelial cell may undergo modulation of its intermediate filament composition and coexpress cytokeratins and mesenchymal markers, including vimentin. Ultrastructural findings support this opinion by demonstrating that the mixed tumor does not consist of distinct cell populations but of cells that show a continuum of cytoplasmic features with both epithelial and mesenchymal characteristics.

The second hypothesis, and the one we favor, proposes that sarcomas arise from pluripotential or uncommitted mesenchymal cells. This concept would explain the origin of certain sarcomas in areas where their normal tissue counterparts are either absent or scanty, such as rhabdomyosarcomas occurring in the urinary bladder, middle ear, nasal cavity, the intrabony compartment of the mandible or other bones, or in major salivary glands.[58, 59] Experimental chemical induction of salivary gland tumors has shown the development of a high proportion of sarcomas relative to carcinomas; this supports the idea that salivary gland regions may contain pluripotential cells.[60, 61] Furthermore, some investigations analyzed salivary gland tumors in children and showed that the combined number of sarcomas occurring in the parotid regions represented about 50 percent of the malignant neoplasms.[4, 23] Similarly, in a report of the Intergroup Rhabdomyosarcoma Study, among the head and neck and nonorbital and nonparameningeal sites, the parotid region was the second most common site involved.[62] It seems likely that sarcomas in these sites arise from undifferentiated mesenchymal cells.

CLINICAL FINDINGS

At present, the AFIP files contain 85 cases of nonlymphoid sarcomas that meet the diagnostic criteria discussed earlier in this chapter. These cases constitute 0.6 percent of all salivary gland tumors and 1.6 percent of all malignant tumors. Clinically, all patients appeared to have a primary salivary gland neoplasm. Furthermore, no evidence of a sarcoma at another site that may have metastasized was present in any patient. Thirteen specific types of sarcomas were represented but 9 cases could not be further classified on the basis of available material (Table 29–1).

The age range of the 85 patients was from 1 to 93 years. The average and median ages were 48.7 and 53.0 years, respectively. On average, female patients were about 2 years older than male patients. A few age differences are noted when these cases are analyzed according to specific sarcoma type (Fig. 29–1), although the number of cases is quite small when analyzed in this manner. The average age of the seven patients with rhabdomyosarcoma was 24.2 years, and the two patients with alveolar soft part sarcomas were 5 and 19 years of age. The relatively young ages of occurrence are in accordance with these types of tumors occurring in other sites.[63, 64] Patients with malig-

Table 29–1. Distribution of Patients with Nonlymphoid Sarcomas from the AFIP Registry by Major Salivary Gland Site and Histologic Type

Sarcoma Type	Parotid Gland	Submandibular Gland	Sublingual Gland	Total
Hemangiopericytoma	11	2	1	14
Malignant schwannoma	11	2	0	13
Fibrosarcoma	11	1	0	12
Malignant fibrous histiocytoma	7	2	0	9
Rhabdomyosarcoma	7	0	0	7
Angiosarcoma	5	0	0	5
Synovial sarcoma	2	2	0	4
Kaposi's sarcoma	2	1	0	3
Leiomyosarcoma	2	1	0	3
Liposarcoma	1	1	0	2
Alveolar soft part sarcoma	2	0	0	2
Epithelioid sarcoma	0	1	0	1
Extraosseous chondrosarcoma	1	0	0	1
Sarcoma, poorly differentiated	7	2	0	9
Total	69	15	1	85

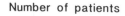

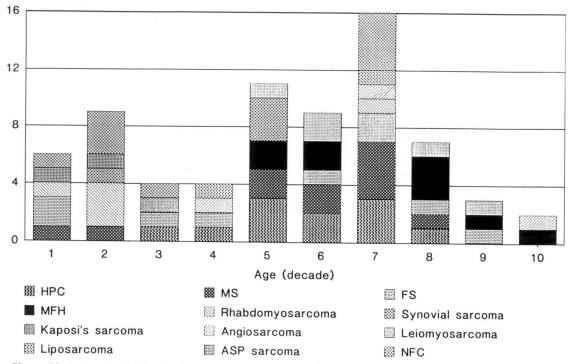

Figure 29–1. Age distribution by decade and histologic type of 72 patients with salivary gland sarcomas from the AFIP registry. (HPC = hemangiopericytoma; MS = malignant schwannoma; FS = fibrosarcoma; MFH = malignant fibrous histiocytoma; ASP = alveolar soft part sarcoma; NFC = not further classified.)

nant fibrous histiocytoma, angiosarcoma, and leiomyosarcoma are about 20 years older than the overall average of 48.7 years, again conforming to the ages of occurrence of these sarcomas in soft tissue sites in general.

There are 41 male patients and 34 female patients, and gender information was not available on the remaining 10 patients. If only the civilian population is considered to eliminate the male bias of the military/veteran population, a negligible predilection for occurrence in female patients (26 women, 24 men) is noted. All patients with rhabdomyosarcoma and Kaposi's sarcoma are male. Of the nine civilian patients with malignant schwannoma, eight are female. Other types of sarcoma affected men and women nearly equally. The race of the patient is known in 34 cases: 30 are white, three Asian, and one black.

The parotid gland dominates as the site of involvement. Sixty-one sarcomas (81.2 percent) occurred in the parotid gland, 15 (17.6 percent) occurred in the submandibular gland, and 1 (1.2 percent) occurred in the sublingual gland.

In the review of 67 cases of sarcomas and sarcomatoid neoplasms by Auclair and colleagues,[52] nearly all tumors occurred as a swelling, nodule, or mass. Nearly 16 percent of the patients complained of pain or tenderness, and 10 percent of the patients suffered facial paralysis. About 10

percent of the patients had noted rapid growth of the tumor in the period just before diagnosis. Tumor duration spanned from two weeks to 18 months, with an average time of 4.3 months. Tumor size varied from 1 to 7 cm in diameter, and the average was 3.1 cm. None of the patients had cervical lymphadenopathy at the time of diagnosis.

PATHOLOGIC FINDINGS

Salivary gland sarcomas are histologically classified according to a modified World Health Organization system[65] used for sarcomas from conventional soft tissue sites. Because the gross and microscopic features of each of the 13 different sarcoma types have been well described by many investigators, our discussion regarding their morphologic appearance is brief.

Among the AFIP cases, the single most common type of sarcoma within the major salivary glands is hemangiopericytoma (Figs. 29–2 and 29–3). Enzinger and Weiss[66] have recognized benign, borderline, and malignant subtypes. They have stated that in the majority of benign hemangiopericytomas two or three mitotic figures per ten high-power fields are present, whereas four or more mitotic figures per ten high-power fields are

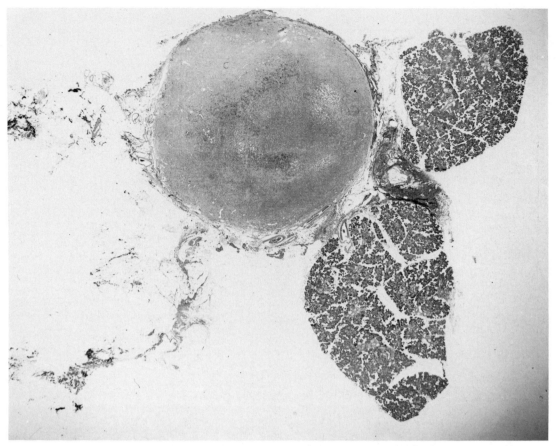

Figure 29–2. Hemangiopericytoma of the parotid replaces nearly the entire involved salivary lobule. A few ductal structures remain (× 3).

indicative of a rapidly growing tumor. Malignant hemangiopericytomas are generally more cellular and demonstrate mild to moderate cellular pleomorphism. Focal hemorrhage and necrosis may also be present. Because of difficulty in predicting the biologic behavior of this group of tumors on a morphologic basis, all hemangiopericytomas of the major salivary glands in the AFIP files have been included in our data (see Table 29–1). In their series of 106 cases, Enzinger and Smith[67] noted that 16 percent of tumors manifested in the head and neck regions and that this tumor was rare in children. In agreement with these findings, only 2 of the patients with hemangiopericytomas in the salivary glands were younger than 40 years, and none were under 20 years of age.

Several investigators[8, 68–70] have reported that in children, benign vascular tumors are among the most common salivary gland tumors, both epithelial and mesenchymal. With this in mind, it is interesting that malignant vascular tumors also predominate among all sarcomas in the AFIP files but in an adult population. Only one patient with a malignant vascular tumor was younger than age 30. In addition to the 14 hemangiopericytomas, there are 5 angiosarcomas (Fig. 29–4) and 3 Kaposi's sarcomas among the 85 cases reviewed. Therefore, 25 percent of all sarcomas were of vascular origin. Hemangiopericytomas are also the most common type of mesenchymal malignancy affecting the salivary glands reported in the literature.[28–43]

There are 13 patients with malignant schwannoma in the AFIP registry. The frequency of these tumors may be attributed to the abundant nerve supply of the major salivary glands and the parotid gland in particular. These tumors consist of cells with wavy nuclei and irregular nuclear contours that are arranged in densely cellular fascicles (Fig. 29–5). Myxoid zones are interspersed between the cellular areas where the parallel orientation of cells is absent. Nuclear palisading is evident focally. Three of the cases were interpreted as epithelioid malignant schwannomas. These are characterized by cords of large, polygonal cells with irregular nuclei, which have prominent nucleoli (Fig. 29–6). Low-power examination reveals a nodular growth pattern (Fig. 29–7) and areas that vary from extremely cellular to myxoid patterns.

Among the 85 AFIP cases, 7 rhabdomyosarco-

Text continued on page 522

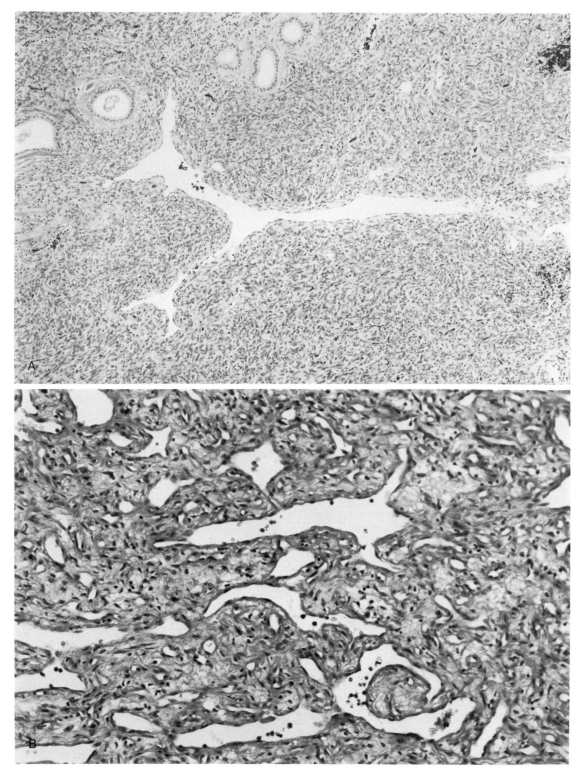

Figure 29–3. Photomicrographs of two different hemangiopericytomas demonstrate formation of ramifying blood channels that are typical within these tumors. The vessels vary in size and are lined by a single row of endothelium. Note a few residual ducts in (A). (A, × 75; B, × 150).

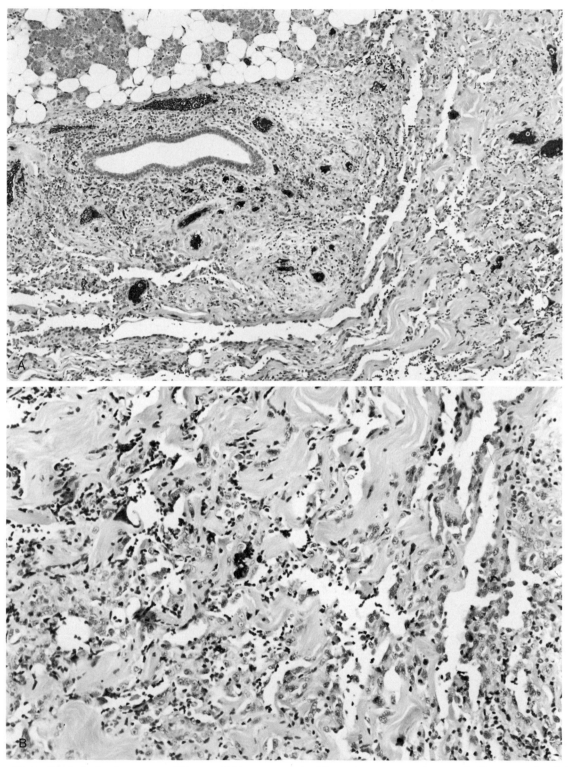

Figure 29–4. *A*, Angiosarcoma of the parotid has a network of irregular, anastomosing vessels (bottom and right) infiltrating the salivary gland (× 75). *B*, Higher magnification illustrates haphazard channels lined by irregular, large neoplastic cells (× 150).

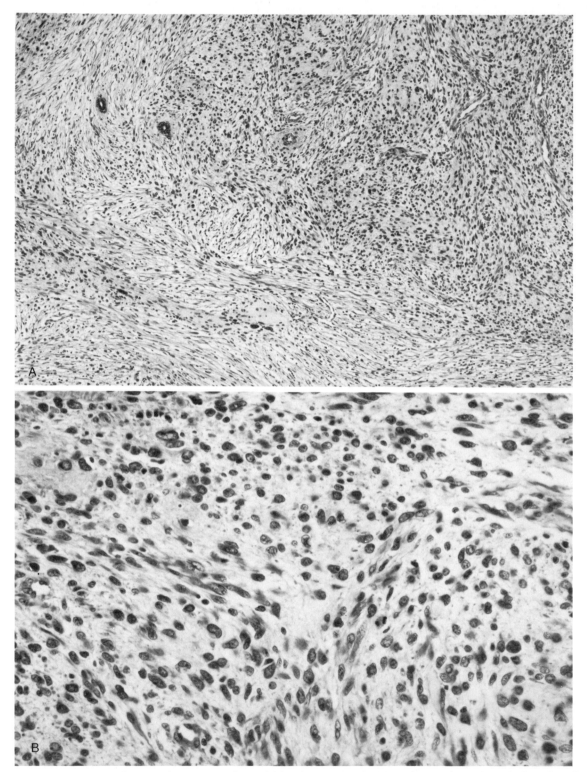

Figure 29–5. *A*, Malignant schwannoma of parotid has intersecting fascicles of wavy, irregular spindle cells. All but two salivary ducts have been replaced by tumor (× 75). *B*, Higher magnification shows a mixture of hyperchromatic ovoid and spindle cells (× 300).

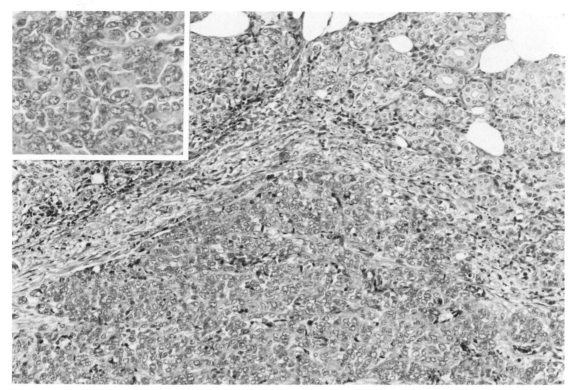

Figure 29–6. A malignant epithelioid schwannoma of the parotid gland is composed of a solid, sheetlike proliferation of cells in this area, but other areas showed tumor cells clustered in small cords. This rare form of malignant schwannoma can casily be misinterpreted as a primary epithelial neoplasm. Residual parotid gland acini and ducts are seen along the top (× 150; *inset*, × 300).

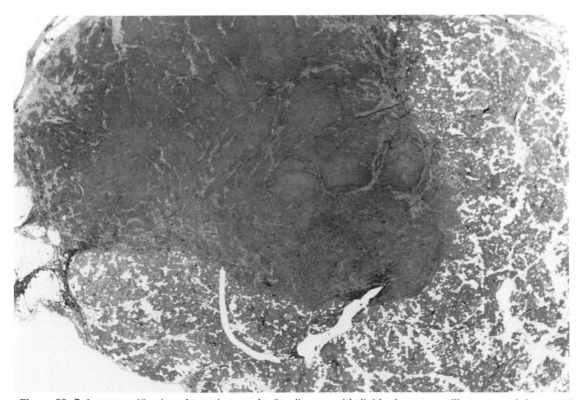

Figure 29–7. Low magnification photomicrograph of malignant epithelioid schwannoma illustrates nodular growth and infiltration through parotid parenchyma (× 7.5).

mas are included. Microscopically, four of the seven cases are the embryonal type, one is alveolar, one is pleomorphic, and one is not classified further. The average age among patients with the embryonal type is 13 years of age. The single patient with the pleomorphic rhabdomyosarcoma is 68 years of age. Other sarcoma types that occur with some frequency include fibrosarcomas and malignant fibrous histiocytomas (Fig. 29–8). The nine sarcomas that cannot be further classified consist of primitive spindled or rounded cells with no morphologic or immunohistochemical evidence of differentiation.

The incidence of occurrence of sarcoma types within the salivary glands is at variance with the reported frequency of occurrence of these tumors in soft tissues. Among sarcomas of traditional soft tissue sites studied at the AFIP from 1970 to 1979, the most common types, in descending order, were malignant fibrous histiocytoma, liposarcoma, fibrosarcoma, rhabdomyosarcoma, and synovial sarcoma. Hemangiopericytomas were considered relatively uncommon, and malignant schwannomas constituted only 10 percent of all sarcomas.[71]

BEHAVIOR AND TREATMENT

In the study by Auclair and colleagues[52] follow-up information was available for 42 patients with sarcomas of the major gland. Overall, about 50 percent of patients either died of disease or were alive with disease, a figure similar to that for high-grade, soft tissue sarcomas. Recurrences occurred in 17 patients (40 percent). The recurrence rates by specific histologic types of sarcomas were five of seven poorly differentiated sarcomas, three of five fibrosarcomas, four of nine malignant schwannomas, and two of five malignant fibrous histiocytomas. In 16 of the patients (38 percent), metastases developed. In ten patients, tumors metastasized to the lung, and other sites, including the brain, small bowel, heart, and pancreas, were often involved. Hematogenous dissemination was common, but lymph node metastasis was unusual, suggesting that lymph node dissection may not be an essential component of standard therapy. Metastases to regional lymph nodes occurred in only three patients, and in two of these patients, metastases to the lung and/or brain also occurred. Exelby[72] has noted that in contrast to many sarcomas, embryonal rhabdomyosarcoma may initially spread to regional lymph nodes. One of our cases with metastasis to lymph nodes was an embryonal rhabdomyosarcoma in a 7-year-old patient, who was also found to have metastatic tumor in the lungs and brain. Auclair and coworkers[52] found that the poorly differentiated sarcomas showed the highest metastatic rate (67 percent), whereas metastases developed in only one of five patients with fibrosarcoma. The metastatic rate was higher for tumors located in the submandib-

ular gland than for those in the parotid gland, and it was higher in patients whose tumors had an extraglandular component that was identified at surgery. In patients who died of disease, death occurred, on average, in 2.4 years, indicating that 5-year patient survival is probably a good indication of cure. Sixteen patients were alive and well with a mean follow-up time of 6.7 years. Patients with extraglandular tumor were more likely to die of disease than those whose tumors were confined to the gland.

Four of seven patients whose treatment consisted of "surgical excision" died of disease. However, of the nine patients treated by superficial or total parotidectomy, only one died of tumor. Similarly, of eight patients treated with a combination of surgery and radiation, tumor-related death occurred in only a single patient. Nearly all patients who received chemotherapy had far advanced disease, which made its efficacy difficult to assess.

Today many sarcomas have vastly improved prognoses as a result of effective combined treatment protocols that involve surgery, radiation, and chemotherapy. Detailed descriptions of current therapeutic modalities and prognoses for each specific type of sarcoma are available in many publications, including *Soft Tissue Tumors*, authored by Enzinger and Weiss.[63]

DIFFERENTIAL DIAGNOSIS

With a sarcomatoid neoplasm of the major salivary glands, the foremost diagnostic considerations are spindle cell carcinoma, carcinosarcoma, and melanoma. Although in our experience sarcomas rarely metastasize to the major glands, this possibility should also be ruled out. Once metastasis is ruled out, correct identification of the tumor as either mesenchymal or epithelial becomes critical to establishing treatment. This identification is more important for determining appropriate therapy than is determining whether the tumor originated in the salivary gland or periglandular tissues. As previously discussed, sarcomas are much less likely to metastasize to regional nodes than are carcinomas and, in general, are more amenable to chemotherapeutic agents.

As shown in our previous assessment of sarcomatoid lesions of the salivary glands,[52] immunohistochemistry plays a significant role in evaluation. Takata and colleagues[50] have discussed its role in the interpretation of undifferentiated tumors of the salivary glands. In many cases, the immunohistochemical studies provide valuable objective evidence for difficult morphologic interpretations. We have studied cases in which sarcomas were favored on the basis of morphologic criteria alone; however, the tumors surprisingly demonstrated diffuse immunoreactivity for cytokeratin and were ultimately interpreted as undifferentiated carci-

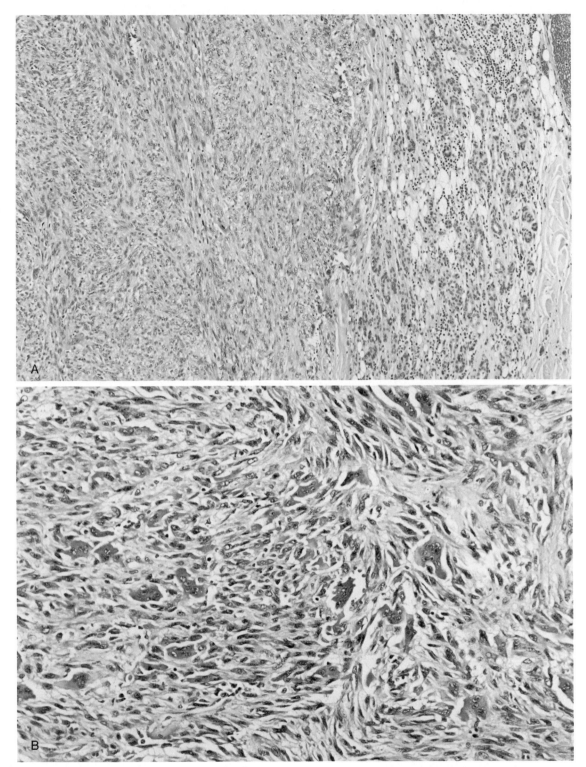

Figure 29–8. A malignant fibrous histiocytoma (left) infiltrates salivary parenchyma (right). Tumor has fascicular growth in some areas (A), but in other areas more pleomorphism and numerous multinucleated giant cells are evident (B). (A, × 75; B, × 150).

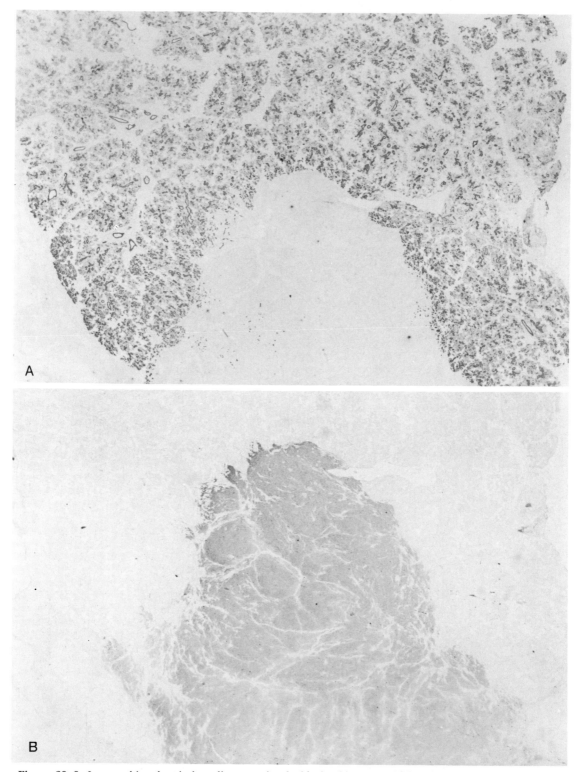

Figure 29–9. Immunohistochemical studies were invaluable in this case, which was submitted for consultative review as a high-grade adenocarcinoma (hematoxylin & eosin stain of tissue shown in Fig. 29–6). These two photomicrographs are of nearly identical fields and are of equal magnification. *A*, A dome-shaped portion of tumor projects upward from the bottom into the center of the field. Strong immunoreactivity with cytokeratin antisera outlines the normal gland occupying the upper half of the photograph, but the epithelioid tumor cells are nonreactive (× 7.5). *B*, Tumor cells are strongly immunoreactive for a neural marker, Leu-7, and the diagnosis of malignant epithelioid schwannoma is confirmed (× 7.5).

nomas. Although it is now recognized that many types of mesenchymal neoplasms may also contain cells immunoreactive for keratin, the reactive cells in these tumors are sparse and only weakly reactive.[73-79] The exceptions are synovial sarcoma and epithelioid sarcoma, discussed below. As suggested by Weiss and colleagues,[74] cytokeratin expression in tumors morphologically suspected to be sarcomas must be considered in the overall context of the case.

We have identified many malignant melanomas in the major glands. In most cases, the morphologic features observed with hematoxylin and eosin staining led us to suspect metastatic melanoma on initial review, and confirmation of the diagnosis was relatively straightforward. However, identification of occasional sarcomatoid melanomas has depended on the absence of cytokeratin immunoreactivity and demonstration of numerous cells that are immunoreactive for S-100 protein. Recently, we have also found HMB-45 monoclonal antibody to help in the identification of melanoma cells. We have reviewed one parotid tumor that had features of both malignant melanoma and malignant schwannoma and was identified as neurotropic melanoma.

Occasionally, sarcomas are misinterpreted as epithelial tumors or as melanomas. Sarcomas that may closely resemble carcinomas include malignant epithelioid schwannoma, synovial sarcoma, and epithelioid hemangioendothelioma. Malignant epithelioid schwannomas, unlike carcinomas but similar to melanomas, may be immunoreactive with Leu-7 and S-100 protein and are unreactive for keratin (Fig 29–9). Support for a diagnosis of malignant schwannoma would include documentation of origin of tumor from a nerve. Demonstration of melanin or immunoreactivity with HMB-45 antibody supports a diagnosis of melanoma, although rare schwannomas may contain small foci of melanin production.

Synovial sarcoma may morphologically and immunohistochemically resemble a carcinosarcomatous type of malignant mixed tumor or spindle cell carcinoma with residual ducts. The spindle cell component of these latter tumors is usually pleomorphic, whereas the spindle cell component of synovial sarcoma is more uniform. The secretions within the intraglandular spaces of synovial sarcoma stain with mucicarmine and are indistinguishable from those found in adenocarcinoma. Both the epithelial and spindle cell elements in synovial sarcoma may be immunoreactive for cytokeratin, although vimentin reactivity is present only in the spindle cells. The mesenchymal component of carcinosarcoma is usually chondrosarcoma[80] or myxosarcoma. In contrast, synovial sarcoma contains a more cellular fibrosarcoma-like spindle cell component, which has only focal myxoid areas. Chondroid differentiation is rarely seen. Calcification and ossification may occur in synovial sarcoma but, if present, are usually most prominent at the periphery rather than in the center of the tumor.

Although we have seen only one case of epithelioid sarcoma in the salivary glands, it is another sarcoma that is typically immunoreactive with cytokeratin. Both the epithelial and spindle cells may show reactivity. A feature that helps identify epithelioid sarcoma is the presence of multiple nodules that have central degeneration and necrosis and are often surrounded by moderately dense collections of chronic inflammatory cells.

Epithelioid hemangioendotheliomas are characterized by strands and solid nests of large, rounded, endothelial cells that show primitive vascular differentiation. This is manifested by the formation of small intracellular lumina, which resemble the mucin-containing vacuoles seen in adenocarcinoma. The stroma may be highly myxoid or hyalinized, imparting a cartilaginous appearance. Tumor cells typically reveal little atypia and few mitoses. Six epithelioid hemangioendotheliomas of the submandibular region have been described by Ellis and Kratochvil.[81] Epithelioid hemangioendotheliomas are mucin-negative, contain reticulin-positive material around both individual cells and groups of cells, are usually immunoreactive for Factor VIII–related antigen and *Ulex europaeus,* are usually unreactive for cytokeratin, and have ultrastructural characteristics of endothelium.

REFERENCES

1. Kauffman SL, Stout AP: Tumors of the major salivary glands in children. Cancer 1963; 16:1317–1331.
2. Hirtzler R, Urbanke A: Rhabdomyosarcoma of the parotid gland. Chir Maxillofac Plast 1967; 6:61–64.
3. Daou RA, Schloss MD: Childhood rhabdomyosarcoma of the head and neck. J Otolaryngol 1982; 11:52–56.
4. Welch KJ, Trump DS: The salivary glands. *In* Ravitch MM, Welch KJ, Benson CD, Aberdeen E, Randolph JG (eds): Pediatric Surgery, 3rd Ed. Chicago, Year Book Medical Publishers, Inc, 1979; 308–323.
5. Postoloff AU, Kaiser FF Jr: Rhabdomyosarcoma of the parotid gland: Report of a case. Cancer 1956; 9:1116–1119.
6. Stobbe GD, Dargeon HW: Embryonal rhabdomyosarcoma of the head and neck in children and adolescents. Cancer 1950; 3:826–836.
7. Archer CR: The radiologic manifestations of intracranial rhabdomyosarcoma. Neuroradiology 1976; 16:131–136.
8. Schuller DE, McCabe BF: Salivary gland neoplasms in children. Otolaryngol Clin North Am 1977; 10:399–412.
9. Sessions DG, Ragab AH, Vietti TJ, Biller HF, Ogura JH: Embryonal rhabdomyosarcoma of the head and neck in children. Laryngoscope 1973; 83:890–897.

10. Seifert G, Oehne H: Mesenchymal (nonepithelial) salivary gland tumors: Analysis of 167 cases of the salivary gland register. Laryngol Rhinol Otol (Stuttg) 1986; 65:485–491.

11. Renick B, Clark RM, Feldman L: Embryonal rhabdomyosarcoma: Presentation as a parotid gland mass. Oral Surg Oral Med Oral Pathol 1988; 65:575–579.

12. Volpe R: Primary sarcomas of the parotid gland: A clinicopathologic report of two cases. Pathologica 1981; 73:541–546.

13. Rawson AJ, Howard JM, Royster HP, Horn RC: Tumors of the salivary glands: A clinicopathologic study of 160 cases. Cancer 1950; 3:445–458.

14. Howard JM, Rawson RJ, Koop CE, Horn RC, Royster HP: Parotid tumors in children. Surg Gynecol Obstet 1950; 90:307–319.

15. Exelby PR, Knapper WH, Huvos AG, Beattie J Jr: Soft-tissue fibrosarcoma in children. J Pediatr Surg 1973; 8:415–420.

16. Gaillard de Collogny L, Delage J, Lafaye M, Lagarde R, Pottecher G, Charbonnel P: Fibrosarcome de la sous-maxillaire. J Fr Otorhinolaryngol 1980; 29:391–396.

17. Sandhyamani S, Mahapatra AK, Kapur BM: Leiomyosarcoma of the parotid gland. Aust NZ J Surg 1983; 53:179–181.

18. Wheelock MC, Madden TJ: Uncommon tumours of the salivary glands. Surg Gynecol Obstet 1949; 88:776–782.

19. O'Brien JE, Stout AP: Malignant fibrous xanthoma. Cancer 1964; 17:1445–1455.

20. Benjamin E, Wells S, Fox H, Reeve NL, Knox F: Malignant fibrous histiocytoma of salivary glands. J Clin Pathol 1982; 35:946–953.

21. Hutchinson JC Jr, Friedberg SA: Fibrous histiocytoma of the head and neck: A case report. Laryngoscope 1978; 88:1950–1955.

22. van Wingerden JJ, van Rensburg PG, Coetzee BP: Malignant fibrous histiocytoma of the parotid gland associated with polycythemia. Head Neck Surg 1986; 8:218–221.

23. Karlan MS, Snyder WH Jr: Salivary gland tumors and sialadenitis in children: Experience at Children's Hospital of Los Angeles. Cal Med 1968; 108:423–429.

24. Welch KJ, Trump DS: The salivary glands. *In* Mustard WT, Ravitch MM, Snyder WH, Welch KJ, Benson (eds): Pediatric Surgery, 2nd Ed. Chicago, Year Book Medical Publishers, Inc, 1969; 215–231.

25. Piscioli F, Antolini M, Pusiol T, Dalri P, Lo-Bello, MD, Mair K: Malignant schwannoma of the submandibular gland: A case report. ORL J Otorhinolaryngol Relat Spec 1986; 48:156–161.

26. Tomec R, Ahmad I, Fu YS, Jaffe S: Malignant hemangioendothelioma (angiosarcoma) of the salivary gland. Cancer 1979; 43:1664–1671.

27. Kirklin JW, McDonald JR, Harrington SW, New GB: Parotid tumours: Histopathology, clinical behaviour, and end results. Surg Gynecol Obstet 1951; 92:721–733.

28. Stout AP: Tumors featuring pericytes. Lab Invest 1956; 5:217–223.

29. Cernea P, Debry D, Laudenbach P, Moreau R, Brocheriou C, Cathelin M, Vaillan JM, Guilbert F, Soubiran JM, Chevallier C, Hosxe G, Peri G: Hémangiopércytome de la parotide. Rev Stomatol Chir Maxillofac 1969; 70:132–135.

30. Pellegrini G, Verdaguer S, Boyre F, de Firmas JL, Philip F: Hémangiopéricytoma parotidien. Rev Laryngol 1967; 28:421–427.

31. Boyre F, Firmas JL de, Philip F: Parotid hemangiopericytoma. Rev Laryngol Otol Rhinol (Bord) 1967; 88:421–427.

32. Leonardelli GB, Bergomi A: Une tumeur rare de la parotide: l'hémangiopéricytome de Murray et Stout. Cah Otorhinolaryngol 1970; 5:37–40.

33. Farr HW, Carandant CM, Huvos AG: Malignant vascular tumors of the head and neck. Am J Surg 1970; 120:501–504.

34. Neal TF, Starke WR: Hemangiopericytoma of the parotid gland: A case report with autopsy. Laryngoscope 1973; 83:1953–1958.

35. Katz AD: Unusual lesions of the parotid gland. J Surg Oncol 1975; 7:219–235.

36. Massarelli G, Tanda F, Fois V, Oppia L: Haemangiopericytoma of the parotid gland: Report of a case and review of the literature. Virchows Arch [A] 1980; 368:81–89.

37. Hubert JC, Drevet D, Gay R: A propos d'un cas d'hémangiopéricytome parotidien. J Fr Otorhinolaryngol 1970; 19:659–661.

38. Yamaguchi KT, Krugman ME, Barr RJ, Reingold IM: Hemangiopericytoma of the parotid gland with a review of the literature. J Otolaryngol 1977; 6:431–435.

39. Peynègre R, Pain F: Un hémangiopéricytome de la parotide chez l'enfant. Ann Otolaryngol Chir Cervicofac 1978; 95:789–793.

40. Auguste LJ, Razack MS, Sako K: Hemangiopericytoma. J Surg Oncol 1982; 20:260–264.

41. Bertrand JC, Guilbert F, Vaillant JM, Szpirglas H, Chomette G, Auriol M, Mercier C: Les hémangiopéricytome de la sphère oro-faciale. Ann Otolaryngol Chir Cervicofac 1984; 101:607–613.

42. Tatum RC, Skinner HG, Adrian J: Hemangiopericytoma of the parotid: Report of a rare case with literature review. Quintessence Int 1986; 17:399–403.

43. Pagliaro G, Poli P, Ralza G, Grandi G: Haemangiopericytoma of the submandibular gland (a case report). J Laryngol Otol 1988; 102:97–99.

44. Puterman M, Goldstein J: Primary lymph nodal Kaposi's sarcoma of the parotid gland. Head Neck Surg 1983; 5:535–538.

45. Yeh C-K, Fox PC, Fox CH, Travis WD, Lane HC, Baum BJ: Kaposi's sarcoma of the parotid gland in acquired immunodeficiency syndrome. Oral Surg Oral Med Oral Pathol 1989; 67:308–312.

46. Manning JT, Raymon AK, Batsakis JG: Extraosseous osteogenic sarcoma of the parotid gland. J Laryngol Otol 1986; 100:239–242.

47. Stimson PG, Valenzuela-Espinoza A, Torteledo ME, Luna MA, Ordonez NG: Primary osteosarcoma of the parotid gland. Oral Surg Oral Med Oral Pathol 1989; 68:80–86.

48. Jones JK, Baker HW: Liposarcoma of the parotid gland: Report of a case. Arch Otolaryngol 1980; 106:497–499.

49. Korentager R, Noyek AM, Chapnik JS, Steinhardt M, Luk SC, Cooter, N: Lipoma and liposarcoma of the parotid gland: High-resolution preoperative imaging diagnosis. Laryngoscope 1988; 98:967–971.

50. Takata T, Caselitz J, Seifert G: Undifferentiated tumours of salivary glands. Pathol Res Pract 1987; 182:161–168.

51. Jaffe BF: Pediatric head and neck tumors: A study of 178 cases. Laryngoscope 1973; 83:1644–1651.

52. Auclair PL, Langloss JM, Weiss SW, Corio RL: Sarcomas and sarcomatoid neoplasms of the major salivary gland regions: A clinicopathologic and immunohistochemical study of 67 cases and review of the literature. Cancer 1986; 58:1305–1315.

53. Caselitz J, Osborn M, Wustrow J, Seifert G, Weber K: The expression of different intermediate-sized filaments in human salivary glands and their tumours. Pathol Res Pract 1982; 175:266–278.

54. Caselitz J, Loning T, Staquet MJ, Seifert G, Thivolet J: Immunocytochemical demonstration of filamentous structures in the parotid gland. J Cancer Res Clin Oncol 1981; 100:59–68.

55. Caselitz J, Osborn M, Seifert G, Weber K: Intermediate-sized filament proteins (prekeratin, vimentin, desmin) in the normal parotid gland and parotid gland tumours. Virchows Arch [A] 1981; 393:273–286.

56. Krepler R, Denk H, Artlieb V, Moll R: Immunocytochemistry of intermediate filament proteins present in pleomorphic adenomas of the human parotid gland: Characterization of different cell types in the same tumor. Differentiation 1982; 21:191–199.

57. Mori M, Sumitomo S, Iwai Y, Meenagham MA: Immunolocalization of keratins in salivary gland pleomorphic adenoma using monoclonal antibodies. Oral Surg Oral Med Oral Pathol 1986; 61:611–616.

58. Peters E, Cohen M, Altini M, Murray J: Rhabdomyosarcoma of the oral and paraoral region. Cancer 1989; 63:963–966.

59. Almanaseer IY, Trujillo YP, Taxy JB, Okuno T: Systemic rhabdomyosarcoma with diffuse bone marrow involvement. Am J Clin Pathol 1984; 82:349–353.

60. Takeuchi J, Miura K, Usizima H, Katoh Y: Histological changes in the submandibular glands of rats after intraductal injection of chemical carcinogens. Acta Pathol Jpn 1975; 25:1–13.

61. Cataldo EF, Reif AE: An explanation for the proportion of carcinomas and sarcomas seen in chemically induced murine submaxillary gland tumors. Cancer 1982; 50:531–542.

62. Wharam MD Jr, Foulkes MA, Lawrence W Jr, Lindberg RD, Maurer HM, Newton WA Jr, Ragab AH, Raney RB Jr, Tefft M: Soft tissue sarcoma of the head and neck in childhood: Nonorbital and nonparameningeal sites. Cancer 1984; 53:1016–1019.

63. Enzinger FM, Weiss SW: Soft Tissue Tumors, 2nd Ed. St. Louis, CV Mosby Co, 1988; 449–450.

64. Lieberman PH, Brennan MF, Kimmel M, Erlandson RA, Garin-Chesa P, Flehinger BY: Alveolar soft-part sarcoma: A clinico-pathologic study of half a century. Cancer 1989; 63:1–13.

65. Enzinger FM, Weiss SW: Soft Tissue Tumors, 2nd Ed. St. Louis, CV Mosby Co, 1988; 4–8.

66. Enzinger FM, Weiss SW: Soft Tissue Tumors, 2nd Ed. St. Louis, CV Mosby Co, 1988; 596–613.

67. Enzinger FM, Smith BH: Hemangiopericytoma: An analysis of 106 cases. Hum Pathol 1976; 7:61–82.

68. Castro EB, Huvos AG, Strong EW, Foote FW JR: Tumors of the major salivary glands in children. Cancer 1972; 29:312–317.

69. Krolls SO, Trodahl JN, Boyers RC: Salivary gland lesions in children: A survey of 430 cases. Cancer 1972; 30:459–469.

70. Lack EE, Upton MP: Histopathologic review of salivary gland tumors in childhood. Arch Otolaryngol Head Neck Surg 1988; 114:898–906.

71. Enzinger FM, Weiss SW: Soft Tissue Tumors, 2nd Ed. St. Louis, CV Mosby Co, 1988; 5, 202, 347, 449, 596, 659, 782.

72. Exelby PR: Management of embryonal rhabdomyosarcoma in children. Surg Clin N Amer 1974; 54:849–857.

73. Brown DC, Theaker JM, Banks PM, Gatter KC, Mason DY: Cytokeratin expression in smooth muscle and smooth muscle tumours. Histopathology 1987; 11:477–486.

74. Weiss SW, Bratthauer GL, Morris PA: Postirradiation malignant fibrous histiocytoma expressing cytokeratin: Implications for the immunodiagnosis of sarcomas. Am J Surg Pathol 1988; 12:554–558.

75. Norton AJ, Thomas JA, Isaacson PG: Cytokeratin-specific monoclonal antibodies are reactive with tumours of smooth muscle derivation: An immunocytochemical and biochemical study using antibodies to intermediate filament cytoskeletal proteins. Histopathology 1987; 11:487–499.

76. Miettinen M, Rapola J: Immunohistochemical spectrum of rhabdomyosarcoma and rhabdomyosarcoma-like tumors. Expression of cytokeratin and the 68-dK neurofilament protein. Am J Surg Pathol 1989; 13:120–132.

77. Miettinen M: Immunoreactivity for cytokeratin and epithelial membrane antigen in leiomyosarcoma. Arch Pathol Lab Med 1988; 112:637–640.

78. Cosgrove M, Fitzgibbons PL, Sherrod A, Chandrasoma PT, Martin SE: Intermediate filament expression in astrocytic neoplasms. Am J Surg Pathol 1989; 13:141–145.

79. Theaker J, Gatter KC, Esiri MM, Fleming KA: Epithelial membrane antigens and cytokeratin expression by meningiomas: An immunohistochemical study. J Clin Pathol 1986; 39:435–439.

80. Stephen J, Batsakis JG, von der Heyden U, Byers RM: True malignant mixed tumors (carcinosarcoma) of salivary glands. Oral Surg Oral Med Oral Pathol 1986; 61:597–602.

81. Ellis GL, Kratochvil FJ: Epithelioid hemangioendothelioma of the head and neck: A clinicopathologic report of twelve cases. Oral Surg Oral Med Oral Pathol 1986; 61:61–68.

30

MALIGNANT LYMPHOMAS

James J. Sciubba, Paul L. Auclair, and Gary L. Ellis

In addition to the production of saliva, the salivary glands have an important immunologic role. The epithelial cells produce receptor proteins for dimeric IgA and pentameric IgM. Furthermore, lymphoid tissue is present within the parotid and submandibular glands. The mesenchyma of the parotid is colonized by numerous lymphocytes by the 12th week of fetal life.[1] Lymphocytes may be individually distributed in small clusters or may be distributed within lymph nodes in the parotid gland.[1] An average of 20, and as many as 32, intraparotid lymph nodes have been found by serial sectioning of the gland.[2] Salivary ductal and acinar epithelium can usually be found within the medullary region of these lymph nodes.

The prevalence of intraparotid lymphoid tissue is reflected by the high proportion of parotid tissue specimens in the salivary gland registry of the Armed Forces Institute of Pathology (AFIP) that have a prominent lymphoid element or are of lymphoid origin. More than 1,600 such parotid lesions exist, including the benign lymphoepithelial lesion, lymphoepithelial cyst, lymphoid hyperplasia, Warthin's tumors, and malignant lymphomas. These cases constitute about 16 percent of all neoplastic and non-neoplastic parotid lesions.

Despite recognition of the close association between salivary glands and lymphoid tissue, some investigators[3, 4] consider all salivary gland lymphomas as extranodal, whereas others distinguish between nodal and extranodal tumors.[5-7] In one of these latter studies, salivary gland lymphomas that arose within previously existing benign lymphoepithelial lesions (BLEL) were classified as extranodal, and the balance were classified as nodal in origin.[6] We have reviewed cases that apparently arose from within intraparotid lymph nodes and others that appeared totally unassociated with nodal tissue. In most cases, it is difficult or impossible to establish nodal or extranodal origin with certainty.

As Gleeson and colleagues[3] have indicated, salivary lymphoma as a primary process may be difficult to classify. These investigators suggested that salivary lymphomas be placed within nodal categories so that comparison with similar lymphomas in other locations might be possible.

A subject related to salivary lymphomas has gained recent attention and may explain some of the problems in classification. It is the unique nature of lymphoid tissue associated with mucosa. Lymphoid tissue of the gastrointestinal mucosa (*gut-associated-lymphoid tissue*, or GALT) has been well described.[8, 9] The lymphoid tissue in the gut wall is integrated into the systemic immune system by preferential migration of some of the system's lymphocytes to other mucosal sites, including the salivary glands.[10] The recognition and understanding of GALT have led to the designation of lymphoid tissue associated with mucosa in other sites, including the stomach, bronchi and genital tract as well as the mammary, thyroid, and salivary glands, as *mucosa-associated lymphoid tissue* (MALT). In the minor salivary glands, this lymphoid tissue has been referred to as duct-associated lymphoid tissue.[11] Apparently, lymphocytes adjacent to the ductal epithelium and within the connective tissue are stimulated by repeated exposure to antigens, resulting in a local immune response.[12] The characteristic cell of MALT is the monocytoid B lymphocyte, or centrocytelike cell, which is so named because of its resemblance to follicular center lymphocytes. These cells are usually slightly larger than small lymphocytes and often have clear cytoplasm and well-defined cell margins.

The lymphoid tissue in these extranodal MALT sites gives rise to a group of lymphomas that often share distinctive clinical, histologic, and immunohistochemical features.[13-16] Isaacson and Spencer[15] have observed that lymphomas developing from this tissue do not fit into any of the categories included in current classifications. Furthermore, many MALT-derived lymphomas tend to remain localized and to evolve slowly. This has led Isaacson and Wright[14] to suggest that the lymphoma cells in these tumors show the specific homing patterns characteristic of MALT-derived lymphocytes or are nonrecirculating cell types.[15] Either concept may explain the regional nature of the disease. Morphologically, it is recognized that lymphomas derived from MALT include small cell lymphocytic lymphoma with plasmacytoid differentiation and monocytoid B-cell lymphoma,[17, 18] which may progress to large cell lymphoma.[15, 19] Furthermore, T-cell and true histiocytic tumors also occur, but less frequently.[20] Lymphomas derived from MALT are characterized by the proliferation of monocytoid B lymphocytes, which tend to invade mucosal epithelium, often in small groups; the formation of lymphoepithelial lesions;[15] and the presence of follicles with reactive germinal centers. In the salivary glands, these lymphomas have usually been associated with BLEL.[21]

Our experience with salivary non-Hodgkin's lymphomas has been that most are readily categorized using current classifications for nodal disease. Yet, our impression is that few show histopathologic evidence of association with nodal tissue. We have reviewed several lymphomas associated with BLEL that demonstrated the features of MALT origin. It is hoped that ongoing studies can provide more accurate histopathologic categorization of these lymphomas and more precise correlation with biologic behavior.

Incidence

The incidence of non-Hodgkin's lymphomas has increased by 123 percent since 1950.[22] Overall, the increase in incidence is greater than the increase in mortality. The increase in the age-adjusted incidence is caused primarily by an increase in incidence among persons aged 65 and over. Although an increase is noted among patients in the 35- to 64-year age group, this increase is of lower magnitude. Within the general group of lymphomas, the reported proportion of tumors presenting as salivary gland masses ranges from 0.06 to 5.00 percent.[3, 23–27] It is interesting to note that Foote and Frazell,[28] in 1954, did not report a single primary malignant lymphoma among 766 parotid tumors. Since that time, however, salivary gland lymphomas, in particular those affecting the parotid region, have appeared with increasing frequency in the literature.[3–6, 16, 26, 27, 29]

The AFIP salivary gland registry contains 455 cases of malignant lymphoma that involved the major salivary glands. Although detailed clinical information is not available for all cases, to our knowledge, the salivary gland enlargement was the first clinical manifestation of disease. On histopathologic examination, all tumors involved the parenchyma. Some parotid tumors possibly arose from intraglandular lymph nodes; however, as discussed, this determination was often very difficult. No submandibular tumors were thought to have originated from lymph nodes in the submandibular area and extended into the gland secondarily. The 455 AFIP cases include 420 non-Hodgkin's lymphomas and 35 Hodgkin's lymphomas. Each of these groups is discussed separately in this chapter. The prognoses and treatments for all groups are discussed at the end of the chapter. Classification of non-Hodgkin's lymphoma and microscopic characteristics of each type are not discussed. Literature on the subject is voluminous, and none of the histologic types are unique to the salivary glands. Furthermore, the salivary gland registry includes cases that were reported more than 40 years ago, and many classification schemes have been applied during that time. Currently, we are using the Working Formulation for classification of non-Hodgkin's lymphomas.[30]

The 420 non-Hodgkin's cases constitute 11.4 percent of all primary malignant tumors of the major salivary glands. The 340 parotid lymphomas constitute 11.1 percent of all primary parotid malignancies in the AFIP files. The proportion of the lymphomas of all parenchymal salivary gland tumors involving the parotid gland has steadily increased during the past 21 years (Fig. 30–1). Schusterman and coworkers[27] have also observed an increase from 1.5 to 6.0 percent of salivary gland tumors during a 34-year period.

BENIGN LYMPHOEPITHELIAL LESION AND LYMPHOMA

In our experience, the vast majority of lymphomas of the major salivary glands arise de novo rather than from pre-existing salivary gland disease. Of the 420 cases of non-Hodgkin's lymphoma in the AFIP salivary gland registry, only 11 were interpreted as having arisen within BLEL. Of those 11 cases, 8 were found within the parotid gland, whereas 3 were within the submandibular gland. The ratio of male to female patients was seven to four, and the average age was 60.4 years, with a range of 50.0 to 73.0 years.

The evolution from BLEL to lymphoma is thought to be a multistep process, with lymphoproliferation leading to emergence of a neoplastic clone that escapes immunologic control and develops into a non-Hodgkin's lymphoma. The initiation may be Sjögren's syndrome, which is an autoimmune disease characterized by xerostomia and xerophthalmia secondary to lymphocytic infiltration (BLEL) that leads to destruction of salivary and lacrimal parenchyma (see Chapter 6).

A high proportion of patients with Sjögren's syndrome demonstrate a paraproteinemia and have a correspondingly high frequency of non-Hodgkin's B-cell lymphomas.[7, 31, 32] Although controversy exists as to the exact risk of lymphoma developing within Sjögren's syndrome, most authorities agree that there is increased risk.[7, 31]

Percent

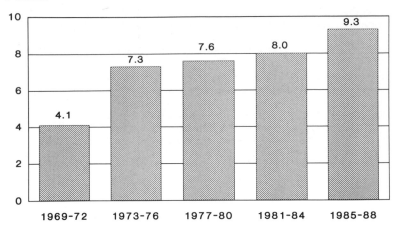

Figure 30–1. Parotid lymphomas as a percentage of the primary epithelial tumors in the AFIP salivary gland registry. An increase in the percentage of lymphomas during each 4-year period over the past 20 years has occurred.

Among 136 Sjögren's patients, Kassan and coworkers[31] noted the occurrence of 7 cases of lymphoma; this amount is 43.8 times higher than the expected number in a control group. This study established the risk of lymphoma among the Sjögren's syndrome population at approximately 6.4 cases per 1,000 patients per year. Furthermore, the risks of lymphoma in primary versus secondary Sjögren's syndrome were roughly similar, although others believe lymphoma to be more common in primary Sjögren's syndrome.[33] Neither age nor duration of Sjögren's syndrome was associated with increased risk of lymphoma; however, lymphoma was more likely to develop in patients with parotid swelling than in those patients without swelling. Additional risk factors affecting this population include lymphadenopathy and splenomegaly. This risk of lymphoma seems peculiar to the Sjögren's syndrome population of patients, since no evidence of oligoclonal rearrangements in tissue biopsies is evident in studies of patients with other autoimmune diseases. This increased risk indicates that individuals with Sjögren's syndrome need to be closely followed.

It can be difficult to distinguish reactive expansions of intrasalivary lymphoid cells from malignant lymphoma. Furthermore, lymphomas may remain relatively dormant over many years, and some low-grade lymphomas appear capable of undergoing spontaneous remission without therapy.[34, 35] Regardless of the ultimate outcome, however, individuals with Sjögren's syndrome and benign lymphoepithelial lesions have a lymphoproliferative disorder that increases the chance of malignant transformation.[36]

The lymphoepithelial lesion is a progressive disorder that begins as a focal lymphoreticular reaction around salivary ducts and progresses to total or near total replacement of glandular parenchyma with disruption and metaplasia of the ductal system. Scattered epimyoepithelial islands develop within a rich stroma of lymphocytes,

plasma cells, and other immunocytes.[37] From limited salivary gland disease, the sialadenopathy progresses to limited exocrine disease, which is clinically characterized by the sicca syndrome (see Chapter 6). The progression from focal periductal lymphocytic sialadenitis to BLEL and then to malignant lymphoma may be traced to an oligoclonal expansion of B and T lymphocytes within the salivary gland tissue. The ultimate event in this multistep process is the development of lymphoma from one or more of these expanded clones.

When lymphoma arises within a benign lymphoepithelial lesion, the process is generally slow and can take as long as 20 years.[33] During this time, immunodysregulation can be roughly separated into three stages. First, autoimmune exocrinopathy manifests as benign lymphoid infiltrates confined to glandular tissue. At this point, hypergammaglobulinemia may be present as well as xerostomia and xerophthalmia. This initial pathologic state progresses to the second stage, pseudolymphoma, during which extraglandular lymphoid infiltrates, hypergammaglobulinemia, and a monoclonal spike are present. Clinically, the patient demonstrates lymphadenopathy, splenomegaly, and lymphoid infiltrates of the lungs and kidneys. The final phase is the development of lymphoma with progressive lymphadenopathy, salivary gland enlargement, and wasting. Pathologically, a B-cell lymphoma is identified. The lymphomatous infiltrate extends beyond the gland and no longer appears confined to individual salivary gland lobules. Extension of the cellular proliferation to interlobular connective tissue results in the appearance of lobular confluence and disruption of the normal salivary gland architecture (Fig. 30–2). High magnification reveals a monotypical infiltrate that surrounds scattered epimyoepithelial islands (Fig. 30–3). Serologically, hypogammaglobulinemia and loss of previously identifiable autoantibodies of the SS-A (anti-Ro) and/or SS-B (anti-La) types occur. Therefore, lym-

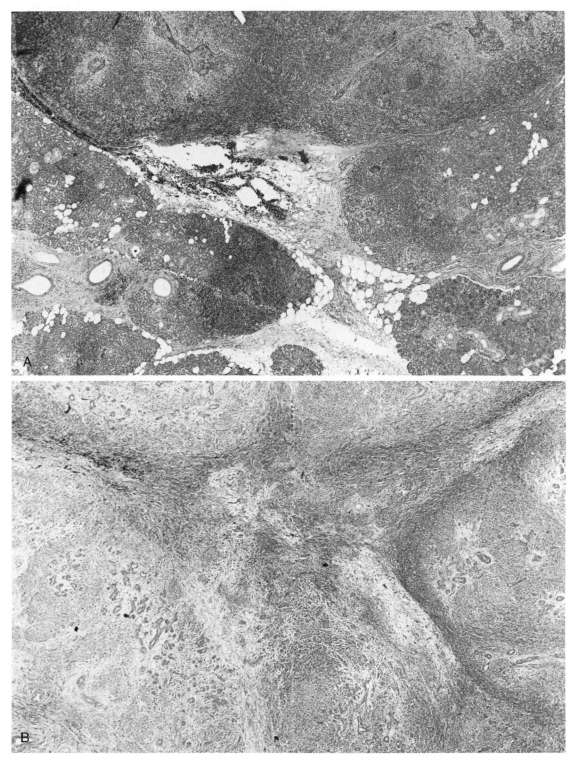

Figure 30–2. *A*, Benign lymphoepithelial lesion shows lymphoid infiltrate confined to salivary gland lobules (× 30). *B*, Lymphomatous infiltrate permeates interlobular connective tissue and destroys the normal lobular glandular architecture (× 30).

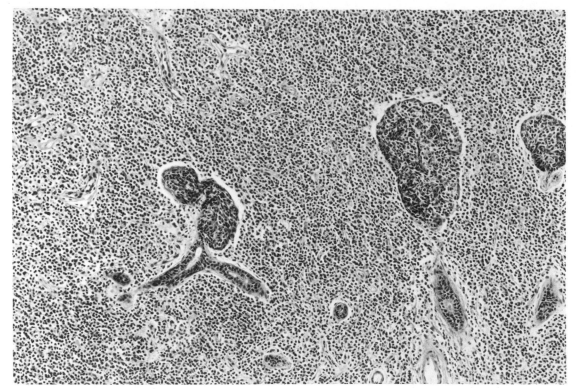

Figure 30–3. Epimyoepithelial islands and residual salivary gland ducts are surrounded by monotypical lymphomatous infiltrate (× 75).

phoma results from aggressive B-cell activation within salivary glands, which evolves to an extraglandular state with potential for malignant transformation during its course.

NON-HODGKIN'S LYMPHOMA (DE NOVO)

Non-Hodgkin's lymphoma arising de novo within salivary glands (409 cases) constitutes the vast majority (97.4 percent) of the 420 primary lymphomas in the AFIP registry seen within these tissues. These lymphomas represent about 3 percent of all salivary gland tumors in the AFIP registry. Of these 409 cases, 305 (75 percent) were in the parotid gland, 93 (23 percent) in the submandibular gland, and 1 in the sublingual gland. The site of occurrence for the remaining 10 cases was stated to be a major salivary gland but was not further specified.

A wide patient age range (1 to 100 years) was noted in the series of 409 patients, with a predominance (61.9 percent) of females affected within the civilian population. The average ages of male and female patients were 59.6 and 64.2 years, respectively. A peak incidence of occurrence was noted among patients in the seventh decade of life (Fig. 30–4). In the overwhelming majority of individuals with malignant lymphoma of major salivary gland origin, the lesion is an asymptomatic

mass within the affected gland. In reviewing the data of Watkin and colleagues,[26] it is interesting that 11 of 17 parotid gland lymphomas exhibited atypical features, such as attachment to skin and bone, facial nerve paresis, pain and rapid growth, multiple masses in the parotid region, multiple bilateral masses, and associated palpable lymph nodes. Of interest is that a single lymphoma within this series was found to have arisen in association with a previously existing Warthin's tumor, and the histologic subtype was a diffuse large cell/ histiocytic lesion similar to those reported by Miller and colleagues[38] and Hall and colleagues.[39] Regardless of the origin of salivary gland lymphoma, such changes within salivary gland tissue mandate a complete staging procedure to determine whether the lymphoma is indeed primary at this location. Staging must include an adequate oral examination as well as lymph node biopsy, if possible, and radiographic imaging. Additionally, peripheral blood studies and bone marrow aspiration should be included. The results of staging impact on treatment and prognosis, which are discussed below.

Pathologic Features

On gross examination, the involved gland is firm, and in tissue sections, it appears tan to white and homogenous (Fig. 30–5). The diagnostic

Percent

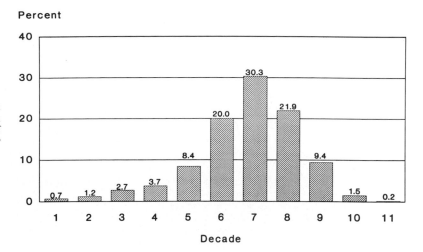

Figure 30–4. Age distribution (by decade) for 406 patients with non-Hodgkin's lymphomas of the salivary glands in the AFIP registry.

problem for the pathologist is the application of conventional histologic criteria to separate reactive lymphoid hyperplasia from nodal or extranodal lymphoma.[40]

The microscopic appearance of malignant lymphomas within the major salivary glands may be identical to that of those malignancies arising in extraglandular lymphoid tissues. In some instances, it is obvious that the tumor arose within an intraparotid lymph node and is beginning to permeate perinodal salivary gland parenchyma. In these cases, alteration of nodal architecture may be an important diagnostic criterion. In most cases, however, no evidence of lymph node in-

volvement is present; thus, the diagnosis depends entirely on assessment of the parenchymal lymphoreticular infiltrate (Fig. 30–6). The lymphomatous infiltrate may replace a large part of the salivary gland parenchyma, destroying its normal lobular organization (Fig. 30–7), and may spread into periglandular tissues. Scattered salivary gland ducts, which are much more resistant to replacement by tumor cells than acini, and epimyoepithelial islands may remain as the only evidence of glandular involvement (Fig. 30–8). Interlobular and periductal fibrosis may be prominent (Fig. 30–9). In salivary lymphomas that are seen at an earlier stage of development, the malignant nature

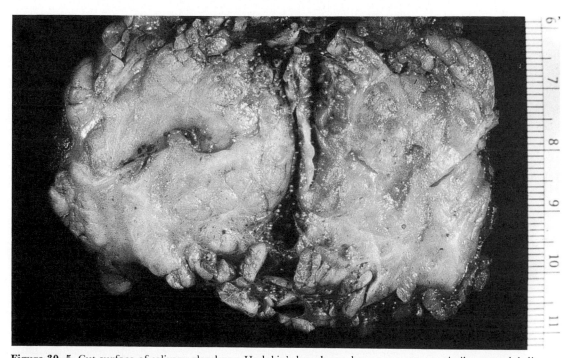

Figure 30–5. Cut surface of salivary gland non-Hodgkin's lymphoma has an appearance similar to nodal disease.

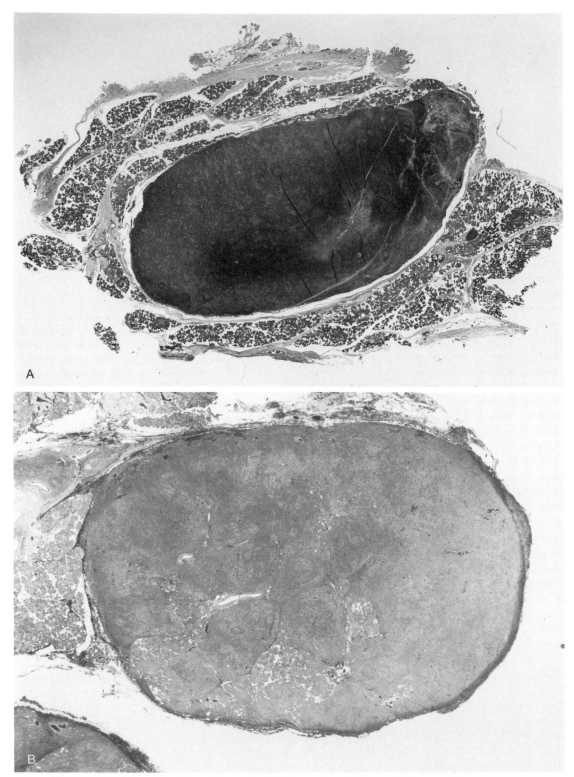

Figure 30–6. *A*, Malignant lymphoma is surrounded by a rim of the remaining parotid gland tissue ($\times$ 1.5). *B*, Malignant lymphoma has replaced majority of parotid gland lobe. Note residual glandular elements within tumor nodule ($\times$ 7.5).

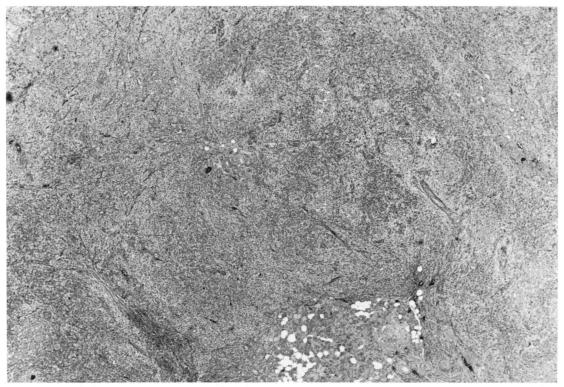

Figure 30–7. Malignant lymphoma in submandibular gland with little remaining parenchyma (lower center) shows loss of normal lobular configuration (× 30).

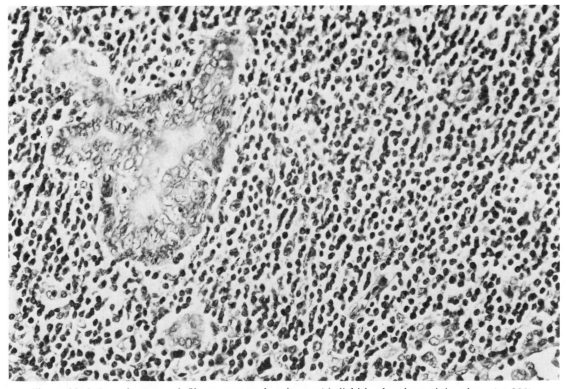

Figure 30–8. Lymphomatous infiltrate surrounds epimyoepithelial island and remaining ducts (× 300).

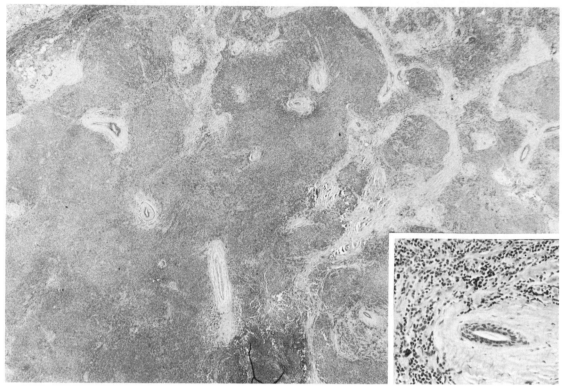

Figure 30–9. Malignant lymphoma shows prominent periductal and interlobular fibrosis (× 15; *inset,* × 75).

of the cellular infiltrate is less obvious. Monotypical tumor cells replace acini (Fig. 30–10) and many ducts and, in some areas of the gland, infiltrate interlobular connective tissue and adjacent lobules. This results in loss of the normal demarcation of lobules and in their eventual confluence.

Of the 409 lymphomas in the AFIP registry, 36 percent were not histologically subclassified. The nodular/follicular lymphomas (Fig. 30–11) constituted the greatest percentage of classified tumors (32 percent), with diffuse (Fig. 30–12) and small lymphocytic variants constituting 13 and 10 percent, respectively. However, clearly many other cytologic types of lymphoma are encountered, and this is in general agreement with the literature on the subject.[5, 6, 41]

Based on categorization of the histologic subtypes within either the Rappaport classification or the Working Formulation, it is clear that salivary gland lymphomas fall into the low-grade category in approximately 60 percent of cases. In our series, the presence of high-grade lymphomas was rare, with only a single case of lymphoblastic lymphoma recorded.

Differential Diagnosis

The distinction between BLEL and lymphoma arising in BLEL, especially in its early develop-

ment, is often difficult. First, it must be recognized that epimyoepithelial islands are not pathognomonic of BLEL. These islands represent hyperplasia and metaplasia of ductal epithelium and may be present in a variety of inflammatory and neoplastic conditions, including malignant lymphoma. Mature lymphocytes, medium-sized lymphocytes with clear cytoplasm (monocytoid B-lymphocytes), and plasma cells are combined to form the lymphoreticular infiltrate in BLEL that replaces, to varying degrees, acinar and ductal elements. The epimyoepithelial islands contain scattered intraepithelial lymphocytes, and the salivary gland lobular architecture is preserved. In contrast, lymphomatous areas are usually composed of infiltrates of monotypic, immature cells that disrupt the normal glandular architecture, invade and eventually replace epimyoepithelial islands, and permeate nerves and periglandular connective tissues. Schmid and coworkers[21] have described so-called "proliferating areas" that, using Giemsa staining, appear as circumscribed or confluent pale zones within the lymphoproliferative region of the BLEL. If the cells in these proliferating areas contained polytypic intracytoplasmic immunoglobulin, the lesion was considered a prelymphomatous process. However, if the cells in these areas were monotypic, the tumors were interpreted as lymphoma.

It is controversial whether or not the diagnosis of malignant lymphoma can be established based

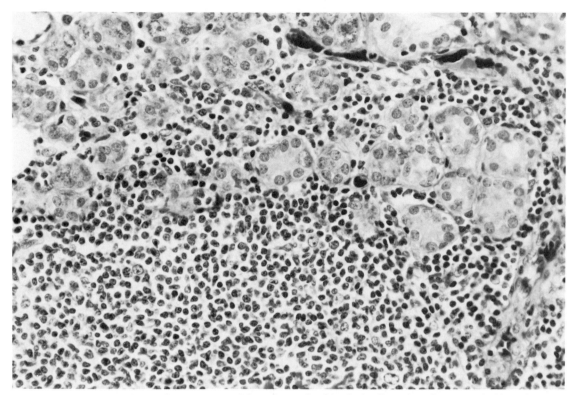

Figure 30–10. Destruction and replacement of the salivary gland by the leading edge of monotypical lymphomatous infiltrate is evident (× 300).

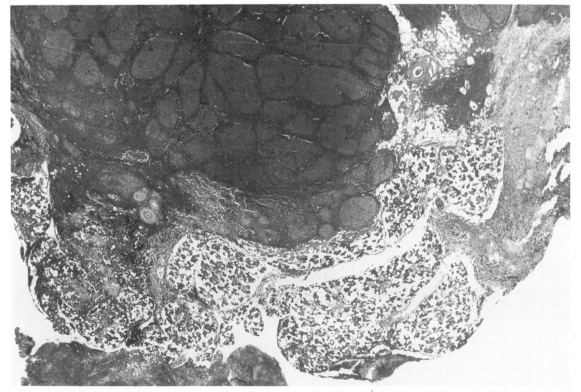

Figure 30–11. This follicular malignant lymphoma leaves virtually no residual parenchyma behind as it spreads through the parotid gland (× 2.5).

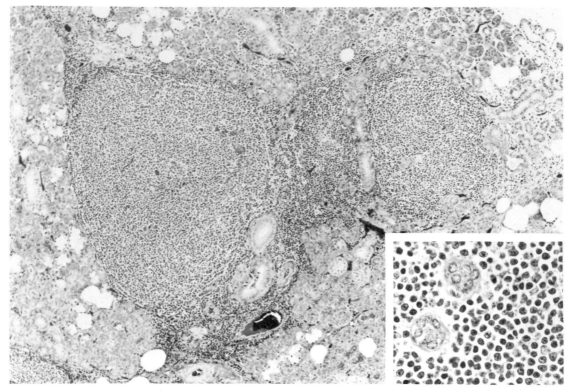

Figure 30–12. Foci of early diffuse lymphoma of parotid gland spread haphazardly through parenchyma (× 75; *inset,* × 300).

only on the presence of a monotypic cellular infiltrate before obtaining evidence of extraglandular infiltration. Fishleder and coworkers[42] suggest that the presence of monotypia is not associated with spread outside the salivary gland. We agree with Hyjek and coworkers,[16] and Schmid and coworkers,[21] who believe it indicates an early stage of lymphoma that may remain localized for prolonged periods. Many of these lymphomas are thought to be derived from monocytoid B cells and could be expected to slowly evolve and respond favorably to local therapy. In contrast to benign or reactive lymphoid infiltrates, lymphoma appears to overrun the salivary gland parenchyma. The acini are destroyed, but many of the more resistant ducts remain embedded in a sea of lymphocytes, especially near the edge of the expanding lymphoid infiltrate.

In general, the differential diagnosis for non-Hodgkin's lymphomas usually involves one of two different situations. In the first, the salivary gland infiltrate is easily recognized as lymphoid, but determination of benignity (reactive state) or malignancy may be problematic. Specific considerations in this situation frequently include benign lymphoepithelial lesion, or lymphadenopathy secondary to an infectious or obstructive sialadenitis. In the infectious category, we have found that the cellular infiltrate in the parotid glands in acquired immunodeficiency syndrome patients may possess morphologically atypical features that are difficult to distinguish from lymphoma, and many times, the human immunodeficiency virus status of the patient is not known at the time of examination of the biopsy material. In human immunodeficiency virus–related lymphadenopathy of the parotid gland, florid follicular hyperplasia is usually evident (see Chapter 4). Unlike follicular lymphoma, the follicles tend to vary in size, and follicle lysis, with mantle lymphocytes extending into and replacing the germinal center cells, may result in irregularly shaped germinal centers with serrated margins. Monocytoid B cells with relatively abundant clear cytoplasm are often numerous and may be misinterpreted as neoplastic. Fortunately, evidence of phagocytosis in the form of tingible bodies is usually present, and neutrophils are typically seen within the cellular infiltrate in addition to histiocytes. These findings should suggest evaluation of the status of the patient regarding human immunodeficiency virus. In obstructive sialadenitis, the lymphoid cell infiltrates are accompanied by prominent sclerosis within the glandular parenchyma. The lobular architecture is usually preserved, and ductal dilatation is often conspicuous.

The second situation involves cases in which the salivary gland tissue contains a poorly differentiated cellular infiltrate whose cell differentiation cannot be determined with routine histologic sections. In these instances, the diagnostic consider-ations often include poorly differentiated adeno-carcinoma, small cell carcinoma, metastatic malig-nant melanoma, and malignant lymphoma. Special stains such as methyl green-pyronine or alpha-naphthol esterase may be useful in identi-fication of the tumor cell population. Immunohis-tochemistry, with a panel of antibodies against such antigens as cytokeratin, chromogranin, S-100 protein, HMB-45, and lymphocyte common anti-gen, can be invaluable in determining the basic differentiation of the infiltrate. If the cell popu-lation shows immunoreactivity with lymphocyte common antigen, further studies may be indicated for light chains and B- and T-cell markers.

In addition to analyzing cell markers, flow cy-tometry may be used to measure DNA ploidy. Although many lymphomas are diploid, the pres-ence of various levels of aneuploidy correlates with the grade of the lymphoma.[43, 44] Levels of aneuploidy are significant, since studies of reactive and normal lymphoid tissues show a normal dip-loid content of DNA.[5]

More recently, molecular techniques have been used in studying MALT lesions including immu-noglobulin and *bcl*-2 gene rearrangement stud-ies.[42, 45] Results of these studies reveal similarity to lymph node–derived follicular center cell lympho-mas.[46]

HODGKIN'S DISEASE

Hodgkin's disease arising in the salivary glands is extremely unusual. The combined experience of Hyman and Wolff[5] and Gleeson and others[3] showed that of 66 salivary gland lymphomas, only 3 were Hodgkin's disease. Of the 455 salivary gland lymphomas in the AFIP files, there are 35 cases of Hodgkin's disease. Therefore, the inci-dence of occurrence of Hodgkin's disease has varied from 3 percent of all salivary gland lym-

phomas as reported in the study of Hyman and Wolff[5] to 7.7 percent as reported in the AFIP files. The AFIP experience closely approximates that of Gleeson and colleagues,[3] who noted a 6.6 percent incidence of occurrence of Hodgkin's lym-phoma.

The AFIP cases show a marked male predomi-nance among civilian patients (78 percent), and an average age of 37.7 years in male patients and 63.1 years in female patients. Although the num-ber of cases is limited, bimodal age peaks are seen; the first peak occurs in the second decade and the second peak occurs in the sixth and seventh dec-ades (Fig. 30–13). The bimodal age distribution of patients with Hodgkin's lymphoma in our series parallels that for patients with Hodgkin's disease in general. A wide patient age range from 6 to 90 years was evident. In terms of site distribution, 27 tumors (77 percent) arose within the parotid gland, and 5 arose (14 percent) in the submandib-ular gland. The three cases of Hodgkin's lym-phoma in the combined studies of Hyman and Wolff[5] and Gleeson and colleagues[3] all arose within the parotid gland.

The clinical manifestation of Hodgkin's lym-phoma is fundamentally identical to that of non-Hodgkin's lymphoma and is typically an asymp-tomatic mass, often presenting as an asymmetry of variable proportion. Although the number of cases is smaller, the site distribution among pa-tients with Hodgkin's lymphoma is similar to that among patients with non-Hodgkin's lymphoma.

It may be generally stated that the morphologic subgroups of Hodgkin's disease have a distinctive histologic pattern and differ relative to the symp-toms they cause, sites of involvement, gender distribution, and stage.[47, 48] Common to all forms and histologic subsets of Hodgkin's disease, of course, is the so-called Reed-Sternberg cell. This diagnostic cell is characterized by a multilobular nucleus with huge, round nucleoli, which domi-nate the nuclear component of the cells (Figs. 30–14 and 30–15). The histologic features of Hodg-

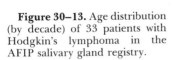

Figure 30–13. Age distribution (by decade) of 33 patients with Hodgkin's lymphoma in the AFIP salivary gland registry.

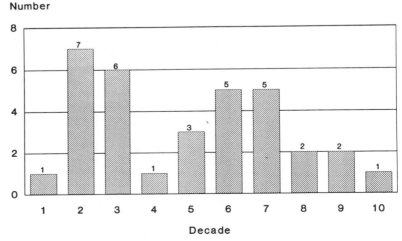

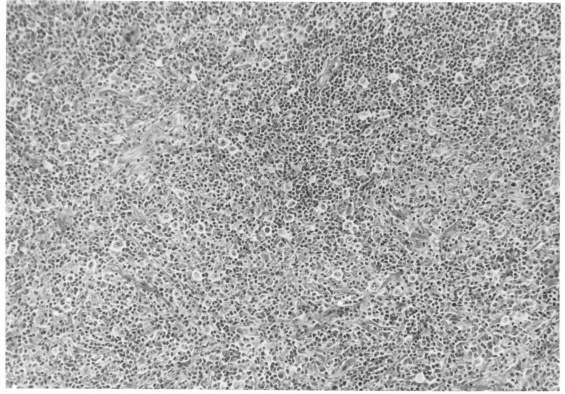

Figure 30–14. Mixed cellularity Hodgkin's lymphoma of parotid gland (× 150).

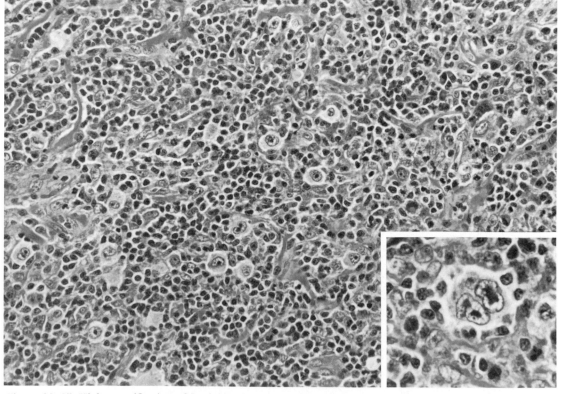

Figure 30–15. High magnification of Hodgkin's lymphoma shows characteristic Reed-Sternberg cell (× 300; *inset*, × 500).

kin's disease vary considerably from one subtype to another. The original Lukes-Butler classification subdivides Hodgkin's disease into four histologic types: lymphocyte predominant, nodular sclerosis, mixed cellularity, and lymphocyte depletion.

The microscopic differential diagnosis of Hodgkin's disease includes diseases for each particular variant[49] and, for the most part, includes entities that involve lymph nodes. The differential diagnosis for the lymphocyte-predominant form of Hodgkin's disease in the salivary gland might consider well-differentiated lymphocytic lymphoma, infectious mononucleosis, progressive transformation of germinal centers,[50] Kimura's disease, and metastases, including malignant melanoma. Of these, metastases to the major salivary gland are far more frequent than Hodgkin's disease of the salivary gland (see Chapter 32) and should always be considered as a possibility. For the nodular sclerosis form of Hodgkin's disease, considerations might include peripheral T-cell, non-Hodgkin's lymphoma with sclerosis and metastatic nasopharyngeal carcinoma. The mixed cellularity form of Hodgkin's disease must be differentiated from Lennert's lymphoma because of the presence of large pleomorphic cells and a mixture of histiocytes, plasma cells, and eosinophils. Finally, the differential diagnosis for the lymphocyte-depleted variant of Hodgkin's disease includes pleomorphic large cell lymphoma and immunoblastic lymphoma. Most important in these considerations is the identification of Reed-Sternberg cells in the characteristic stromal setting. In difficult cases of the nodular sclerosis, mixed cellularity and lymphocyte-depleted subtypes, immunohistochemical studies with antisera for Leu M-1 and Ki-1 facilitate identification of Reed-Sternberg cells.[51] Similarly, recognition of metastatic malignant melanoma is augmented by immunoreactivity of tumor cells with S-100 protein and HMB-45.

PROGNOSIS AND TREATMENT

Important to the prognosis for all forms of malignant lymphoma is clinical staging, which affects treatment more than does the histologic subtype. Radiation therapy for localized lymphomas remains a mainstay in many institutions. However, a better understanding of biologic principles has had a dramatic impact on overall management strategies. Management considerations beyond radiation therapy include chemotherapeutic regimens with proven clinical results.

In a study of 1,467 nondisseminated extranodal lymphomas, including 69 within the salivary glands, Freeman and colleagues[4] found a 5-year survival rate of 67 percent. However, unlike patients with lymphomas of most extranodal sites, the survival rate of those patients with salivary gland lymphoma continued to decline, and at 10 years, it was only 21 percent. The prognosis was affected by extent of disease (localized or regional) at the time of diagnosis. Hyman and Wolff[5] reported that 6 of their 15 patients were alive and well at 8 years, and Gleeson and coworkers[3] found that 52 percent of their patients survived 5 years. Schmid and colleagues[6] reported that survival in patients without immunosialadenitis was 83 percent at 5 years and 40 percent at 10 years. A better prognosis would be expected for patients with many of the MALT lymphomas.[15, 17, 20, 21]

So few cases of Hodgkin's lymphoma in the salivary glands have been reported that no comment can be made regarding any possible site-related effect on patient prognosis or treatment. In the past, the prognosis for patients with Hodgkin's disease was well correlated with the histologic subclassification of the disease. The best prognosis was found in patients with the lymphocyte-predominant and nodular sclerosis forms. Correspondingly, the worst prognosis included the lymphocyte depletion form of the disease, including the lymphocyte depletion subcategory of the nodular sclerosis variant. Average 5-year survival rates for patients with the lymphocyte-predominant form ranged from 47 to 55 percent, whereas those with the mixed cellularity form had 5 to 18 percent 5-year survival rates. Dismal prognoses were seen in patients with the lymphocyte depletion form, with 0 to 8 percent 5-year survival rates. More recently, the prognostic differentiation between the various subtypes of Hodgkin's disease has become less important because of the effectiveness of modern therapy.

Schusterman and colleagues[27] have observed that in contrast to surgical procedures for most other salivary gland tumors, those for lymphomas are reserved for diagnosis and not for treatment. Frozen section diagnosis may allow identification of a mass as a lymphoid rather than an epithelial malignancy, which may consequently prevent unnecessary surgery. As with lymphomas in other sites, radiotherapy or chemotherapy or both have been used. In addition, monoclonal antibodies and lymphokines, such as interferon, interleukin 2, and tumor necrosis factor, are assuming a greater level of importance.

REFERENCES

1. Martinez-Madrigal F, Micheau C: Histology of the major salivary glands. Am J Surg Pathol 1989; 13:879–899.
2. Feind CR: The head and neck. *In* Haagensen CD, Feind CR, Herter FP (eds): The Lymphatics in Cancer. Philadelphia, WB Saunders Co, 1972; 63–64.
3. Gleeson MJ, Bennett MH, Cawson RA: Lymphomas of salivary glands. Cancer 1986; 58:699–704.
4. Freeman C, Berg JW, Cutler SJ: Occurrence and prognosis of extranodal lymphomas. Cancer 1972; 29:252–260.

5. Hyman GA, Wolff M: Malignant lymphomas of the salivary glands: Review of the literature and report of 33 new cases, including four cases associated with the lymphoepithelial lesion. Am J Clin Pathol 1976; 65:421–438.

6. Schmid U, Helbron D, Lennert K: Primary malignant lymphomas localized in salivary glands. Histopathology 1982; 6:673–687.

7. Schmid U, Helbron D, Lennert K: Development of malignant lymphoma in myoepithelial sialadenitis (Sjögren's syndrome). Virchows Arch [A] 1982; 395:11–43.

8. Bienenstock J: Gut and bronchus associated lymphoid tissue: An overview. Adv Exp Med Biol 1982; 149:471–477.

9. Pabst R: The anatomical basis for the immune function of the gut. Anat Embryol 1987; 176:135–144.

10. Brandtzaeg P: Mucosal immunology—with special reference to specific immune defense of the upper respiratory tract. ORL 1988; 50:225–235.

11. Nair PNR, Schroeder HE: Duct-associated lymphoid tissue (DALT) of minor salivary glands and mucosal immunity. Immunology 1986; 57:171–180.

12. Nair PNR, Schroeder HE: Local immune response to repeated topical antigen application in the simian labial mucosa. Infect Immunol 1983; 41:399–409.

13. Isaacson P, Wright DH: Malignant lymphoma of mucosa-associated lymphoid tissue: A distinctive type of B-cell lymphoma. Cancer 1983; 52:1410–1416.

14. Isaacson P, Wright DH: Extranodal malignant lymphoma arising from mucosa-associated lymphoid tissue. Cancer 1984; 53:2515–2524.

15. Isaacson PG, Spencer J: Malignant lymphoma of mucosa-associated lymphoid tissue. Histopathology 1987; 11:445–462.

16. Hyjek E, Smith WJ, Isaacson PG: Primary B-cell lymphoma of salivary glands and its relationship to myoepithelial sialadenitis. Hum Pathol 1988; 19:766–776.

17. Sheibani K, Burke JS, Swartz WG, Nademanee A, Winberg CD: Monocytoid B-cell lymphoma: Clinicopathologic study of 21 cases of a unique type of low-grade lymphoma. Cancer 1988; 62:1531–1538.

18. Shin S, Sheibani K, Fishleder A, Ben-Ezra J, Bailey A, Koo CH, Burke JS, Tubbs R, Rappaport H: Monocytoid B-cell lymphoma in patients with Sjögren's syndrome: Clinicopathologic study of twelve patients. (Abstr.) Lab Invest 1990; 62:93A.

19. Sheibani K, Koo C, Bailey A, Ben-Ezra J, Winberg C: Progression of monocytoid B-cell lymphoma to large cell lymphoma: Report of six cases. (Abstr.) Lab Invest 1990; 62:92A.

20. Van Der Valk P, Meijer CJ: The non-Hodgkin's lymphomas: Old and new thinking. Histopathology 1988; 13:367–384.

21. Schmid U, Lennert K, Gloor F: Immunosialadenitis (Sjögren's syndrome) and lymphoproliferation. Clin Exp Rheumatol 1989; 7:175–180.

22. Devesa SS, Silverman DT, Young JS Jr, Pollack ES, Brown CC, Horm JW, Percy CL, Myers MH, McKay FW, Fraumeni JF Jr: Cancer incidence and mortality trends among Whites in the United States, 1947–84. J Natl Cancer Inst 1987; 79:701–770.

23. Patey DH, Thackray AC, Keeling DH: Malignant disease of the parotid. Br J Cancer 1965; 19:712–737.

24. Boddie AW Jr, Mullin JD, West G, Bouda D: Extranodal lymphoma: Surgical and other therapeutic alternatives. Curr Probl Cancer 1982; 6:1–64.

25. Beahrs OH, Woolner LB, Carveth SW, Devine KD: Surgical management of parotid lesions: Review of seven hundred cases. Arch Surg 1960; 80:890–904.

26. Watkin GT, MacLennan KA, Hobsley M: Lymphomas presenting as lumps in the parotid region. Br J Surg 1984; 71:701–702.

27. Schusterman MA, Granick MS, Erickson ER, Newton ED, Hanna DC, Bragdon RW: Lymphoma presenting as a salivary gland mass. Head Neck Surg 1988; 10:411–415.

28. Foote FW Jr, Frazell EL: Tumors of the major salivary glands, Section IV, Fascicle 11. Atlas of Tumor Pathology, Washington, DC, Armed Forces Institute of Pathology, 1954.

29. Nichols RD, Rebuck JW, Sullivan JC: Lymphoma and the parotid gland. Laryngoscope 1982; 92:365–369.

30. National Cancer Institute sponsored study of classifications of non-Hodgkin's lymphomas. Summary and description of a working formulation for clinical usage. Cancer 1982; 49:2112–2135.

31. Kassan S, Thomas T, Moutsopoulos HM, Hoover R, Kimberly RP, Budman DR, Costa J, Decker JL, Chused TM: Increased risk of lymphoma in sicca syndrome. Ann Intern Med 1978; 89:888–892.

32. Fox RT, Adamson TC, Fong S, Young C, Howell FV: Characterization of the phenotype and function of lymphocytes infiltrating the salivary gland in patients with primary Sjögren's syndrome. Diag Immunol 1983; 1:233–239.

33. Tzioufas AG, Moutsopoulos HM, Talal N: Lymphoid malignancy and monoclonal proteins. *In* Talal N, Moutsopoulos HM, Kassan SS (eds): Sjögren's syndrome, Clinical and Immunological Aspects. Berlin, Springer-Verlag, 1987; 129–136.

34. Krikorian JG, Portlock CS, Cooney P, Rosenberg SA: Spontaneous regression of non-Hodgkin's lymphoma: A report of nine cases. Cancer 1980; 46:2093–2099.

35. Horning SJ, Rosenberg SA: The natural history of initially untreated low grade non-Hodgkin's lymphoma. N Engl J Med 1981; 311:1471–1475.

36. Freimark B, Fantozzi R, Bone R, Bordin G, Fox R: Detection of clonally expanded salivary gland lymphocytes in Sjögren's syndrome. Arthritis Rheum 1989; 32:859–869.

37. Ferlito A, Cattai N: The so-called "benign lymphoepithelial lesion." Part I—explanation of the term and of its synonymous and related terms. J Laryngol Otol 1980; 94:1189–1197.

38. Miller R, Yanagihara ET, Dubrow AA, Lukes RJ: Malignant lymphoma in a Warthin's tumor. Cancer 1982; 50:2948–2950.

39. Hall G, Tesluk H, Baron S: Lymphoma arising in an adenolymphoma. Hum Pathol 1985; 16:424–426.

40. Evans HL: Extranodal small lymphocytic proliferation. Cancer 1982; 49:84–96.

41. Colby TV, Dorfman RF: Malignant lymphomas involving the salivary glands. Pathol Ann 1979; 14:307–324.

42. Fishleder A, Tubbs R, Hesse B, Levine H: Uniform detection of immunoglobulin-gene rearrangements in benign lymphoepithelial lesions. N Engl J Med 1987; 316:1118–1121.

43. Costa A, Mazzini G, DelBino G, Silvestrini R: DNA content and proliferative kinetic characteristics of non-Hodgkin's lymphoma: Determined by flow cytometry and autoradiography. Cytometry 1981; 2:185–191.

44. Shackney SE, Skramstad RE, Cunningham DJ, Dugas DJ, Lincoln TL, Lukes RJ: Dual parameter flow cytometry studies in human lymphomas. J Clin Invest 1980; 66:1281–1294.

45. Kerrigan DP, Irons J, Chen I-M: bcl-2 gene rearrangement in salivary gland lymphoma. Am J Surg Pathol 1990; 14:1133–1138.

46. Weiss LM, Warnke RA, Sklar J, Cleary ML: Molecular analysis of the t(14:18) chromosomal translocation in malignant lymphoma. N Engl J Med 1987; 317:1185–1189.

47. Grogan TM: Hodgkin's disease. *In* Jaffe ES, (ed): Surgical Pathology of Lymph Nodes and Related Organs. Philadelphia, WB Saunders Co, 1985; 86–134.

48. Kaplan HS: Hodgkin's Disease, 2nd ed. Cambridge, Mass, Harvard University Press, 1980.

49. Burns BF, Colby TV, Dorfman RF: Differential diagnostic features of nodular L & H Hodgkin's disease, including progressive transformation of germinal centers. Am J Surg Pathol 1984; 8:253–261.

50. Poppem S, Kaiserling E, Lennert K: Hodgkin's disease with lymphocyte predominance nodular type (nodular paraganglioma) and progressively transformed germinal center: A cytohistological study. Histopathology 1979; 3:295–308.

51. Davey FR, Elghetany MT, Kurec AS: Immunophenotyping of hematologic neoplasms in paraffin-embedded tissue sections. Am J Clin Pathol 1990; 93(Suppl 1):S17–S26.

31

SINONASAL AND LARYNGEAL SALIVARY GLAND LESIONS

Dennis K. Heffner

Histoanatomic Considerations

The nasal cavity and paranasal sinuses are collectively referred to as the "sinonasal tract" in this chapter. The inferoanterior portions of the nasal cavities (the nostrils or nares) have been called the nasal vestibules and are lined with skin and associated skin adnexal structures. The remaining portions of the sinonasal cavities are lined by respiratory mucosa, except for the upper portion of the nasal cavities, which is lined by specialized olfactory epithelium. All of the sinonasal epithelium embryologically develops from ectoderm.

Specific Gland Sites

Mucosal seromucous glands (Fig. 31–1) are most abundant in the lateral nasal cavity walls; they are particularly numerous in the convex edges of the turbinate projections but are also found in the concave meatus. The nasal septum has moderately abundant glands. The nasal mucosa of the superolateral nasoethmoid area has many glands, although the air cells themselves (ethmoid sinuses) have a dearth of glands. Likewise, the maxillary, frontal, and sphenoid sinuses normally have only meager evidence of glands. Some glands are found within the maxillary sinuses near the ostia,[1] but most sinus areas have almost no seromucous glands.

Although it might seem logical that sinonasal glandular neoplasms would arise more frequently from the regions that have higher concentrations of glands, this correlation is questionable. For example, a relatively large percentage of sinonasal adenoid cystic carcinomas seem to arise in the maxillary sinus. Although the exact histologic site of origin of most of these tumors is difficult to

discern, an appreciable number of glandular tumors of this area may arise directly from the surface mucosal epithelium.[2]

Laryngeal seromucous glands are present throughout the supraglottic areas, but they are especially prominent in the false vocal cord area.[3] These glands are absent from the true vocal cords; however, just below the true cords, the subglottic mucosa manifests some glands as does, of course, the tracheal mucosa.

The piriform sinus is part of the hypopharynx, but the medial portions of this "laryngeal hypopharynx" give rise to carcinomas that are clinically considered to be essentially supraglottic laryngeal tumors.

Seromucous Glands Versus Minor Salivary Glands

Histologically, the seromucous glands in the sinonasal tract and larynx markedly resemble minor salivary glands, and most pathologists refer to them as such. From a physiologic standpoint, since we generally do not refer to secretions from the nose as saliva, an argument can be made for not referring to nasal (or laryngotracheal) glands as minor salivary glands. However, this is a minor semantic point, and although the term *seromucous glands* is used in this chapter, from a histologic and tumorigenic standpoint, it is understood that these glands are tantamount to minor salivary glands.

Nonsialoid Glandular Neoplasms

Although many sinonasal and laryngeal glandular tumors are either identical or at least similar

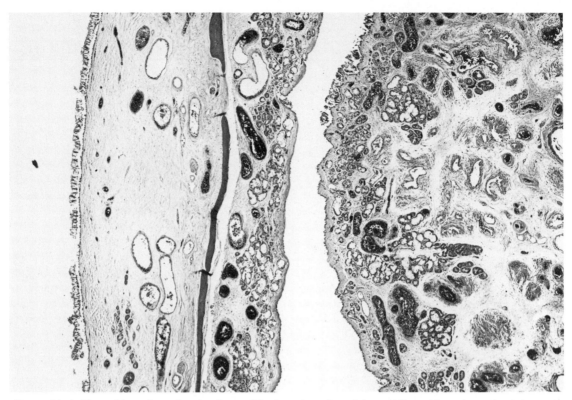

Figure 31–1. Normal lateral nasal cavity tissues. The lateral portion of the middle turbinate is on the right, and to the left is the combined lateral nasal cavity and medial maxillary sinus wall, with its thin plate of bone. Note the dearth of glands in the maxillary sinus lining compared with the abundance of glands in the nasal cavity tissues ($\times$ 24) (Artifactual degenerative erosion of respiratory epithelium is present in this autopsy specimen.)

to salivary gland tumors histologically, it is important to remember that many others are not and have patterns different from those seen among the spectrum of salivary neoplasias. Sometimes, however, it is difficult to draw a sharp line of separation between these two groups. Most of the tumors that are not of the salivary gland type probably arise from the surface mucosal epithelium and are unrelated to seromucous glands in histogenesis, although salivary gland type tumors of these anatomic regions also may occasionally appear to arise from the surface mucosal epithelium. Not surprisingly, it may be impossible to decide whether or not some poorly differentiated carcinomas are analogous to salivary gland tumors.

Statistics on Neoplasm Incidence (AFIP)

Cited statistics are based on cases in the Registry of Otolaryngic Pathology, Otolaryngic Tumor Registry (OTR), from the Armed Forces Institute of Pathology (AFIP), that have been received for diagnostic consultation during a 10-year period (1976–1985). Although these figures may reflect some biases as a result of the types of cases that

are sent to the AFIP (for example, squamous cell carcinomas are probably underrepresented in Table 31–1), the data are useful.

Table 31–1 compares the numbers of cases in general categories of sinonasal neoplasms in the OTR. The last category in this table is glandular tumors, many of which are of the salivary gland type. This category is subdivided in Table 31–2. The subdivisions of low- and high-grade adenocarcinomas that are not otherwise specified con-

Table 31–1. Sinonasal Neoplasia
Reported by the AFIP from 1976 to 1985

General Tumor Types	Number of Cases
Papillomas (schneiderian membrane; inverted type)	545
Soft tissue tumors	332
Skeletal tumors	124
Undifferentiated malignancies	84
Keratinizing squamous cell carcinomas	61
Nonkeratinizing squamous cell carcinomas	178
Glandular tumors	311
Total	1635

Table 31–2. Sinonasal Glandular Tumors
Reported by the AFIP from 1976 to 1985

Tumor Type	Number of Cases
Mixed tumors (pleomorphic adenomas)	73
Oncocytic tumors	7
Low-grade adenocarcinomas (including acinic cell)	67
Mucoepidermoid carcinomas	17
Adenoid cystic carcinomas	54
High-grade adenocarcinomas and miscellaneous types	93
Total	311

Table 31–4. Laryngeal Glandular Tumors
Reported by the AFIP from 1976 to 1985

General Tumor Types	Number of Cases
Mixed tumors (pleomorphic adenomas)	3
Malignant mixed tumor	1
Oncocytic tumors	12
Cystadenoma	1
Mucoepidermoid carcinomas	11
Adenoid cystic carcinomas	11
Adenosquamous carcinomas	19
Adenocarcinomas (mostly neuroendocrine)	45
Total	103

tain tumors of variable resemblance to salivary neoplasia.

Tables 31–3 and 31–4 contain similar information for laryngeal tumors.

SINONASAL LESIONS

Benign Mixed Tumor (Pleomorphic Adenoma)

Clinical Findings

Nasal cavity mixed tumors are found in patients of all ages, although they are most frequent in patients ranging from 20 to 60 years. Patients' symptoms or complaints commonly involve unilateral nasal obstruction, presence of a mass, or epistaxis. Most patients have had symptoms for a year or less when they seek treatment.

The clinical examination typically reveals a polypoid, firm, gray mass that is often covered with an intact mucosa. Radiographic studies often demonstrate a mass that is larger than expected and that may be eroding bone. Although occasionally extending into the maxillary sinus, these tumors are generally limited in origin to the nasal cavity. About three fourths of these tumors arise from the septum, and one fourth arise from the lateral nasal cavity wall. Apparently, rare mixed tumors arise in the paranasal sinuses.

Table 31–3. Laryngeal Neoplasia
Reported by the AFIP from 1976 to 1985

General Tumor Types	Number of Cases
Papillomas	219
Soft tissue tumors	185
Skeletal tumors	68
Undifferentiated carcinomas	8
Squamous cell carcinomas	1188
Spindle cell (sarcomatoid) carcinomas	241
Verrucous carcinomas	118
Glandular tumors	103
Total	2130

Pathologic Findings

These tumors range from 0.5 to 7.0 cm in diameter, with a mean of 2.6 cm.[4] They are lobular, polypoid masses with a firm to friable consistency and are gray-white to gray-pink, occasionally with foci of hemorrhage.

The histologic appearance of sinonasal mixed tumors is similar to that of benign mixed tumors as described in Chapter 10, except that stromal elements are usually sparse and may be meager or absent. Thus, nasal cavity mixed tumors are generally "cellular" mixed tumors. They usually are not encapsulated and often are not well circumscribed at all margins. In this respect, they are similar to palatal mixed tumors.

Immunostaining of these tumors produces results similar to those for salivary gland mixed tumors.

Behavior and Treatment

Nasal cavity mixed tumors are treated by wide local or total surgical excisions. Although the tumors are often rather large and are removed piecemeal, recurrences are infrequent. If a recurrence should happen, additional conservative (but complete) removal is usually curative.

The incidence of carcinoma arising in nasal cavity mixed tumors is not accurately known, but it probably is less than that for the major salivary glands. One nasal cavity mixed tumor in the AFIP files that was not overtly cytologically malignant but that was atypical recurred multiple times during a period of several years and eventually escaped surgical control. Two adenocarcinomas had some features resembling those of mixed tumors, but whether or not they were definitely carcinomas arising from benign mixed tumors was unclear, because no areas of typical benign mixed tumor were clearly present. Several high grade sinonasal malignancies have had carcinoma and malignant chondroid elements, but these were classified as sinonasal teratocarcinomas.[5] This peculiar type of tumor may be considered in the differential diagnosis.

Differential Diagnosis

Because nasal cavity mixed tumors are usually highly cellular and are often biopsied or removed piecemeal, the diagnosis can be difficult. An additional factor predisposing to misdiagnosis is the rarity with which these tumors are seen in most general surgical pathology laboratories. A diagnosis of mixed tumor may not come readily to mind when examining a cellular nasal cavity neoplasm. Other diagnoses that have been considered by pathologists who have submitted mixed tumors of the nasal cavity to the AFIP have included papilloma, angiofibroma, chondromyxoid fibroma, hemangiopericytoma, low-grade fibrosarcoma, adenoid cystic carcinoma, mucoepidermoid carcinoma, chondrosarcoma, malignant mixed tumor, and alveolar rhabdomyosarcoma.

Because of the somewhat "rhabdoid" appearance that plasmacytoid myoepithelial cells may have (Fig. 31–2), it is understandable why the misdiagnosis of rhabdomyosarcoma can occur. The cellularity and cartilaginous areas explain why chondrosarcoma might be considered. Careful attention to nuclear detail helps to avoid these misdiagnoses, since benign mixed tumors lack malignant nuclear features.

Because mixed tumors can have a preponderance of spindled myoepithelial cells (Fig. 31–3), various soft tissue tumors may be simulated. Palisading of nuclei may suggest a neural or smooth muscle tumor. Distinction from hemangiopericytoma sometimes can be difficult, since nasal cavity hemangiopericytomas usually have plump spindle cells and often do not have a prominent vascular pattern.[6] Finding ductal or glandular formations, which may require careful searching, usually allows recognition of a mixed tumor (Fig. 31–3).

Of course, immunohistochemistry can be helpful in diagnosis. Keratin immunostaining can be especially helpful in distinguishing mixed tumors from a number of mesenchymal tumors. However, recognition of mixed tumor depends on considering it in the differential diagnosis in the first place, and this remains an important fundamental step in the evaluation. Mixed tumor should be included on the list of diagnostic possibilities when the pathologist is confronted with a cellular tumor from the nasal cavity, unless the tumor is obviously malignant.

Excluding the possibility of sinonasal adenoid cystic carcinoma or mucoepidermoid carcinoma is just as important in this instance as it is in other anatomic locations. The frequent piecemeal removal of nasal mixed tumors, coupled with a dearth of normal tissue in the biopsy or excision specimen, can complicate the evaluation of tumor

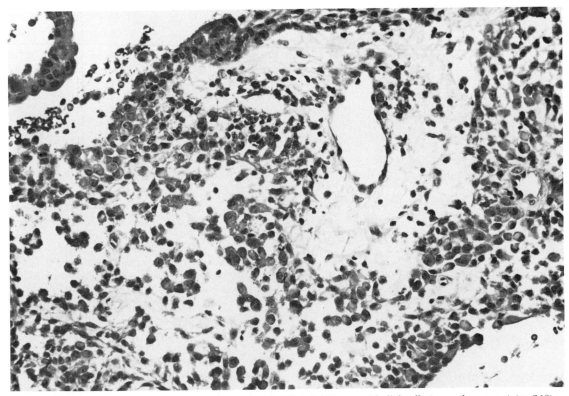

Figure 31–2. A nasal cavity benign mixed tumor with "rhabdoid" myoepithelial cells (near the center) (× 240).

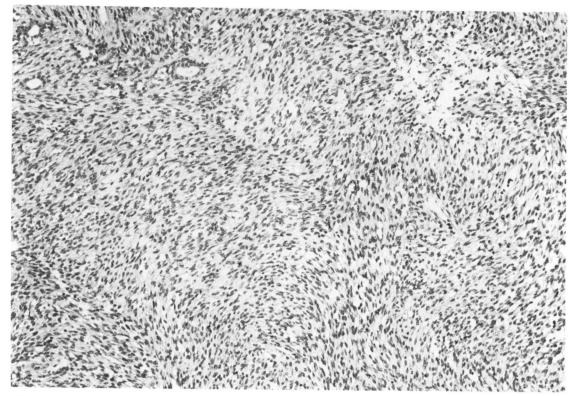

Figure 31–3. A nasal cavity benign mixed tumor composed predominantly of spindled myoepithelial cells and resembling a mesenchymal tumor. Slight palisading is present, which could cause this lesion to be misinterpreted as a schwannoma or a smooth muscle tumor. A few ductal structures in the upper left corner serve as a clue to the correct diagnosis (× 99).

borders. Otherwise, criteria for distinction from these two carcinomas are similar to those described for the same problem in other locations.

Some very cellular mixed tumors of the nasal cavity might be considered monomorphous adenomas, but typically uniform monomorphous patterns were absent from the AFIP cases (see Table 31–2). If a uniform basaloid tumor is encountered in this location, an unusual basaloid carcinoma should be carefully excluded before considering a diagnosis of monomorphous adenoma.

Oncocytic Neoplasms

Clinical Findings

Oncocytic neoplasms (oncocytomas) of the sinonasal tract are rare. They may manifest as small nasal cavity lesions, particularly if present on the nasal septum,[7] or may occur as extensive masses involving the paranasal sinuses that manifest considerable bone erosion.[8]

Microscopic Findings

Sinonasal oncocytomas are generally relatively solid proliferations. They are often composed of nests, cords, or tubules of oncocytes but may have a more sheetlike growth pattern.

Although nasal septal oncocytic tumors are usually referred to as minor salivary gland tumors, examination of several of these tumors in the AFIP files has suggested that they originated from the surface mucosal epithelium.

Behavior and Treatment

Large oncocytic neoplasms of the sinonasal tract can behave rather aggressively.[8] It has been suggested that in this location they can be essentially regarded as low-grade adenocarcinomas.[7] Although small oncocytic tumors of the nasal septum should be readily curable by conservative (although complete) surgical removal, larger tumors require more extensive surgery to ensure complete removal and to prevent recurrences.[9]

Differential Diagnosis

Oncocytic neoplasms should be distinguished from oncocytic metaplasias with hyperplasia. The latter lesions are small and often appear as multifocal oncocytic transformation and proliferation of non-neoplastic ductal or acinar elements. In contrast to those lesions occurring in the nasopharynx and supraglottic larynx, sinonasal onco-cytic metaplasia seems to be quite rare.

Cylindric cell papillomas are variants of inverted papillomas and often have a prominent oncocytoid appearance. Their oncocytoid nature has been substantiated by the demonstration of increased mitochondria with electron microscopy.[10] Although a diagnosis of oncocytic papillary cystadenoma might seem appropriate, the thicker epithelium and the presence of mucus-containing microcysts give cylindric cell papilloma a different appearance from that of Warthin's tumors and oncocytic papillary cystadenomas of salivary glands. In any case, these sinonasal oncocytoid papillomas are readily distinguished from the more solid oncocytic neoplasms referred to earlier.

The eosinophilic granular cells of a maxillary granular cell ameloblastoma that has extended into the sinonasal cavities may have a superficial resemblance to oncocytoma. However, the ameloblastoma is easily distinguished by the ameloblastic histologic features of proliferating columnar odontogenic epithelium, which has palisaded and frequently polarized nuclei.

Low-Grade Adenocarcinomas Resembling Acinic Cell Adenocarcinoma

Clinical Findings

Low-grade adenocarcinomas of the sinonasal tract can occur in patients of a wide age range that extends at least from 9 to 75 years.[7] Nasal obstruction or epistaxis is the most common symptom, and only occasional patients have some pain. The nasal cavity, ethmoid sinuses, maxillary sinus, or combinations of these cavities are the areas of tumor occurrence.

Microscopic Findings

These tumors have various histomorphologic patterns, but they are all characterized by uniform cytologic characteristics and a glandular architecture. The majority of these tumors are composed of small glands formed by a single row of cuboidal or columnar cells (Fig. 31–4). A back-to-back arrangement of glands is a frequent feature. Sometimes, irregular, large spaces produce a cystadenomatous appearance, and papillary infoldings are present in varying degrees. A few of these tumors (Fig. 31–5) bear a rather striking resemblance to salivary gland acinic cell adenocarcinomas, with well-formed follicular or papillary-cystic patterns and well-differentiated acinar-type cells. Other tumors have a lesser resemblance, and it is often difficult to know where to draw the line when making an analogy.

Some of these low-grade adenocarcinomas may be of seromucous gland origin, but many seem to arise from the surface mucosal epithelium.[2]

Behavior and Treatment

These tumors have a very low metastatic rate of less than 5 percent, and if assured surgical removal were applied in all cases, the incidence of metastatic disease would probably be even lower. Sinonasal carcinomas, in general, have a lower metastatic potential (for a given stage or size of tumor) than similar carcinomas in the pharynx. (This might be related to differences in richness of lymphatic drainage in these different areas.) This site-related factor and the low histologic grade of these adenocarcinomas probably contribute to the very low metastatic rate.

However, local recurrences of these tumors are frequent. Probably because of the well-differentiated and bland cytologic features of these tumors, initial treatment is often too conservative and inadequate. Although surgical treatment should certainly be conservative in comparison with that performed for a high-grade carcinoma, assured complete removal is indicated. This therapy has a good chance of being completely curative and prevents recurrences that sometimes can become extensive and troublesome.

Differential Diagnosis

Because the nuclear features of many of these tumors are so uniform and bland, the question of benignancy versus malignancy often arises. An analogy can be made with acinic cell adenocarcinomas of the major salivary glands, for which even the extremely well-differentiated and histologically "benign-appearing" tumors have some metastatic potential and are therefore low-grade carcinomas.

Most important in differential diagnosis is the distinction of these low-grade tumors from the high-grade adenocarcinomas that require more radical therapy and that have a much poorer prognosis for the patient. This is not difficult for the higher grade sinonasal adenocarcinomas that have obvious malignant cytologic and histologic features (e.g., nuclear anaplasia, necrosis, solid patterns). However, some sinonasal adenocarcinomas are moderately well differentiated but clinically behave as high-grade tumors. Histologically, these adenocarcinomas usually resemble moderately well-differentiated colon carcinomas, and this feature aids in their recognition. Although moderately well differentiated, they manifest more malignant nuclear features than those seen in low-grade adenocarcinomas.

Mucoepidermoid Carcinoma

Clinical Findings

Tumors that appear analogous to mucoepidermoid carcinomas of the salivary gland occur in the sinonasal tract, but they are rare. The only

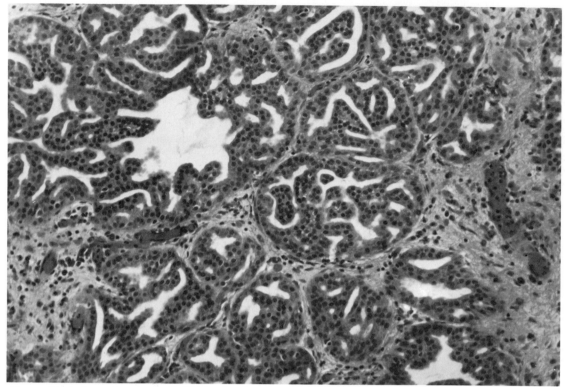

Figure 31–4. A nasal cavity, well-differentiated, low-grade adenocarcinoma with cytologic uniformity (× 180). (From Heffner, D.K., Hyams, V.J., Hauck, K.W., and Lingeman, C.: Low grade adenocarcinoma of the nasal cavity and paranasal sinuses. Cancer 50:312–322, 1982.)

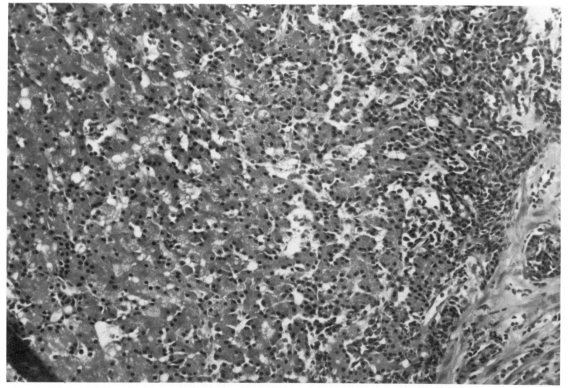

Figure 31–5. A nasal cavity low-grade adenocarcinoma with cytologic similarity to salivary acinic cell adenocarcinoma (× 150). (From Heffner, D.K., Hyams, V.J., Hauck, K.W., and Lingeman, C.: Low grade adenocarcinoma of the nasal cavity and paranasal sinuses. Cancer 50:312–322, 1982.)

noteworthy clinical point is that two of these tumors (and a possible third one) from the AFIP files slowly developed after nasal cosmetic plastic surgery. The initial pathologic specimens of the lesions (1 to 2 years after cosmetic surgery) were interpreted as probable multiple inclusion cysts that occurred as complications of the cosmetic procedures. After the proliferations recurred and became more extensively invasive (Fig. 31–6), the lesions were interpreted as neoplasms that resembled mucoepidermoid carcinoma of the type seen in the salivary glands.

Microscopic Findings

These sinonasal tumors resemble low-grade mucoepidermoid carcinomas of salivary glands. They have appreciable mucocytes that contain abundant cytoplasmic mucus and many bland, slightly epidermoid cells. A multicystic growth pattern may be present. In spite of having these features in common with salivary mucoepidermoid carcinoma, histological evidence for some of these tumors suggests that they originate from the surface mucosal epithelium.

Differential Diagnosis

In various inflammatory conditions of the sinonasal tract, especially conditions involving in-flammatory polyps, the respiratory epithelium invaginates from the surface and forms inclusion or "entrapment" cysts. Squamous metaplasia of this epithelium, coupled with reactive mucous cell hyperplasia, can be confused with low-grade mucoepidermoid carcinoma. Histologic distinction from mucoepidermoid carcinoma can be difficult, but awareness of this phenomenon and appreciation of the general inflammatory features of the bulk of the tissue (sometimes including the general architecture of inflammatory polyps) can usually prevent misdiagnosis.

A condition resembling necrotizing sialometaplasia occurs in the nasal cavity, particularly the nasal septum (Figs. 31–7, 31–8). Just as has occurred in the oral cavity, this condition has been mistaken for mucoepidermoid carcinoma. Preservation of the general size and shape of the seromucous gland lobules aids in recognition of this metaplastic lesion. As with other pitfalls in histopathologic diagnosis, awareness of the various possibilities goes a long way toward avoiding misdiagnosis. In this particular situation, clinical history may also be of some help, since clinical evidence of trauma to the nasal mucosa, such as silver nitrate cautery for epistaxis a week or two previously, is often, although not always, present.

The diagnosis of poorly differentiated, high-grade mucoepidermoid carcinoma in the sinonasal tract is usually difficult. Poorly differentiated carcinomas with some squamoid and adenoid fea-

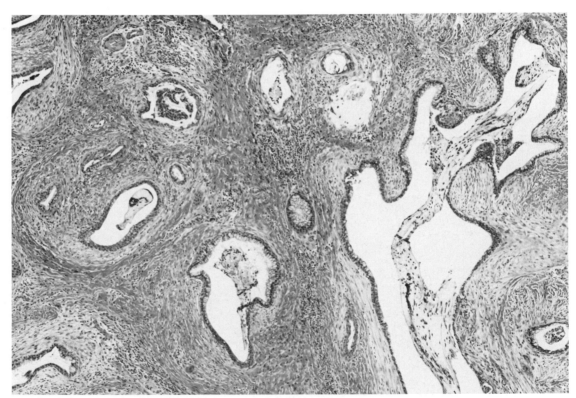

Figure 31–6. A nasal cavity proliferation of cystic epithelium composed of mucocytes and some epidermoid cells similar to salivary gland low grade mucoepidermoid carcinoma (× 48).

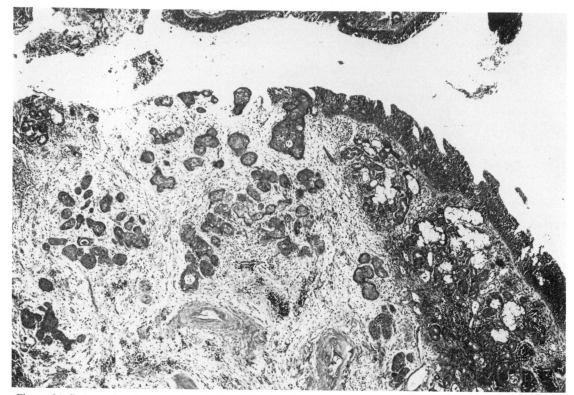

Figure 31–7. A nasal cavity metaplastic lesion (following silver nitrate cautery for epistaxis) analogous to necrotizing sialometaplasia found in the oral cavity. The lobular pattern of the seromucous units, from which the metaplastic lesion is derived, tends to be maintained (× 39).

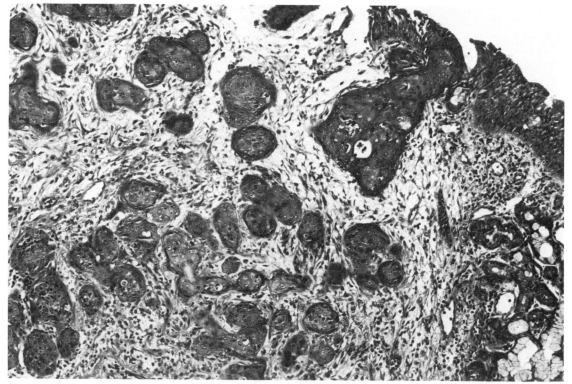

Figure 31–8. A higher magnification of Figure 31–7 demonstrates the appearance of metaplastic squamoid nests that could be mistaken for invasive well-differentiated carcinoma (× 99).

tures are probably best diagnosed as poorly differentiated adenosquamous carcinomas. This has the advantage of helping surgeons avoid evaluating such a tumor in terms of their general experience with mucoepidermoid carcinomas, many of which, of course, are less malignant than poorly differentiated adenosquamous carcinomas of mucosal origin.

Adenoid Cystic Carcinoma

Clinical Features

Adenoid cystic carcinoma is an important neoplasm of the sinonasal area, being the most frequently occurring malignant salivary gland type of neoplasm. In the AFIP cases, the patient age range was from 20 to 91 years, with a median age of 48 years, and 60 percent of the patients were male. The location of the tumor was described as nasal cavity in 40 percent of the cases, maxillary sinus in 30 percent, nasomaxilla in 12 percent, ethmoid or nasoethmoid in 6 percent, and frontal and sphenoid sinuses in 2 percent (one case) each. The remaining 10 percent of tumors occurred in various combinations of multiple cavities.

The primary symptom associated with these tumors was nasal obstruction in 40 percent of patients, epistaxis in 26 percent, pain (including neuralgia) in 20 percent, and deformity (usually facial asymmetry or swelling) in 14 percent. Many patients had combinations of these symptoms. It is well known that adenoid cystic carcinoma virtually always invades nerves; however, pain was not significantly more frequent in this carcinoma than it is with other sinonasal malignancies. Duration of symptoms ranged from 2 months to 2 years, with an average of about 1 year.

Pathologic Findings

These tumors are almost always larger than 2 cm by the time they are discovered, and some are quite large and extensive, as judged by radiographic findings. Imaging studies usually reveal significant degrees of bone destruction and infiltrative growth. At surgery, it is often difficult to determine the margins or limits of the cancer.

The cytologic features and histologic patterns of sinonasal adenoid cystic carcinoma are the same as those of adenoid cystic carcinoma that occur in other locations. The pathologist is often presented with only a small biopsy or portions of a fragmented tumor; therefore, evaluation of the growth pattern of the tumor at its edges is impossible. This obviously complicates diagnosis, particularly when the biopsy includes only a relatively solid pattern.

The histologic features of a portion of an adenoid cystic carcinoma may not be typical, and yet, when additional tumor is obtained and examined, the diagnosis becomes clear. For this reason, a high index of suspicion for adenoid cystic carcinoma should be maintained when examining a sinonasal glandular tumor. At the same time, caution should be exercised against overdiagnosis of this tumor as the result of insufficient material.

Behavior and Treatment

Adenoid cystic carcinomas in the sinonasal tract are even more egregious in terms of their virtual incurability and threat to life than when this carcinoma type arises in other locations. This increased severity is probably related to the extensive growth of these tumors that usually occurs before they are discovered and their relative closeness to vital structures (e.g., the brain). Spiro and coinvestigators[11] suggest an approximate 10-year cure rate of 7 percent for sinonasal tumors as compared with 29 percent for parotid lesions, 23 percent for oral cavity lesions, and 10 percent for those of the submandibular gland. Follow-up information on the AFIP cases indicates that a majority of patients die of disease in less than 5 years. Given the very poor prognosis for these patients and the fact that radiation therapy has been indicated to have some beneficial effect on this tumor,[12] combined surgery/radiation therapy is warranted in most cases. Hematogenous metastases from this tumor are not uncommon, which may support use of chemotherapy.

Differential Diagnosis

Not uncommonly, sinonasal adenocarcinomas have a pattern resembling adenoid cystic carcinoma (such as some vague cribriform areas), but they have cytologic features that are uncharacteristic for adenoid cystic carcinoma. The nuclei may be larger than usual, and the cytoplasm may be more abundant than expected. I usually diagnose such a tumor as adenocarcinoma, not otherwise specified, but separation from adenoid cystic carcinoma can be difficult or impossible. Adequate sampling of the tumor is obviously important. Sometimes the diagnosis of "adenocarcinoma with adenoid cystic features" has been used to connote uncertainty in classification.

As in other locations, distinction from mixed tumor is extremely important. As indicated earlier, surgery often requires fragmentation of a sinonasal tumor, and the edges of the tumor frequently are not sufficiently intact to reliably evaluate the growth patterns at the tumor's margins. A thorough search for evidence of invasive growth is necessary. Obviously, nerve invasion is an important indicator of malignancy. Another important indicator is evidence of invasion by neoplastic epithelium into preexisting connective tissue rather than the neoplastic epithelium lying within the integral "stroma" formed by a mixed tumor. This judgment about stromal invasion can be difficult, but the presence of normal structures, such as seromucous glands, aids in making this determination.

Monomorphous adenomas and polymorphous low-grade adenocarcinomas are so rare in this location that they are not a problem in differential diagnosis.

Miscellaneous and Rare Neoplasms

High-Grade Adenocarcinomas

Some clinically aggressive sinonasal adenocarcinomas are histologically moderately differentiated, but, generally, their histomorphologic character is not typical of any of the recognized salivary gland neoplasms. Many resemble colon adenocarcinomas and often suggest origin from the surface epithelium. Other adenocarcinomas are poorly differentiated and have nonspecific patterns. Since some salivary gland adenocarcinomas are also poorly differentiated, it seems logical that some sinonasal poorly differentiated adenocarcinomas could be of seromucous gland origin. However, it is usually impossible to determine the specific histogenesis. If such carcinomas included some tumor cells that are immunoreactive for S-100 protein, this might indicate seromucous gland origin. However, by itself, this finding would offer meager support, and it is reasonable to withhold a salivary gland analogy for most high-grade, poorly differentiated adenocarcinomas of the sinonasal tract.

Clear Cell Carcinomas

Rarely, a sinonasal carcinoma is composed predominantly of clear cells and may be similar to clear cell tumors of salivary gland origin. If the tumor has foci that resemble the typical features of one of the salivary tumors that may have a large clear cell component (e.g., mucoepidermoid carcinoma, oncocytic tumors, or acinic cell adenocarcinoma), then an analogy to salivary gland tumors can be made. Like clear cell carcinoma elsewhere, metastasis from a distal primary site (e.g., renal cell adenocarcinoma) should be considered.

Polymorphous Low-Grade Adenocarcinoma

Although quite rare, this tumor has been reported in the sinonasal tract.[13]

Metastatic (Secondary) Neoplasms

Sinonasal tract tumors with unusual or nonspecific histologic appearances for the anatomic location should be investigated for the possibility of a metastasis from an undiscovered primary malignancy elsewhere. This holds true for tumors with only a slight "salivary appearance," since tumors arising from many different locations or organs can sometimes resemble salivary gland neoplasia.

LARYNGEAL LESIONS

Mixed Tumors

As can be seen in Table 31–4, mixed tumors of the larynx are quite uncommon. Some of the laryngeal mixed tumors in the OTR from the AFIP were atypical, and their classification was difficult. Certainly, the diagnosis of benign mixed tumor in this anatomic location should be entertained cautiously, and distinction from the many tumors that occur more frequently (e.g., adenoid cystic carcinoma, mucoepidermoid carcinoma, and low-grade chondrosarcoma) should be foremost in the mind of the pathologist.

One case of malignant mixed tumor of the carcinosarcoma type (see Chapter 20) is present in the OTR, but the classification of this tumor was also difficult and somewhat equivocal.

Oncocytic Lesions (Metaplasia, Hyperplasia, Oncocytoma)

Clinical Findings

Oncocytic lesions of the larynx occur most often in patients from ages 50 to 80 years. A slight predominance of male patients exists. The lesions may be associated with hoarseness, but in many instances they are relatively asymptomatic and may be an incidental finding during laryngoscopy. In a few cases in the OTR, the lesion was present in the patient for several years, with little growth.

These lesions are most often located in the false vocal cord or laryngeal ventricle areas, and they arise from the seromucous glands of these areas.[14] Very rarely, they may be in the subglottic area.

Pathologic Findings

The lesions vary in size from 0.1 to 3.0 cm, and most lesions are closer to the smaller end of this range. They are usually polypoid and cystic.

The microscopic findings in most cases suggest oncocytic metaplasia and cystic hyperplasia rather than neoplasia. Well-defined, columnar, oncocytic epithelium arises from seromucous ducts or acini and subsequently expands into cystic structures. Papillary growths into the cystic spaces are common. The process seems to be multifocal in the large majority of cases, and this contributes to the impression that this is a metaplastic process. Very rarely, a solitary, solid, large nodule of oncocytes with large nuclei, moderately prominent nucleoli, and slightly increased nuclear-cytoplasmic ratios is encountered that can be reasonably interpreted as an oncocytic adenoma or oncocytoma.[14]

Behavior and Treatment

These lesions are usually quite small, and their growth potential seems limited, which also favors a metaplastic-hyperplastic interpretation over that of a neoplastic one. Simple excisional biopsy is usually sufficient treatment. Occasionally, patients may have an apparent recurrence, but at least some instances probably represent the enlargement of a previously occult lesion that was separate from the originally excised lesion. This is reasonable, since the lesions are so frequently multifocal.

Differential Diagnosis

Granular cell tumors, which are eosinophilic and occur in the larynx, must be distinguished from oncocytic lesions. The well-defined ribbons of columnar epithelium present in most of the oncocytic lesions allow easy distinction from a granular cell tumor. In the rare solid oncocytoma, the cells are more closely packed, and the edges of the tumor are better demarcated than in a granular cell tumor. If there is any uncertainty about the diagnosis, the immunoreactivity of granular cell tumors with anti–S-100 protein can be very helpful.

Acinic Cell Adenocarcinoma

Although a few cases of laryngeal acinic cell adenocarcinoma have been reported,[15] no examples are contained in the OTR. This is an extremely rare tumor in this anatomic location. This diagnosis should be approached with caution, and everything reasonable should be considered to exclude another type of tumor. Acinic cell adenocarcinoma involving the anterior subglottic region in a patient with a history of thyroid gland disease has been reported,[16] but certainly this situation is quite suggestive of a thyroid carcinoma (although one with perhaps a less than typical appearance) invading the subglottic larynx.

Mucoepidermoid Carcinoma

Clinical Findings

The presenting signs and symptoms of laryngeal mucoepidermoid carcinomas mimic those of squamous cell carcinoma of the larynx.[17] Hoarseness is common, and some patients have hemoptysis, foreign body sensation, dysphagia, or a neck mass.

Pathologic Findings

Reported lesions have varied in size from about 0.5 to 5.0 cm. Nothing in their gross appearance distinguishes them from squamous cell carcinomas.

Microscopically, low-grade mucoepidermoid carcinomas of the larynx resemble the same type of tumor found in other sites, and recognition is usually not too difficult. Rarely, these tumors may appear to arise from the surface epithelium rather than from the mucous glands or ducts, and this may be confusing to the pathologist who is unaware of the possibility. High-grade mucoepidermoid carcinomas may resemble poorly differentiated squamous cell carcinomas. A clear cell variant of mucoepidermoid carcinoma in the larynx has been reported.[18]

Behavior and Treatment

The behavior of these laryngeal tumors has been referred to as unpredictable.[19] This may partly result from analyses that contain different numbers of high-grade adenosquamous carcinomas, which often are difficult to separate from mucoepidermoid carcinomas (see the discussion of differential diagnosis that follows). Although histologic grading influences treatment, the most important factor in therapy is the clinical stage. Total laryngectomy has been the most frequently employed treatment, but appropriately small or limited lesions have been treated with vertical hemilaryngectomy or supraglottic laryngectomy. In the presence of clinically enlarged neck lymph nodes, neck dissection should generally be performed. Elective neck dissection is controversial, but histologic grade is a factor in this decision. Radiation therapy is more appropriate for high-grade lesions, and decisions for the use of this modality are based on factors similar to those for poorly differentiated squamous cell carcinomas.

Differential Diagnosis

Occasionally, benign hamartomatous mucous gland proliferations occur in the larynx. Some have ectatic ductal structures that mimic the cystic patterns of low-grade mucoepidermoid carcinoma. Generally, however, the mucous glands are well formed, and the lesions lack foci of epidermoid or intermediate cells that are found in the carcinomas.

A metaplastic alteration similar to necrotizing sialometaplasia is rarely found in the larynx and must be differentiated from mucoepidermoid carcinoma, just as it is for other sites of occurrence (see Chapter 5).

The most troublesome and frequent diagnostic problem is the differentiation of high-grade mucoepidermoid carcinoma from adenosquamous carcinoma. The literature indicates that a majority of laryngeal mucoepidermoid carcinomas behave like rather high-grade carcinomas. This experience may partly result from the inclusion of some cases of adenosquamous carcinoma, which is more frequent in the supraglottic larynx than is mucoepidermoid carcinoma. Adenosquamous carcinomas of this location are poorly differentiated carcinomas that arise from the surface mucosal epithelium just as do squamous cell carcinomas. Although, rarely, a mucoepidermoid carcinoma might arise from the surface, significant areas of surface carcinoma favor the diagnosis of adenosquamous carcinoma (see Chapter 27). Adenosquamous carcinomas have duct formations (Fig. 31–9) but usually do not have mucocytes.

Adenoid Cystic Carcinoma

Clinical Findings

Adenoid cystic carcinomas of the larynx comprise only about 0.25 percent of laryngeal carcinomas.[20] The age range of occurrence is fairly wide, but they are found most often in the fourth to the sixth decades of life. The sex incidence is approximately equal. These laryngeal tumors most often occur in the subglottic area, but a substantial proportion are found supraglottically. Tumors of glottic origin are even less common.

Hoarseness or other voice change, pain, and dysphagia (from large tumors) are the most common symptoms caused by supraglottic tumors. Subglottic tumors may cause shortness of breath, dyspnea on exertion, hoarseness, or pain.[20] Durations of symptoms have ranged from 3 weeks to 3 years, with a mean time period of 20 months.[21]

Pathologic Findings

Laryngeal adenoid cystic carcinomas are usually widely infiltrative at the time of discovery. The extent of the tumor, as judged by clinical or radiographic means, can be deceptive; consequently, frozen sections during surgery are quite important for judging the required extent of resection.

The histologic features are the same as those seen with adenoid cystic carcinomas found at other sites.

Behavior and Treatment

Total laryngectomy has generally been employed for treatment. Not unexpectedly, a high incidence (greater than 50 percent) of local treat-

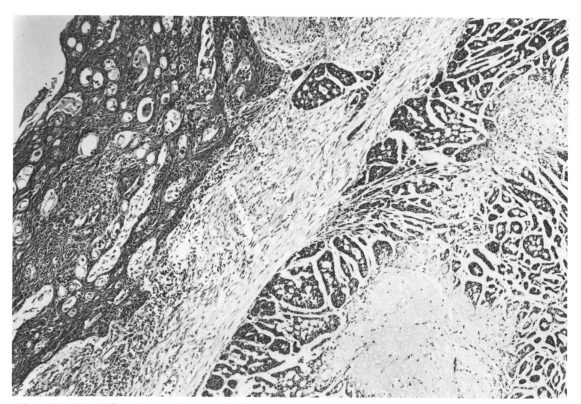

Figure 31–9. A piriform sinus and laryngeal adenosquamous carcinoma derived from the surface epithelium shows a moderately differentiated squamous area at the left and an adenocarcinomatous component, which could be mistaken for adenoid cystic carcinoma, on the right (× 75).

ment failure does occur; thus postoperative radiotherapy may be beneficial.[20] Because the reported incidence of lymph node metastasis is higher than that for adenoid cystic carcinomas elsewhere, some have recommended elective neck dissection.[20] This relatively high incidence of neck metastases may be misleading, however. Some reported cases of adenoid cystic carcinoma may, in fact, be poorly differentiated adenosquamous or basaloid squamous cell carcinomas that are sometimes misdiagnosed as adenoid cystic carcinoma (see the discussion of differential diagnosis that follows). These poorly differentiated variants of squamous cell carcinoma have a more aggressive metastatic behavior (particularly to lymph nodes) than that seen in adenoid cystic carcinoma.

Differential Diagnosis

Just as in other anatomic locations, laryngeal adenoid cystic carcinoma has to be distinguished from benign mixed tumor, and the histologic features that are important for the distinction are the same as those used for other locations.

In the subglottic area, invasive thyroid carcinoma needs to be kept in mind, but usually, the histologic distinction from adenoid cystic carcinoma is not too difficult. Immunostaining for thyroglobulin (or, rarely, calcitonin) obviously can be quite helpful in the rare difficult case.

It is not uncommon for the supraglottic larynx or piriform sinus area to give rise to poorly differentiated variants of squamous cell carcinoma that have heterogenous patterns. Generally, they have been called either adenosquamous carcinomas or basaloid squamous cell carcinomas.[22] Some of these tumors can have an adenoid pattern (see Fig. 31–9) that is suggestive of adenoid cystic carcinoma, which has led to misdiagnosis.[23] Although classic cribriform patterns are generally not found, cytologic similarities can make the distinction between these squamous cell carcinoma variants and adenoid cystic carcinoma difficult. The cells are generally cytologically more malignant than expected for adenoid cystic carcinoma. Perhaps even more helpful, squamoid differentiation is not found in the latter tumor.

Miscellaneous Carcinomas

A majority of tumors in the larynx that have a slight adenocarcinomatous appearance are neuroendocrine carcinomas of intermediate differentiation that are not comparable to salivary gland neoplasia.[24] Small cell undifferentiated neuroendocrine carcinoma occurs in the larynx,[25] and conceivably, it is analogous to small cell carcinoma of salivary gland origin (see Chapter 25).

Epithelial-myoepithelial carcinoma has been reported in the subglottic region.[26]

SALIVARY GLAND TYPES OF TUMORS OF MISCELLANEOUS HEAD AND NECK SITES

Nasopharynx

Oncocytic metaplasia and hyperplasia of seromucous glands, similar to that described earlier for the larynx, are not rare in the nasopharynx (Fig. 31–10). Although this condition has, in rare instances, produced a nodule large enough (about 1.0 to 1.5 cm) to cause some dysfunction of the eustachian tube opening, usually these lesions are quite small and asymptomatic. They are usually found coincidentally in "random" biopsies of the nasopharynx that are performed during endoscopic evaluation of patients with neck masses that are clinically suspected of being metastatic carcinoma. The OTR files contain several cases of small, non-neoplastic oncocytic lesions that were found in nasopharyngeal biopsies, and the neck masses, which were subsequently surgically excised, proved to be Warthin's tumors near the tail of the parotid glands. Since the normal lymphoid tissue around the nasopharyngeal oncocytic metaplasias creates some resemblance to Warthin's tumors, these patients were thought (by the case contributors) to have "metastatic Warthin's tumor from the nasopharynx." One patient was actually given radiation therapy before the correct diagnosis was established. This error in interpretation is clearly one to be avoided.

Mixed tumors of the nasopharynx are quite scarce. It is important not to mistake chordoma (a malignancy) for a benign mixed tumor. The bone involvement that is usually present with a chordoma is a useful radiographic finding. Histologically, the multivacuolated "physaliphorous" cells of the chordoma are a diagnostic aid, and well-formed ducts or cells with myoepithelial features are not found in chordoma as they usually are in mixed tumor. Immunohistochemistry is often not helpful, since both lesions are immunoreactive for keratin and S-100 protein. Glial fibrillary acidic protein or abundant actin reactivity lends support to the diagnosis of mixed tumor.

Polymorphous low-grade adenocarcinoma of the nasopharynx has been reported.[27]

Ear

The ceruminal glands of the external ear canal can give rise to both benign mixed tumors and adenoid cystic carcinomas.[28] With adenoid cystic carcinomas, clinical information may be necessary to determine whether the carcinoma arose from ceruminal glands or, instead, from the parotid gland, with invasion of the external ear canal.

Small salivary gland choristomas are occasionally found in the middle ear space.

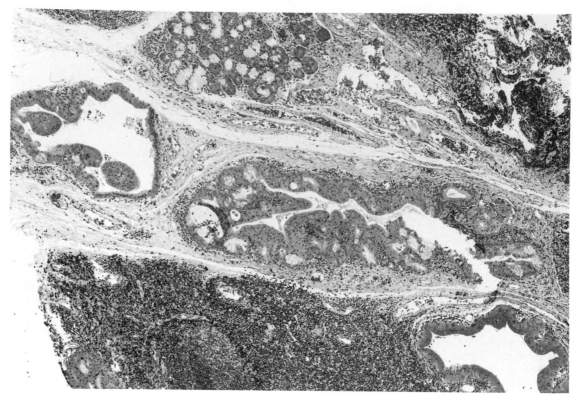

Figure 31–10. Small foci of oncocytic metaplasia and hyperplasia that developed in nasopharyngeal ducts and that were incidentally discovered in a biopsy specimen (× 48).

Trachea

Tracheal tumors, in general, are uncommon, but adenoid cystic carcinoma is the second most frequent malignancy (after squamous cell carcinoma) of the trachea.[29] It can occur in any portion of the trachea, but it is most common in the upper one third. Because reanastomosis of the trachea is necessary, this carcinoma is difficult to adequately resect in this anatomic location. Since the histologic extent of invasion is often much greater than what is judged clinically, frozen section control of margins during surgery is obviously important.

Although the chance of curing tracheal adenoid cystic carcinoma is not good, recurrent growth may be slow, and survival is better than that for squamous cell carcinoma of this same site. Two thirds of patients have survived an average of 7 years.[28] Subsequent metastases to the lungs are not uncommon, but death is usually due to the consequences of local recurrence in the obviously vital airway.

Benign mixed tumors of the trachea are rare, with barely more than a dozen reported cases. Mucoepidermoid carcinomas are even more rare, with about one-half dozen reported cases.[28] Most of these cases have occurred in teenagers or young adults.

REFERENCES

1. Toppozada HH, Talaat MA: The normal human maxillary sinus mucosa. Acta Otolaryngol 1980; 89:204–213.
2. Gnepp DR, Heffner DK: Mucosal origin of sinonasal adenomatous neoplasms. Modern Pathol 1989; 2:365–371.
3. Nassar VH, Bridges GP: Topography of the laryngeal mucous glands. Arch Otolaryngol 1971; 94:490–498.
4. Compagno J, Wong RT: Intranasal mixed tumors (pleomorphic adenomas): A clinicopathologic study of 40 cases. Am J Clin Pathol 1977; 68:213–218.
5. Heffner DK, Hyams VJ: Teratocarcinosarcoma (malignant teratoma?) of the nasal cavity and paranasal sinuses: A clinicopathologic study of 20 cases. Cancer 1984; 53:2140–2154.
6. Compagno J, Hyams VJ: Hemangiopericytoma-like intranasal tumors: A clinicopathologic study of 23 cases. Am J Clin Pathol 1976; 66:672–683.
7. Heffner DK, Hyams VJ, Hauck KW, Lingeman C: Low-grade adenocarcinoma of the nasal cavity and paranasal sinuses. Cancer 1982; 50:312–322.
8. Cohen MA, Batsakis JG: Oncocytic tumors (oncocytomas) of minor salivary glands. Arch Otolaryngol 1968; 88:97–99.
9. Handler SD, Ward PH: Oncocytoma of maxillary sinus. Laryngoscope 1979; 89:372–376.

10. Barnes L, Bedetti C: Oncocytic schneiderian papilloma: A reappraisal of cylindrical cell papilloma of the sinonasal tract. Hum Pathol 1984; 15:344–351.

11. Spiro RH, Huvos AG, Strong EW: Adenoid cystic carcinoma of salivary gland origin: A clinicopathologic study of 242 cases. Am J Surg 1974; 128:512–520.

12. Rounthwaite FJ, Wallace AC, Watson TA: The effect of radiotherapy in the treatment of adenoid cystic carcinoma of the head and neck arising in minor salivary glands. J Otolaryngol 1977; 6:297–308.

13. Dardick I, van Nostrand AWP: Polymorphous low-grade adenocarcinoma: A case report with ultrastructural findings. Oral Surg Oral Med Oral Pathol 1988; 66:459–465.

14. Gallagher JC, Puzon BQ: Oncocytic lesions of the larynx. Ann Otol Rhinol Laryngol 1969; 78:307–318.

15. Crissman JD, Rosenblatt A: Acinous cell carcinoma of the larynx. Arch Pathol 1978; 102:233–236.

16. Reibel JF, McLean WC, Cantrell RW: Laryngeal acinic cell carcinoma following thyroid irradiation. Otolaryngol Head Neck Surg 1981; 89:398–401.

17. Damiani JM, Damiani KK, Hauck K, Hyams VJ: Mucoepidermoid-adenosquamous carcinoma of the larynx and hypopharynx: A report of 21 cases and a review of the literature. Otolaryngol Head Neck Surg 1981; 89:235–243.

18. Seo IS, Tomich CE, Warfel KA, Hull MT: Clear cell carcinoma of the larynx: A variant of mucoepidermoid carcinoma. Ann Otol Rhinol Laryngol 1980; 89:168–172.

19. Binder WJ, Som P, Kaneko M, Biller HF: Mucoepidermoid carcinoma of the larynx: A case report and review of the literature. Ann Otol Rhinol Laryngol 1980; 89:103–107.

20. Stillwagon GB, Smith RRL, Highstein C, Lee DJ: Adenoid cystic carcinoma of the supraglottic larynx: Report of a case and review of the literature. Am J Otolaryngol 1985; 6:309–314.

21. Olofsson J, van Nostrand AWP: Adenoid cystic carcinoma of the larynx: A report of four cases and a review of the literature. Cancer 1977; 40:1307–1313.

22. Wain SL, Kier R, Vollmer RT, Bossen EH: Basaloid-squamous carcinoma of the tongue, hypopharynx and larynx: Report of ten cases. Hum Pathol 1986; 17:1158–1166.

23. McKay MJ, Bilous AM: Basaloid-squamous carcinoma of the hypopharynx. Cancer 1989; 63:2528–2531.

24. Wenig BM, Hyams VJ, Heffner DK: Moderately differentiated neuroendocrine carcinoma of the larynx: A clinicopathologic study of 54 cases. Cancer 1988; 62:2658–2676.

25. Gnepp DR, Ferlito A, Hyams V: Primary anaplastic small cell (oat cell) carcinoma of the larynx. Cancer 1983; 51:1731–1745.

26. Mikaelian DO, Contrucci RB, Batsakis JG: Epithelial-myoepithelial carcinoma of the subglottic region: A case presentation and review of the literature. Otolaryngol Head Neck Surg 1986; 95:104–106.

27. Wenig BM, Harpaz N, DelBridge C: Polymorphous low-grade adenocarcinoma of seromucous glands of the nasopharynx. Am J Clin Pathol 1989; 92:104–109.

28. Perzin KH, Gullane P, Conley J: Adenoid cystic carcinoma involving the external auditory canal. Cancer 1982; 50:2873–2883.

29. Heffner DK: Diseases of the trachea. In Barnes L (ed): Surgical Pathology of the Head and Neck with Clinical Correlations, Vol. 1. Marcel Dekker, New York, 1985; 509–518.

32

METASTATIC DISEASE TO THE MAJOR SALIVARY GLANDS

Douglas R. Gnepp

Secondary involvement of the major salivary glands by a nonsalivary gland malignancy is relatively common. Tumors may directly infiltrate the parotid gland or submandibular salivary gland parenchyma from adjacent areas, or they may spread by hematogenous or lymphogenous routes to the gland proper, to the intraparotid or periparotid lymph nodes, or to the lymph nodes adjacent to the submandibular gland. This chapter reviews metastatic lesions to the parotid region and to the submandibular gland. No cases of metastatic tumors in the sublingual gland have been found in the literature[1-107] or in any of the 490 cases of major salivary gland metastases on file at the Armed Forces Institute of Pathology (AFIP).

In reviewing the literature, it was usually easy to separate tumors metastasizing to the submandibular gland from those in the adjacent lymph nodes; however, in the parotid gland, it was more difficult to separate tumors metastatic to the periparotid or intraparotid lymph nodes from those actually metastasizing to the parotid gland parenchyma. Therefore, in the review of the literature, all tumors metastatic to the parotid gland or its adjacent lymph nodes were included, but only tumors metastatic to the submandibular gland proper were included.

ANATOMIC CONSIDERATIONS

The periparotid soft tissues and parotid gland contain numerous lymph nodes that function as a single unit, although anatomically, these lymph nodes are divided into intraglandular and extraglandular groups. The parotid gland proper contains 3 to 32 intraglandular lymph nodes (average 20), most of which are located in the superficial lobe and are connected by a rich interconnecting plexus of lymph vessels.[93, 108, 109] This plexus of vessels drains the skin of the side of the head above the parotid gland (frontal, temporal, scalp, ear, posterior cheek and preauricular regions), the lateral aspects of the eyelids, the lacrimal gland, the conjunctiva, the root of the nose, the upper lip, the external auditory canal, the eustachian tube, and the tympanic membrane.[109] The submandibular gland, on the other hand, does not appear to contain lymph nodes within the parenchyma proper, although considerable controversy exists about the presence of a rare intracapsular or subcapsular lymph node.[110, 111] This subcapsular lymph node may actually represent a lymph node protruding from or partially embedded in an interlobar fissure on the deep side of the submandibular gland[109] rather than an actual intraglandular lymph node.

INCIDENCE

Tumor metastasis to the submandibular gland or parotid region is fairly common, accounting for between 1 and 42 percent of various published series of salivary gland tumors (Table 32–1). All but one series had an incidence rate that ranged between 1 and 4 percent, which is consistent with the incidence in the AFIP material of 3.3 percent of all tumors. The only exception to this incidence range was the series published by Bergersen and colleagues,[45] who found 51 (42 percent) metastatic tumors among 121 total tumors. They attributed this higher incidence rate to patient selection (a

Table 32–1. Incidence of Metastasis to Parotid and Submandibular Salivary Glands from Selected Reports in the Literature and from the AFIP Registry

Series (Year)	Number of Metastases	Number of Malignant Tumors	Percent of Malignant Tumors	Total Number of Tumors
Beahrs and coworkers[31] (1960)	9	162	5	760*
Grage and Lober[23] (1962)	9	68	13	210
Patey and coworkers (1965)	6	95	6	95†
Katz[15] (1975)	2	63	3	318*
Nussbaum and coworkers[30] (1976)	5	—	—	700*
Gleave and coworkers[101] (1979)	24	149	16	977§
Yarington[92] (1981)	10	—	25	251*
Rees and coworkers[83] (1981)	52	545	9.5	545*†
Seifert and coworkers[4, 112] (1986)	108	—	—	3,850‡
Bergersen and coworkers[45] (1987)	51	71	72	121*
Gnepp and coworkers[113] (1987)	6	72	8	234
Bouquot and coworkers[10] (1989)	4	28	14	28†
AFIP registry (1990)	490	6,083††	8.1	15,070‖

*Parotid gland only.
†Malignant tumors only.
‡Estimated.
§Includes periparotid and adjacent submandibular lymph nodes.
‖Includes major and minor salivary glands.

large percentage of elderly male war veterans constituted their patient population) and to the incidence of skin cancer among the Australian population (39 of 51 patients in their series had metastatic skin cancer from anatomic sites that normally drain into the parotid nodal system).

The percentage of salivary gland malignancies that result from secondary involvement of the parotid and submandibular glands is quite variable, accounting for 3 to 72 percent of all epithelial malignancies in various series (see Table 32–1). If the series by Bergersen and coworkers[45] is excluded because of the biases previously mentioned, the overall incidence rate ranged up to 25 percent of malignant lesions, suggesting that metastases to the parotid gland may be significantly more commonplace than previously recognized. In addition, there is considerable variance in incidence of metastases, depending on the histologic type of the primary neoplasm. Conley and Sebastian[93] found that 37 of 175 (21 percent) head and neck melanomas metastasized to the parotid region, whereas Ridenhour and Spratt[20] noted that 43 of 2,802 (1.5 percent) patients with squamous carcinoma of the head and neck metastasized to the parotid region.

CLINICAL FINDINGS

Analysis of the 490 patients in the AFIP files demonstrates a steady linear increase in incidence among patients from the second to the sixth decade of life, with a peak incidence in the seventh decade (Fig. 32–1). Metastatic disease is unusual in the first 2 decades of life. Only nine patients were under 20 years of age. The mean age of the 423 patients whose ages were known is 59.3 years;

the mean age for men and that for women are similar. The youngest patient, who suffered from a metastatic retinoblastoma, was 1 year of age; the oldest patient, who had a metastatic cutaneous squamous cell carcinoma, was 98 years old at the time of the initial diagnosis.

Data on gender show a male to female ratio of almost 3 to 1. Racial data were supplied for 310 cases; 288 patients were white, 11 black, 8 Asian, 2 Malaysian, and 1 Native American.

Data on site of occurrence from the AFIP and the literature are summarized in Tables 32–2 to 32–4. Four cases in the literature[1] and 19 cases in the AFIP material did not state the exact salivary gland. There were 1,309 patients with 1,316 tumors in the combined review. About 90 percent of metastases involved the parotid region, whereas about 8 percent involved the submandibular gland. Two of the AFIP cases manifested synchronous unilateral parotid and submandibular metastases, and bilateral parotid metastases occurred in five patients in the literature.

HISTOLOGIC FEATURES

Squamous carcinoma is the most common tumor, accounting for 27 percent of the cases in the AFIP series (25 percent of parotid tumors and 33 percent of submandibular tumors) and 60 percent of the cases in the literature (61 percent of parotid tumors and 23 percent of submandibular tumors). This difference in percentages between the literature and the AFIP files may be due to the referral pattern to the AFIP, which receives a large number of diagnostically difficult lesions. Since squamous carcinoma is usually not diagnostically difficult, a lower percentage of squamous carcinoma

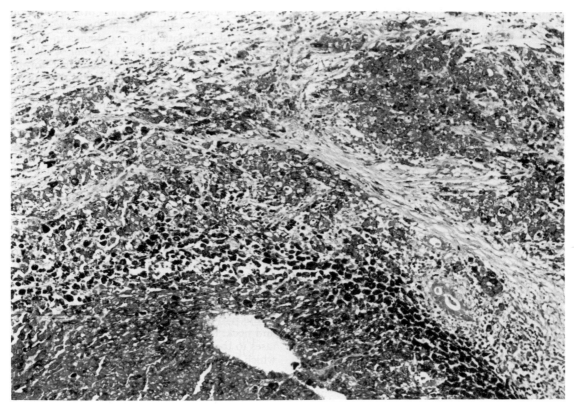

Figure 32–2. Malignant melanoma metastatic to parotid gland. Note irregular collections of tumor replacing normal tissue (× 100).

moid carcinoma, and one retinoblastoma. Two were located on the face, two on the tongue, two in the tonsillar region, two in the central nervous system, and one each on the scalp, in the thyroid gland, in the paranasal sinuses, and in the ear. Distant tumor sites that metastasized to the parotid gland included the breast (eight tumors) (Fig. 32–3), the lung (five tumors), and the kidney (three tumors). Of the 14 submandibular primary tumors 43 percent arose in the head and neck, including three thyroid tumors, and one each from the face, the eye, and the eyelid. Distant sites that metastasized to the submandibular gland were the breast (four tumors), the lung (three tumors), and the kidney (one tumor).

The primary sites of tumors metastatic to the parotid area and to the submandibular gland were available in 86 percent of patients in the literature reviewed. A total of 85 percent of parotid tumors with known primary sites (excluding the 84 skin, not otherwise specified, cases; see Table 32–3) and 15 percent of the submandibular tumors (see Table 32–4) arose in the head and neck region. The most common locations of primary tumors with parotid area metastases were the skin regions with lymphatics that drain into the parotid and periparotid lymph nodes. In decreasing order of incidence, these sites include the preauricular and ear region, face, temple, forehead and eyebrow,

cheek, eyelid, neck, and scalp. Other sites of primary tumors were the oral cavity, all the areas of the pharynx, the thyroid gland, the paranasal sinuses, the central nervous system, and, rarely, the submandibular and lacrimal glands. Only four primary head and neck tumors metastasized to the submandibular gland; three were from the upper and lower lips, and one was from the hypopharynx. Distant metastases to the submandibular gland arose, with almost equal frequency, from the lung, kidney, and breast, and, less commonly, from the colorectal areas, prostate, skin (not from the head and neck), stomach, bladder, pancreas, and uterus (see Tables 32–3, 32–4).

DIFFERENTIAL DIAGNOSIS

The most important differential diagnostic consideration is the separation of a primary from a metastatic neoplasm. A careful history and physical examination is of vital importance in this regard and should eliminate most of the potential pitfalls. However, several primary salivary gland tumors have histologic features similar to those of tumors occurring in other regions of the body. Therefore, in certain instances, it is imperative to rule out a metastasis from another source before

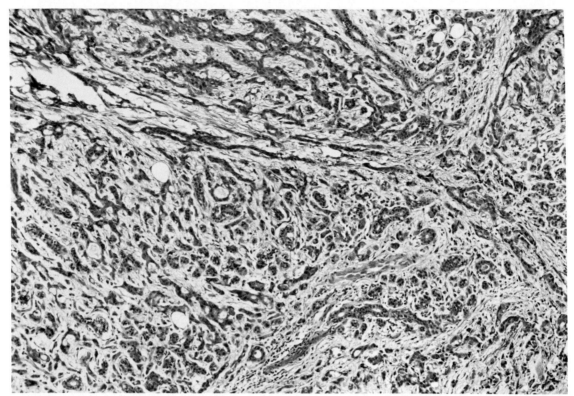

Figure 32–3. Breast carcinoma metastatic to parotid gland. Note infiltrating cords of tumor typical of a breast primary (× 100).

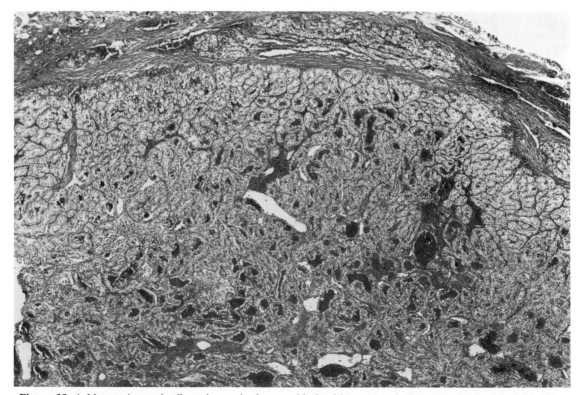

Figure 32–4. Metastatic renal cell carcinoma in the parotid gland is composed of tumor cells with clear cytoplasm. Note prominent vascularity that aids in the differential diagnosis with a primary clear cell carcinoma of salivary gland origin (× 30).

considering a tumor as primary. Specific conflicts in differential diagnosis include metastatic breast carcinoma versus primary ductal carcinoma, metastatic squamous carcinoma versus primary squamous carcinoma, metastatic small cell carcinoma versus primary small cell carcinoma, metastatic undifferentiated carcinoma from the nasopharynx or tonsillar region versus primary lymphoepithelial or undifferentiated carcinoma, and metastatic renal cell carcinoma versus primary clear cell carcinoma. Certain features may help distinguish a primary tumor from a metastasis. If the tumor appears to be localized predominantly in lymph nodes with only secondary invasion of parenchymal tissues, it is most likely metastatic. If a clear cell tumor is clinically pulsatile[41, 51] and/or has a histologically prominent vascular pattern (Fig. 32–4), it should be considered metastatic renal cell carcinoma until it is proved otherwise. Lastly, ductal carcinomas of the breast that metastasize to the salivary glands usually do not have an intraductal component; therefore, ductal carcinomas with foci of intraductal carcinoma are most likely primary tumors.

PROGNOSIS AND TREATMENT

Conley and Sebastian[93] stated that once a tumor had metastasized to the parotid gland area, the prognosis was grave. Their 5-year patient survival rates were 11.5 percent for metastatic melanoma, 14.5 percent for metastatic squamous carcinoma, and 11.1 percent for other malignant tumors. Ridenhour and Spratt[20] reported a 67.4 percent 3-year patient survival rate for epidermoid carcinoma metastatic to the parotid area. Rees and coworkers[83] found that patient survival depended on histologic cell type. The absolute survival rate was 100 percent for basal cell carcinoma, 67 percent for cutaneous squamous carcinoma, 43 percent for melanoma, and only 9 percent for tumors of a noncutaneous origin. Bergersen and colleagues[45] found that 21 of 51 (41 percent) patients with parotid area metastases died of causes related to their tumors, usually within 2 years of diagnosis. However, Jackson and Ballantyne[78] had a local control rate of 84 percent with squamous cell carcinoma of the skin that metastasized to the parotid area in patients in whom the primary skin cancer site was free of disease at the time of parotidectomy.

Storm and colleagues[88] recommended that patients with deeply invasive melanomas and large anaplastic squamous carcinomas that arose in skin sites with a high metastatic potential to the parotid area (ipsilateral eyelid, frontal, temporal, posterior cheek, and anterior ear) undergo ipsilateral wide excision of the primary lesion and superficial parotidectomy, with a radical neck dissection, whether or not lymph nodes were clinically involved. They recommended this because in 45 percent of their patients with tumors in these anatomic areas, metastases developed even though these patients had clinically negative parotid lymph nodes at the time of diagnosis.

From the preceding, we may conclude two things. First, in the group of patients in whom salivary gland metastases are a manifestation of distant spread, survival is poor; and second, in the group of patients in whom metastases indicate only locoregional spread (certain cutaneous sites previously outlined) more aggressive surgical treatment may be beneficial.

REFERENCES

1. Hui KK, Luna MA, Batsakis JG, Ordonez NG, Weber R: Undifferentiated carcinomas of the major salivary glands. Oral Surg Oral Med Oral Pathol 1990; 69:76–83.
2. Lippi L, DeMeester W, Norberti A, Porzio P: Malignant parotid tumors: Diagnostic considerations and therapeutic suggestions. Tumori 1989; 75:53–56.
3. Thackray AC, Lucas RB: Tumors of the Major Salivary Glands, Fascicle 10, 2nd Series. Atlas of Tumor Pathology. Washington, DC, Armed Forces Institute of Pathology, 1974; 123–124.
4. Seifert G, Hennings K, Caselitz J: Metastatic tumors to the parotid and submandibular glands—analysis and differential diagnosis of 108 cases. Pathol Res Pract 1986; 181:684–692.
5. Yoel J: Pathology and Surgery of the Salivary Glands. Springfield, Illinois, Charles C Thomas, 1975; 582–595.
6. Meyers AD, Arm RN, Potsic W: Adenocarcinoma of the rectum with metastasis to the parotid. Trans Am Acad Ophthalmol Otolaryngol 1977; 84:102–104.
7. Hirshowitz B, Mahler D: Unusual case of multiple basal cell carcinoma with metastasis to the parotid lymph gland. Cancer 1968; 22:654–657.
8. Nassif AC: Metastatic tumors in the parotid gland. Harper Hospital Bulletin 1962; 20:69–78.
9. Herrmann JB, Adair FE: Unusual metastatic manifestations of breast carcinoma. Ann Surg 1949; 129:137–141.
10. Bouquot JE, Weiland LH, Kurland LT: Metastases to and from the upper aerodigestive tract in the population of Rochester, Minnesota, 1935–1984. Head Neck 1989; 11:212–218.
11. Margo CE, Horton MB: Malignant fibrous histiocytoma of the conjunctiva with metastasis. Am J Ophthalmol 1989; 107:433–434.
12. Solomon MP, Rosen Y, Gardner B: Metastatic malignancy in the submandibular gland. Oral Surg Oral Med Oral Pathol 1975; 39:469–473.
13. Coulthard SW: Metastatic disease of the parotid gland. Otolaryngol Clin North Am 1977; 10:437–442.
14. Soni NK, Arora HL, Chatterji P: Massive metastatic retinoblastoma of the parotid gland. J Laryngol Otol 1978; 92:1049–1052.
15. Katz AD: Unusual lesions of the parotid gland. J Surg Oncol 1975; 7:219–235.
16. Graham JW: Metastatic cancer in the parotid lymph nodes. Med J Aust 1965; 2:8–12.

17. Mallett SP: A renal-cell metastatic carcinoma involving the mandible and submaxillary gland. Oral Surg Oral Med Oral Pathol 1961; 14:4–7.

18. Parkin JL, Stevens MH: Unusual parotid tumors. Laryngoscope 1977; 87:317–325.

19. Moghtader A: Cervical and parotid metastasis secondary to cerebral astrocytoma. Laryngoscope 1966; 76:1834–1841.

20. Ridenhour CE, Spratt JS: Epidermoid carcinoma of the skin involving the parotid gland. Am J Surg 1966; 112:504–507.

21. Bissett D, Bessell EM, Bradley PJ, Morgan DAL, McKenzie CG: Parotid metastases from carcinoma of the breast. Clin Radiol 1989; 40:309–310.

22. Megele R, Grub P, Buhrmann K: Das extrakraniell metastasierende maligne gliomiatrogen? Neurochirurgia 1989; 32:157–159.

23. Grage TB, Lober PH: Malignant tumors of the major salivary glands. Surgery 1962; 52:284–294.

24. Gunbay MU, Ceryan K, Kupelioglu AA: Metastatic renal carcinoma to the parotid gland. J Laryngol Otol 1989; 103:417–418.

25. Moul JW, Paulson DF, Fuller G, Gottfried MR, Floyd WL: Prostate cancer with solitary parotid metastasis correctly diagnosed with immunohistochemical stains. J Urol 1989; 142:1328–1329.

26. Gruber B, Moran WJ, Pearle MS, Strauss FF, Chodak G: Prostate cancer presenting as facial paralysis. Otolaryngol Head Neck Surg 1989; 100:333–338.

27. Abrams HL, Spiro R, Goldstein N: Metastases in carcinoma analysis of 1000 autopsied cases. Cancer 1950; 3:74–85.

28. Smith RL, Davis TS, Kennedy TJ, Graham WP, Miller SH: Metastatic malignancies of the parotid gland. Am Fam Physician 1977; 16:139–140.

29. Patey DH, Thackray AC, Keeling DH: Malignant disease of the parotid. Br J Cancer 1965; 19:712–737.

30. Nussbaum M, Cho HT, Som ML: Parotid space tumors of non-salivary origin. Ann Surg 1976; 183:10–12.

31. Beahrs OH, Woolner LB, Carveth SW, Devine KD: Surgical management of parotid lesions. Arch Surg 1960; 80:890–904.

32. Gairin JM, Cortez LL, Canonge RS, Molins JB, Rosell MTV: Hipernefroma: metastasis tardias infrecuentes y sindrome paraneoplasico. Med Clin (Barc) 1986; 87:374–376.

33. Gandon J, Trotoux J, Marandas P, Calmette Y: Les métastases des cancers du rein au niveau des glandes salivaires. A propos d'un cas de métastase intraparotidienne. Ann Otolaryngol Chir Cervicofac (Paris) 1977; 94:485–490.

34. Melnick SJ, Amazon K, Dembrow V: Metastatic renal cell carcinoma presenting as a parotid tumor: A case report with immunohistochemical findings and a review of the literature. Hum Pathol 1989; 20:195–197.

35. Ord RA, Ward-Booth RP, Avery BS: Parotid lymph node metastases from primary intra-oral squamous carcinomas. Int J Oral Maxillofac Surg 1989; 18:104–106.

36. Ord RA: Metastatic melanoma of the parotid lymph nodes. Int J Oral Maxillofac Surg 1989; 18:165–167.

37. Shalowitz JI, Cassidy C, Anders CB: Parotid metastasis of small cell carcinoma of the lung causing facial nerve paralysis. J Oral Maxillofac Surg 1988; 46:404–406.

38. Jordan DR, Addison DJ, Watson AG, McLeish WA: Adenocarcinoma of the lacrimal gland with metastasis to the preauricular lymph nodes and parotid gland. Can J Ophthalmol 1988; 23:136–140.

39. Lopez-Cedrun JL, Aguirre Urizar JM, Martinez-Conde Llamosas R, Prieta Rodriguez A: Melanome metastatique de la parotide a propos de 5 cas. Rev Stomatol Chir Maxillofac 1988; 89:44–48.

40. Marks MW, Ryan RF, Litwin MS, Sonntag BV: Squamous cell carcinoma of the parotid gland. Plast Reconstr Surg 1987; 79:550–554.

41. Owens RM, Friedman CD, Becker SP: Renal cell carcinoma with metastasis to the parotid gland: Case reports and review of the literature. Head Neck 1989; 11:174–178.

42. Tabbara KF, Kersten R, Daouk N, Blodi FC: Metastatic squamous cell carcinoma of the conjunctiva. Ophthalmology 1988; 95:318–321.

43. Gattuso P, Castelli MJ, Shah PA, Kron T: Fine needle aspiration cytologic diagnosis of metastatic Merkel cell carcinoma in the parotid gland. Acta Cytol 1988; 32:576–578.

44. Harrison DJ, McLaren K, Tennant W: A clear cell tumour of the parotid. J Laryngol Otol 1987; 101:633–635.

45. Bergersen PJ, Kennedy PJ, Kneale KL: Metastatic tumours of the parotid region. Aust N Z J Surg 1987; 57:23–26.

46. Rosti G, Callea A, Merendi R, Beccati D, Tienghi A, Turci D, Marangolo M: Metastases to the submaxillary gland from breast cancer: Case report. Tumori 1987; 73:413–416.

47. da Costa SA, Kampschoer GH: Metastasering van huidtumoren van gelaat en behaard hoofd naar het parotisgebied. Ned Tijdschr Geneeskd 1986; 130:1395–1397.

48. Markitziu A, Fisher D, Marmary Y: Thyroid papillary carcinoma presenting as jaw and parotid gland metastases. Int J Oral Maxillofac Surg 1986; 15:648–653.

49. Halczy-Kowalik L, Saldziun D, Gorczyca W: Przerzuty guzow nowotworowych do przyusznic. Czas Stomat 1986; 39:25–29.

50. Orget J, Ollivier H, Dore B, Grange P, Aubert J: Les metastases parotidiennes de l'adenocarcinome a cellules claires du rein. A propos de 2 observations. J d'Urologie 1986; 92:543–544.

51. Zoltie N: Pulsatile secondary from renal cell carcinoma presenting in the submandibular gland. J R Coll Surg Edinb 1986; 31:236.

52. Storey DW, McGowan B: Renal carcinoma metastasis in salivary gland. Br J Urol 1986; 58(2):227.

53. Mehlum DL, Parker GS, Strom CG, Marx DW, Burris TE: Conjunctival squamous cell carcinoma with parotid gland metastasis. Otolaryngol Head Neck Surg 1986; 94:246–249.

54. Shimm DS: Parotid lymph node metastases from squamous cell carcinoma of the skin. J Surg Oncol 1988; 37:56–59.

55. Mendenhall NP, Million RR, Cassisi NJ: Parotid area lymph node metastases from carcinoma of the skin. Int J Radiat Oncol Biol Phys 1985; 11:707–714.

56. Saw D, Ho JHC, Lau WH, Chan J: Parotid swelling

as the first manifestation of nasopharyngeal carcinoma: A report of two cases. Eur J Surg Oncol 1986; 12:71–75.

57. Lee K, McKean ME, McGregor IA: Metastatic patterns of squamous carcinoma in the parotid lymph nodes. Br J Plast Surg 1985; 38:6–10.

58. Velez A, Petrelli N, Herrera L, Lopez C, Mittelman A: Metastasis to the parotid gland from colorectal adenocarcinoma. Dis Colon Rectum 1985; 28:190–192.

59. Wagner W, Böttcher HD, Korinthenberg R, Schadel A: Extraneurale Medulloblastommetastase nach nicht operiertem Medulloblastom. Klin Padiatr 1985; 197:135–137.

60. Brodsky G, Rabson AB: Metastasis to the submandibular gland as the initial presentation of small cell ("oat cell") lung carcinoma. Oral Surg Oral Med Oral Pathol 1984; 58:76–80.

61. Smits JG, Slootweg PJ: Renal cell carcinoma with metastasis to the submandibular and parotid glands: A case report. J Maxillofac Surg 1984; 12:235–236.

62. Bedrosian SA, Goldman RL, Dekelboum AM: Renal carcinoma presenting as a primary submandibular gland tumor. Oral Surg Oral Med Oral Pathol 1984; 58:699–701.

63. Anonsen C, Patterson HC: Facial squamous carcinoma with parotid metastasis—closure with cheek-neck rotation. J Otolaryngol 1984; 13:137–140.

64. Laudadio P, Ceroni AR, Cerasoli PT: Metastatic malignant melanoma in the parotid gland. ORL J 1984; 46:42–49.

65. Pean CE, Smith WI Jr: Metastasizing cerebral germinoma. Ann Neurol 1984; 16:94–95.

66. Smith JM, Irons GB: Metastatic basal cell carcinoma: Review of the literature and report of three cases. Ann Plast Surg 1983; 11:551–553.

67. Moss ALH: Metastatic tumour in the submandibular salivary gland. Br J Plast Surg 1983; 36:79–80.

68. Bela Z, Andor K, Mihaly IB: Metastatizalo basalsejtes carcinoma. Orvosi Hetilap 1984; 125:1669–1670.

69. Luna MA: The occult primary and metastatic tumors to and from the head and neck. In Barnes L (ed): Surgical Pathology of the Head and Neck. New York, Marcel Dekker, Inc., 1985; 1211–1232.

70. Percival RC, Curt JRN: Metastatic hypernephroma of the parotid gland. Postgrad Med J 1982; 58:167–168.

71. Sist TC Jr, Marchetta FC, Milley PC: Renal cell carcinoma presenting as a primary parotid gland tumor. Oral Surg Oral Med Oral Pathol 1982; 53:499–502.

72. Wiesel JM, Weshler Z, Sherman Y, Gay I: Parotid gland metastatic carcinoma of breast origin. J Surg Oncol 1982; 20:227–230.

73. Currens HS, Sajjad SM, Lukeman JM: Aspiration cytology of oat-cell carcinoma metastatic to the parotid gland. Acta Cytol 1982; 26:566–567.

74. Edwab RR, Roberts MJ, Sole MS, Mahoney WD, Rappaport SC: Metastasis of a transitional cell carcinoma of the bladder to the submandibular gland. J Oral Surg 1981; 39:972–974.

75. Kucan JO, Frank DH, Robson MC: Tumours metastatic to the parotid gland. Br J Plast Surg 1981; 34:299–301.

76. Jarchow RC, Rhodes MF: Metastatic basal cell carcinoma: Report of a case. Laryngoscope 1983; 93:481–482.

77. Berryhill BH, Armstrong BW: Extracranial presentation of craniocervical chordoma. Laryngoscope 1984; 94:1063–1065.

78. Jackson GL, Ballantyne AJ: Role of parotidectomy for skin cancer of the head and neck. Am J Surg 1981; 142:464–469.

79. Meyers AD, Olshock R: Metastasis to the submaxillary gland from the breast: A case report and literature review. J Otolaryngol 1981; 10:278–282.

80. Eitschberger E, Wangemann HH, Weidner F, Stolte M: Metastasierendes Schläfenbasaliom oder Ausbreitung per continuitatem? Operatives Vorgehen und Ergebnis. HNO 1982; 30:346–349.

81. Vollrath M, Droese M, Hinney B: Die Parotis als Zielorgan von Nah—und Fernmetastasen. Laryngol Rhinol Otol (Stuttg) 1981; 60:39–41.

82. Nichols RD, Pinnock LA, Szymanowski RT: Metastases to parotid nodes. Laryngoscope 1980; 90:1324–1328.

83. Rees, R, Maples M, Lynch JB, Rosenfeld L: Malignant secondary parotid tumors. South Med J 1981; 74:1050–1052.

84. Selman JW: Pathologic case quiz I. Arch Otolaryngol 1981; 107:194–196.

85. Kline TS, Merriam JM, Shapshay SM: Aspiration biopsy cytology of the salivary gland. Am J Clin Pathol 1981; 76:263–269.

86. Tommerup AB: Overlaebecancer. Ugeskr Laeger 1981; 143:3232–3233.

87. LiVolsi VA: Prostatic carcinoma presenting as a primary parotid tumor. Oral Surg Oral Med Oral Pathol 1979; 48:447–450.

88. Storm FK, Eilber FR, Sparks FC, Morton DL: A prospective study of parotid metastases from head and neck cancer. Am J Surg 1977; 134:115–119.

89. Cassisi NJ, Dickerson DR, Million RR: Squamous cell carcinoma of the skin metastatic to parotid nodes. Arch Otolaryngol 1978; 104:336–339.

90. Ballanger R, Ballanger P: Une forme rare de metastase du cancer du rein, la metastase parotidienne. Societe Francaise d'Urologie du Sud-Ouest 1978; 85:548–550.

91. Pope TH Jr, Lehmann WB: Regional metastasis to parotid nodes. Arch Otolaryngol 1967; 86:91–93.

92. Yarington CT Jr: Metastatic malignant disease to the parotid gland. Laryngoscope 1981; 91:517–519.

93. Conley J, Sebastian A: Parotid gland as a focus of metastasis. Arch Surg 1963; 7:757–764.

94. Katsantonis GP, Friedman WH, Rosenblum BN: The surgical management of advanced malignancies of the parotid gland. Otolaryngol Head Neck Surg 1989; 10:633–640.

95. Januska JR, Leban SG, Orange E: Pulmonary metastasis to the submandibular gland. J Oral Surg 1978; 36:50–51.

96. Casolino D, Vitelli N, Bergonzoni C: Localizzazioni metastatiche parotidee da tumore primitivo in altri distretti. Acta Otorhinolaryngol Ital 1988; 8:175–182.

97. Feinmesser R, Lahovitzki G, Wexler MR, Peled IG: Metastatic carcinoma to the submandibular sali-

vary gland. J Oral Maxillofac Surg 1982; 40:592–593.

98. Cantera JMC, Hernandez AV: Bilateral parotid gland metastasis as the initial presentation of a small cell lung carcinoma. J Oral Maxillofac Surg 1989; 47:1199–1201.

99. Abramson AL: The submaxillary gland as a site for distant metastasis. Laryngoscope 1971; 81:793–795.

100. Hansson L-G, Johansen CC, Biorklund A: CT sialography and conventional sialography in the evaluation of parotid gland neoplasms. J Laryngol Otol 1988; 102:163–168.

101. Gleave EN, Whittaker JS, Nicholson A: Salivary tumours—experience over thirty years. Clin Otolaryngol 1979; 4:247–257.

102. Gaillard J, Haguenauer JP, Dubreuil C, Pignal JL: Tuméfaction parotidienne au cours d'une maladie auto-immune (syndrome de Sjögren). Métastase tardive d'un adéno-carcinome du rein. J Fr Otorhinolaryngol 1982; 31:275–278, 281–283.

103. Watarai J, Akutsu T, Kubota H, Komatani A, Tsukamoto M, Suzuki S: [Case of skin cancer with unusual sites of metastasis]. Rinsho Hoshasen 1983; 28:1013–1015.

104. Albahary A, Auffret J, Ripault J, Rigault J, Roisin L, Aubry G, Fleury JE: Bilateral intra-parotid metastasis of a small cell bronchial epithelioma. Revue de Stomatologie (Paris) 1972; 73:229–234.

105. Forster: Ein fall von markschwamm mit unge-wohnlich vielfacher metastatischer verbreitung. Virchow Arch [A] 1858; 13:271–274.

106. McWhorter GL: Operation on two cases of secondary carcinoma and on one case of primary cystadenoma of the parotid gland: Relation of the lobes of the parotid gland to the facial nerve. Surg Clin North Am 1927; 7:489–505.

107. Godtfredsen E: Malignant nasopharyngeal tumours manifesting themselves as parotid tumours. Acta Chirurgica Scand 1947; 95:205–214.

108. McKean ME, Lee K, McGregor IA: The distribution of lymph nodes in and around the parotid gland: An anatomical study. Br J Plast Surg 1985; 38:1–5.

109. Feind CR: The head and neck. *In* Haagensen CD, Feind CR, Herter FP, Slanetz CA Jr, Weinberg FA: The Lymphatics in Cancer. Philadelphia, WB Saunders Co, 1972; 63–74.

110. Stanley CJ, Kaupp HA, Fischer E: The submandibular salivary gland in radical neck dissection specimens. Am J Surg 1963; 106:831–834.

111. Martin H, Del Valle B, Ehrlich H, Cahan WG: Neck dissection. Cancer 1951; 4:441–499.

112. Seifert G, Miehlke A, Haubrich J, Chilla R: Diseases of the Salivary Glands: Pathology-Diagnosis-Treatment-Facial Nerve Surgery. Stuttgart, Georg Thieme Verlag, 1986; 171.

113. Gnepp DR, Rader WR, Cramer SF, Cook LL, Sciubba JJ: Accuracy of frozen section diagnosis of the salivary gland. Otolaryngol Head Neck Surg 1987; 96:325–330.

Index

Note: Page numbers in *italics* indicate figures; those followed by t indicate tables.

MAJOR PROBLEMS IN PATHOLOGY

- **Pathology of AIDS and the HIV Infection** *(Nash & Said)* Order #W1540-6
- **Disorders of the Spleen** *(Wolf & Neiman)* Order #W2503-7
- **Immunomicroscopy: A Diagnostic Tool for the Surgical Pathologist** *(Taylor)* Order #W8770-9
- **Mucosal Biopsy of the Gastrointestinal Tract, 4th Edition** *(Whitehead)* Order #W3287-4
- **Pathology of Neoplasia in Children and Adolescents** *(Finegold)* Order #W1337-3
- **Pathology of the Uterine Cervix, Vagina, and Vulva** *(Fu & Reagan)* Order #W7493-3
- **Problems in Breast Pathology** *(Azzopardi)* Order #W1463-9
- **Surgical Pathology of Bone Marrow: Core Biopsy Diagnosis** *(Wittels)* Order #W1434-5
- **Cardiovascular Pathology** *(Virmani, Atkinson & Fenoglio)* Order #W3232-7
- **Surgical Pathology of the Lymph Nodes and Related Organs** *(Jaffe)* Order #W1027-7
- **Surgical Pathology of Non-Neoplastic Lung Disease, 2nd Edition** *(Katzenstein & Askin)* Order #W1852-9
- **Surgical Pathology of the Thyroid** *(LiVolsi)* Order #W5782-6
- **Surgical Pathology of the Uterine Corpus, 2nd Edition** *(Hendrickson & Kempson)* Order #W1224-5
- **The Renal Biopsy, 2nd Edition** *(Striker, Olson & Striker)* Order #W3040-5
- **Thin-Needle Aspiration Biopsy** *(Frable)* Order #W3835-X
- **Tumors of the Lung** *(MacKay, Lukeman & Ordóñez)* Order #W5807-5

Enroll today!
See reverse side for details.

BUSINESS REPLY MAIL
FIRST CLASS MAIL   PERMIT NO 7135   ORLANDO, FL
POSTAGE WILL BE PAID BY ADDRESSEE

ORDER FULFILLMENT DEPARTMENT
WB SAUNDERS COMPANY
Harcourt Brace Jovanovich, Inc.
6277 SEA HARBOR DRIVE
ORLANDO FL 32821-9989

NO POSTAGE
NECESSARY
IF MAILED
IN THE
UNITED STATES

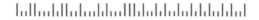